A Quick Guide to Essential Orthopedics

Vishal Kumar • Sitanshu Barik
Sarvdeep Singh Dhatt
Editors

A Quick Guide to Essential Orthopedics

Springer

Editors
Vishal Kumar
Department of Orthopaedics
PGIMER
Chandigarh, Chandigarh, India

Sitanshu Barik
Department of Orthopaedics
AIIMS Nagpur
Nagpur, Maharashtra, India

Sarvdeep Singh Dhatt
Department of Orthopaedics
PGIMER
Chandigarh, Chandigarh, India

ISBN 978-981-95-2675-8 ISBN 978-981-95-2676-5 (eBook)
https://doi.org/10.1007/978-981-95-2676-5

This Springer imprint is published by the registered company Springer Nature Singapore Pte Ltd.
The registered company address is: 152 Beach Road, #21-01/04 Gateway East, Singapore 189721, Singapore

Foreword

It is with great pleasure that I introduce *A Quick Guide to Essential Orthopedics*, a comprehensive resource tailored specifically for undergraduate medical students in India. The book has been edited by faculty of Institute of National Importance, namely, Post Graduate Institute of Medical Education and Research, Chandigarh, and All India Institute of Medical Sciences, Nagpur. It has been authored by various orthopedic surgeons who are currently involved in active medical teaching in various medical colleges of India. This book marks a significant contribution to the field of orthopedic education.

Orthopedics is a cornerstone of medical practice, encompassing the diagnosis, treatment, and rehabilitation of musculoskeletal disorders—a discipline crucial for any aspiring physician. In this meticulously crafted guide, the author distils years of expertise and practical insights into a concise yet thorough overview designed to meet the unique needs of undergraduate students.

This book not only covers fundamental concepts but also addresses common clinical scenarios encountered in orthopedic practice. From fractures to joint disorders, from spinal conditions to sports injuries, each chapter provides clear explanations supported by illustrative diagrams and case studies. By emphasizing key principles and practical applications, it equips students with the essential knowledge and skills necessary for their clinical journey.

Moreover, the publication by Springer underscores its commitment to fostering excellence in medical education. Springer's reputation for academic rigor and global reach ensures that this guide will reach a wide audience of aspiring healthcare professionals, enriching their learning experience and preparing them for the challenges of modern orthopedic practice.

As such, I recommend this book to all undergraduate medical students. May it serve as a valuable companion throughout your academic and professional endeavors, guiding you toward a deeper understanding of orthopedic principles and instilling confidence in your clinical practice.

Prashant P. Joshi

Executive Director & CEO
All India Institute of Medical Sciences, Nagpur
Nagpur, Maharashtra, India

Preface

The idea for this book was born from a simple observation: while orthopedics has always been a vital part of medical education, undergraduate students in India have long lacked a concise, theory-oriented text tailored to their needs. With orthopedics now gradually being recognized as a distinct subject in the MBBS curriculum—often taught and examined separately during the third or fourth year—the demand for a structured, accessible, and evidence-based resource has never been greater.

A Quick Guide to Essential Orthopedics was conceptualized to address this gap. Our aim has been to provide students with a clear conceptual foundation, supported by scientific reasoning and updated with recent advances, while retaining the clinical relevance that makes orthopedics both challenging and fascinating. This text is designed to serve as a first point of reference for MBBS students preparing for university examinations, NEXT/NEET assessments, and beyond. At the same time, we hope it will also be useful to postgraduates, residents, and allied health professionals who seek a compact yet reliable source of knowledge.

As editors, we are deeply grateful to our contributors and reviewers who have worked tirelessly to maintain academic rigor while ensuring clarity of presentation. We also acknowledge the students and teachers whose feedback and encouragement inspired the creation of this book.

We hope this work will not only aid in examination preparation but also spark a genuine interest in orthopedics, laying the foundation for lifelong learning and better patient care.

Chandigarh, India — Vishal Kumar
Nagpur, Maharashtra, India — Sitanshu Barik
Chandigarh, India — Sarvdeep Singh Dhatt

Acknowledgments

The completion of this book has been possible only through the encouragement, guidance, and support of many individuals to whom I remain deeply grateful.

I am indebted to Dr. Vishal Kumar, my mentor at AIIMS Deoghar, whose constant encouragement and vision promoted the very idea of this book and provided the inspiration to pursue it to completion. I also extend my heartfelt thanks to my colleagues and friends from AIIMS Rishikesh and other institutes, who not only contributed chapters with dedication and punctuality but also tolerated my occasional tantrums with patience and good humor.

I owe much to my postgraduate teachers, Dr. Muhammed Nazeer and Dr. Ranjith Unnikrishnan at the Kerala Institute of Medical Sciences, Trivandrum, for their foundational training and mentorship. I would also like to acknowledge Dr. Anil Agarwal from Chacha Nehru Bal Chikitsalaya, Delhi, who provided me with my first hands-on training in orthopedics after junior residency.

My deepest gratitude goes to my MCh teachers at AIIMS Rishikesh—Prof. Shobha Arora, Prof. Pankaj Kandwal, and Dr. Vivek Singh—whose encouragement and training not only refined my clinical skills but also nurtured in me the discipline and confidence to write academically.

On a personal note, I am blessed with the constant support of my siblings and cousins—Ritanshu, Shivani, Shikha, Neha, and Rohit—whose encouragement and affection kept me grounded throughout this journey. I am equally fortunate to have the unwavering friendship of **Tapas Mishra and Dr. Richa**, whose companionship, motivation, and belief in me have been a source of strength through every stage of this project.

Finally, I thank Neeraja Padmanabhan from Springer Publishing House for her guidance, patience, and support in shaping this manuscript into its final form.

To all of you, I remain sincerely grateful.

Sitanshu Barik

Key Features – A Quick Guide to Essential Orthopedics

A Quick Guide to Essential Orthopedics is a vital resource tailored specifically for undergraduate medical students in India. This book provides a comprehensive overview of orthopedic principles essential for your academic and professional journey.

Key Features:

- *Comprehensive Coverage*: From basic anatomy to advanced surgical techniques, this guide covers a wide array of orthopedic topics, ensuring a thorough understanding of the field.
- *Clinical Relevance*: Each chapter includes practical insights and case studies that bridge theoretical knowledge with real-world applications, preparing you for clinical practice.
- *Clear Illustrations*: Richly illustrated diagrams and images enhance comprehension of complex anatomical structures and surgical procedures.
- *Student-Friendly Format*: Concise and structured chapters facilitate efficient learning, making complex concepts accessible and understandable.
- *Exam Preparation*: Designed to align with undergraduate medical curricula in India, this guide serves as an invaluable aid for exams and assessments.

Contents

Part I

Basic Sciences in Orthopaedics

1 Anatomy of Bone

S. Lakshmana Das and Aman Kumar

1.1 Introduction

The human skeleton serves as a framework that supports our bodies, protects vital organs, and facilitates movement. The human skeleton is composed of 206 bones, which are divided into two main categories: axial bones and appendicular bones.

1. *Axial Bones:*
   These bones make up the axial skeleton, which includes the skull, vertebral column (spine), rib cage, and breastbone.
2. *Appendicular Bones:*
   These bones make up the appendicular skeleton, which includes the bones of the arms, legs, scapula, and pelvis.

1.2 Histological Classification

Microscopically, bone can be divided into woven and lamellar types.

1.2.1 Woven Bone

Woven bone is found in areas of rapid bone growth or repair, such as the callus formed during fracture healing or the fetal skeleton. Its presence indicates an active bone formation. Woven bone is considered less structurally strong and more susceptible to fractures compared to mature bone tissue. The defining feature of woven bone or immature bone is the haphazard arrangement of collagen fibers and bone cells. During the development of fetal bones, woven bone forms the initial framework that is later replaced by mature bone tissue. During fracture healing, woven bone is initially formed as a temporary scaffold to stabilize the injured area to provide mechanical support and initiate the healing process. As bone remodeling progresses, the woven bone is gradually replaced by lamellar bone, resulting in a stronger and more organized bone structure.

1.2.2 Lamellar Bone

Lamellar bone is highly structured and provides strength, stability, and resilience to the skeletal system. The collagen fibers and bone cells of lamellar bone, or mature bone, are arranged in a systematic way, i.e., parallel sheets or lamellae of mineralized collagen fibers. All bones, including cortical and cancellous, are made of lamellar bone. The lamellae in cancellous bone are loosely

S. Lakshmana Das (✉)
Department of Orthopedics, All India Institute of Medical Sciences, Bathinda, Punjab, India

A. Kumar
Department of Orthopedics, All India Institute of Medical Sciences, Deoghar, Jharkhand, India

V. Kumar et al. (eds.), *A Quick Guide to Essential Orthopedics*,
https://doi.org/10.1007/978-981-95-2676-5_1

Fig. 1.1 Osteon

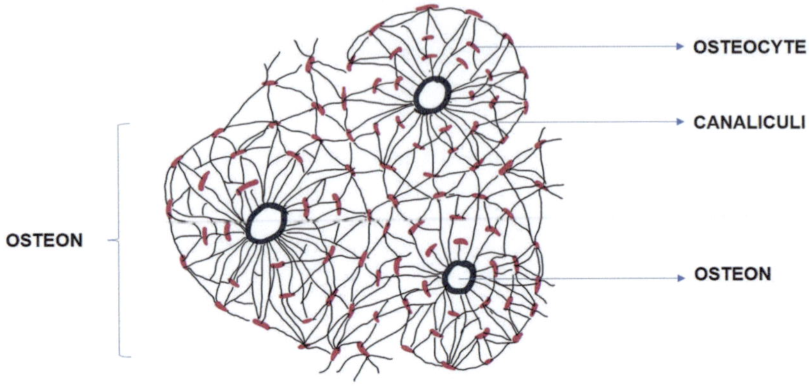

packed, whereas in cortical bone, they are tightly packed. The lamellar structure of bone provides mechanical strength, makes the bone resistant to fractures, and is capable of withstanding various forces and stresses during weight-bearing activities.

The osteon is the fundamental structural component of lamellar bone (Fig. 1.1). It is made up of a central Haversian canal with encircling lamellae or concentric laminations. These canals have a longitudinal course and are freely connected to one another and with Volkmann's canals. Volkmann's canals run horizontally from endosteal to periosteal surfaces.

1.3 Development of Bones

Bones develop through a process called ossification or osteogenesis, which involves the formation of bone tissue by the action of specialized cells called osteoblasts. There are two main types of ossification:

Intramembranous Ossification: This process occurs in the flat bones of the skull and involves the direct transformation of embryonic connective tissue into bone tissue. Osteoblasts secrete mineralized matrix, which then hardens and forms bone tissue.

Endochondral Ossification: This process occurs in most other bones in the body and involves the replacement of cartilage with bone tissue. The process begins with the formation of a cartilage model, which is gradually replaced by bone tissue through the action of osteoblasts and osteoclasts.

1.3.1 Ossification Center

Ossification centers are areas of developing bone tissue where ossification, or bone formation, begins. These centers represent the early stages of bone development and are typically visible on X-rays or other imaging studies.

1.3.2 Types of Ossification Center

Primary Ossification Center: These are the first centers of ossification to form in developing bones. They appear during fetal development and are responsible for the formation of the shaft or diaphysis of long bones and the main part of flat bones.

Secondary Ossification Center: These are the later centers of ossification that appear in certain bones after birth. Secondary ossification centers typically appear in the epiphyses, i.e., the ends of the bone. They are mainly responsible for the longitudinal growth of the long bones.

The developmental process of the clavicle is unique; it involves the formation of two separate bony ossification centers, which eventually fuse together to form a single bone.

1.3.3 Importance of Ossification Center

Ossification center are important because they represent the early stages of bone development and provide important information for the diagnosis of various bone disorders and developmental abnormalities. The timing and sequence of ossification center appearance can help determine the developmental age of a fetus or child, while the presence or absence of certain center can provide clues to the presence of bone disorders.

1.4 Blood Supply

The blood supply of bone is critical for the growth, repair, and maintenance of bone tissue. The blood supply of long bone is shown in Fig. 1.2. Bones have a rich blood supply, which is essential for delivering oxygen, nutrients, and immune cells to bone tissue, as well as removing waste products and metabolic by-products. Blood supply to the inner two-thirds of the bone comes from the nutrient artery, and the outer one-third from the periosteal vessels.

Nutrient Arteries—These are the main arteries that supply blood to the diaphysis, or the shaft of long bones. These arteries enter the bone through nutrient foramina and branch out to form a network of smaller vessels called periosteal arteries, which supply blood to the outer surface of the bone.

Metaphyseal and Epiphyseal Arteries—These arteries supply blood to the metaphysis and epiphysis, which are the growing ends of long bones. The metaphyseal arteries supply blood to the region where bone growth occurs, while the epiphyseal arteries supply blood to the articular cartilage and other tissues in the joint.

Periosteal Vessels—The periosteum is highly vascularized, meaning it contains a rich network of blood vessels that supply nutrients, oxygen, and immune cells to the underlying bone tissue.

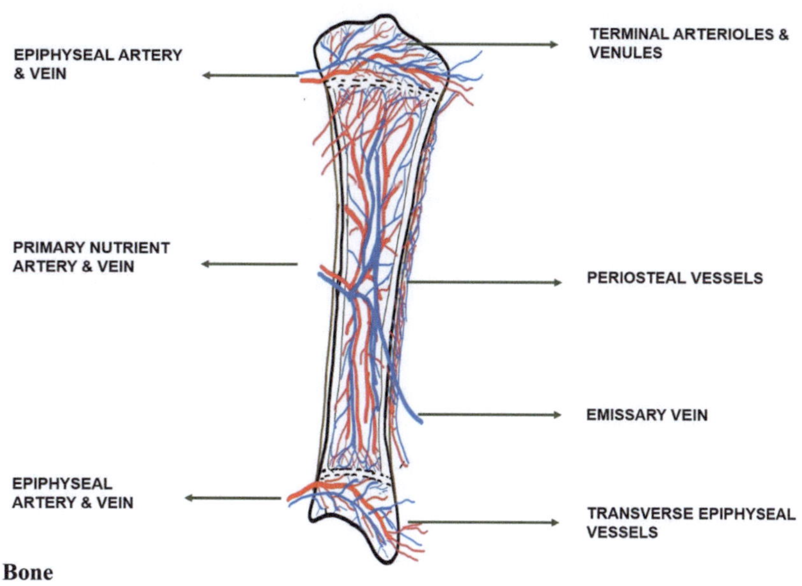

Fig. 1.2 Blood supply of bone

1.5 Bone

Bone is a complex tissue that has a unique structure and function. Its histology can be divided into two main parts: the organic matrix and the inorganic matrix.

1. *Organic Matrix*—This is composed of living cells, collagen fibers (Type 1), and ground substance and is responsible for the growth and repair of bones. The main cells found in the organic matrix include osteocytes (mature bone cells), osteoblasts (bone-forming cells), and osteoclasts (bone-resorbing cells). The organic matrix constitutes 30–35% of dry weight of a bone.
2. *Inorganic Matrix*—This is composed of minerals, primarily calcium and phosphorus, and provides bones their hardness and strength. Especially hydroxyapatite [Ca10(PO4)6(OH)2]. The minerals are deposited in a matrix of collagen fibers, forming a complex network that provides the mechanical support needed for bones to carry the weight of the body. It constitutes about 65–70% of dry weight of a bone.

1.6 Classification of Human Bones

Human bones can be classified into five main types based on their shape:

1. *Long Bones*—These bones are longer than they are wide and are characterized by a shaft or diaphysis and two rounded ends or epiphyses. Examples of long bones include the femur, humerus, tibia, and fibula.
2. *Short Bones*—These bones are roughly equal in length, width, and thickness and are generally cube-shaped or round. Examples of short bones include the bones of the wrist (carpals) and ankle (tarsals).
3. *Flat Bones*—These bones are thin and flat and are composed of two layers of compact bone surrounding a layer of spongy bone. Examples of flat bones include the scapula, ribs, and skull bones.
4. *Irregular Bones*—These bones have complex, irregular shapes and do not fit into any of the other categories. Examples of irregular bones include the vertebrae, facial bones, and hip bones.
5. *Sesamoid Bones*—These are small, round bones that are embedded within tendons and are typically found near joints. The most well-known example of a sesamoid bone is the patella or kneecap.

1.6.1 Long Bones

Long bones are bones that are longer than they are wide and have a cylindrical shape. They have a shaft (diaphysis) and two rounded ends (epiphyses) separated by a growth plate (epiphyseal plate). Long bones are found in the arms (humerus, radius, and ulna), legs (femur, tibia, and fibula), fingers (metacarpals), and toes (metatarsals). Long bones consist of several parts, as shown in Fig. 1.3, including:

Diaphysis—This is the shaft of the long bone, which is composed of dense, hard, compact bone. The diaphysis contains the medullary cavity, which is filled with yellow bone marrow.

Epiphyses—These are the rounded ends of the long bone and are composed of spongy bone. They are covered by a thin layer of articular cartilage, which provides a smooth surface for joints to move on.

Metaphysis—It is the portion of a long bone between the diaphysis (the shaft) and the epiphysis (the rounded end). In a growing bone, the metaphysis is the site of active growth and the transition between the dense, hard compact bone of the diaphysis and the spongy bone of the epiphysis. The metaphysis contains the epiphyseal plate. The metaphysis is also an important site for nutrient exchange between the bone and surrounding tissues, as well as for the growth of blood vessels and

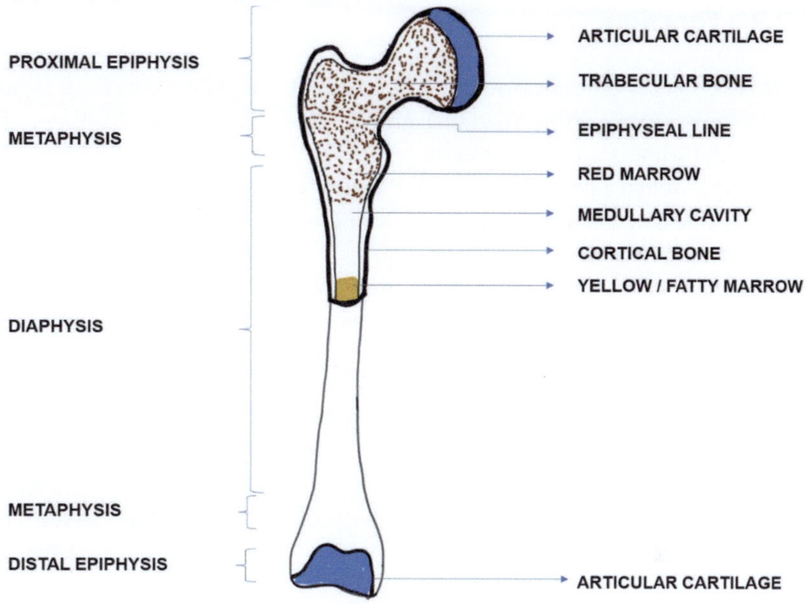

Fig. 1.3 Long bone

nerve fibers that supply the bone. The metaphysis is often involved in certain types of bone injuries, such as fractures and osteochondritis dissecans, and is an important area to consider in the evaluation and management of bone conditions.

Epiphyseal Plate—A thin plate of hyaline cartilage found between the diaphysis and epiphyses in growing bones. It allows for growth in length during childhood and adolescence. In adults, it becomes the epiphyseal line.

Long bones provide structural support, serving as levers for movement and storing minerals such as calcium and phosphorus. They also play an important role in the formation of red blood cells in the bone marrow.

1.7 Periosteum

The periosteum is a fibrous membrane covers the entire surface of long bones, except at the joints, and also covers the surface of flat bones and short bones. It helps in their growth, repair, and nutrition. The strands of fibrous tissue connecting the bone to the periosteum are called Sharpey's fibers. It is composed of two layers: the outer fibrous layer and the inner cambium layer. Based on its location and function, there are two types of periosteum.

Fibrous Periosteum—This is the outer layer of the periosteum that consists of dense irregular connective tissue. It serves as a protective layer for the bone and provides attachment sites for tendons and ligaments.

Cambium Periosteum—This is the inner layer of the periosteum that is composed of osteoblasts and chondroblasts. It is responsible for bone growth and repair, as it forms new bone tissue in response to injury or stress.

1.7.1 Physiology

The periosteum plays a vital role in the growth and repair of bones. When a bone is damaged, the periosteum releases growth factors that stimulate the formation of new bone tissue. In addition, the blood vessels in the inner layer of the periosteum provide oxygen and nutrients to the bone, while the nerves in the inner layer regulate bone growth and sensation.

1.7.2 Function

1. *Bone Growth*—The periosteum plays a crucial role in bone growth by secreting growth factors that stimulate bone formation.
2. *Repair*—When a bone is damaged, the periosteum releases growth factors that stimulate the formation of new bone tissue.
3. *Nutrition*—The blood vessels in the inner layer of the periosteum provide oxygen and nutrients to the bone.
4. *Sensory Function*—The nerves in the inner layer of the periosteum regulate bone growth and sensation.

1.8 Cartilage

Cartilage is a type of connective tissue that provides support, stability, and cushioning in the body. It is composed of cells called chondrocytes, which produce and maintain the extracellular matrix (ECM), the material that gives cartilage its unique properties. The ECM is composed of collagen fibers, proteoglycans (large molecules made up of protein and carbohydrates), and a small amount of fluid. It is composed of the following components:

Chondrocytes—These are the cells that produce and maintain the extracellular matrix (ECM) of hyaline cartilage.

Extracellular Matrix (ECM)—The ECM of hyaline cartilage is composed of collagen fibers, proteoglycans (large molecules made up of protein and carbohydrates), and a small amount of fluid. The proteoglycans help to maintain the hydration of the ECM, giving hyaline cartilage its elasticity and resilience.

Ground Substance—The ground substance is a gel-like material that surrounds the chondrocytes and helps to lubricate and cushion the joint.

1.9 Types of Cartilage

There are three main types of cartilage: hyaline, fibrocartilage, and elastic cartilage.

1.9.1 Hyaline Cartilage

Hyaline cartilage is also known as glassy or translucent cartilage. This type of cartilage is smooth and transparent, and covers the ends of bones in joints to reduce friction and absorb shock. It is also found in the trachea, bronchi, and larynx.

Histology—Hyaline cartilage has a relatively uniform appearance with chondrocytes located within lacunae (small cavities) within the ECM. The ECM of hyaline cartilage is composed of type II collagen fibers and a dense mesh of proteoglycans, which give the tissue its smooth, translucent appearance. The chondrocytes are well-spaced within the lacunae, allowing for adequate nutrition and waste exchange. Hyaline cartilage is an important component of joints, and its proper functioning is crucial for smooth joint movement.

Example—The rounded ends of long bones in joints such as the shoulder, hip, and knee are covered in hyaline cartilage.

1.9.2 Fibrocartilage

Fibrocartilage is cartilage that is tougher and more dense than hyaline cartilage. Fibrocartilage is found in areas of high stress and tension, such as the intervertebral discs, the pubic symphysis, and the menisci of the knee. It is able to withstand compressive and tensile forces, making it well-suited for its role in supporting and stabilizing joints.

Histology—Fibrocartilage has a more fibrous appearance compared to hyaline and elastic cartilage. The chondrocytes are spread out and fewer in number, with the ECM being dominated by collagen fibers and fibrous tissue. The ECM of fibrocartilage is composed of collagen fibers, proteoglycans, and fibrous tissue. The fibrous tissue gives fibrocartilage its strength, while proteoglycans provide resilience and hydration. The ground substance is similar to that of hyaline and elastic cartilage.

Example—The intervertebral discs in the spine and the knee menisci are examples of fibrocartilage.

1.9.3 Elastic Cartilage

Elastic cartilage is flexible and resilient, allowing it to quickly return to its original shape after being stretched. It is found in the external ear, epiglottis, and larynx.

Histology—Elastic cartilage has a more organized appearance than hyaline cartilage. The chondrocytes are arranged in rows along the elastic fibers, which run in parallel to each other. The ECM is denser and contains more elastic fibers compared to hyaline cartilage, giving the tissue its distinctive yellow color. The ground substance is similar to that of hyaline cartilage.

Example—The external ear and epiglottis in the larynx are examples of elastic cartilage.

1.10 Collagen

Collagen is a fibrous protein that is the main component of connective tissue in the body, including bone, cartilage, tendons, ligaments, and skin. It is the most abundant protein in the human body, making up around one-third of the total protein.

1.10.1 Structure

Collagen is composed of three polypeptide chains that form a triple helix, which gives collagen its characteristic strength and flexibility. The triple helix is stabilized by hydrogen bonds between the amino acid residues in the chains.

1.10.2 Biochemical Composition

Collagen is composed of amino acids, mainly glycine, proline, and hydroxyproline. Collagen is a polypeptide chain composed of a triple helix of two alpha-1 chains and one alpha-2 chain. These amino acids are arranged in a unique sequence that varies between the different types of collagens.

1.10.3 Formation

Collagen is formed by fibroblasts. Collagen synthesis occurs both inside and outside the cell.

3 Alpha chains → Procollagen → Tropocollagen → Collagen fibril → Collagen fiber

1.10.4 Types

There are over 25 types of collagens, each with a unique structure and function. The most common types are:

Type of collagen	Component of	Related clinical condition
Type- I most abundant type (90% of total collagen)	Bone, ligament, tendon, nerves, meniscus, annulus of intervertebral disc, skin	Osteogenesis imperfecta Ehlers-Danlos syndrome
Type II	Hyaline cartilage, nucleus pulposus of intervertebral disc	
Type III	Skin and blood vessels	Ehlers-Danlos syndrome Dupuytren's contracture
Type IV	Basement membrane	Goodpasture's and Alport syndrome
Type IX	Articular cartilage	Multiple epiphyseal dysplasia

Multiple Choice Questions

1. What is the process of development of bones called?
   (a) Osteogenesis
   (b) Osteoclasis
   (c) Chondrogenesis
   (d) Endogenesis
2. The major blood supply to the inner second/third of the cortical part of the long bone comes from
   (a) Metaphyseal vessels
   (b) Epiphyseal vessels
   (c) Nutrient artery
   (d) Periosteal artery
3. What is the major collagen type in bone
   (a) Type II
   (b) Type IV
   (c) Type IX
   (d) Type I
4. Patella is an example of
   (a) Long bone
   (b) Sesamoid bone
   (c) Flat bone
   (d) Innominate bone
5. The type of cartilage in articular cartilage is
   (a) Hyaline cartilage
   (b) Elastic cartilage
   (c) Fibro cartilage
   (d) None of the above

Answers: 1. (a), 2. (c), 3. (d) 4. (b), 5. (a)

Biochemistry of Bone

2

S. Lakshmana Das and Sitanshu Barik

2.1 Introduction

Bone is a dynamic tissue that undergoes constant remodelling through a process called bone metabolism. Bone metabolism is a complex sequence of osteoblastogenesis (bone formation) and osteoclastogenesis (bone resorption). The process involves two major types of cells: osteoblasts and osteoclasts, which work together to maintain a balance between bone formation and bone resorption, respectively.

2.2 Osteoblasts and Osteoclasts

Osteoblasts and osteoclasts are two types of cells that play important roles in bone metabolism.

Osteoblasts—Osteoblasts are bone-forming cells that are responsible for building new bone tissue. They have a flat, spindle-shaped appearance and are typically found along the edges of bone tissue. Osteoblasts secrete a mixture of proteins and minerals, including collagen and hydroxyapatite, that form the extracellular matrix of new bone tissue.

Osteoclasts—Osteoclasts are bone-resorbing cells that are responsible for breaking down old or damaged bone tissue. They have a multi-nucleated appearance and are typically found on the surface of bone tissue. Osteoclasts secrete enzymes and acids that dissolve the mineralized bone matrix and release calcium into the bloodstream.

Both osteoblasts and osteoclasts are regulated by hormones and growth factors, such as parathyroid hormone (PTH), calcitonin, and vitamin D, that help to maintain the proper balance between bone formation and resorption. The balance between bone formation and bone resorption is essential for maintaining healthy bones. When there is more bone resorption than bone formation, bones become weaker, which can lead to osteoporosis. When there is more bone formation than bone resorption, bones become denser, which can lead to conditions such as osteopetrosis.

2.3 Osteoblastogenesis

Osteoblastogenesis is the process by which osteoblasts, which are cells responsible for bone formation, are formed. This process involves a series of molecular and cellular events that lead to the differentiation of mesenchymal stem cells (MSCs) into mature osteoblasts.

S. Lakshmana Das (✉)
Department of Orthopedics, All India Institute of Medical Sciences, Bathinda, Punjab, India

S. Barik
Department of Orthopaedics, AIIMS Nagpur, Nagpur, Maharashtra, India

V. Kumar et al. (eds.), *A Quick Guide to Essential Orthopedics*,
https://doi.org/10.1007/978-981-95-2676-5_2

2.3.1 Key Steps of Osteoblastogenesis

1. *MSCs Differentiate into Pre-osteoblasts*
   MSCs are multipotent stem cells that can differentiate into various cell types, including osteoblasts. Under the influence of various factors, such as bone morphogenetic proteins (BMPs), MSCs differentiate into pre-osteoblasts.
2. *Pre-osteoblasts Proliferate and Differentiate into Mature Osteoblasts*
   Pre-osteoblasts are immature cells that can differentiate into mature osteoblasts under the influence of various factors, including BMPs, Wnt signalling, and parathyroid hormone (PTH) signalling. These factors promote the proliferation and differentiation of pre-osteoblasts into mature osteoblasts.
3. *Osteoblasts Synthesize and Deposit Bone Matrix*
   Mature osteoblasts synthesize and deposit extracellular matrix, including collagen and various proteins, which forms the bone matrix. The matrix is then mineralized with calcium and phosphate to form new bone tissue.
4. *Osteoblastic Regulation of Bone Resorption*
   Osteoblasts secrete various factors that regulate osteoclast activity, such as osteoprotegerin (OPG) and receptor activator of nuclear factor kappa-B ligand (RANKL). OPG acts as a decoy receptor for RANKL and inhibits osteoclastogenesis, while RANKL promotes osteoclast differentiation and activation.

2.4 Osteoclastogenesis

Osteoclastogenesis is the process by which osteoclasts, which are cells responsible for breaking down and resorbing bone tissue, are formed. It involves a complex series of signalling pathways and interactions between various cells and molecules, including osteoblasts (cells that form new bone tissue), osteoclast precursors, cytokines, growth factors, and hormones.

During osteoclastogenesis, osteoclast precursors differentiate into mature osteoclasts under the influence of various factors, including Receptor Activator of Nuclear Factor Kappa-B Ligand (RANKL), macrophage colony-stimulating factor (M-CSF), and osteoprotegerin (OPG). RANKL, which is produced by osteoblasts and other cells, binds to its receptor RANK on osteoclast precursors and triggers their differentiation into mature osteoclasts. Macrophage colony-stimulating factor (M-CSF) signalling stimulates the proliferation and survival of osteoclast precursors. Osteoprotegerin (OPG) acts as a decoy receptor for RANKL and inhibits osteoclastogenesis.

Osteoclastogenesis plays a crucial role in bone remodelling, which is the process by which old bone tissue is replaced by new bone tissue. Imbalances in osteoclastogenesis can lead to various bone diseases, including osteoporosis, Paget's disease, and bone metastasis.

2.5 Pathways Involved in Osteoblastogenesis and Osteoclastogenesis

Osteoblastogenesis and osteoclastogenesis are two essential processes involved in bone remodelling. Here are the main pathways involved in these processes:

2.5.1 Osteoblastogenesis Signalling Pathways

1. *Bone Morphogenetic Protein (BMP) Signalling*
   BMPs are a family of growth factors that play a critical role in bone development and regeneration. BMP signalling stimulates the differentiation of mesenchymal stem cells (MSCs) into pre-osteoblasts and further into mature osteoblasts.
2. *Wnt Signalling*
   The Wnt signalling pathway is also crucial for bone formation. It stimulates the prolifera-

tion and differentiation of osteoblast progenitors and enhances the activity of mature osteoblasts.

3. *Parathyroid Hormone (PTH) Signalling*

   PTH is a hormone that regulates calcium and phosphate metabolism. It also stimulates the proliferation and differentiation of osteoblasts.

2.5.2 Osteoclastogenesis Pathways

1. *Receptor Activator of Nuclear Factor Kappa-B Ligand (RANKL) Signalling*

   RANKL is a cytokine produced by osteoblasts, T cells, and other cells. It binds to its receptor RANK on osteoclast precursors and stimulates their differentiation into mature osteoclasts.
2. *Macrophage Colony-Stimulating Factor (M-CSF) Signalling*

   M-CSF is a cytokine that stimulates the proliferation and survival of osteoclast precursors.
3. *Osteoprotegerin (OPG) Signalling*

   OPG is a protein that acts as a decoy receptor for RANKL. It blocks the binding of RANKL to RANK, preventing osteoclastogenesis.

2.6 Key Steps of Bone Metabolism

1. Bone resorption by osteoclasts
2. Bone formation by osteoblasts
3. Mineralization of osteoid matrix
4. Remodelling

   Remodelling is regulated by various hormones, such as parathyroid hormone (PTH), vitamin D, and calcitonin, as well as other factors, such as growth factors and cytokines.

2.7 Metabolic Functions of Bone

In addition to providing structural support for the body, bone also has several important metabolic functions.

1. *Calcium and Phosphorus Homeostasis*—Bone tissue serves as a major reservoir for calcium and phosphorus ions, which are essential for many physiological processes. When blood levels of calcium and phosphorus are low, osteoclasts break down bone tissue to release these ions into the bloodstream. Conversely, when blood levels of calcium and phosphorus are high, osteoblasts deposit these ions back into the bone tissue.
2. *Hematopoiesis*—Bone marrow, which is located in the central cavity of bones, is responsible for producing blood cells, including red blood cells, white blood cells, and platelets. Hematopoietic stem cells differentiate into these specialized cells in response to various growth factors and cytokines.
3. *Fat Storage*—Yellow bone marrow, which is located in the central cavity of long bones, serves as a storage site for adipose tissue. This adipose tissue can be used as an energy source when needed.
4. *Acid-Base Balance*—Bone tissue helps to maintain the pH balance of the body by buffering excess acid or base ions. Osteoclasts release calcium ions into the bloodstream to neutralize excess acid, while osteoblasts deposit calcium ions into bone tissue to neutralize excess base.

2.8 Regulators of Bone Metabolism

Bone metabolism is regulated by various hormones, growth factors, and signalling molecules that interact with bone cells to maintain the balance between bone formation and resorption. The key regulators are

1. *Calcium and Phosphorus*—These minerals are essential for the proper mineralization of new bone tissue and for maintaining the strength and integrity of bones.
2. *Hormones*—The primary hormones involved in bone metabolism are parathyroid hormone (PTH), vitamin D, and calcitonin.

2.8.1 Calcium

Calcium is a critical component of bone mineral, which makes up the majority of the weight and strength of bone tissue. Approximately 99% of the body's calcium is stored in bone, where it is constantly being deposited and resorbed as part of the bone remodelling process. Calcium also plays a vital role in many cellular processes, including muscle contraction, nerve impulse transmission, and blood clotting. Majority of calcium in the bone is seen in the form of hydroxyapatite.

Hydroxyapatite (HA) is a mineral compound that is the main component of bone and teeth in mammals. It has a chemical formula of $Ca_{10}(PO_4)_6(OH)_2$ and a crystalline structure that resembles the mineral apatite. HA crystals are formed in the extracellular matrix of bone tissue, where they provide the structure and rigidity that give bones their strength. In addition to its role as a structural component, hydroxyapatite also plays a key role in mineral metabolism. It is constantly being formed and reabsorbed in bone tissue as part of the process of bone remodelling, which involves the coordinated action of osteoblasts and osteoclasts.

2.8.2 Phosphorus

Phosphorus is the second most abundant mineral in the bone. It is a major component of hydroxyapatite, the mineral that gives bone its hardness and strength. Like calcium, phosphorus is constantly being deposited and resorbed in bone tissue as part of the bone remodelling process. Phosphorus also plays important roles in energy metabolism, DNA and RNA synthesis and intracellular cell signalling. In the blood, phosphorus is mostly in the form of inorganic phosphate. Phosphate is absorbed in the intestines and excreted by the kidneys.

2.8.3 Parathyroid Hormone (PTH)

PTH is produced by the parathyroid glands in response to low serum calcium levels. PTH is the major regulator of extracellular calcium. Secretion of PTH is regulated by plasma ionized calcium. Reduced plasma ionized calcium increases the secretion of PTH, which increases the levels of calcium in the blood by increasing the activity of osteoclasts, leading to increased bone resorption and release of calcium into the bloodstream, leading to increased serum calcium and fall in serum phosphorus levels.

Action of PTH

1. *In bone cells:* PTH stimulates the activity of osteoclasts, cells that break down bone tissue and release calcium and phosphorus into the bloodstream. This process is known as bone resorption.
2. *In the kidneys:* PTH increases the reabsorption of calcium from the urine back into the bloodstream. PTH also stimulates the production of calcitriol, the active form of vitamin D, which increases the absorption of calcium from the gut.
3. *In the gut:* PTH indirectly increases the absorption of calcium from the gut by stimulating the production of calcitriol, which promotes the uptake of calcium from the diet.

Negative feedback High levels of calcium in the blood can inhibit PTH secretion, which in turn reduces bone resorption and calcitriol production. This negative feedback loop helps to maintain calcium homeostasis in the body.

2.8.4 Vitamin D

Vitamin D is a fat-soluble vitamin. It plays an important role in the absorption and transport of calcium and phosphate from the intestines, which are necessary for bone formation. When the levels of calcium in the blood are low, vitamin D is activated in the kidneys, which in turn increases the absorption of calcium and phosphate from the intestines. It helps ensure that there is an adequate supply of calcium for new bone formation. Calcitriol also works with PTH to increase the release of calcium from bone tissue when blood calcium levels are low.

In addition to its role in calcium and phosphorus metabolism, vitamin D also plays a role in immune function, cell growth, and gene expression.

2.8.5 Vitamin D Pathway

1. Vitamin D production: The skin produces vitamin D3 (cholecalciferol) in response to exposure to UVB radiation from the sun. Vitamin D2 (ergocalciferol) can also be obtained from dietary sources.
2. Vitamin D transport: Vitamin D3 and D2 are transported to the liver, where they are converted to 25-hydroxyvitamin D (25(OH)D), the major circulating form of vitamin D.
3. Activation of vitamin D: 25(OH)D is transported to the kidneys, where it is converted to its active form, 1,25-dihydroxyvitamin D ($1,25(OH)_2D$), also known as calcitriol. This conversion is regulated by parathyroid hormone (PTH) and calcium levels in the blood.
4. Vitamin D receptor activation: Calcitriol binds to vitamin D receptors (VDRs) on target tissues, such as the small intestine, bone, and kidneys. This binding stimulates the expression of genes that are involved in calcium and phosphorus absorption, bone remodelling, and mineralization.
5. Negative feedback: High levels of calcium and phosphorus in the blood can inhibit PTH secretion, which in turn reduces the production of calcitriol. This negative feedback loop helps to maintain calcium and phosphorus homeostasis in the body.

2.8.6 Calcitonin

Calcitonin is produced by the parafollicular C cells of thyroid gland and works to decrease the levels of calcium in the blood. Calcitonin inhibits bone resorption by decreasing the activity of osteoclasts. Calcitonin also increases the excretion of calcium by the kidneys.

Other hormones and growth factors

1. *Estrogen*—Estrogen is a sex steroid important for peak bone mass attainment in both the sexes. It prevents bone loss by decreasing the rate of bone turnover (reduced frequency bone resorption and remodelling). Reduced estrogen levels in postmenopausal women leading to increased risk of osteoporotic fractures.
2. *Growth Hormone*—Growth hormone increases the serum calcium by increasing intestinal absorption and decreasing urinary excretion.
3. *Thyroid Hormone*—Thyroid hormone stimulates the growth of chondrocytes and collagen synthesis. Thyroid hormone also increases bone resorption by increasing alkaline phosphatase activity, which can cause osteoporosis.
4. *Steroids*—Steroids reduce bone mass by decreasing calcium absorption, decreasing collagen synthesis, and inhibiting osteoblastic new bone formation.
5. *Osteoprotegerin (OPG)*—OPG is a protein that regulates osteoclast activity and helps to maintain the balance between new bone formation and resorption.
6. *Bone Morphogenetic Proteins (BMPs)*—BMPs belong to transforming growth factor-beta (TGF-B) superfamily. BMPs 2,4,6, and 7 are the most important osteoinductive BMPs that promote the differentiation of mesenchymal stem cells into osteoblasts and new bone formation.
7. *Cytokines and Growth Factors*—

   Various cytokines and growth factors, such as transforming growth factor-beta (TGF-β), fibroblast growth factor (FGF), platelet-derived growth factor (PDGF) and insulin-like growth factors 1 & 2 (IGF), also play important roles in bone metabolism by regulating osteoblast and osteoclast activity.

   (i) *TGF-B*: Both osteoblasts and osteoclasts synthesize and respond to TGF-B. It stimulates the production of collagen and proteoglycans.

(ii) *IGF*-1: It is the most abundant growth factor in bone. It causes proliferation of growth plate without maturation, leading to linear growth.
(iii) *IGF*-2: It is more potent than IGF-1. It stimulates the production of type-I collagen and cartilage matrix synthesis.
(iv) *Fibroblast Growth Factor (FGF)*: It promotes growth and differentiation of epithelial cells, myocytes, osteoblasts, and chondrocytes.

8. *Mechanical Loading*—Mechanical loading, such as through exercise or weight-bearing activities, can stimulate bone formation by promoting osteoblast activity and inhibiting osteoclast activity.
9. Nutrition—Adequate intake of nutrients such as calcium, phosphorus, vitamin D, and protein is essential for bone health and metabolism.

Multiple Choice Questions

1. The cell responsible for bone resorption is
   (a) Osteoblast
   (b) Osteoclast
   (c) Osteocyte
   (d) Pericytes
2. Secretion of parathyroid hormone acts on bone and
   (a) Increases blood calcium level
   (b) Decreases blood calcium level
   (c) No effect on blood calcium level
   (d) Increases urinary excretion of calcium
3. The major minerals in bone are
   (a) Phosphorus and iron
   (b) Calcium and phosphorus
   (c) Calcium and iron
   (d) Calcium and magnesium
4. Osteoblasts are responsible for
   (a) New bone formation
   (b) Bone resorption
   (c) Calcium storage
   (d) Collagen synthesis
5. Calcitonin is produced by
   (a) Osteoblasts
   (b) Kidneys
   (c) Parafollicular C cells of thyroid
   (d) Parathyroid gland

Answers: 1. (b), 2. (a), 3. (b), 4. (a), 5. (c)

3 Fracture Healing

S. Lakshmana Das and Vishal Kumar

3.1 Introduction

A fracture is a breach in structural continuity of bone cortex with variable degree of surrounding soft tissue injury. Bone is capable of undergoing spontaneous regeneration following injury. Fracture healing is a complex sequential series of events to restore the structural integrity. The stability of the fracture decides the mode of fracture healing.

3.2 Modes of Fracture Healing

There are two modes of fracture healing (Fig. 3.1).

(a) *Primary Bone Healing (Direct)*

Direct fracture healing occurs through intramembranous bone formation by Haversian remodeling. Direct fracture healing requires good vascular supply, anatomical fracture reduction, and absolute stability (no motion at fracture site). Primary healing can be gap healing or contact healing. The hallmark feature of Direct bone healing is the absence of callus formation as it requires only the remodeling of lamellar bone by osteoblastic cutting cone formation. The cutting cones tunnel across the fracture site, which creates a path for blood vessels and laying of lamellar bone by osteoblasts.

Example: Compression plating—In Compression plating, the fracture ends are anatomically aligned, approximated without any gap, and stabilised with a compression plate. The interfragmentary compression and absolute stability achieved through compression plating promote primary bone healing without any need for external callus formation, also known as contact healing.

(b) *Secondary Bone Healing (Indirect)*

Secondary or indirect fracture healing occurs mainly through endochondral bone ossification by callus formation. It is the most common mode of fracture healing. This type of fracture healing occurs when there is relative stability at the fracture site. Periosteum and surrounding soft tissue play the major role in this type of fracture healing.

S. Lakshmana Das (✉)
Department of Orthopedics, All India Institute of Medical Sciences, Bathinda, Punjab, India

V. Kumar
Department of Orthopaedics, PGIMER, Chandigarh, Chandigarh, India

V. Kumar et al. (eds.), *A Quick Guide to Essential Orthopedics*,
https://doi.org/10.1007/978-981-95-2676-5_3

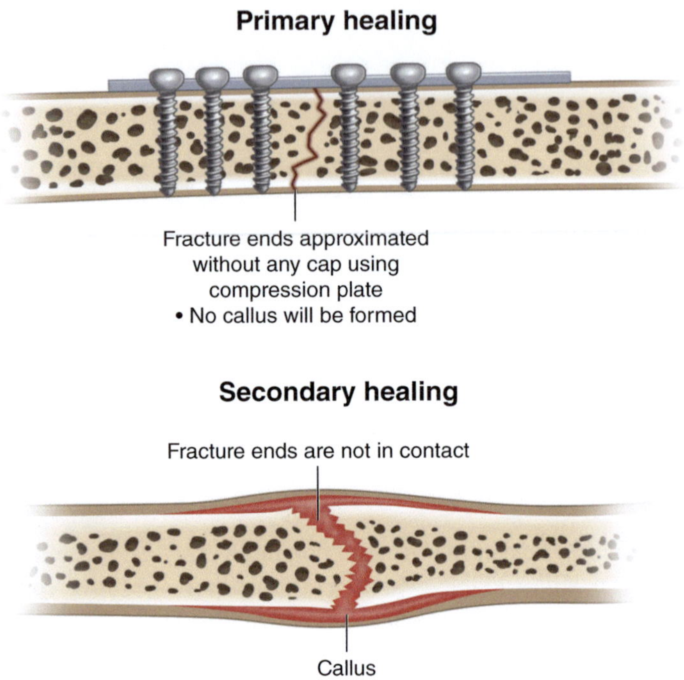

Fig. 3.1 Primary & secondary fracture healing

3.3 Callus

Callus is the regenerative bone tissue that forms in response to bony injury and aims at naturally uniting the fracture ends. Callus is a combination of fibrous tissue, cartilage, and woven bone. Formation of callus reduces interfragmentary strain by increasing the surface area and helps in healing.

There are three types of callus formation that occur at fracture site (Fig. 3.2). They are

1. *Intramembranous Callus (Bony/Periosteal)*
   This primary callus response is promoted by the cambium layer of the periosteum. The osteoprogenitor cells produce bone directly without cartilage formation. This callus does not bridge the fracture ends.
2. *Endochondral/Briding Callus (Fibrocartilagenous)*
   This is the predominant type of callus that forms during the stage of soft callus formation.
3. *Endosteal or Medullary Callus*
   This type of callus formation happens during later stages of fracture healing. This helps in uniting the fracture.

Examples:

1. Conservative management of fractures by slab and cast—The fracture ends are reduced, and relative stability is provided by the slab or cast. There will be some motion at the fracture site.
2. External fixator—External fixator acts as external splint, and relative stability is provided.
3. Intramedullary nailing—Intramedullary nail acts as internal splint. Though the fracture is reduced, the stability provided by the nail is relative stability; thus, some degree of motion always occurs at the fracture site, leading to secondary fracture healing.

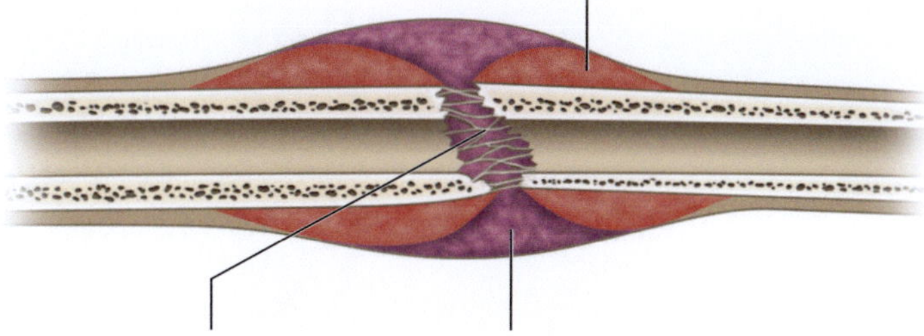

Fig. 3.2 Types of callus

3.4 Stages of Fracture Healing

Secondary fracture healing happens through four stages (Fig. 3.3), namely the stage of

1. Hematoma formation (inflammation) and angiogenesis
2. Fibrocartilaginous callus (soft callus) formation
3. Bony callus (hard callus) formation
4. Bone remodeling

3.4.1 Stage I: Hematoma Formation (Day 0–7)

The stage of hematoma formation begins immediately following the fracture. Bleeding from ruptured blood vessels at fracture site leading to hematoma and subsequent fibrin clot formation. Hematoma is the source of hematopoietic stem cells and proinflammatory cytokines (platelet-derived growth factor, TNF-alpha, TGF-beta, IL-1, 6, 10, and 12). These cytokines recruit inflammatory cells (monocytes, macrophages, and lymphocytes) to remove dead and necrotic cells and to secrete cytokines like Vascular Endothelial Growth Factor (VEGF). VEGF helps in angiogenesis and recruitment of mesenchymal stem cells. The periosteum plays an important role in this stage. Osteoblast progenitors are recruited by osteogenic induction by undifferentiated cells from bone marrow and mesenchymal cells from cambium layer of periosteum. Gradually the hematoma is replaced by granulation tissue due to cellular proliferation, differentiation, and matrix synthesis.

3.4.2 Stage II: Fibrocartilaginous Callus Formation (Days 7–28)

The recruited mesenchymal stem cells differentiate (driven by Bone Morphogenic Protein (BMPs)) into fibroblasts, chondroblasts, and osteoblasts. The fracture hematoma becomes organised and is infiltrated by fibrovascular tissue and collagen fibres are laid, which acts as a Framework for primary callus formation. Some mesenchymal cells transform into Chondroblasts that form hyaline cartilage and some cells into osteoblasts and deposit organic matrix (disorganised collagen fibers). At the same time, adjacent to the periosteal layers, a layer of woven bone is laid down by the osteoprogenitor cells. The initial callus acts as a good internal splint against bending and rotational forces but weak on shear and compression forces. Clinically the fracture becomes sticky in this stage.

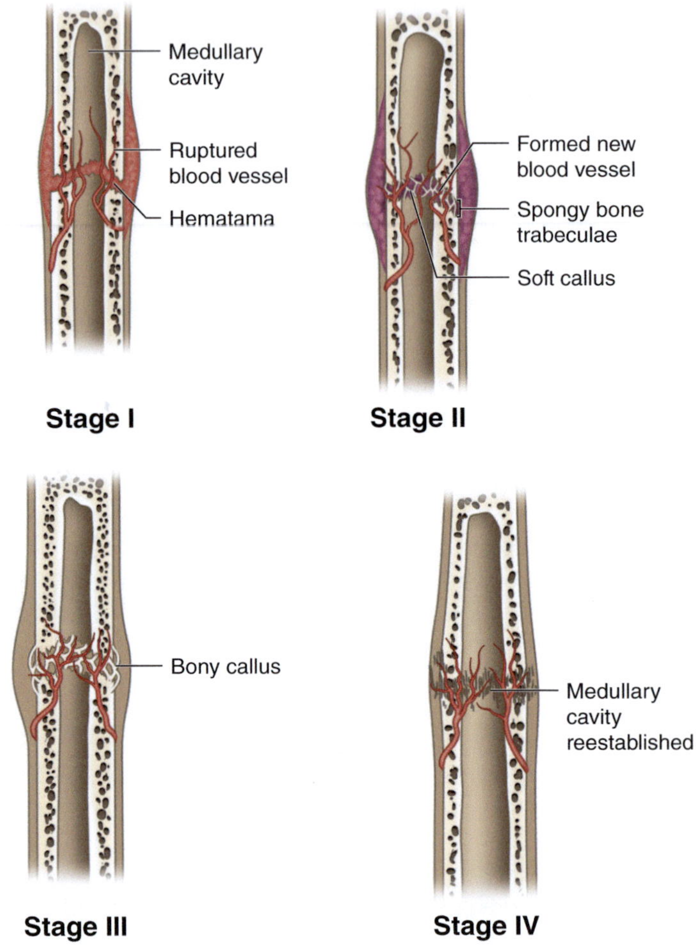

Fig. 3.3 Stages of fracture healing

3.4.3 Stage III: Bony Callus Formation (Days 28–120)

The cartilaginous callus begins to undergo endochondral ossification, i.e., conversion of cartilage to bone. Receptor Activator of Nuclear Factor-Ligand (RANK-L) is expressed, stimulating further differentiation of chondroblasts, chondroclasts, osteoblasts, and osteoclasts. As a result, the cartilaginous callus is resorbed and begins to calcify. Subperiosteally, woven bone continues to be laid down. The newly formed blood vessels continue to proliferate, allowing further migration of mesenchymal stem cells. At the end of this phase, a hard, consolidated, calcified callus of immature woven bone forms. Clinically the fracture is united, stable, and pain free.

3.4.4 Stage IV: Bone Remodeling (Day 120 Onwards, Lasting Months to Years)

After fracture union, the hard callus undergoes repeated remodeling—termed "coupled remodeling." This "coupled remodeling" is a balance of osteoclastic resorption followed by osteoblastic new bone formation. The center of the callus is ultimately replaced by compact bone, while the callus edges become replaced by lamellar bone. This stage lasts for many months, ultimately resulting in the regeneration of the normal bone structure. The medullary canal reforms at the end of this stage.

3.5 Factors Influencing Fracture Healing

The factors influencing fracture healing can be local and systemic factors:

3.5.1 Local Factors

1. *Blood Supply*—The most important factor that promotes fracture healing. Good vascular supply promotes healing by migration of mesenchymal cells. Thus, preservation of periosteum and soft tissue coverage is of paramount importance in case of open reduction and fixation of fractures.
2. *Site of Fracture (Metaphyseal Versus Diaphyseal)*—The healing of cancellous and cortical bone is different from each other due to differences in cellularity, surface area, and vascularity. Metaphyseal areas mainly consist of cancellous bone, thus metaphyseal fractures have good healing potential due to large surface area and good vascularity.
3. *Degree of Soft Tissue Trauma*—High-velocity traumas have significant soft tissue injury and periosteal stripping, which adversely impacts fracture healing (vascularity is disrupted).
4. *Associated Neurovascular Injury*
5. *Fracture Pattern*—Segmental fracture of long bones disrupts the intramedullary blood supply to the middle fragment. The probability of delayed union or nonunion involving the middle fragment, proximally or distally is increased.
6. *Reduction and Stability at Fracture Site*—Approximation of fracture without any gap decreases the volume of tissue needed to repair the fracture. Providing stability to the fracture reduces the motion at the fracture site and promotes healing and union. Absolute fracture stability is particularly important for fractures with associated extensive soft tissue injury, intra-articular fractures like neck of femur due to presence of synovial fluid.
7. *Open Fracture*—Adversely impacts fracture healing as the fracture hematoma is lost and the fracture ends are exposed to the environment due to loss of soft tissue coverage. This leads to higher chance of infection and nonunion.
8. *Pathological Fracture Due to Infection (Osteomyelitis), Tumour, and Radiation Therapy*—It adversely impacts fracture healing due to reduced osteogenic cellularity at fracture site.
9. *Soft Tissue Interposition*—Interposition of soft tissues including muscles, fascia tendon, etc., adversely impacts fracture healing due to loss of bone contact at fracture end.

3.5.2 Systemic Factors

1. *Smoking*—Adversely impacts fracture healing. Nicotine affects the function of osteoblasts and inhibits neovascularization and angiogenesis. Smokers have higher risk of fracture nonunion than non-smokers.
2. *Diabetes Mellitus*—Affects fracture repair and remodeling of bone by reduced cellularity of fracture callus, delayed endochondral ossification, and reduced strength of fracture callus.
3. *Age*—The rate of healing decreases with increasing age due to multiple factors. The children have good fracture healing and remodeling potential than older adults.
4. *Poor Nutritional Status*—Deficiency of calcium and Vitamin D has higher risk of fracture nonunion. Protein malnourishment decreases the strength of fracture callus.
5. *Drugs*
   (a) *Non-steroidal Anti-inflammatory Drugs (NSAIDS)*—Increases the time of fracture healing.
   (b) *Steroids*—Compromise fracture healing by inhibiting differentiation of mesenchymal cells and synthesis of bone matrix. Prolonged use of steroids also decreases bone density.
6. *Hormones*
   (a) *Growth hormone*—Increases callus volume

(b) *Corticosteroids*—Decreases callus formation due to microvascular osteonecrosis.
(c) *Thyroid, Estrogen, Androgen*—Promotes fracture healing and remodeling.

7. *Associated Head Injury* (Enhanced fracture healing by exuberant callus formation)

Multiple Choice Questions

1. Primary bone healing happens by
   (a) Intramembranous bone formation
   (b) Endochondral bone ossification
   (c) Callus formation
   (d) Indirect new bone formation
2. What is the most common mode of fracture healing
   (a) Primary bone healing
   (b) Intramembranous bone formation
   (c) Secondary or Indirect fracture healing
   (d) Fibrous healing
3. Combination of fibrous tissue, cartilage and woven bone that forms at the fracture site is called
   (a) Primary bone healing
   (b) Haversian remodeling
   (c) Callus
   (d) Osteon
4. Fracture hematoma is rich in
   (a) Hematopoietic stem cells and proinflammatory cytokines
   (b) Calcium
   (c) Vitamin D
   (d) Calcitonin
5. All are risk factors of nonunion except
   (a) Smoking
   (b) Diabetes mellitus
   (c) Metaphyseal fractures
   (d) Steroid use

Answers: 1. (a), 2. (c), 3. (c), 4. (a), 5. (c)

Amputation

4

S. Lakshmana Das

4.1 Introduction

Amputation is defined as surgical removal of part or whole of the limb. Amputation is one of the oldest surgical procedures to be performed. Amputation is a reconstructive procedure performed when the part of the limb is not salvageable.

Amputation has a long and varied history that spans across different civilizations and eras. Throughout the centuries, amputation has been performed for various reasons, including medical conditions, traumatic injuries, and warfare. Egyptians and Greeks practiced amputation as early as 2600 BCE. The Edwin Smith Surgical Papyrus, an ancient Egyptian medical text, contains descriptions of amputations. In ancient Greece, renowned physician Hippocrates wrote about the indications and techniques for limb amputation. Galen, a renowned Greek physician who practiced in Rome, developed techniques and instruments for performing amputations. He employed cauterization, using a heated iron or a caustic substance to control bleeding during the procedure. The invention of ligatures and tourniquets by Ambroise Paré in the sixteenth century revolutionized amputation surgery, reducing bleeding and increasing the chances of survival. Paré also emphasized the importance of wound care and the use of antiseptics to prevent infection.

The advent of anesthesia in the nineteenth century further transformed amputation surgery. With the discovery and widespread use of ether and chloroform, patients could undergo amputations without experiencing excruciating pain. Additionally, the development of aseptic techniques by Joseph Lister significantly reduced postoperative infections. During World War I (1914–1918) and World War II (1939–1945), amputation took on a different significance as it became a necessary procedure for soldiers injured in battle. The advancements in military weaponry led to severe limb injuries that often required immediate amputation to save lives. Because of aseptic techniques, the survival rate of amputees increased significantly during these conflicts. Prosthetic limbs also underwent significant developments to aid in the rehabilitation and restoration of functionality for amputees. While the reasons for amputation and techniques have changed, the goal remains consistent: to alleviate suffering, save lives, and provide individuals with the opportunity to regain mobility and independence through advancements in surgical techniques, prosthetics, and rehabilitation.

S. Lakshmana Das (✉)
Department of Orthopedics, All India Institute of Medical Sciences, Bathinda, Punjab, India

V. Kumar et al. (eds.), *A Quick Guide to Essential Orthopedics*,
https://doi.org/10.1007/978-981-95-2676-5_4

4.2 Indications

The indication for amputations can be remembered using the pneumonic 6Ds

Dead limb—Wet and dry gangrene, frostbite
Dying limb—Ischemic limb, crush injury and severely mangled nonsalvageable limb
Deadly limb—Malignancy and infections threatening to the limb and life (Necrotizing fasciitis and gas gangrene)
Damn useless limb—Congenital limb deficiencies
Damn painful limb—Neuropathic limb
Damn nuisance limb—Diabetic and neuropathic foot, chronic nonhealing ulcer

4.3 Principles of Amputation

The principles of amputation are

1. Removing the diseased or nonfunctioning limb
2. Restoring the function of the limb to enable the patient for independent functioning
3. Preserving the length and strength of the residual limb for early prosthetic fitting
4. Providing a stable residual limb by balancing the muscle forces
5. Tapering of the bone edges to avoid sharp edges
6. The amputation stump should be cylindrical or conical to enable better prosthetic fitting
7. Prevention of hematoma formation and post-surgical edema formation
8. Postoperative analgesia for pain control

4.4 Preoperative Evaluation and Preparation

The preoperative evaluation includes assessment of the generational physiological status of the patient and assessment of the affected limb for vascularity, joint mobility, neurology, and skin integrity.

Before an amputation, it is necessary to optimize the patient. Focus should be given to the glycemic control, presence of infection or sepsis, and nutritional status of the patient. All these factors play an important role in the wound healing and recovery of the patient.

Vascular status is critical in deciding the level of amputation. The preferred modality for vascular assessment is by arterial doppler ultrasonography. Other assessment techniques are transcutaneous oxygen tension, toe systolic blood pressure, arteriography, and skin blood flow measurement.

Patient and family counselling is an important step before performing an amputation. They should be educated to view amputation as a step towards recovery, early prosthetic fitting, and return to function.

Lower limb amputations are more common than upper limb amputations. The most common cause of lower limb amputation is limb ischemia (peripheral vascular disease with or without diabetes).

4.5 Levels of Amputation (Fig. 4.1)

1. **Lower Limb Amputations**

   The levels of lower limb amputation from proximal to distal are as follows:

   (a) *Above knee amputation*

   Above knee amputations can be hemipelvectomy, hip disarticulation, short transfemoral, medium transfemoral, long transfemoral, supracondylar, and knee disarticulation.

   (b) *Below knee amputations*

   Below knee amputations include short transtibial, standard transtibial, low transtibial and symes amputation (ankle disarticulation).

   (c) *Foot and ankle amputations* (Fig. 4.2)

   This includes Boyd, Pirogoff, Chopart, Lisfranc, Transmetatarsal, Metatarsophalangeal disarticulation and toe disarticulation.

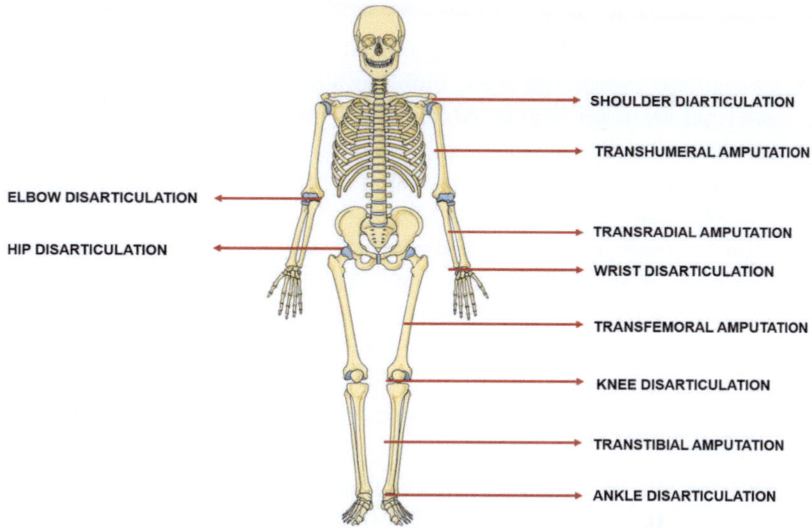

Fig. 4.1 Levels of amputation

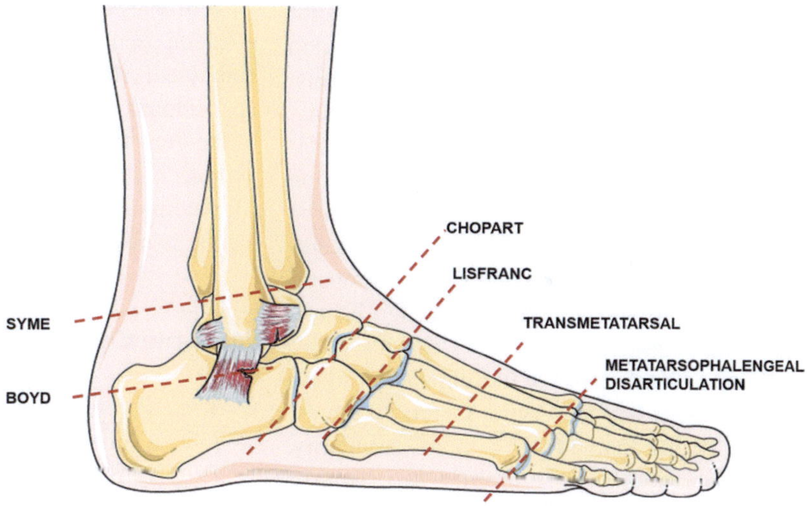

Fig. 4.2 Levels of foot and ankle amputation

2. **Upper Limb Amputations**

   The upper limb amputations include

   (a) *Forequarter amputation*
   (b) *Shoulder disarticulation*
   (c) *Transhumeral amputations—Short and standard*
   (d) *Elbow disarticulation*
   (e) *Transradial amputation*
   (f) *Wrist disarticulation*
   (g) *Transcarpal amputation*
   (h) *Ray resection*

4.6 Complications

1. *Hematoma formation*—One of the major complications following an amputation. It may be due to inadequate ligation of vessels or presence of dead space. It can be prevented by thorough ligation of the transected vessels, ensuring hemostasis and soft tissue apposition before closure of the wound, and rigid postoperative dressings with soft compression padding.

2. *Edema*—Postoperative edema may impede wound healing by placing a significant tension on the tissues. Residual limb elevation and rigid dressings help in avoiding this condition. Edema after the maturation of stump is mostly due to poor socket fit and other medical conditions.
3. *Phantom limb pain*—It is a burning painful sensation in the part of the limb that is removed. It usually diminishes over time. Treatment modalities include early prosthetic fit, use of neuromodulators like gabapentin, physical therapy, and transcutaneous nerve stimulation.
4. *Phantom limb sensation*—It is a feeling that all or a part of the amputated limb is still present. It usually decreases with time.
5. *Joint contractures*—The most common joint contractures seen are hip and knee flexion contractures. They usually develop between the time of amputation and prosthetic fitting. It may be due to improper intraoperative balancing of the muscles with the joint in flexion or lack of postoperative splinting. It can be prevented by proper positioning of the residual limb during closure, immediate postoperative rigid splinting, adequate analgesia, and early rehabilitation.
6. *Infection*—Infections of the amputation stump can happen due to varying factors like presence of residual infection, poor vascularity, and poor local hygiene. It can be superficial or deep. Treatment options include intravenous antibiotics and regular sterile dressings with or without debridement.
7. *Wound necrosis*—It may be due to insufficient blood supply, infection or errors in surgical technique and planning.

4.7 Amputation in Children

The amputation in children is different from that of the adults. The child's skeleton is immature and growing. The cause of amputation in children can be broadly divided into two categories. Congenital (60%) and acquired (40%).

Congenital: Congenital limb anomalies and deficiencies.
Acquired: Trauma, neoplasm, and infection.

The general principles of childhood amputation as summarized by Krajbich are

1. Length preservation—It is crucial
2. Growth plate preservation—Helps in preserving the length of the stump.
3. Disarticulation is better than trans-osseous amputation—Because it provides a sturdy stump for well-balanced weight bearing
4. Knee joint preservation whenever possible
5. Stabilizing the proximal part of the limb/ amputation stump

Terminal bone overgrowth is an important complication occurs in children mostly following trans-diaphyseal amputations. The bone growth is due to appositional new bone formation and not because of the growth of the physis. It is most common in younger children following traumatic amputations. Most commonly seen in humerus and fibula. It may lead to swelling, pain, and bursa formation.

Multiple Choice Questions

1. The surgical removal of the limb through the joint is called
   (a) Disarticulation
   (b) Amputation
   (c) Auto-amputation
   (d) Excision
2. The most common cause of lower limb amputation is
   (a) Trauma
   (b) Tumour
   (c) Limb ischemia
   (d) Iatrogenic
3. The specific complication following amputation in children is
   (a) Hematoma formation
   (b) Seroma formation
   (c) Pain
   (d) Terminal bone overgrowth

4. Amputation through the tarso-metatarsal joint is called
   (a) Chopart amputation
   (b) Lisfranc amputation
   (c) Boyd amputation
   (d) Syme amputation
5. Amputation through the mid-tarsal joint is called
   (a) Chopart amputation
   (b) Lisfranc amputation
   (c) Boyd amputation
   (d) Syme amputation

Answers: 1. (a), 2. (c), 3. (d), 4. (b), 5. (a)

Prosthetics and Orthosis

5

S. Lakshmana Das, Kshitij Gupta,
and Sant Prakash Gautam

5.1 Prosthesis

5.1.1 Definition

Prosthesis is a device designed to replace either the function or appearance of a limb or body part. Removal of a part or whole of a limb is called amputation. Amputations are done when all other modalities are explored, evaluated, and rejected, and removal of the limb is considered as the best solution for the patient.

5.1.2 Classification of Prostheses

1. *End-bearing prostheses*—These are designed to transfer weight directly through the prosthetic limb to the ground. They are often used for lower limb amputations, such as below-the-knee or above-the-knee amputations.
2. Suspension prostheses—These are designed to keep the prosthetic limb attached to the residual limb without transferring weight directly through the limb. They are often used for upper limb amputations, such as below-the-elbow or above-the-elbow amputations.

5.1.2.1 Criteria for Good Prosthesis

- One which fulfils its function
- Light weight
- Compliant to the patient
- Cosmetically acceptable

5.1.3 Parts of Prostheses

Prosthesis can be grossly divided into the following parts:

- Socket—Socket is the part of prosthesis that encloses the stump and forms union between stump and artificial limb.
- Suspension—Suspension is how the socket is kept on the residual limb, preventing it from falling while moving. Suspension is achieved either by using bands and straps or by using suction-fitted sockets.

S. Lakshmana Das (✉)
Department of Orthopedics, All India Institute of Medical Sciences, Bathinda, Punjab, India

K. Gupta
Department of Orthopedics, All India Institute of Medical Sciences, Rishikesh, Uttarakhand, India

S. P. Gautam
Department of Prosthetics and Orthotics, Dr Shakuntala Misra National Rehabilitation University, Lucknow, Uttar Pradesh, India

V. Kumar et al. (eds.), *A Quick Guide to Essential Orthopedics*,
https://doi.org/10.1007/978-981-95-2676-5_5

- Joint—Various joints are provided based on the level of amputation to replicate the normal movements of the limb as much as possible.
- Terminal appliance—It includes the foot and ankle for lower limb prosthesis and hand and wrist for upper limb prosthesis.

5.1.4 Types of Prostheses

1. *Lower limb prostheses*—They are designed based on the amputation level to replace missing or damaged legs and feet. They include below-the-knee, above-the-knee, and hip disarticulation prostheses.

   Lower limb prostheses are categorised as exoskeletal or endoskeletal.

   Exoskeletal prosthesis—The exoskeletal prosthesis has a rigid outer shell to provide strength and shape (Fig. 5.1).

   Endoskeletal prosthesis—The endoskeletal prosthesis has a tubular structure connecting the components and is covered by cosmetic foam. The primary components of the prosthesis are the socket, suspension system, foot, and knee unit (Fig. 5.2).
2. *Upper limb prostheses*—These are designed to replace missing or damaged arms and hands. They include below-the-elbow, above-the-elbow, wrist disarticulation, and shoulder disarticulation prostheses (Fig. 5.3).
3. *Cranial prostheses*—These are designed to replace missing or damaged parts of the skull.
4. *Facial prostheses*—These are designed to replace missing or damaged parts of the face, such as the nose, ears, and eyes.
5. *Prosthetic Foot*—Prosthetic feet can be classified into:
   - *Non articulating*
     - Non-energy storing—It is most commonly used because it is light, durable and economic. It is best for juvenile and geriatric population. E.g., SACH foot and Jaipur foot
     - Energy storing—It is indicated for active individuals

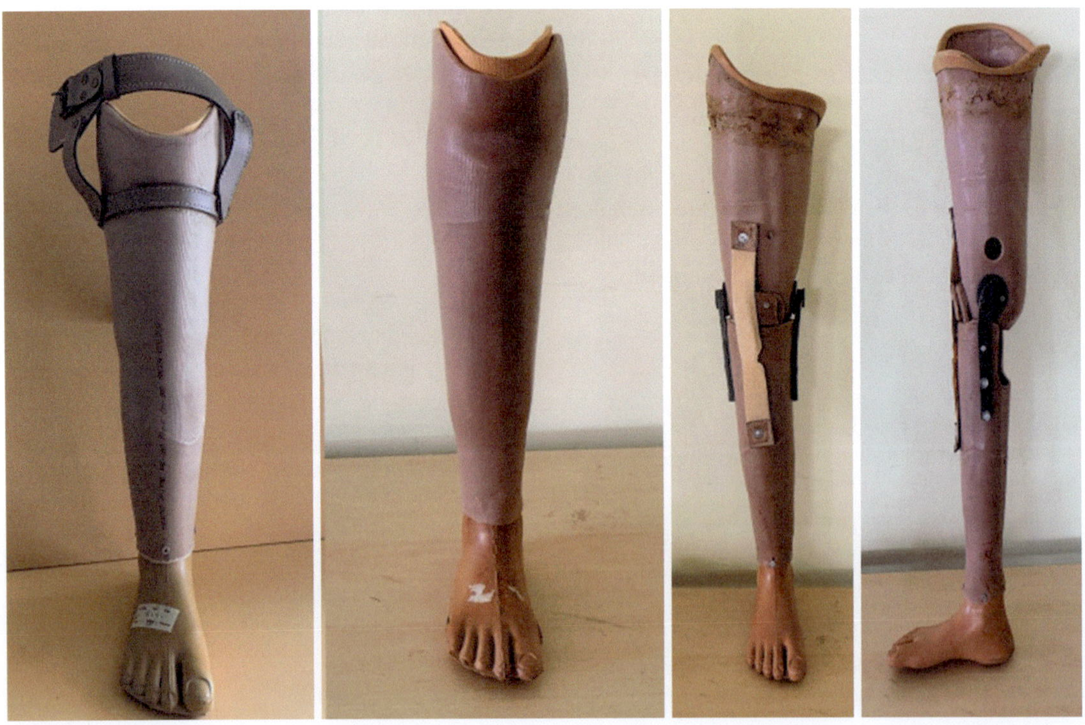

Fig. 5.1 Exoskeletal below knee and above knee prosthesis

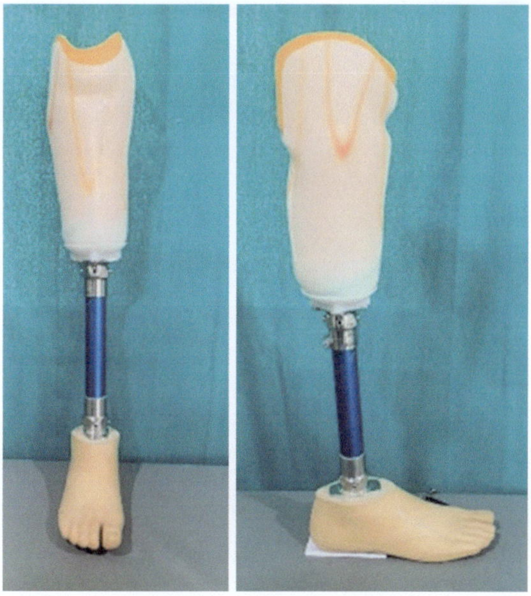

Fig. 5.2 Endoskeletal below knee prosthesis

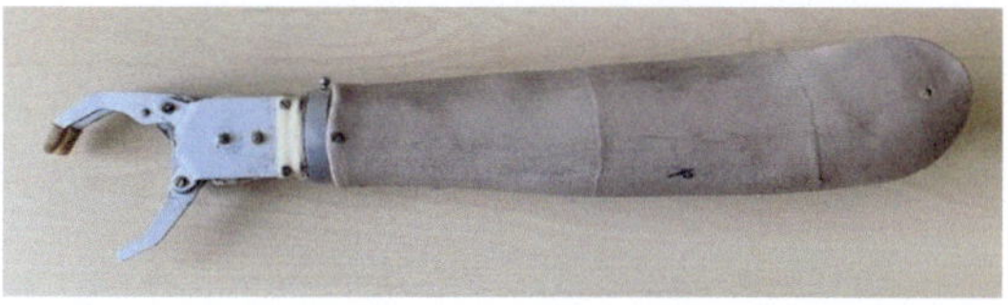

Fig. 5.3 Below elbow prosthesis

- *Articulating*
  - Single axis—It has an ankle joint that moves only in one up and down plane. It is commonly used in transfemoral amputees.
  - Multiple axes—Its joint is more versatile and allows both up and down and side-to-side movements. It is more compatible for walking on uneven surfaces.

5.1.5 Solid Ankle Cushion Heel (SACH) Foot

It consists of a solid wooden keel, high-density rubber for dorsum, and low-density rubber for toes and plantar aspect. It has no true ankle joint but contains a 'simulated ankle joint' by compressed wedge-shaped rubber heel.

5.1.6 Jaipur Foot

It was developed by Prof P.K. Sethi. It contains two wooden keels (broken keel and there is provision of toe break (Fig. 5.4 and Table 5.1).

5.1.7 Note

- *Myoelectric Prosthesis*—This is a type of prosthesis that uses electrical signals from the residual limb to control the movement of the prosthetic limb.
- *Osseointegration Prosthesis*—This is a type of prosthesis that is anchored directly to the bone, providing a more secure and stable connection between the residual limb and the prosthetic limb.

5.1.8 Immediate Post-operative Prosthesis Fitting (IPOPF)

This concept was described by Berlemont in 1961 but popularised by Weiss in 1966. A temporary prosthesis was applied in operating room at the conclusion of amputation. The most commonly used IPOP consists of a rigid plaster cast carefully moulded to a patellar tendon-bearing configuration to which pylon and foot are attached. Patient starts touchdown weight bearing within 24–48 h after surgery. Gradually weight bearing is increased with crutches and walkers.

5.1.8.1 Advantages

1. Reduces pain and edema
2. Prevents muscular atrophy
3. Prevents contracture
4. Provides good motivation
5. Reduces chances of phantom pain
6. Speeds up rehabilitation

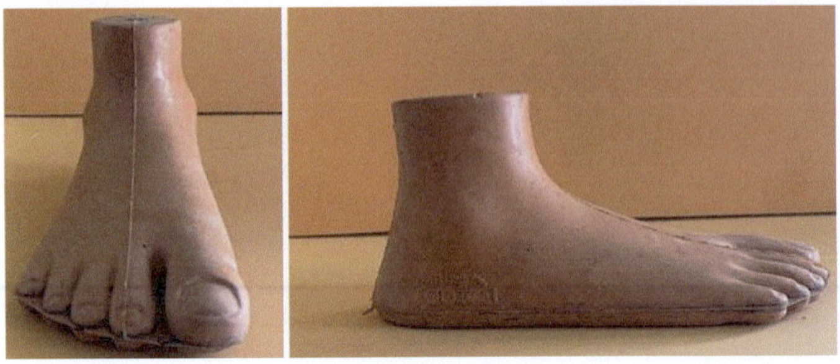

Fig. 5.4 Jaipur foot

Table 5.1 Comparison of Jaipur foot and SACH foot

Jaipur foot	SACH foot
Appearance similar to normal foot	Dissimilar to normal foot
Can be worn without shoe but if someone wishes to wear one he can use a flat heel shoe.	Requires a closed shoe to protect and hide it.
No restriction of movements at ankle as the metallic keel (carriage bolt) is confined to ankle only and all movements take place at natural site	Solid ankle consisting of long wooden keel restricts movements in nearly all directions
Squatting possible (adequate dorsiflexion)	Not possible
Cross-legged sitting is possible (adequate forefoot adduction and internal rotation possible)	Not possible
Walking on uneven ground possible (good inversion and eversion)	Suitable for walking only on level ground
Barefoot walking possible (cosmetic skin colour, no heel and toe height difference)	Not possible

5.1.8.2 Disadvantages

1. Increased incidence of wound gaping
2. Delayed wound healing
3. Infection of wound

5.1.9 Definitive Prosthesis

It is the one applied 3–6 months post-surgery once the wound has healed and the skin has matured.

5.2 Orthosis

5.2.1 Definition

An orthosis is defined as an externally applied device used to modify structural and functional characteristics of neuromusculoskeletal system. It is designed to supplement or augment the function of an existing limb or body part. It controls the abnormal movements or allows restricted normal movements.

Orthoses are given to the following conditions:

1. Post-polio paralysis
2. Nerve injuries
3. Stroke and traumatic brain injury
4. Spinal cord injury
5. Arthritis and soft tissue rheumatism
6. Deformities
7. Congenital limb deficiency
8. Burns
9. Sports

5.2.2 Functions of Orthosis

Orthosis are of two types with both having different functions.

1. *Static orthosis*
   - Protection
   - To put joints to rest
   - To decrease inflammation and pain
   - To prevent undesired motion
   - To correct deformities (e.g. serial casting)
   - Maintain limb in functional position preventing contractures
2. *Dynamic orthosis*
   - Support the segment of extremity.
   - Preventing stiffness of joint.
   - Strengthen and re-educate the muscle.
   - Mobilize the joint in desired position.
   - Assist in activities of daily living.

5.3 Spinal Orthosis

5.3.1 Cervical Orthosis

5.3.1.1 Cervical Collar

It extends from base of mandible and superior nuchal line to manubrium and C7 spine inferiorly. Functions:

1. Restricts movements of neck
2. Heat retention allowing pain relief
3. Reminder to the patient to limit cervical motion- relieves inflammation

It is of 2 types-a soft and a hard collar. Both have same function with hard collar providing more restriction of movements. Indications:

- Mild soft tissue sprains
- Spasms of cervical muscles
- Spondylosis
- Disc diseases

5.3.1.2 Philadelphia Collar

It is a semi-rigid collar made up of foam and plastic sheets. It consists of 2 separate pieces which fit around the neck using velcrow straps. It is used for temporary immobilization in cases of cervical spine injury.

5.3.2 Thoracolumbar Orthosis

5.3.2.1 Taylor's Brace

It is a semi rigid brace composed of:

- Abdominal corset with thoracic extension
- Paraspinal bars
- Shoulder harness
- Straps

Functions: It acts by limiting thoracolumbar spinal motion.

Indications:

1. Spinal osteoporosis
2. Spinal trauma
3. Degenerative disc disease
4. Pott's spine
5. Postoperative rehabilitation

5.3.2.2 Anterior Spinal Hyperextension (ASH) Brace (Fig. 5.5)

It is also a semi-rigid brace. It consists of a cruciate frame with attached pads- sternal, suprapubic, 2 lateral thoracolumbar and 1 posterior thoracolumbar pad connected with straps. It acts on principle of 3-point pressure and limits spinal flexion and provides hyperextension. It is commonly used for pathologies involving T4-L2 vertebra.

5.3.3 Lumbosacral Orthosis

5.3.3.1 Lumbosacral (LS) Corset

It is a fabric garment or thermoplastic mould that wraps around the lower abdomen and lumbosacral spine. It limits the terminal motion in lumbosacral spine, preventing further damage and provides support to the LS spine. It is commonly used for pathologies at L1-L4 levels. Indications:

1. Spinal sprain and strain
2. Degenerative spine disease
3. Prolapsed intervertebral disc (PIVD)
4. Sciatica

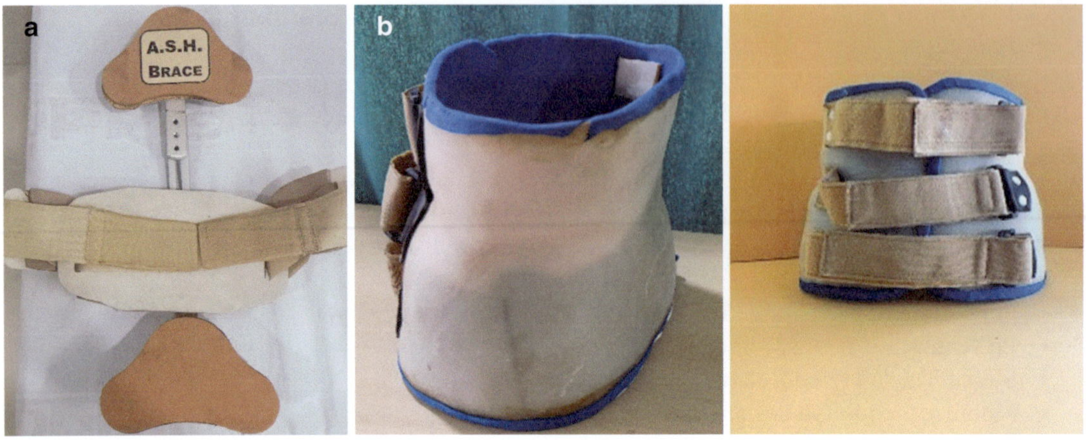

Fig. 5.5 Images of (**a**) ASH brace, (**b**) LS corset

5.3.4 Scoliosis Orthosis

Scoliosis orthosis refers to a type of spinal orthosis specifically designed for individuals with scoliosis, a condition characterised by an abnormal curvature of the spine. The goal of scoliosis orthosis is to prevent further progression of the spinal curvature and to maintain the spine in its corrected position. Bracing is used in the conservative management of mild to moderate scoliosis. Braces are typically made of plastic and are worn for several hours each day. There are several types of scoliosis orthoses, each designed to treat a specific type of scoliosis curvature.

5.3.4.1 Boston Brace

This is the most commonly used orthosis for treating scoliosis, and it is designed to correct a variety of scoliosis curves. The Boston Brace is a custom-made, rigid plastic brace that is worn around the torso and applies corrective pressure to the spine.

5.3.4.2 Milwaukee Brace (Fig. 5.6)

This type of orthosis is used to treat patients with a severe scoliosis curve that affects the entire spine. The Milwaukee Brace is a full-torso brace that extends from the neck to the hips and is designed to apply corrective pressure to the spine.

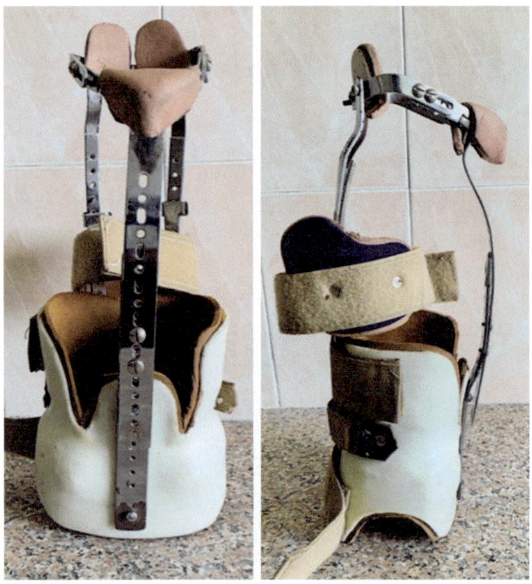

Fig. 5.6 Images of Milwaukee brace

5.3.4.3 TLSO (Thoracic-Lumbar-Sacral Orthosis)

This is a type of brace that is used to treat a variety of spinal conditions, including scoliosis. The TLSO is a custom-made, rigid plastic brace that is worn around the torso and applies corrective pressure to the spine.

5.4 Upper Limb Orthosis

5.4.1 Hand Orthosis

These are made of metal, thermoplastics, leather, or rubber. It can be either static or dynamic. Functions of hand orthosis are:

1. Restrict movement of interphalangeal joints or metacarpophalangeal joints.
2. It can be used as a corrective splint.
3. Jointed splints can also allow guarded movements of joints.

Some common hand orthosis are:

- *Finger cot*—It is used to immobilise interphalangeal joint in cases of sprains and fractures.
- *Mallet finger splint*—It immobilises the DIP joint in extension to correct finger flexion deformity seen in mallet finger (Fig. 5.7).

5.4.2 Wrist Orthosis

Functions of wrist orthosis:
1. Immobilization of wrist and metacarpophalangeal joint (MCP joint)
2. Correction of wrist deformity and MCP joints
3. Provides guarded movement at wrist and MCP joint

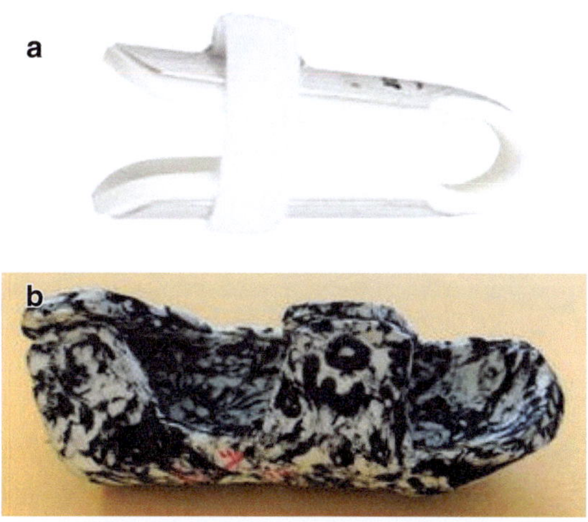

Fig. 5.7 (**a**) Finger cot, (**b**) Mallet finger splint

Some common wrist orthosis are (Fig. 5.8):

- *Static cockup splint*—This is an immobilisation splint, which maintains the wrist in extension using a volar support. Common indications are wrist and MCP joint sprain and fracture of radiocarpal and metacarpal bones.
- *Dynamic cockup splint*—This is a functional splint which maintains the wrist in 45° of extension, and fingers are extended using elastic bands, allowing active finger flexion. It is used in wrist drop.
- *Thumb spica*—It is an immobilisatiion splint which maintains the wrist in 10–20° extension with thumb in slight flexion and palmar abduction. It is used for thumb immobilisation in various traumatic and non-traumatic cases of thumb.
- *Knuckle bender splint*—This is a deformity correcting splint used in claw hand deformity.

5.4.3 Elbow Orthosis

5.4.3.1 Elbow ROM Brace

It is made of metal bars, plastics, or fabrics. It includes pieces for arm and forearm jointed at elbow to allow for movement. Functions:

1. Postoperative mobilisation of elbow
2. For sprain, strain, fractures around elbow
3. For stabilisation of unstable joint
4. Provide mediolateral stability to elbow

5.4.3.2 Turn Buckle Splint

It is a dynamic splint used to correct deformity in elbow and wrist in cases such as VIC. It is made of thermoplastics fitted around the arm and forearm or wrist. The two pieces are connected using a turnbuckle system which can be utilized to gradually correct the deformity.

5.4.4 Shoulder Orthosis

5.4.4.1 Air Plane Splint (Fig. 5.9)

It is a shoulder abduction brace. It is composed of a trunk piece with arm and forearm support. The

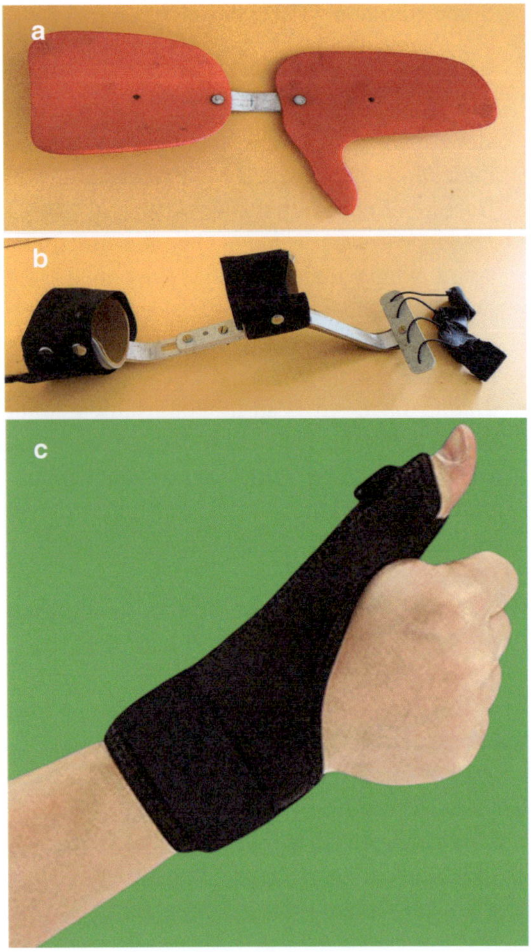

Fig. 5.8 Images of (**a**) static cockup splint (attached), (**b**) dynamic cockup splint, (**c**) thumb spica

whole splint is fixed to the body using straps. It maintains the shoulder in 90–120° abduction and 15–20° forward flexion. Functions:

1. Brachial plexus injury
2. After shoulder surgeries
3. Burn cases
4. Adduction contracture

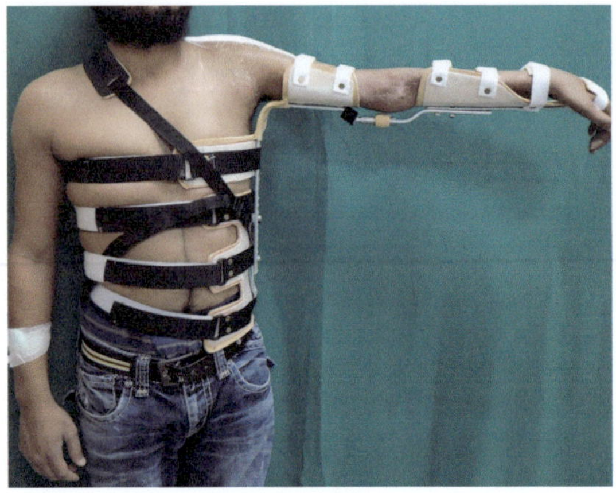

Fig. 5.9 Image of airplane splint

5.5 Lower Limb Orthosis

5.5.1 Surgical Shoe (Fig. 5.10)

Components of surgical shoe:

- Toe box
- Vamp-anterior
- Quarter-posterior
- Sole insole and outsole
- Counter
- Heel

5.5.1.1 Shoe Modifications

The function of shoe modification is (Table 5.2):

1. Restoration of normal gait
2. Proper distribution of body weight
3. Balance
4. Management of flexible deformities of foot

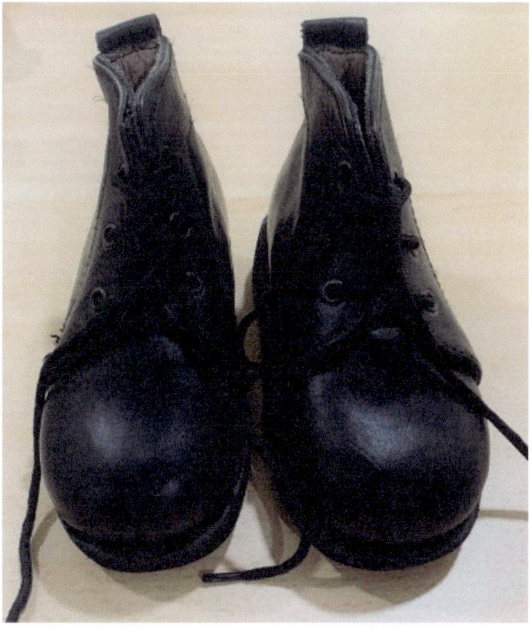

Fig. 5.10 Surgical shoe

Table 5.2 Various shoe modifications

External shoe modification	Internal shoe modification
Shoe wedging	Shoe wedging
Heel flare	Heel elevation
Heel elevation	Medial arch support
Metatarsal bar	Metatarsal pad
	Heel cushion

5.5.2 Ankle Foot Orthosis (AFO) (Fig. 5.11)

Functions of AFO:

1. Support foot and ankle, e.g., foot drop
2. Prevent equines contracture, e.g., post-surgery
3. Maintain ankle stability, e.g., paralysis

5.5.2.1 Conventional AFO

It consists of a surgical shoe with a stirrup and ankle joints. Shoe is connected to a calf band using metal uprights.

5.5.2.2 Total Contact AFO

It is thermoplastic made AFO which is placed on the posterior aspect of calf and plantar aspect of foot. It is moulded over a negative POP foot cast. It maybe of articulating or non- articulating type based on the required function.

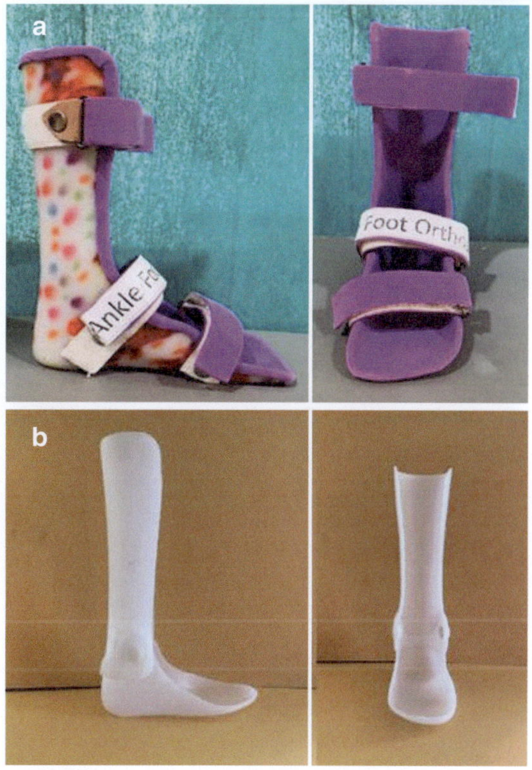

Fig. 5.11 (**a**) Static AFO, (**b**) Dynamic AFO

5.5.3 Floor Reaction AFO

This is a special type of total contact AFO. Its functioning is based on the Newton's third law. It is made of flexible polypropylene or carbonfiber with ankle kept in 3–5° of plantar flexion. The AFO is closed circumferentially proximally to encircle the proximal leg and knee. It holds the ankle in equines preventing heel from touching the ground. As the body weight forces the heel downwards, the proximal portion of AFO forces the knee into extension preventing knee buckling. It allows knee bending during the swing phase.

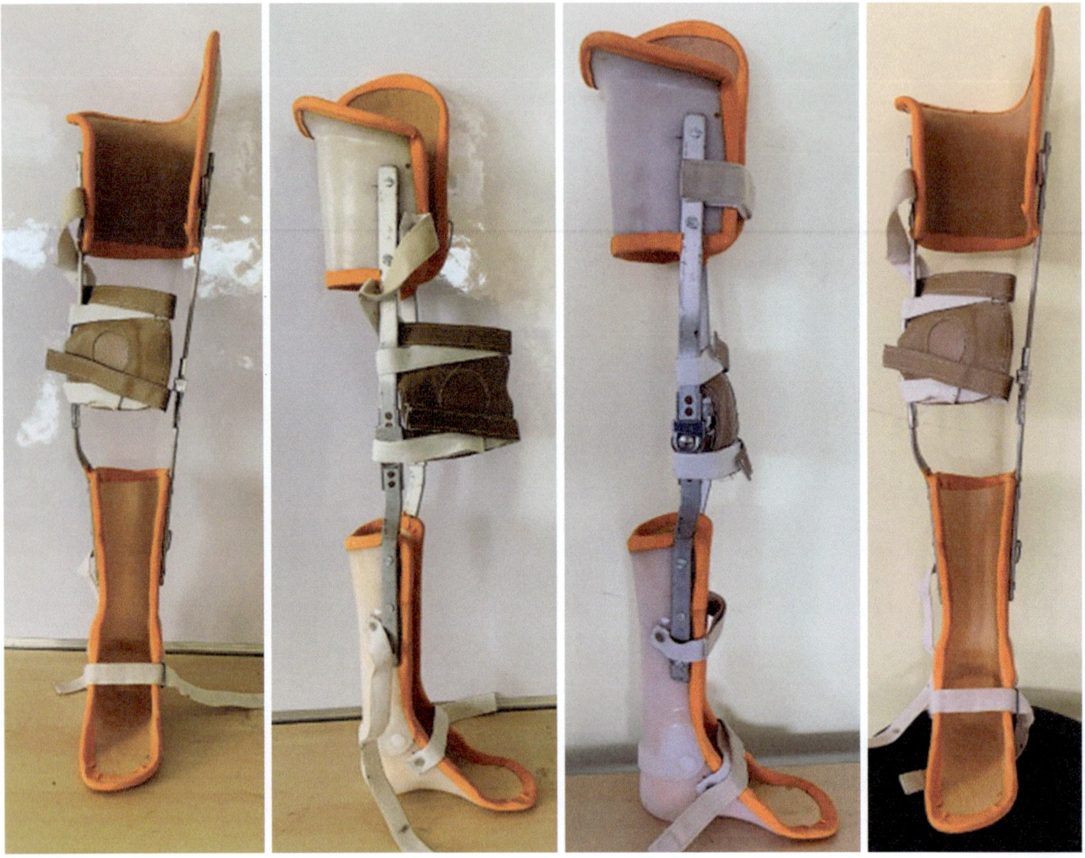

Fig. 5.12 KAFO

5.5.4 Knee Ankle Foot Orthosis (KAFO)

Functions of KAFO:

1. Prevent buckling in case like postpolio residual paralysis
2. Stabilize the knee, e.g., charcot knee
3. Relieve weight on bone and joints of lower limbs
4. Provides medio-lateral stability at ankle

There are various types of KAFOs available. The simplest is the conventional KAFO which includes a surgical shoe with an ankle joint and stirrup mounted with metal uprights. It includes a knee joint with calf and thigh bands to hold the limb in place. While total contact KAFO is made of thermoplastic pieces held with a knee joint (Fig. 5.12).

5.5.5 Hip Knee Ankle Foot Orthosis (HKAFO)

It is given when the hip muscles are weak; especially hip abductors and with hip instability. It has external hip joint and in addition pelvic band to stabilize the hip. Functions of HKAFO:

1. Maintain standing position of person and ensure mobility
2. Stabilize the hip joint

5.5.5.1 Components of HKAFO

- Surgical shoes
- Ankle joint with stirrup
- Metal uprights
- Knee and hip joints
- Calf, thigh, and pelvic bands

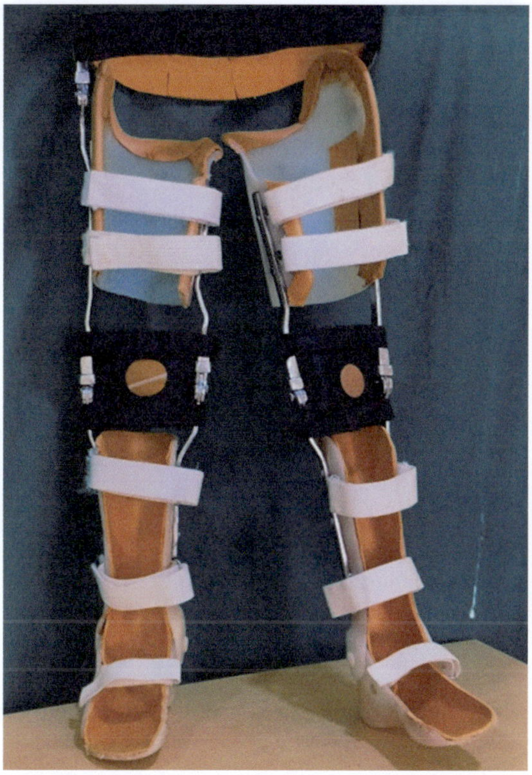

Fig. 5.13 HKAFO

A total contact HKAFO is made of thermoplastics with attached hip and knee joints. A variant of total contact HKAFO is reciprocating gait orthosis which is a bilateral HKAFO. In this orthosis, hip flexion of side is utilized to aid the extension of contralateral hip (Fig. 5.13).

5.5.6 Orthoses for Special Conditions

(a) *Developmental dysplasia of Hip (DDH)*—Pavlik harness, Von-Rosen splint, hip abduction brace (Fig 5.14)
(b) *Perthes disease—Hip abduction brace,* Trilateral orthosis, Toronto orthosis, and Newington orthosis.
(c) *Congenital talipes equinovafrus (CTEV)*—CTEV shoes. Dennis brown splint and steinbeck foot abduction brace (Fig. 5.15).

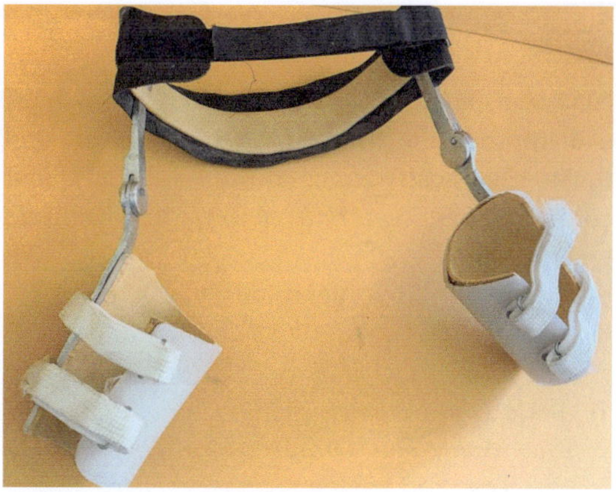

Fig. 5.14 Hip abduction brace

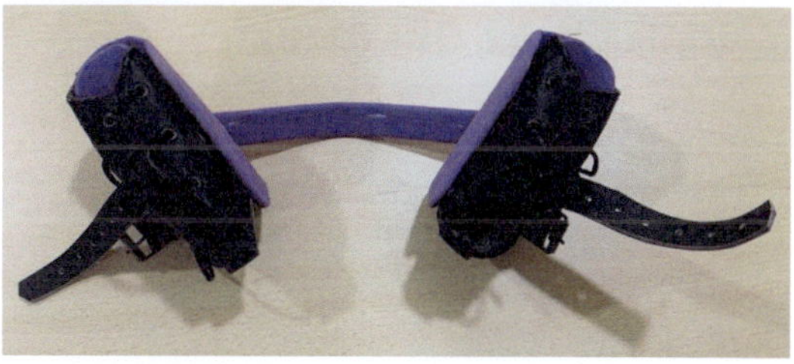

Fig. 5.15 Dennis brown splint

5.5.7 Cranial Orthoses

Cranial orthoses, also known as cranial helmets, are used to protect and shape the head, in conditions like head shape deformities and cranial vault asymmetry.

There are several types of cranial orthoses, including:

1. *Infant Helmets*—Used to treat infant head shape deformities such as plagiocephaly and brachycephaly.
2. *Scaphocephaly Helmets*—Used to treat scaphocephaly.
3. *Complex Cranial Remolding Orthoses*—Used to treat more complex cranial shape deformities, such as craniosynostosis and skull deformities.

5.5.8 Neuromuscular Orthoses

Neuromuscular orthoses are used to support and improve the function of the muscles and limbs, specifically for conditions such as spinal cord injuries, cerebral palsy, and muscle weakness.

Examples of neuromuscular orthoses, including:

1. *Ankle-Foot Orthoses (AFOs).*
2. *Knee-Ankle-Foot Orthoses (KAFOs).*
3. *Hip-Knee-Ankle-Foot Orthoses (HKAFOS).*
4. *Spinal Orthoses*

Multiple Choice Questions

1. Which material is commonly used in the fabrication of orthotic devices?
   (a) Wood
   (b) Glass
   (c) Rubber
   (d) Thermoplastics
2. What is the primary purpose of orthosis?
   (a) To treat infectious diseases
   (b) To provide support and correct deformities
   (c) To perform surgical procedures
   (d) To diagnose medical conditions
3. An orthosis designed to control motion and provide stability to the spine is called:
   (a) Spinal orthosis
   (b) Elbow orthosis
   (c) Hip orthosis
   (d) Shoulder orthosis
4. What is the main difference between orthosis and prosthesis?
   (a) Orthosis is for supporting and correcting deformities, while prosthesis replaces missing body parts.
   (b) Orthosis is used internally, while prosthesis is used externally.
   (c) Orthosis is only for the upper body, while prosthesis is for the lower body.
   (d) Orthosis is a newer medical technology compared to prosthesis.
5. Osseointegration is a technique used in prosthesis that involves:
   (a) Replacing the entire limb with a robotic device
   (b) Fusing the prosthesis with the remaining bone
   (c) Creating a wearable exoskeleton for the body
   (d) Stimulating nerve regeneration around the amputation site

Answers: 1. (d), 2. (b), 3. (a), 4. (a), 5. (b)

6 Introduction to Evidence-Based Medicine

Kshitij Gupta

6.1 Definition

Evidence-based medicine (EBM) was originally defined as the conscientious, explicit, and judicious use of current best evidence in making decisions about the care of individual patients. The practice of evidence-based medicine means integrating individual clinical expertise with the best available external clinical evidence from systematic research.

The revised and improved definition of evidence-based medicine is a systematic approach to clinical problem solving, which allows the integration of the best available research evidence with clinical expertise and patient values. EBM practitioners must combine their clinical expertise, the best available evidence and their patient's personal characteristics and preferences when making decisions (Fig. 6.1).

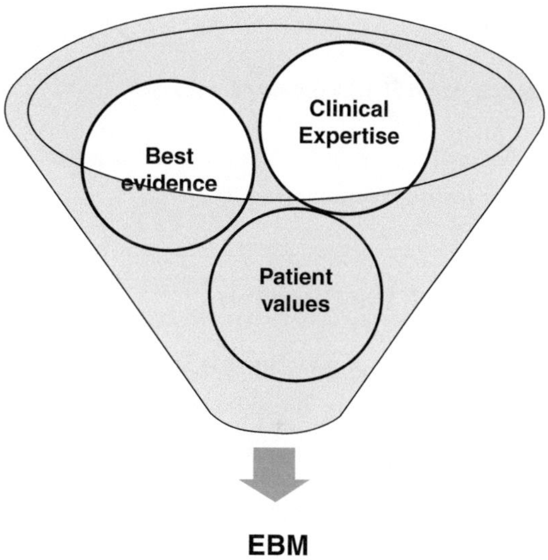

Fig. 6.1 Definition of evidence-based medicine

6.2 Steps of Evidence-Based Medicine (EBM)

The EBM cycle begins when a question arises in the course of caring for a patient. How do you practice EBM? Here is the five-step approach for practicing EBM for physicians.

1. Ask the question
2. Acquire the evidence
3. Appraise the evidence
4. Apply to the patient
5. Evaluate your performance

K. Gupta (✉)
Department of Orthopedics, All India Institute of Medical Sciences, Rishikesh, Uttarakhand, India

V. Kumar et al. (eds.), *A Quick Guide to Essential Orthopedics*,
https://doi.org/10.1007/978-981-95-2676-5_6

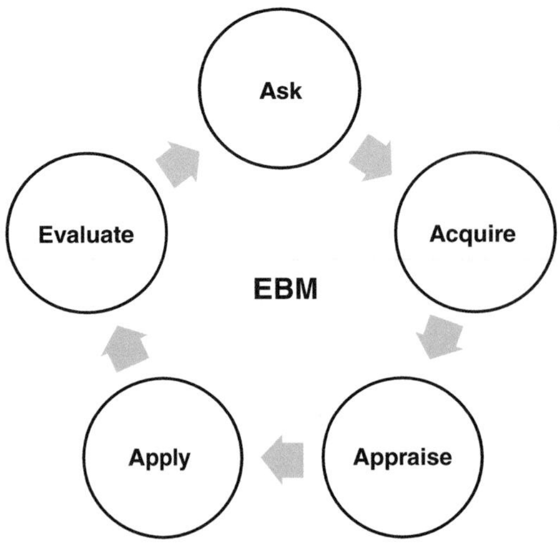

Fig. 6.2 Steps of evidence-based medicine

We will go through all of these steps individually in further sections (Fig. 6.2).

6.2.1 Ask the Question

Clinicians are posed with problems in patient care on a daily basis. It can be pertaining to diagnostics, therapeutics or cost-effectiveness of a particular test or treatment. A clinician starts his or her search for the best and newest data needed to solve individual patient's problem by formulating an answerable clinical question. Good clinical question must be clear, directly focused on the problem, and answerable by searching the medical literature.

6.2.1.1 PICO Format

A good clinical question should have four essential components structured in the PICO format

P—Patient population or the problem: who are our relevant patients, and what problem are we trying to solve?
Intervention—It can be a diagnostic test or therapeutic modality—drug or surgery
C—Comparison—What is our alternate management strategy against which we are comparing our current intervention?
O—Outcomes—What are the consequences of our intervention that we are interested in?

6.2.2 Acquire the Evidence

The next step is to search for relevant evidence that will provide the answer to the question. The ideal information source is valid, relevant, comprehensive, and user-friendly. The sheer vastness of information available can be perplexing to the clinician. Because searching the primary literature is challenging and time consuming, a number of resources exist to help clinicians identify the most relevant evidence to answer their clinical questions. These include clinical practice guidelines from professional organizations and commercial resources which aim to collect and synthesize all available literature on a topic. Figure 6.3 shows the pyramid depicting the hierarchy of evidence available to us. Though the hierarchy is not absolute. For e.g., a well-designed cohort study with a large sample size might hold more credibility than a poorly designed and poorly executed RCT. That's where the role of critically appraising the evidence comes into play.

6.2.3 Appraise the Evidence

In the critical appraisal process, you are seeking to determine what accounts for a study's results. In critically analyzing a study, we aim to determine whether a study's results are most likely due to bias, chance, confounding, or truth. The questions needed to critically appraise a specific study will depend on the study design but, broadly speaking, should include the following:

1. Validity: Are the study results valid? Was an appropriate research method used, and how were biases handled?
2. Significance: What are the results, and are they statistically significant? What is the clinical importance of the findings?
3. Generalizability: Are the results of the study generalizable to your patient or population?

The ability to critically appraisal a study requires an understanding of epidemiology and

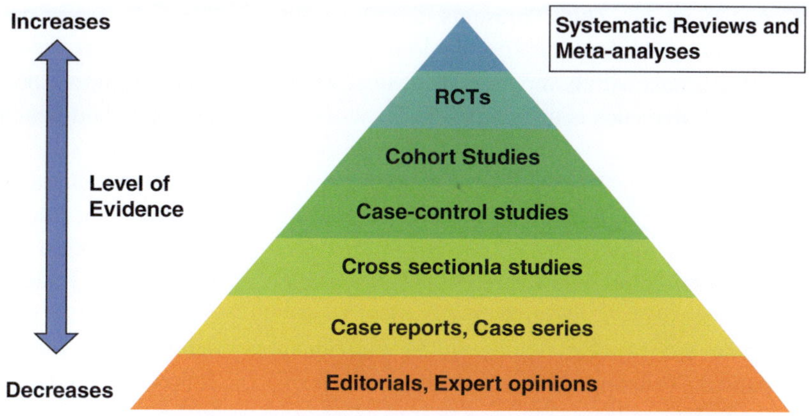

Fig. 6.3 Hierarchy of evidence

biostatistical concepts such as clinical study designs, biases and confounders and common measures of association in biomedical studies.

6.2.4 Apply to the Patient

The most crucial step in practice of EBM is to apply the acquired information to our patient. We need to take into account special circumstances pertaining to each patient. We need to be aware if there is something in relation to our patient because of which we need to discard the acquired information. The questions that we should ask before the decision to apply the results of the study are:

(a) Are the participants in the study similar enough to my patient?
(b) Is the treatment available, and is healthcare system prepared to fund it?
(c) What alternatives are available?
(d) Do the potential side effects of the drug or procedure outweigh the benefits?
(e) Are the outcomes appropriate to the patient? Does the treatment conflict with the patient's values and expectations?

Eliciting a patient's values and preferences and taking them into account when making decisions is a complex skill set. Evidence-based medicine requires that clinical decisions be consistent with the informed values and preferences of the patient.

6.2.5 Evaluate Your Performance

The final step is the evaluation of your evidence-based approach and the efficiency of its application to your patient. During this process it is important to assess whether the evidence-based intervention worked as expected. If not, what could be the cause for the deviation of results in our patient compared to the evidence? EBM is constantly evolving, and thus it becomes necessary to evaluate the performance of EBM, whether positive or negative. A clinician need to find the cause of EBM not working the way it was expected and also find ways that it can be made to work as expected.

Evidence-based medicine (EBM) is the conscious, reasonable, and specific use of the best available evidence in making the best possible decisions in the management of individual patients. It is not a medical cookbook of recipes. It requires time and a skillset in the use of computers, biostatistics, and epidemiology on part of the clinician, but its good use brings about cost-effective and better health-care for the patient.

Multiple Choice Questions

1. Which of the following study designs represent a level III evidence study?
   (a) Prospective, randomized controlled trial
   (b) Retrospective case-control study
   (c) Retrospective case series
   (d) Prospective cohort study

2. A therapeutic study presents a systematic review of 15 high-quality randomized controlled trials with homogeneous results. What level of evidence is this considered?
   (a) I
   (b) II
   (c) III
   (d) IV
3. Evidence-based medicine (EBM) is a systematic approach to identifying the most appropriate strategy for managing an individual patient. This approach is based on which of the following?
   (a) Advice given by mentors and colleagues
   (b) Analysis of relevant medical literature
   (c) Advice derived from recently published literature
   (d) Strategies based of your personal opinions
4. The first step in practicing EBM is formulating a clinical question. A well-designed question specifies the population under study, outcome, and which of the following?
   (a) Costs
   (b) Patient characteristics
   (c) Relevant studies
   (d) Intervention
5. Good clinical question must be clear, directly focused on the problem, and answerable by searching the medical literature. Which of the following is not the component of a good clinical question?
   (a) Patient population
   (b) Outcome
   (c) Cost
   (d) Intervention

Answers: 1. (b), 2. (a), 3. (b), 4. (d), 5. (c)

Part II

Basic Traumatology

7 Common Terminologies and Classification of Fractures

Syed Ifthekar

7.1 Fracture

A bone is said to be fractured when there is a break in the cortical continuity which is visible radiologically as a breach in at least one of the cortices.

For the sake of better understanding and nomenclature, the fractures are classified based on the

1. Displacement of fracture fragment
2. Segment/part of the bone involved
3. Completeness of fracture
4. Morphology of fracture
5. Relation with the exterior
6. Etiology of fracture

7.2 Displacement of Fracture Fragment

- **Undisplaced fractures:** The fractures are said to be undisplaced when the fractured segments of bone remain aligned to each other (Fig. 7.1a)
- **Displaced fractures**: The fractures are said to be displaced when the alignment between the fracture segments is lost. Displacement of the fracture occurs due to one or combined effects of the following factors (Fig. 7.1b)
  (a) Primary force of the injury
  (b) Gravitational force acting on fragments
  (c) Due to the powerful pull of muscles attached to the bony fragments

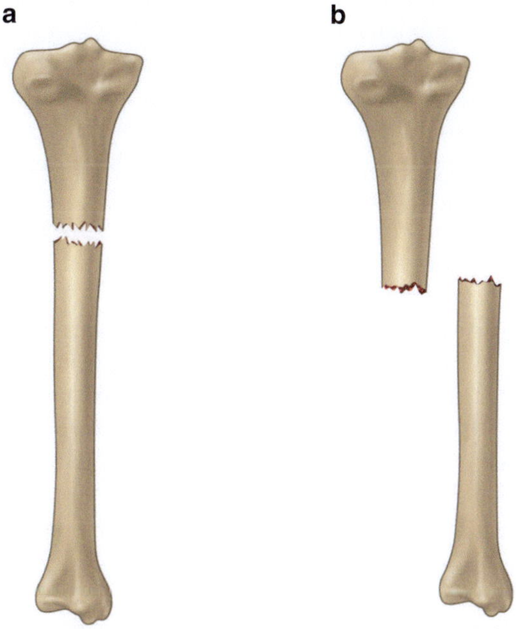

Fig. 7.1 (**a**) Undisplaced fracture, (**b**) Displaced fracture

The displacement of the fractured fragments is usually described in relation to the direction of distal fragment. There are various types of dis-

S. Ifthekar (✉)
Department of Orthopedics, All India Institute of Medical Sciences, Bibinagar, Telangana, India

V. Kumar et al. (eds.), *A Quick Guide to Essential Orthopedics*,
https://doi.org/10.1007/978-981-95-2676-5_7

placements routinely observed in orthopedic trauma. They are,

(a) *Medial displacement*—The distal fragment is displaced medially with reference to proximal fragment.
(b) *Lateral displacement*—The distal fragment is displaced laterally with reference to proximal fragment.
(c) *Anterior displacement*—The distal fragment is displaced anteriorly with reference to proximal fragment.
(d) *Posterior displacement*—The distal fragment is displaced posteriorly with reference to proximal fragment.
(e) *Dorsal displacement*: This nomenclature is usually used in relation to wrist fractures when the distal fragment is dorsally(extension) displaced with reference to proximal fragment.
(f) *Volar displacement*: The distal fragment is volarly (flexion) displaced with reference to proximal fragment.
(g) *Avulsion fractures*: These fractures are a type of displaced fracture which occur when the tendon/ligament attached to the bone undergoes violent contraction, causing a fracture.

Displacement is also described in terms of translation, rotation, angulation and shortening or lengthening.

Translation (shift): The fracture is said to be translated when there is a simple shift of the fracture fragments in anteroposterior or mediolateral planes.

Rotation (twist): When the fractured fragment is twisted along its long axis, the fracture is said to be rotated.

Angulation: When the fracture fragments are oriented to each other at a specific angle, the fracture is said to be angulated.

Shortening: There may be apposition of fracture fragments leading to shortening or distraction leading to lengthening.

7.3 Segment/Part of the Bone Involved

The classical long bone has three parts. The epiphysis, metaphysis, and diaphysis. The fractures involving the bone can be named as epiphyseal, metaphyseal, or diaphyseal fractures. The classification can further be made accurate by using proximal and distal in addition to the above nomenclature.

7.4 Completeness of Fracture

7.4.1 Complete Fractures

In these fractures, the bone is distinctively divided into a minimum of two fragments. When there are numerous small fragments in the fracture, such fractures are called comminuted fractures. These are usually unstable fractures and require stabilization.

7.4.2 Incomplete Fractures

These fractures are usually seen in children who have thick periosteum. The bone is not completely separated after the fracture due to thick and intact periosteum. These fractures are named as greenstick fractures as they resemble a broken fresh green twig. There can also be buckling in the metaphysis of the children after injury. These fractures are called as torus fractures.

In adults, the incomplete fractures are usually seen in cancellous bones like vertebral bodies (compression fractures) and calcaneum.

7.5 Morphology of Fracture

Based on the morphological appearance, the fractures can be classified into following patterns (Fig. 7.2).

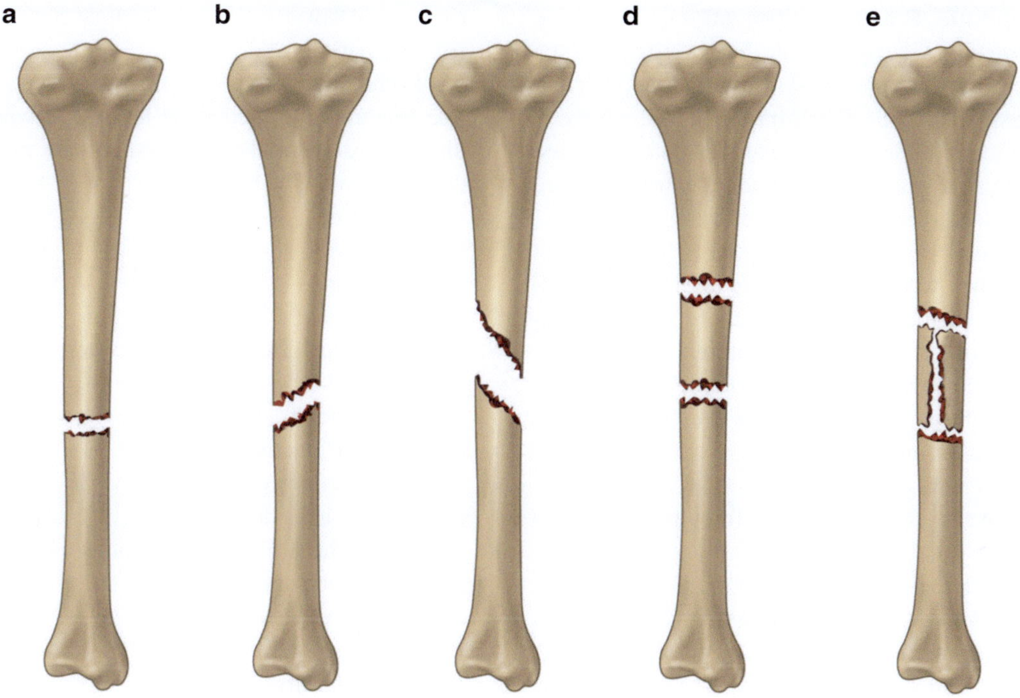

Fig. 7.2 (**a**) Transverse fracture, (**b**) Oblique fracture, (**c**) Spiral fracture, (**d**) Segmental fracture, (**e**) Comminuted fracture

Transverse fracture: When the fracture line is either perpendicular or less than 30 degrees tilted to the long axis of the bone, the fracture is named as transverse fracture.

Oblique fractures: When the fracture line is tilted more than 30 degrees to the long axis of the bone, the fracture is named as an oblique fracture.

Spiral fractures: These fractures are commonly seen in rotational injuries where the fracture line runs spirally in more than one plane.

Segmental fractures: When the fracture of the long bone results in more than two large fragments, the fracture is said to be segmental.

Comminuted fractures: These fractures are usually caused by crushing and high-velocity injuries where the bone is crushed into multiple small fragments.

7.6 Relation with the Exterior

Based on the communication of the fracture hematoma with the external environment, the fractures are classified into following types.

Closed Fractures: The fracture hematoma in these types of fractures does not communicate with the external environment.

Open Fractures: When the fracture hematoma is in communication with the external environment, the fracture is labelled as open fracture.

7.7 Etiology of Fracture

Based on the cause or etiology that leads to fracture, the fractures are classified into following types.

Traumatic Fractures: The etiology in these fractures is significant direct injury to the bone.

Stress or Fatigue Fractures: When the bone is fractured due to abnormal and unaccustomed physical stresses on bone, the fractures are classified as stress fractures.

Pathologic Fractures: If a fracture occurs in an already weakened bone due to disease/pathology of the bone, that fracture is termed as pathologic fracture. The patient comes to the hospital with the history of inability to bear weight or inability to use the limbs after a trivial trauma.

The causes for pathologic fractures can be

(a) *Congenital causes*: Osteogenesis imperfecta
(b) *Inflammatory/Infective causes*: Osteomyelitis
(c) *Neoplastic*: Osteoclastoma, Osteosarcoma
(d) *Systemic*: Osteoporosis, Osteomalacia, Rickets
(e) *Miscellaneous*: Aneurysmal bone cyst, Simple bone cyst

Multiple Choice Questions

1. Which of the following displacements are not seen in Colles fracture?
   (a) Dorsal displacement
   (b) Dorsal Tilt
   (c) Supination
   (d) Pronation
2. The fracture is termed to be transverse when the fracture line makes an angulation of more than ____ with the horizontal.
   (a) 30 degrees
   (b) 10 degrees
   (c) 20 degrees
   (d) 15 degrees
3. The children often experience incomplete fractures and they are called
   (a) Greenstick fractures
   (b) Rolando fractures
   (c) Essex Lopresti fractures
   (d) Malgaignes fractures
4. Which of the following is not a cause of pathologic fracture?
   (a) Fall from 10 feet height
   (b) Osteomyelitis
   (c) Pagets disease
   (d) Osteoporosis
5. A military recruit had pain in the foot after prolonged drills; the most probable etiology after x rays would be
   (a) Stress fractures
   (b) Osteosarcoma of metatarsal
   (c) Osteomyelitis of metatarsal
   (d) Tendon rupture

Answers: 1. (d), 2. (a), 3. (a), 4. (a), 5. (a)

8 Open Fractures

Syed Ifthekar and Vishal Kumar

8.1 Definition

When a fracture is exposed to the external environment due to disruption of the soft tissues and overlying skin, such fractures are called open fractures (Fig. 8.1).

These are usually caused due to high-energy injuries, which are associated with varying degrees of soft tissue damage, compromised vascular supply and contamination in most of the cases. These injuries pose a significant challenge to the treating surgeon because of the compromise in the blood supply, overlying skin/soft tissue cover and associated infection.

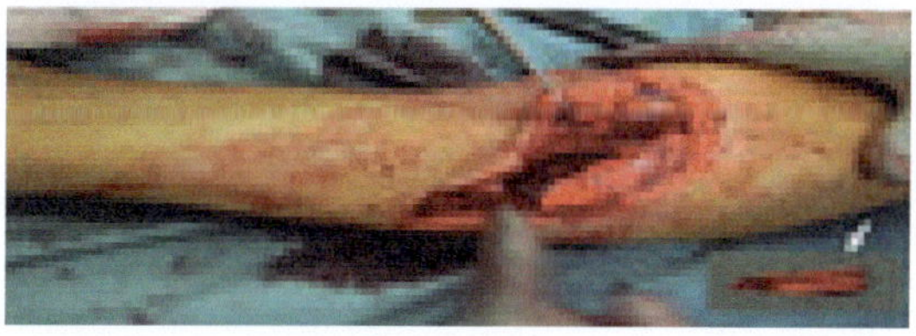

Fig. 8.1 Open fracture of Tibia

S. Ifthekar (✉)
Department of Orthopedics, All India Institute of Medical Sciences, Bibinagar, Telangana, India

V. Kumar
Department of Orthopaedics, PGIMER, Chandigarh, Chandigarh, India

8.2 Clinical Features of Open Fractures

When a patient comes to emergency room with an open fracture, usually the injury will be associated with high-energy trauma. This concept should be kept in mind while evaluating the patients with open fractures. All the patients should be evaluated initially with the established principles of Advanced Trauma Life Support (ATLS). The priority should be set accordingly, and airway, breathing and circulation should be evaluated in the initial period of arrival.

Once the steps of ATLS are followed and the patient is stabilised, the local wound must be packed by a sterile compression bandage, the fracture must be splinted and the limb must be elevated.

A quick evaluation of the examination of the wound to assess the extent of soft tissue injury and thorough clinical evaluation for distal neural and vascular deficits, if any, should be noted. Neural status can be evaluated by asking the patient to move the fingers/toes of the extremity, and vascular status can be evaluated by assessing the distal pulses, colour of the skin and warmth of the skin. Oozing should be controlled by sterile saline packing, and an attempt to tie a bleeding vessel should only be considered when a large bleeding vessel is confirmed.

V. Kumar et al. (eds.), *A Quick Guide to Essential Orthopedics*,
https://doi.org/10.1007/978-981-95-2676-5_8

8.3 Investigations

The investigations should be requested according to the nature of the injury and associated systemic injuries.

Ordering Xrays of the involved extremity in two perpendicular planes is a standard investigation—This gives the idea regarding the severity, comminution or bone loss at fracture site and also helps in planning the treatment.

CT scan—If the fractures are periarticular or intra-articular, the CT scan gives accurate information regarding the morphology of the fracture and is vital in preoperative planning.

Doppler scan—If the peripheral vessels are not palpable after injury, a doppler examination reveals the site of vessel injury and extent of vessel injury.

8.4 Classification of Open Fractures

Gustilo-Anderson classification of open fractures is by far the most commonly used open fracture classification system. It considers the open skin wound, the extent of soft tissue injury, the type of bony injury and the level of contamination. The classification system has three grades, with the third grade further divided into three categories. The classification system is as follows.

Grade	Skin wound	Soft tissue status	Bone fracture	Contamination
I	Less than 1 cm in length	Minimal muscle contusion. Inside out injuries	Simple transverse or oblique pattern	Usually clean wound
II	Length between 1–10 cms	Minimal to moderate crushing component/periosteal stripping	Short transverse/oblique with minimal contamination	Minimal contamination
IIIA	>10 cms	Severe crush but no need of flap	Comminuted fracture	High contamination
IIIB	>10 cms	Very severe crush, requires flaps	Severely comminuted, bone loss/tissue loss	High contamination
IIIC	>10 cms	Very severe crush with vascular injury requiring repair.	Severe comminuted, bone / tissue loss	High contamination

8.4.1 Few Exceptions to This Classification

IIIC—Irrespective of the size of the wound, vascular compromise will make the injury IIIC

IIIB—Irrespective of the size of the wound, following characteristics in an injury will make it IIIB

1. Farm injuries with severe contamination with faecal matter or sewage.
2. Severe crush injury with extensive devitalisation of soft tissues.
3. Extensive degloving of the skin or deep abrasions requiring debridement of the skin.
4. High-energy injuries with severe comminution of the bone or primary bone loss at accident site.
5. Delay in treatment for more than 12 h.

IIIA—Gunshot injuries are grouped as type IIIA injuries irrespective of the skin loss.

Gustilo-Anderson classification has a value in prognosticating the injury and guiding towards the treatment based on the grades of the classification. However, this classification does not help the treating surgeon to decide regarding the salvage of the injured limb. So other scoring systems like Mangled extremity severity score and Ganga Hospital Open Injury Severity Score were designed.

8.5 Mangled Extremity Severity Score (MESS)

Modality	Definition	Points
A	*Skeletal/soft tissue injury*	
	Low energy (stab; simple fracture; civilian GSW)	1
	Medium energy (open or multiple fractures; dislocation)	2
	High energy (close-range shotgun or 'military' GSW; crush injury	3
	Very high energy (above and gross contamination; soft-tissue avulsion)	4
B	*Limb ischemia (*Score doubled for ischemia > 6 h)*	
	Pulse reduced or absent but perfusion normal	1
	Pulseless; paraesthesia; diminished capillary refill	2
	Cool; paralyzed; insensate; numb.	3
C	*Shock*	
	Systolic BP always >90 mm Hg	0
	Hypotensive transiently	1
	Persistent hypotension	2
D	*Age (years)*	
	<30	0
	30–50	1
	>50	2

8.6 Total Score in a Patient and Its Interpretation

<7: Salvage
≥7: Amputation

8.7 Ganga Hospital Open Injury Severity Score

This score was evaluated based on injury to the covering structures (skin), structural tissues (bone) and functional tissues (muscles, tendons and nerves).

One to five points are allocated, according to the severity of injury, to each of the three components of the limb. Systemic factors, which may influence treatment and outcome, are given two points each, and the final score is derived by adding the individual scores together.

Ganga Hospital Open Injury Severity Score	
Covering Structures: Skin and Fascia	
Wound with no skin loss and not over the fracture site	1
Wound with no skin loss and over the fracture site	2
Wound with skin loss and not over the fracture site	3
Wound with skin loss and over the fracture site	4
Wound with circumferential skin loss	5
Functional Tissues: Musculotendinous and Nerve Units	
Partial injury to musculotendinous unit	1
Complete but repairable injury to musculotendinous units	2
Irreparable injury to musculotendinous units, partial loss of a compartment, or complete injury to posterior tibial nerve	3
Loss of one compartment of musculotendinous units	4
Loss of two or more compartments or subtotal amputation	5
Skeletal Structures: Bone and Joints	
Transverse or oblique fracture or butterfly fragment	1
Large butterfly fragment >50% circumference:	2
Comminution or segmental fractures without bone loss	3
Bone loss <4 cm	4
Bone loss >4 cm	5
Comorbid Conditions: Add 2 Points for Each Condition Present	
Injury leading to debridement interval >12 h	
Sewage or organic contamination or farmyard injuries	
Age >65 years	
Drug-dependent diabetes mellitus or cardiorespiratory diseases leading to increased anaesthetic risk	
Polytrauma involving chest or abdomen with injury severity score >25 or fat embolism	
Hypotension with systolic blood pressure	
Another major injury to the same limb or compartment syndrome	

8.7.1 Interpretation of the Score

≤14: Salvage
≥17: Amputation

Injuries with scores of 15 and 16 are in borderline, and decision can be made on patient-to-patient basis.

8.8 Treatment

All the patients should be resuscitated in the casualty according to ATLS guidelines and once stabilised, the treatment of the injured extremity should begin.

The salvage of the injured extremity in question can be decided by the above scores.

Once the extremity is decided to be salvaged,

1. The extremity should be immobilised with a well-padded splint over the sterile dressing. Exploration and debridement should be avoided in emergency department.
2. Antibiotic prophylaxis according to the institutional protocol should be administered as soon as possible to decrease the risk of infection.
3. Tetanus toxoid prophylaxis should be administered if the last booster dose is administered more than 5 years ago.
4. Parenteral analgesics should be administered to relieve the patient of pain.
5. Complete and adequate imaging of the extremity is obtained before definitive planning is done.

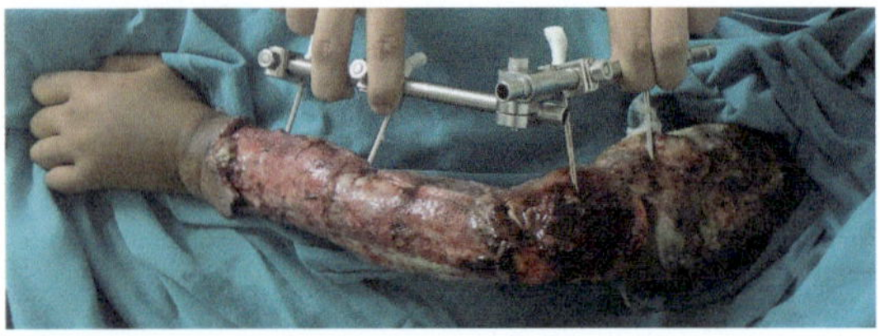

Fig. 8.2 Before debridement

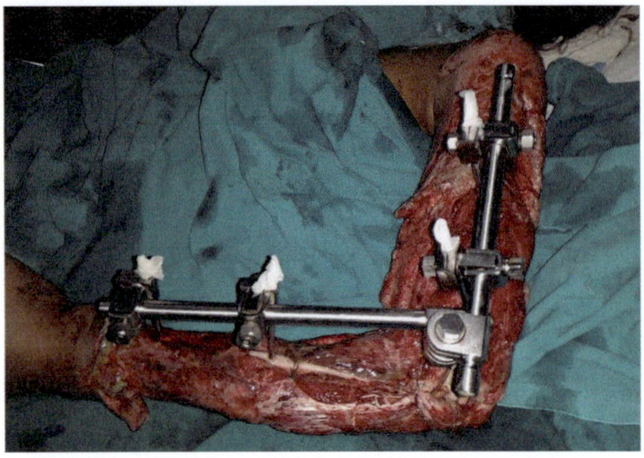

Fig. 8.3 After debridement

8.8.1 Debridement

After a definitive plan is documented and the salvage is decided, the patient should be taken to operating room, and a thorough debridement should be done under anaesthesia as soon as possible (Figs. 8.2 and 8.3).

The dead skin and muscles should be removed. Muscles are evaluated for viability using 4C (colour, consistency, contractility and capacity to bleed) formula. Dead bone pieces devoid of periosteum and soft tissues should also be removed from the wound.

8.8.2 Wound Cover

The wound can be covered by sterile dressings if adequate soft tissue cover is available, or VAC (vacuum assisted closure)/LAD (Limited access dressing) can be used depending on the case.

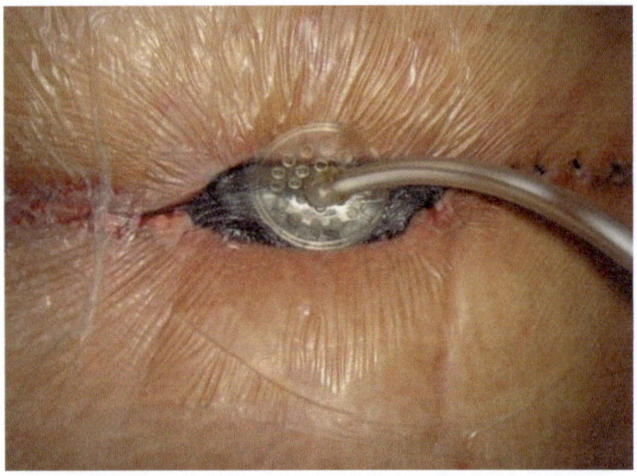

Fig. 8.4 Showing VAC application on wound

Once the infection subsides and the wound is healthy, flaps or grafts can be planned (Fig. 8.4).

8.9 Topical Oxygen

Topical oxygen therapy can be considered as an adjunctive modality for the treatment and management of wound care. The various modalities of delivery of oxygen can be classified as topical, intermittent or continuous. An example of intermittent, topical oxygen is hyperbaric oxygen (HBO) therapy. The oxygen is supplied in a high-pressure chamber (>1.4 atm) for about 90 min a day, 3–5 days a week. Flaps or skin covers can be planned once the infection subsides and wound heals.

Bone Stabilisation Usually, external fixators play an important role in stabilising the fractured bone. Ilizarov ring fixator can also be used in treating intraarticular/metaphyseal fractures (Fig. 8.5).

Definitive fixation like interlocking nails/plates can also be considered if the wound after debridement is healthy (usually in grade 1 and 2 open fractures).

Amputation Primary amputation is considered if the limb is non-viable and salvage is impossible according to the MESS and Ganga hospital scores. The examination should be documented by two different surgeons independently. Written informed consent should be taken before amputation is attempted.

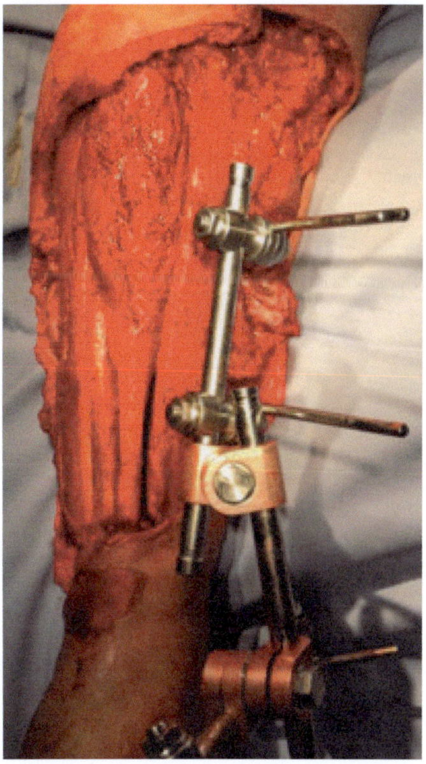

Fig. 8.5 Showing an external fixator applied to an open fracture

The open fractures are always complex injuries, and treatment of these injuries is challenging. Multimodality approach involving different fields like plastic surgery, rehabilitation medicine, and microbiology should be considered for the best outcome of the patient.

Multiple Choice Questions

1. The mangled extremity severity score (MESS) utilises all of the following variables EXCEPT:
   (a) Shock
   (b) Age
   (c) Skeletal injury
   (d) Time from admission to surgery
2. In open fractures stabilised with external fixators, which is the better dressing system?
   (a) Daily dressing
   (b) Limited access dressing
   (c) VAC dressing
   (d) Antibiotic solution dressings
3. Intra-articular grade 3 open tibial fractures are best treated by
   (a) Plating of fracture
   (b) Ilizarov fixation
   (c) Amputation
   (d) Nailing of fracture
4. Muscles are evaluated for viability using all of the following except:
   (a) Colour
   (b) Contractility
   (c) Consistency
   (d) Swelling
5. Open fractures are prognosticated according to the Ganga Hospital Open Injury Severity Score (GHOIS). Which of the following scores indicate amputation?
   (a) 8
   (b) 3
   (c) 10
   (d) 11

Answers: 1. (d), 2. (b), 3. (b), 4. (d), 5. (a)

Pathological Fractures

9

Syed Ifthekar and Sitanshu Barik

9.1 Definition

When a fracture occurs in a bone which is already weakened by some diseases, such fractures are termed pathological fractures.

9.2 Etiology

The bone strength may be compromised due to various causes. Some of these can be limited to a single bone, whereas few disorders may be generalised bone disorders. The various causes are enlisted in the below table.

9.3 Generalised Diseases

9.3.1 Genetic

Osteopetrosis
Osteogenesis imperfecta

9.3.2 Metabolic/Deficiency Disorders

Rickets
Scurvy
Osteoporosis
Osteomalacia

9.3.3 Malignancy

Multiple myeloma
Metastasis

9.3.4 Miscellaneous

Paget's disease

9.4 Localised Diseases

9.4.1 Tumours

Benign—Chondromas, Osteoclastoma
Malignant
- Primary—Osteosarcoma, Ewing's tumour
- Secondary—Lung, Breast, Prostate, Cervix, Ovaries

Infective:
- Pyogenic Osteomyelitis
- Tubercular Osteomyelitis

S. Ifthekar (✉)
Department of Orthopedics, All India Institute of Medical Sciences, Bibinagar, Telangana, India

S. Barik
Department of Orthopaedics, AIIMS Nagpur, Nagpur, Maharashtra, India

V. Kumar et al. (eds.), *A Quick Guide to Essential Orthopedics*,
https://doi.org/10.1007/978-981-95-2676-5_9

9.5 Clinical Features

The patients with pathological fractures often complain of pain, deformity and inability to bear weight following trivial trauma or sometimes spontaneously while sleeping. Few patients may have a history of genetic diseases or previous malignancy.

9.6 Examination

Tell-tale signs of previously healed fractures and deformities, as in genetic causes, can be seen. All the signs of fracture, like visible deformity of the extremity, swelling, tenderness, and crepitus while handling the fracture are present.

9.7 Investigations

The investigations of a pathological fracture depend on the suspected etiology. The initial investigation in any pathological fracture is plain x-ray of the involved bone in two perpendicular planes.

Following the x-ray examination and complete history, further investigations are performed in the form of

1. MRI.
2. CT scan.
3. PET CT scan.
4. Skeletal survey.
5. In suspected cases of metastasis, investigations like chest x-ray, mammogram, tumour markers like Carcinoembryonic antigen (CEA), CA-125 etc can be done to find out the primary tumour.

9.8 Treatment

The treatment in pathological fractures depends on

(a) Etiology of fracture (generalised/local etiology)
(b) Ability of the fracture to heal
(c) Survivability of the patient with fracture

In localised pathological fractures, like bone cysts, the fractures are treated with definitive intention and immediate stabilisation.

In systemic metabolic conditions like osteomalacia and rickets, the underlying etiology is corrected along with the treatment of fracture. The outcomes are satisfactory in these conditions.

In metastatic bone disease, the treatment should be tailor made on patient-to-patient basis with due consideration to the primary tumour, age of the patient and 5-year survival rate.

9.9 Prophylactic Treatment of Fractures in Suspected Metastasis

If the patient presents very early in the disease or if an impending pathological fracture is diagnosed incidentally, prophylactic stabilisation of those fractures is considered based on a criteria given by Mirel et al.

The complete criteria are as below.

Component	1	2	3
Site	Upper limb	Lower limb	Peritrochanteric
Pain	Mild	Moderate	Functional
Lesion	Blastic	Mixed	Lytic
Size	<1/3rd	1/3rd to 2/3rd	>2/3rd

If the overall score is ≥9, then prophylactic fixation is considered.

If the overall score is 7 or less, then the lesion can be managed conservatively.

While treating pathological fractures, consideration should be given to the quality of the bone and the bone that's already destroyed. So, various adjuvants like bone cement, bone allografts, bone substitutes should be kept as a backup. The implants used for fixation should also be versatile to support the weak bone like locking plates.

Multiple Choice Questions

1. The lytic lesion of the bone is seen on an x-ray, when the destruction is more than _____% of bone
   (a) 30
   (b) 40
   (c) 20
   (d) 50
2. Mirels criteria has all the following components except
   (a) Site
   (b) Pain
   (c) Lesion
   (d) Fever
3. Prophylactic fixation is required in impending pathologic fractures when the Mirels score is
   (a) 9
   (b) 6
   (c) 5
   (d) 4
4. All of the following malignancies lead to lytic lesions in bone except
   (a) Prostate
   (b) Renal Cell Carcinoma
   (c) Lung Carcinoma
   (d) Thyroid carcinoma
5. Involvement of which area of the bone among the following has maximum chances of ending up in a pathological fracture?
   (a) Peritrochanteric area
   (b) Radial Shaft
   (c) Humerus shaft
   (d) Tibia diaphysis

Answers: 1. (a), 2. (d), 3. (a), 4. (a), 5. (a)

10 Dislocations and Subluxations

Ritesh Runu and Vishal Kumar

Learning Objectives
Definition, Types—Traumatic, Congenital, Pathological, Clinical features, Investigations, Emergency Management, Definitive Management, Complications, Preventions.

10.1 Definition and Types

Complete loss of articular contact between two joint surfaces is known as dislocation while partial loss of articular contact as subluxation (Fig. 10.1).

- Types—depending on the etiology, it may be divided into traumatic and nontraumatic.
- Traumatic dislocations—may be
  - Acute
  - Chronic/unreduced
  - Missed
- Non traumatic dislocations—may be
  - Congenital—neonate born with dislocated or dislocatable joint.
    - Ligament laxity
    - Abnormal joint formations
  - Developmental—a dysplastic joint may present with frank dislocation if diagnosed late or improperly managed.
  - Pathological
    - Ligament laxity
    - Infective lesions
    - Neurological conditions
    - Muscular dystrophy
    - Neuromuscular
    - Dysplasia

10.2 Clinical Features, Diagnosis and Management

10.2.1 Traumatic Dislocations

- Acute traumatic dislocation presents with pain and swelling over the affected joint and inability to perform normal joint movements.
- The attitude of the limb is usually diagnostic of dislocation. —Arm hanging by the side of body or supported by the other limb and flattened shoulder contour suggests—anterior dislocation of shoulder, abducted and externally rotated upper limb is found in luxatio erecta or inferior dislocation of humeral head. —Abnormally protruded point of elbow posteriorly is seen in elbow dislocation. —Abnormal bony hard swelling on the palmar aspect at metacarpophalangeal joint with

R. Runu (✉)
IGIMS, Patna, Bihar, India

V. Kumar
Department of Orthopaedics, PGIMER, Chandigarh, Chandigarh, India

V. Kumar et al. (eds.), *A Quick Guide to Essential Orthopedics*,
https://doi.org/10.1007/978-981-95-2676-5_10

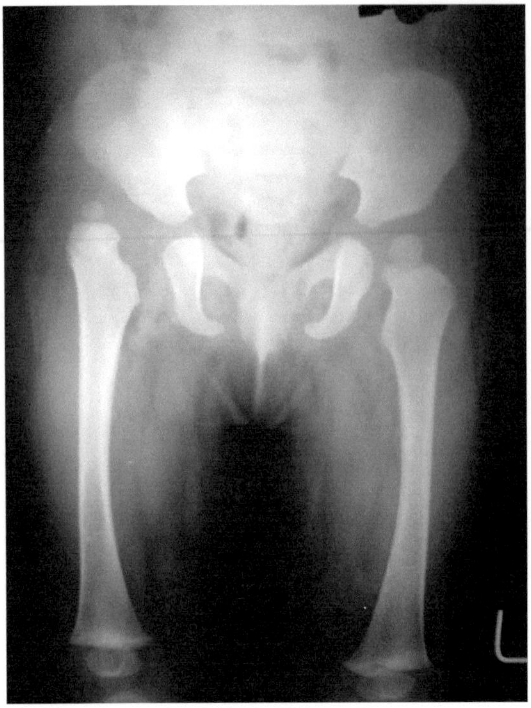

Fig. 10.1 Right hip dislocation

hyperextension at the same joint is seen in metacarpophalangeal dislocation.

- Posterior dislocation of hip presents with Flexion ADDuction and INTernal rotation of lower limb.
- Anterior dislocation of hip presents with Flexion ABDuction and EXTernal rotation of lower limb.
- Apart from typical attitude of limb, abnormal bony hard tender swelling is palpable in the gluteal region (posterior hip dislocation), groin (anterior hip dislocation), infraclavicular pre-glenoid area (anterior dislocation of shoulder), and popliteal fossa (knee dislocation). These injuries may present with associated neurological and vascular complications (Boxes 10.1 and 10.2).

Box 10.1 Neurological complications

Shoulder dislocation—Axillary nerve palsy
Elbow dislocation—Median nerve injury
Lunate dislocation—Median nerve injury
Hip dislocation—Sciatic nerve injury
Knee dislocation—Posterior Tibial nerve injury

Box 10.2 Vascular complications

Shoulder dislocation—Axillary artery injury
Elbow dislocations—Brachial artery injury
Knee dislocations—Popliteal artery injury

- Chronic or unreduced dislocations may present with minimal pain and deformity. Example—posterior dislocation of shoulder, anterior radial head dislocations.
- Missed traumatic dislocations are usually diagnosed during investigation for other clinical conditions. The joint function may be compromised, but activities of daily living may not be compromised. Example—missed radial head dislocation after missed Monteggia fracture (Fig. 10.2).
- These dislocations are diagnosed on X rays—anteroposterior and lateral views. Oblique views and stress views are required for diagnosis of bony defects and ligament injuries. Example—Hill Sach's lesion of proximal humerus in shoulder dislocation, collateral ligament injury in knee dislocation (Figs. 10.3 and 10.4).
- CT scan and MRI scans are required to define the bony defects and soft tissue defects in older children (Fig. 10.5).

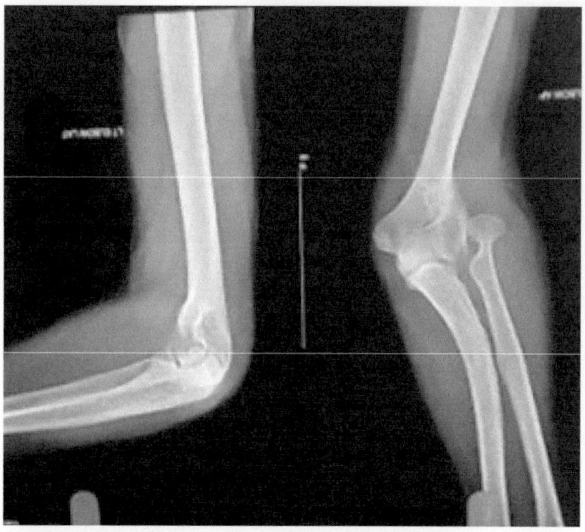

Fig. 10.2 Missed monteggia with radial head dislocation

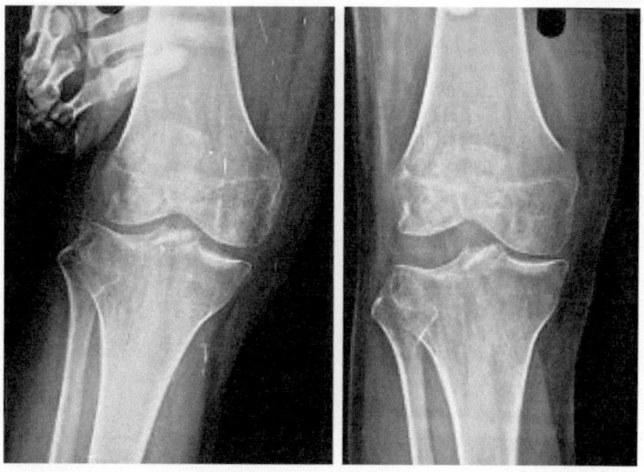

Fig. 10.4 Knee Stress x ray showing collateral ligament injury

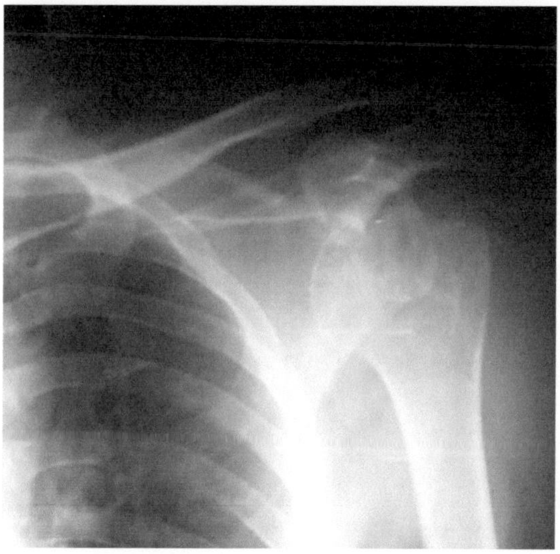

Fig. 10.3 Shoulder dislocation with Hill Sachs lesion

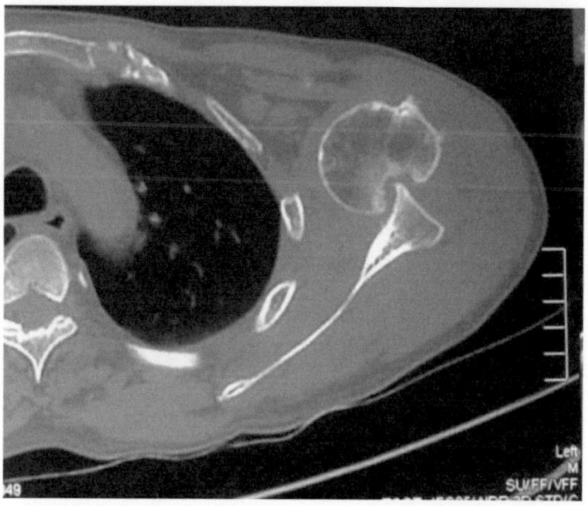

Fig. 10.5 CT scan showing Hill sach's lesion in proximal humerus

- Ultrasound as noninvasive, radiation free investigation is used in younger children.
- Treatment—Early closed reduction under conscious sedation is the treatment of choice. Proper reduction of dislocation or subluxation reduces the pain, and function is regained. After reduction the joint is immobilized for soft tissue healing. Joint mobilization is started early to prevent joint stiffness (Figs. 10.6 and 10.7).

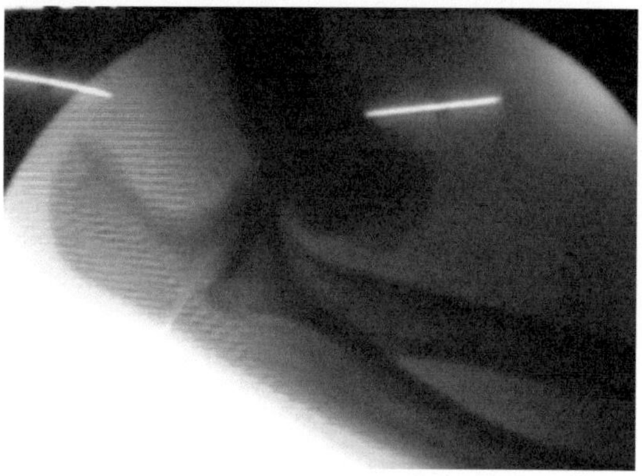

Fig. 10.6 Elbow dislocation

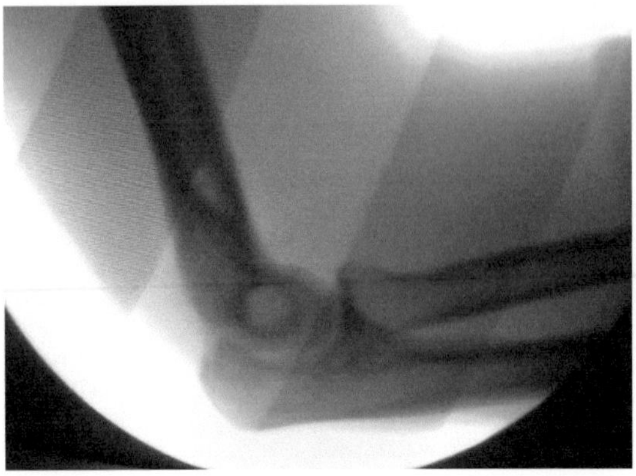

Fig. 10.7 Reduction of elbow dislocation

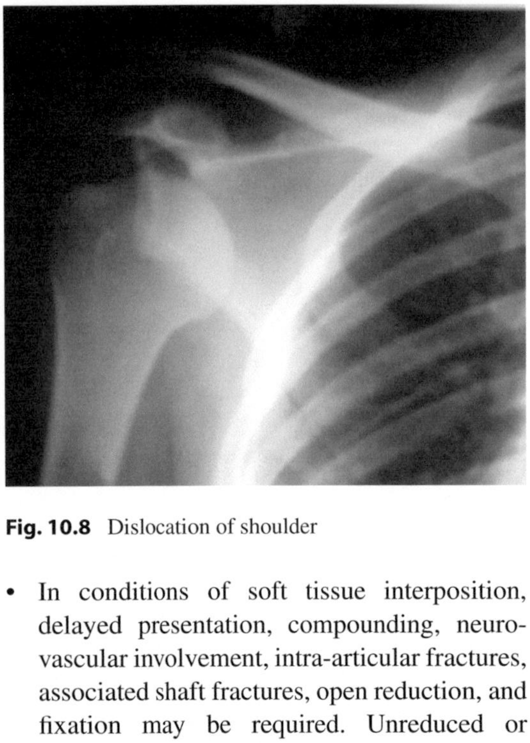

Fig. 10.8 Dislocation of shoulder

- In conditions of soft tissue interposition, delayed presentation, compounding, neurovascular involvement, intra-articular fractures, associated shaft fractures, open reduction, and fixation may be required. Unreduced or missed radial head dislocations are treated by ulnar osteotomy, open reduction of radial head, and annular ligament reconstruction (Figs. 10.8 and 10.9).
- Complications of traumatic dislocations may be—osteochondral fractures, myositis ossificans, and recurrent dislocations. In pediatric age group, physeal injury, avascular necrosis, chondrolysis, and heterotrophic ossifications may occur.

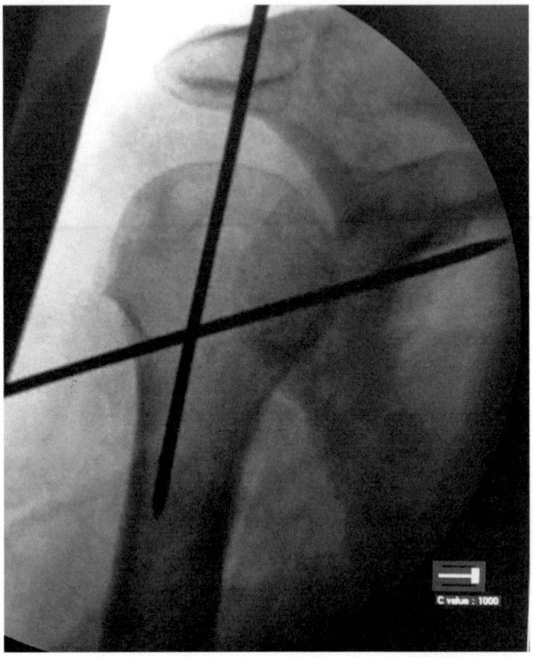

Fig. 10.9 Reduction and k wire fixation of shoulder joint

- Recurrent dislocations are due to ligament laxity, inadequate immobilization after injury, dysplastic joint anatomy, undiagnosed articular fractures, and psychiatric disorders. It is managed by soft tissue tightening and redirectional surgery of the joint.

10.2.2 Congenital Dislocations

- Congenital dislocations are usually diagnosed at the time of birth or during infancy. Antenatal diagnosis can be done at level II examinations after 5 months of intrauterine life. It is due to dysplastic joints/syndromic conditions. Common congenital dislocations are patella and hip.
- Nontraumatic hip dislocation in children is known as developmental dysplasia of hip (DDH). It is due to dynamic changes occurring in the infants' hips. The acetabular and femoral head cartilaginous part gradually ossifies to end up as normal adult hip. Any defect or dysplastic changes will end up with dysplastic dislocated hip. Since the process of

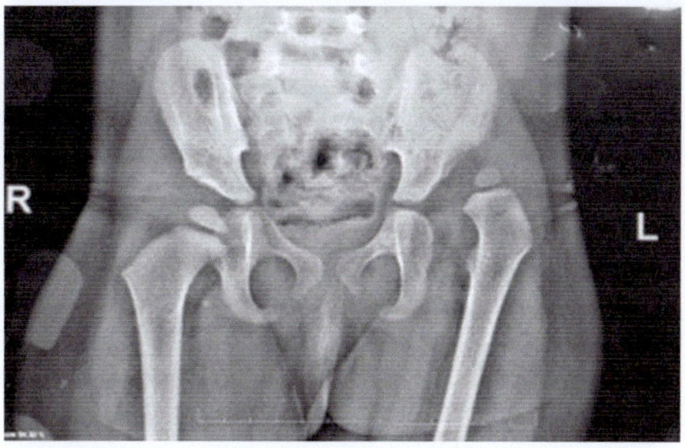

Fig. 10.10 Dislocated left femoral head with acetabular changes

hip development continues even after birth, which can be affected by our intervention; hence, it is known as developmental dysplasia (Fig. 10.10).

- The clinical tests done to confirm DDH are Barlow's test and Ortolani's test. Barlow's test confirms the dislocatable hips. It is done by flexion of both hips and knees and gently adducting the hips with posterior push. The femoral head may move out in case of dislocatable hip.
- Ortolani's test is done by gently abducting the hips with anterior pull in a supine patient. The femoral head may get reduced with a clunk sound. The test is considered positive. In case of stable hip, dislocated hip, irreducible hip, this test is negative.
- Developmental dysplasia of hip is treated by Pavlik harness (Fig. 10.11) or abduction pads in infancy up to 3–4 months of age. Those not responding to bracing therapy may require adductor tenotomy, open reduction, bony surgery, and hip spica (Fig. 10.12).
- *Congenital dislocation of the patella* is usually familial and bilateral. It may be an isolated entity or associated with arthrogryposis multiplex congenita and Down syndrome. On examination, the patella is poorly developed, reduced in femoral trochlea on extension, and slips out laterally on knee flexion. The lateral band of quadriceps is tight, and knee flexion contractures are seen. If unreduced, it may lead to flattening of lateral femoral condyle, valgus, flexion, and external rotation deformity of knee.

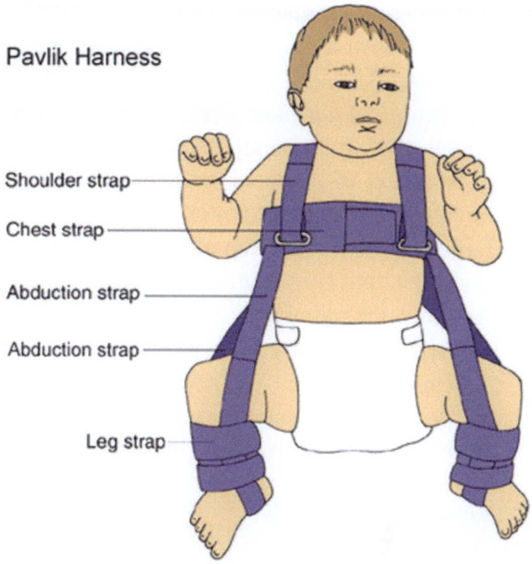

Fig. 10.11 Pavlik harness

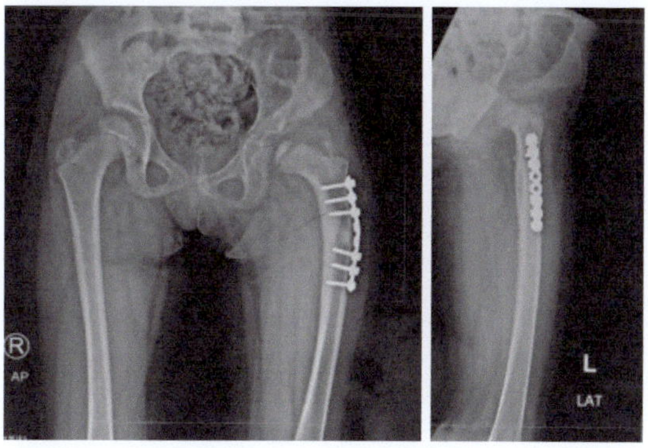

Fig. 10.12 Reduced femoral head with proximal femur osteotomy fixed with plate

- On X-ray, diagnosis is done by 3–4 years of age due to ossification of patella. The patella is seen lying out of femoral trochlea. The lateral femoral condyle is flattened compared to the normal side (Fig. 10.13).
- Early diagnosis is possible with MRI of knee.
- It is treated by surgical release of lateral tight structures, medial plication of soft tissue, advancement of vastus medialis, and distal realignment of ligamentum patellae (Fig. 10.14).

- In older children, medial patello-femoral ligament reconstruction is done in case it is deficient.
- *Congenital radial head* dislocations are usually bilateral. It is usually palpable on the posterior aspect of elbow as bony hard swelling moving with forearm rotations (Fig. 10.15).
- It is associated with achondroplasia, Larsen syndrome, and Nail Patella syndrome.
- On X-ray, the radial head is small, misshapen, long ulna and poorly formed radial notch on proximal ulna.
- Active surgical intervention is delayed till maturity. After growth completion, if the elbow is painful and arthritic, then radial head excision is suggested.

10.2.3 Pathological Dislocations

- Ligament laxity, infections, dysplasia of joints, muscular imbalance, and neuromuscular conditions are few of the causes where joint dislocates.
- Ligament laxity as seen in Marfan's syndrome, Ehlers Danlos syndrome the joints are unstable and dislocate. These patients are managed by proper splinting.
- Infective arthritis of the hip, shoulder, or elbow may dislocate due to erosion of joint surfaces, effusion, and pathological ligament laxity. These patients usually present with history of fever, joint swelling, and discharge of pus. Hemogram shows raised leukocyte

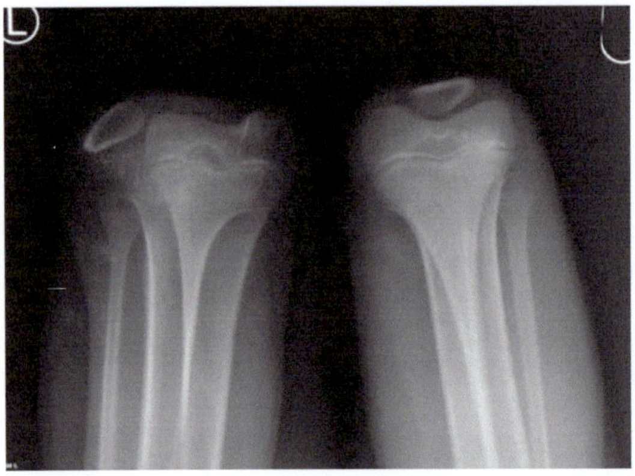

Fig. 10.13 Lateral dislocation of patella

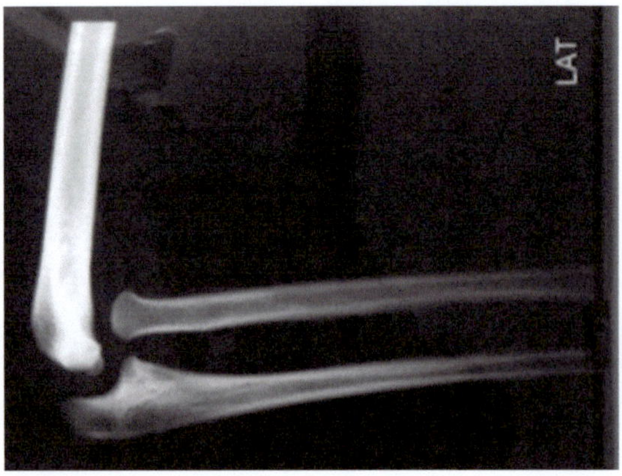

Fig. 10.15 Dislocated radial head

Fig. 10.14 Open reduction and soft tissue realignment procedures

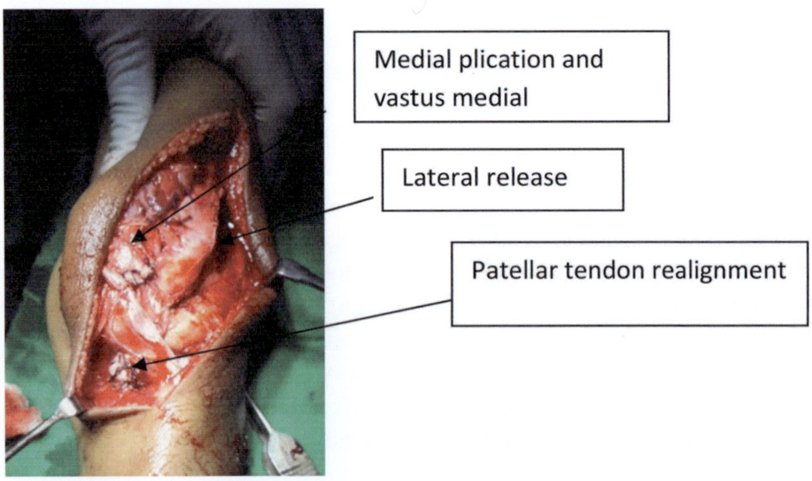

counts along with ESR and CRP titers. Ultrasound-guided joint aspiration and synovial fluid examination confirm the diagnosis. These patients are managed by joint debridement, traction or splintage of joints, antibiotic therapy, and analgesics (Fig. 10.16).

- Neuromuscular problems lead to joint instability due to unbalanced forces across the joint, causing dislocation. Example—dislocation of hip joint in cerebral palsy child. Due to hyperactive flexors and adductors, the hip joint dislocates posterosuperiorly. Management includes tendon release, tendon transfer, derotation bony surgery, joint reorientation surgery, and total joint replacements in adolescence (Fig. 10.17).

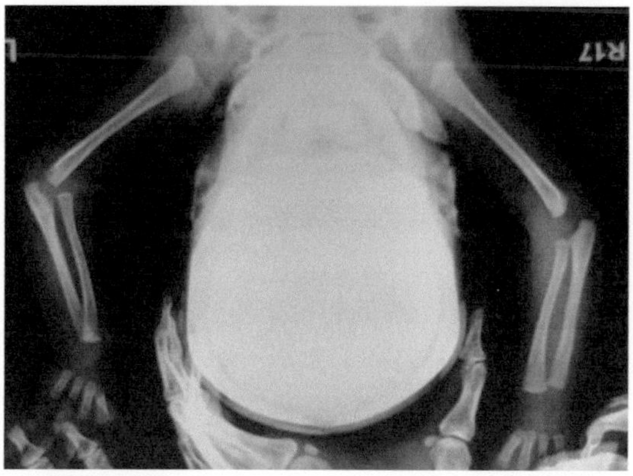

Fig. 10.16 Dislocation of right radial head

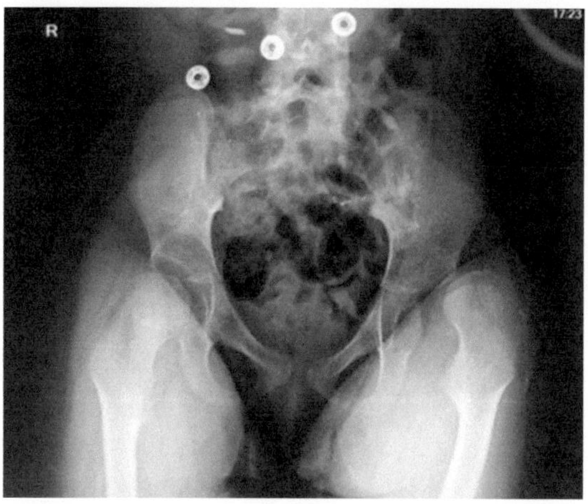

Fig. 10.17 left femoral head subluxation

10.3 Prevention from Dislocations and Subluxations

During infancy, on regular examination, the dislocatable joints are detected and evaluated. To maintain the anatomical position, the joints are reduced and kept in that position with braces. For hip dysplasias, Pavlik harness, abduction pillow, or double diaper is used. For knee and elbow—patient-specific braces are made. Shoulder joint is maintained by collar and cuff sling.

Multiple Choice Questions

1. Dislocation of joint is associated with all except
   (a) Trauma
   (b) Infection
   (c) Hereditary
   (d) Neuromuscular
2. An acute dislocation is reduced
   (a) Immediately
   (b) After 48 h
   (c) Aafter complete evaluation
   (d) Never reduced
3. Barlows test is done for
   (a) Shoulder dislocation
   (b) Eelbow dislocation
   (c) Hip dislocations
   (d) Knee dislocations
4. Pavlik harness is used for
   (a) Ttraumatic dislocations
   (b) Infective dislocations
   (c) Developmental hip dysplasias
   (d) Neuromuscular hip dysplasias
5. Congenital dislocation of patella presents in
   (a) Infants
   (b) School going children
   (c) Adolescents
   (d) Adults

Answers: 1. (c), 2. (a), 3. (c), 4. (c), 5. (b)

11 Injuries to Ligaments, Muscles and Tendons

Ritesh Runu

Learning Objectives
Mechaism, of injury, types of injury, healing mechanism of muscle injuries, clinical presentation, diagnosis, investigation, management, complications.

(a) Anatomical details of ligament
- Ligaments are collagenous structures connecting bones across the joint, providing stability to the joints.
- It comprises water and type I collagen (70–80%). The collagen fibrils' longitudinal and spiral organization provides strength to it
- It is directly attached over the bone or indirectly over the periosteum.
- On immobilization, the strength and mass of ligaments reduce in animal models.
- Exercises increase the strength of ligament without increasing its size.
- The healing potential of ligament depends on its size, location, attachment, vascularity, and type of injury.

(b) Mechanism of ligament injury
- Extrinsic factors—by sharp instruments, during operation, sports activity (stretching, twisting, pivoting)
- Intrinsic factors—collagen disorder, calcium metabolism disorder, dietary changes, female gender (less muscle mass, more loading over the ligaments)
- The most common joint affected is knee then hips, shoulder, ankle, elbow, and wrist.

(c) Types of ligament injuries—strain, sprain, and rupture.

(d) Healing mechanism of ligaments
- A torn ligament induces an inflammatory response. More so if injury is near the bony attachment. Due to the involvement of platelet-derived growth factor (PDGF), transforming growth factor B (TGF-B), vascular endothelial growth factor (VEGF), and fibroblast growth factor (FGF) the inflammatory changes occur.
- Fibroblasts deposit collagen, proteoglycans, glycoproteins, and other proteins.
- The collagen formed is type III, smaller fibrils, disorganized, and weaker compared to original collagen.

R. Runu (✉)
IGIMS, Patna, Bihar, India

V. Kumar et al. (eds.), *A Quick Guide to Essential Orthopedics*,
https://doi.org/10.1007/978-981-95-2676-5_11

(e) Presentation
- Injury to ligaments, muscles, and tendons is common in children due to sports-related injuries, farmyard injuries, conflicts, and self-inflicting injuries. Due to stretching force over the ligaments, either they may tear to various degrees, or they can avulse from the bony end with or without bony fragments.
- A sprain is stretching of ligament without any rupture of fiber. The affected joint is painful and swollen. The joint motion is preserved with minimal restriction. Clinico-radiologically, the joint is stable, and no bony injury is evident. MRI may show hyperintensity in the area of affected ligament.
- Strain occurs due to higher force over the joint, causing rupture of a few fibers. Clinically the joint is painful and swollen with restriction of motion. The joint is stable. X-ray may not show any bony changes, but MRI reveals hyperintensity along the injured ligament.
- Due to high force across the joint, a ligament may be partially or completely torn, causing ligament rupture. It may cause joint instability. The joint movement is restricted, and instability is noted. It can be confirmed by stress x-ray. MRI is diagnostic (Fig. 11.1 and 11.2).

(f) Diagnosis
- X ray—the joint x-ray is usually normal. On stress x-ray, abnormal joint opening is seen in ligament rupture (Figs. 11.3 and 11.4).
- Ultrasound is a noninvasive and cheaper tool to examine ligament integrity. In acute conditions, the ligament appears thickened, with diffuse hypoechogenicity and surrounding fluid. It is due to interruption of fibers continuity. It is also a dynamic test, which can show the abnormal joint motions.
- MRI is more accurate. It shows the inflamed soft tissues, torn ligaments, and evidence of bone contusion or edema. A normal ligament appears as low intensity signal in T1- and T2-weighted images. After injury, hyperintense signals are seen on the T2-weighted images.

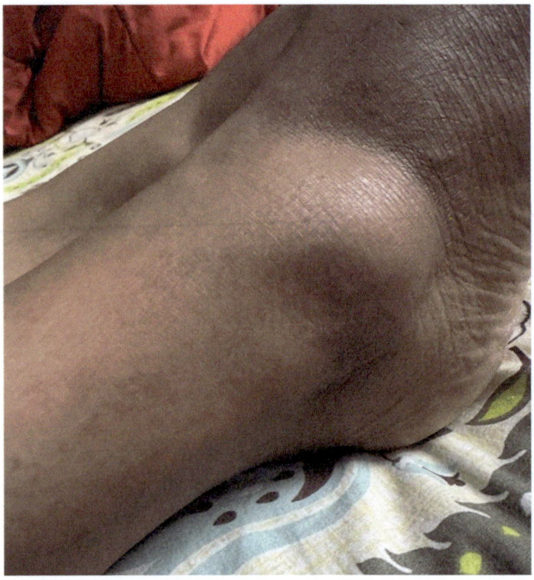

Fig. 11.1 Swelling over anterolateral aspect of right ankle due to anterior talofibular ligament injury

(g) Management (RICE = Rest, Ice fomentation, Compression bandaging, Elevation of limb)
- Ligament injury is managed by rest, elevation, analgesics, cold compression, splints, and plasters.
- Ice fomentation reduces swelling and pain when done intermittently.
- Plaster slabs are used to immobilize the joint for the shortest period of time till pain subsides, then non-weight-bearing exercises are advised.
- Partial or complete rupture of ligament is treated by surgical repair or reconstruction of ligament. It provides stability to joint and prevents future arthritic changes.
- Prolotherapy—It is injection of either platelet-rich plasma, hypertonic dextrose, or sodium morrhuate. It proliferates the cells for ligament healing.

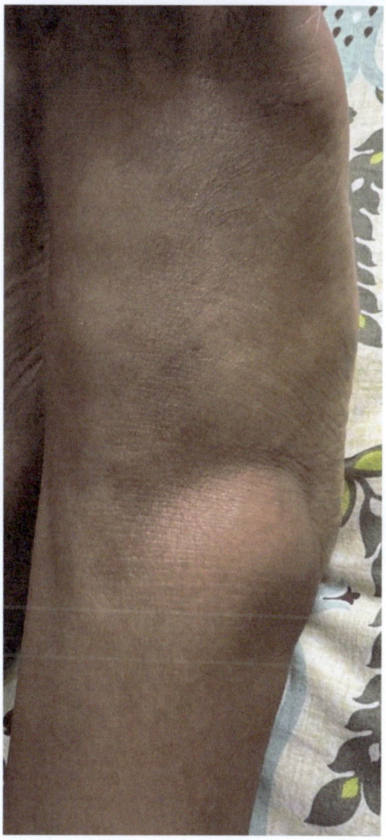

Fig. 11.2 Dorsal view of swelling over the anterolateral aspect of right ankle due to anterior talofibular ligament injury

- Exercises—They should be started early to prevent shrinking of ligament and to maintain the strength and bulk of ligament intact.
- Physiotherapy devices are used to maintain the joint motion and ligament length

(h) Complications
- Missed, neglected, or inadequately treated ligament injury leads to joint instability.
- Articular cartilage injury and arthritic changes.
- Painful joint.
- Recurrent instability and joint damage.

(i) Prevention
- Missed, neglected, or inadequately treated ligament injury leads to joint instability.

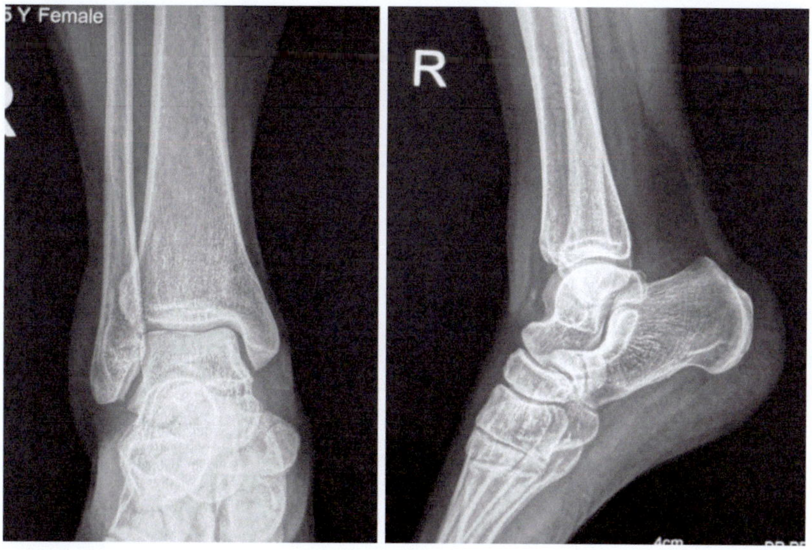

Figs. 11.3 and 11.4 AP and Lateral radiograph of right ankle showing intact bony structures

11.1 Muscle Injuries

(a) Mechanism of injury
- A muscle can be injured by direct trauma due to impact. It can be blunt trauma or penetrating trauma. Penetrating trauma may injure the muscle either partially or completely. It can be due to sharp pointed object or knife-like object. Example: khukhri.
- Muscle can be injured indirectly by sudden pulls during sports activities, riots, fear responses, emotional responses, or psychiatric or neurological disorders.
- Repetitive trauma to muscle is common with persons involved in jobs over computers, construction activity, military activities, etc.

(b) Types of injuries
- Bruises, sprains, and Lacerations
- Bruise is due to direct impact over the muscle. Occasional localized hematoma is seen. The muscle contractility and strength are not affected.
- Sprains are common sports injuries due to sudden or excessive stretching; the muscle fibers are torn, causing hematoma formation and ecchymosis. Palpable gap may be found during examination. The muscle contractility is reduced.
- Lacerated muscle injuries lead to tears of muscle fibers, either exposed or unexposed. The injured area is ecchymosed with underlying hematoma.

(c) Healing mechanism of muscle injury
- First phase of healing after injury is destruction of myofibrils. The myofibrils are necrosed and locally inflammatory cell concentration increases.
- Second phase consists of repair and remodeling. At this stage, the necrosed myofibrils are phagocytosed, and the space created is filled by regeneration of myofibrils and connective tissue. Neovascularization at this stage is the first sign of regeneration.
- Third phase is maturation of myofibrils, contraction, and reorganization of scar tissue. Gradually the muscles recover their contractility and strength.

(d) Clinical presentation
- Pain over the injured area is the commonest presentation. It can be in the neck, arm, back, thigh, calf, forearm, or the area of injury.
- Deformity after trauma may be another presentation due to abnormal muscle spasm. For example, wry neck may be due to cervical muscle spasm, flexion deformity of the knee may be due to hamstring spasm, and scoliosis may be due to thoracolumbar muscle spasm.
- Due to high-energy blunt impact, localized hematoma may be formed and seen as ecchymosis. An example of this is Morel-Lavallée lesion which forms around the posterior aspect of pelvis secondary to inner degloving.
- Muscle tear is visible in case of open injury (Fig. 11.5).
- Penetrating injury may cause severe muscle damage with minimal external signs.
- On palpation, the muscle in spasm appears as cord along the long axis. It may be firm

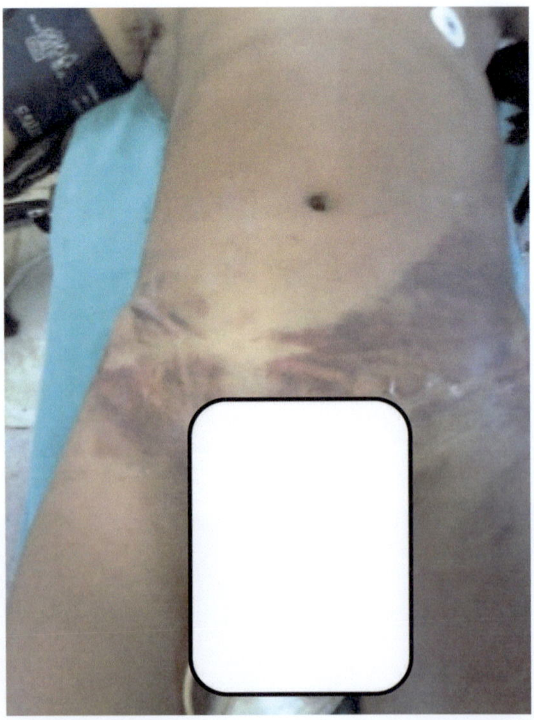

Fig. 11.5 Internal degloving and muscle tear over the pelvic region

and tender. In case of full thickness tear, palpable gap is present.
- In open wounds, the lacerated muscle edges are noncontractile, and they need debridement.
- Range of motion of joints is reduced. The power of muscle is reduced.

(e) Diagnosis
- The diagnosis of muscle injury is confirmed by clinical examination and investigations. Being a soft tissue injury, MRI is investigation of choice. It shows the details of injury. But it doesn't show the functional status of muscle. For functional status, ultrasound is the investigation of choice. It can show the muscle contractility and the area of injury.

(f) Management (RICE—Rest, Ice, Compression, and Elevation)
- Rest to the part and splinting of limb or body part reduces the pain and further injury to the muscles. Splints for neck area—cervical collar, for shoulder and arm—broad arm sling, for knee–knee brace, for back–spine braces, and for leg–ankle foot orthosis works.
- Ice fomentation for 15 min every 2–4 h helps in reducing vascularity, swelling, and pain. It works in early inflammatory phase. Later, warm saline fomentation improves vascularity and healing.
- NSAIDs and glucocorticoids for pain relief and to reduce the inflammatory swelling.
- Muscle relaxation reduces the spasm and improves the vascularity of the muscle.
- Early mobilization and gradual weight bearing are started for better healing of muscle. Isotonic exercises are range of motion exercises. It maintains the joint motion and muscle length. Isometric exercises improve the strength of the muscles. It is done after regaining the joint range of motion. Also for muscle trauma due to repetitive activity, the muscle strength improvement is essential.
- Surgical intervention is required for more than half or complete tear of muscle. The muscle repaired is splinted for healing, which may require rest for 6 weeks. The strength of muscle is gradually regained by progressive loading.
- Pulsed electromagnetic field therapy, transcutaneous electric nerve stimulation, and ultrasonic therapy are tools for muscle rehabilitation.
- Newer approaches are on growth factors, gene therapy, and stem cell therapy. Inhibition of myostatin gene promotes healing of skeletal tissue in mice. Follistatin gene expression increases strength and muscle mass. Shh gene is related to increased expression of vascular and myogenic factors, which increases the muscle regeneration. IGF-1 (Insuline-Like Growth Factor) gene at injury site attracts bone marrow stem cells, which accelerates tissue and muscle repair. VEGF (Vascular Endothelial Growth Factor) is related to faster muscle regeneration.
- Cells involved in muscle regeneration are mesenchymal stem cells, satellite cells, muscle-derived stem cells, and adipose-derived stem cells. These have shown accelerated muscle regeneration in animals. Combined therapy of genes and cells has promising results in treatment of muscle injury by reducing fibrosis and improving functional recovery of the muscles.

(g) Complications of muscle injury can be divided as early, intermediate, and late.
- Compartment syndrome is major and serious early complication of blunt muscle trauma. It can occur due to large hematoma in the muscle belly causing tight myofascial compartment. Any sign of tight compartment requires early myofascial release and early coverage of wound.
- Deep venous thrombosis is also serious complication that can occur due to blunt trauma. The vascular channels may be compromised with minimal clinical features. Suspicion due to persistent pain and

distal swelling of limb should be investigated and treated by anticoagulant therapy.

- Myositis Ossificans—The traumatized muscle with large hematoma may develop heterotrophic calcification in the muscle or adjacent to it. It is due to mesenchymal cell proliferation in the degenerated necrotic muscle mass. It affects the function of muscle and hence should be removed once it matures. Risk of recurrence after excision is high.
- Infection in the hematoma after muscle injury causes pyomyositis or pyogenic myositis. It should be drained early to prevent the damage of other intact muscle mass.
- Rhabdomyolysis—This is loss of muscle fibers following crush syndrome and infections; the rapid loss of muscle may cause acute renal failure, hyperkalemia, disseminated intravascular coagulopathy, myoglobinuria, and raised creatine kinase and serum creatinine.
- Calcific myonecrosis is mostly seen in large muscle compartments where the fusiform muscle mass has central liquefaction with peripheral plaque-like calcification.
- Muscle herniation can occur in condition where the epimysial sheath has defect causing muscle herniation. It can lead to chronic compartment syndrome. Hence, the defect needs repair.

Multiple Choice Questions

1. Moral Leville Lesion is seen in
   (a) Shoulder region
   (b) Pelvic region
   (c) Back region
   (d) Abdominal region
2. Investigation of choice for muscle lesions—
   (a) Ultrasound
   (b) MRI
   (c) X ray
   (d) None
3. Isotonic exercises are done for
   (a) Range of motion of joints
   (b) Strengthening of muscle
   (c) Stiff joints
   (d) Deformed joint
4. Isometric exercises are done for
   (a) Strengthening of muscles
   (b) Increasing joint range of motion
   (c) Correction of joint deformity
   (d) Stiff joint correction
5. Myositis Ossficans is due to
   (a) Ossification of muscles
   (b) Inflammation of muscles
   (c) Calcification of hematoma
   (d) Periosteal reaction to trauma
6. Rhabdomyolysis causes all except
   (a) Myoglobinuria
   (b) Acute renal failure
   (c) Hypokalemia
   (d) Raised creatine kinase
7. Muscle herniation is due to defect in
   (a) Epimysium
   (b) Perimysium
   (c) Endomysium
   (d) None

Answers: 1. (b), 2. (b), 3. (b), 4. (a), 5. (c), 6. (c), 7. (b)

Polytrauma 12

Vikash Raj and Ranjit Kumar Singh

The term 'polytrauma' refers to injuries to multiple organs, some of which may be life threatening or cause disability to the patient.

12.1 Causes

Road traffic accidents, fall from height, bullet injuries, blast injuries, etc.

This condition puts a considerable strain over the healthcare system as specialised centres are needed for handling of polytrauma patients and the results are often poor with high morbidity and mortality.

12.2 Golden Hour

Professor Richard Cowley coined the phrase 'The Golden Hour'.

It has been observed that the vast majority of deaths occurred in the first 60 minutes following injury and rapid interventions in this time period improves outcomes significantly.

12.3 Causes of Death in Polytrauma Patients

The deaths in polytrauma patients can be either.

Immediate or early—occurring within a few hours of injury. They account for 80% of polytrauma related deaths. Brain injury or major blood loss are the main causes of death in these cases.

Late—occurring after a few days or weeks following trauma. They are mainly due to sepsis or multi organ failure.

12.4 High-Risk Cases

The morbidity and mortality in trauma patients increase if they have co-morbid conditions like old age, obesity, diabetes, cardiac diseases, renal diseases, malignancy, etc. or if the GCS (Glasgow coma scale) score is less than 8.

12.5 Management of Polytrauma Patients

An organised approach with a pre designed management protocol helps to improve outcomes in the polytrauma scenario. A universal protocol namely *ATLS (advanced trauma life support)* is available. It consists of primary survey, adjunct measures, secondary survey and tertiary survey.

V. Raj (✉)
Department of Orthopedics, All India Institute of Medical Sciences, Deoghar, Jharkhand, India

R. K. Singh
Department of Orthopaedics, Nalanda Medical College & Hospital, Patna, Bihar, India

V. Kumar et al. (eds.), *A Quick Guide to Essential Orthopedics*,
https://doi.org/10.1007/978-981-95-2676-5_12

- The *primary survey* is carried out by a trauma team comprising of members from emergency department, orthopaedic surgery, general surgery, neurosurgery, intensive care, radiology, nursing and laboratory. All trauma centres have a trauma protocol which has to be activated whenever a trauma patient arrives. All the patients of polytrauma are subjected to a 'Primary survey' in the trauma care centre as soon as the patient arrives. It is very prompt and quick. The primary survey is completed rapidly to identify and treat any life-threatening injury in the patient.

The ABCDE of assessment are performed

1. Airway—it is ensured that the airway is patent and no foreign object or body fluids are blocking it. An adequate verbal response by patient indicates airway patency. Manoeuvres like chin lift and jaw thrust assist in keeping airway patent. If one fears cervical spine injury, then the cervical spine should be immobilised using a Philadelphia collar.

Unresponsive patients or patients with GCS (Glasgow coma scale) < 8 should be intubated to keep airway patent. Patients in whom intubation is not possible may be considered for tracheostomy.

2. Breathing—Chest auscultation and observation of breathing movements help us to know that the patient is breathing. The chest and axilla should be adequately exposed and examined for any signs of injury. Any pneumothorax or haemothorax should be excluded.
3. Circulation—The carotid and peripheral pulses are checked for rhythm and volume to ensure adequate blood supply. The patient is examined to look for signs of hypovolemic shock i.e. tachycardia, cool periphery, decreased consciousness and feeble pulses. If the patient is in hypovolemic shock, appropriate fluid replacement therapy is started after getting intravenous access. Blood transfusion may be considered if the patient is not responding to fluid therapy. Any obvious source of bleeding is identified, and steps are taken to stop blood loss.
4. Disability—All the patients are examined using the Glasgow coma scale, pupil's reaction to light and peripheral neurological examination. Cervical spine injuries are looked for and spine immobilized.
5. Exposure/Environment—Patient should be kept warm by removing all soiled and wet clothing and applying blankets or warmers to prevent hypothermia.

The patient is subjected to appropriate investigations like ABG, blood investigation, X-rays, USG, CT scans and ECG as per the primary assessment by the trauma team at the earliest after the patient has been stabilised by fluid replacement, pH correction, neck stabilisation, etc.

- After the patient is stabilised and resuscitated based on the primary survey, the *secondary survey* is done. A detailed history of the patient is taken, which reveals mode of injury, allergies, drug history, medical co-morbidities and surgical treatment history. He is examined from head to toe in detail to look for any injury which has been missed in the primary survey. Appropriate diagnostic tests are ordered.

Many occult injuries may not be apparent immediately in patients with multiple trauma or patients with a potentially life-threatening condition. They may add to the morbidity and mortality of the patient if left undiagnosed and not treated. The common ones are abdominal injuries, penetrating injuries, bowel injuries, thoracic injuries, pelvic injuries, compartment syndrome, etc., which can be identified and treated by secondary survey.

- The *tertiary survey* is a delayed evaluation of a polytrauma patient once he is fully alert. It is important in patients who are confused or comatose after trauma and cannot communicate with the trauma team. These patients are treated and stabilised based on initial survey and once the patient is alert enough, he is subjected to further examinations and investigations.

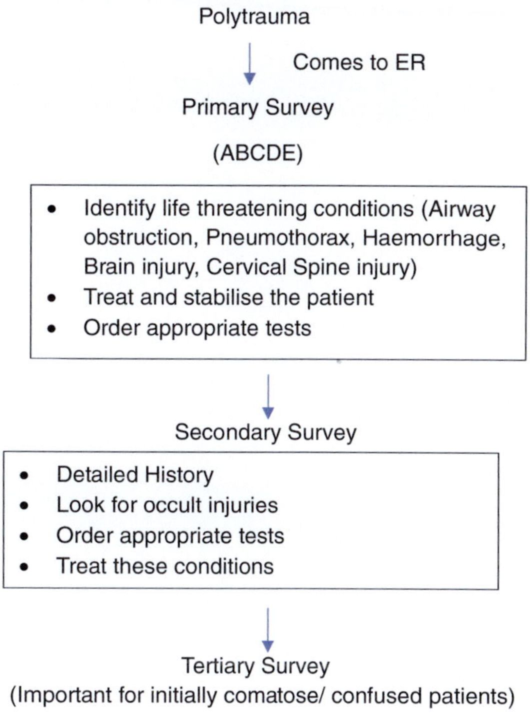

Multiple Choice Questions

1. ATLS refers to
   (a) Advanced trauma life support
   (b) Approach to life saving
   (c) Advancement in treatment and life support
   (d) None of the above
2. The concept of 'golden hour' was proposed by
   (a) Sir HO Thomas
   (b) Sir Joseph Charnley
   (c) Prof Richard Cowley
   (d) Prof J Bado
3. BLS stands for
   (a) Basic Life support
   (b) British life support
   (c) Bring life support
   (d) Bureau of life support
4. Primary survey involves the inspection of
   (a) Airway patency
   (b) Breathing efforts
   (c) Blood pressure
   (d) All of the above
5. Secondary survey involves
   (a) Examination of injury site after initial stabilisation
   (b) Ordering relevant investigations to confirm diagnosis
   (c) Planning of treatment of the injury
   (d) All of the above

Answers: 1. (a), 2. (c), 3. (a), 4. (d), 5. (d)

References for Further Reading

1. American College of Surgeons Committee on Trauma. Advanced trauma life support program for doctors. 7th ed. Chicago: American College of Surgeons; 2004.
2. Cowley RA. A total emergency medical system for the State of Maryland. Md State Med J. 1975;24(7):37–45.
3. Rogers FB, Rittenhouse KJ, Gross BW. The golden hour in trauma: dogma or medical folklore? Injury. 2015;46(4):525–7. https://doi.org/10.1016/j.injury.2014.08.043.

13 Recent Concepts in Fracture Treatment

Vikash Raj and Ranjit Kumar Singh

The efforts to treat a fracture are age old and can be traced back to the first human settlements. There has been evidence of splinting of fractures of limbs in the Egyptian and Indus valley civilisations. The earliest splints were made of sticks, bamboo pieces or reeds tied together around the limb.

Various different materials like egg white, gum, resins, etc. soaked on cloth/linen were used for fracture splinting. The use of 'Plaster of Paris' for immobilisation of fractured limbs marks a major development in the process. Nowadays POP is used as a standard material for applying casts or slabs for fracture cases.

Plaster of Paris (POP) also known as gypsum is chemically calcium sulfate hemihydrate. It has an exothermic reaction when mixed with water and hardens. The plaster is smooth and mouldable and does not shrink or crack, making it ideal for cast application. They are also radioluscent, and X ray can be taken over them to see for fracture reduction.

Other conservative means besides immobilisation were application of traction over the fractured limb to keep it immobilised and to reduce the fracture until it unites. This prolonged period of immobilisation caused muscle wasting and stiffness of joints.

Examples of tractions

1. Buck's skin traction
2. Russel Traction
3. 90–90 traction

Various functional braces were developed to overcome the problem of prolonged immobilisation on tractions. These braces were applied after an initial period of immobilisation for 2–3 weeks until the fracture ends became sticky due to soft callus and the swelling subsided. Thus, the patient could be mobilised early without loss of reduction. Sarmiento came up with one of the largest series of successful outcomes using functional braces for fractures of tibia, humerus and femur.

The attempts for surgical treatment of fractures, especially the open fractures, started in eighteenth century. Although the early results were not good because of lack of anaesthesia or antiseptics. The field of operative orthopaedics progressed along with the development of better implants, anaesthesia, surgical techniques and imaging modalities.

V. Raj (✉)
Department of Orthopedics, All India Institute of Medical Sciences, Deoghar, Jharkhand, India

R. K. Singh
Department of Orthopaedics, Nalanda Medical College & Hospital, Patna, Bihar, India

V. Kumar et al. (eds.), *A Quick Guide to Essential Orthopedics*,
https://doi.org/10.1007/978-981-95-2676-5_13

13.1 AO Concept of Fracture Treatment

AO (Arbeitsgemeinschaft für Osteosynthesefragen) was established in 1958 with its headquarters in Switzerland.

It is a non-profit organisation committed to research and development in the field of musculoskeletal injuries. They have been involved in educating surgeons and operating personnel worldwide about the principle of management of trauma and fractures. They have developed various instrument sets and implants for improved fracture treatment.

The standardisation of techniques of fracture fixation and implant design with propagation of the orthopaedic surgical procedures was done by AO (Arbeitsgemeinschaft für Osteosynthesefragen) or Association of the Study of Internal Fixation (ASIF) in 1960s.

13.2 AO Principles

The basic principles propagated by AO are

- Fracture treatment aims to *achieve the preoperative length and near-normal anatomical alignment and rotation* of the bone being treated and maintain it till the fracture unites.
- *A Fracture needs to be stabilised* for uneventful healing. It can be done by use of appropriate methods of casting/bracing during conservative treatment and adequate fixation during surgical treatment.

  The choice of intervention, conservative or operative is guided by the bone involved, fracture location and morphology, along with the associated factors like wound over fracture site, injury to neurovascular structures, other fractures, general condition of the patient, etc. The treatment is based on the overall assessment of the patient and classification of the fracture based on the images (X-rays and CT scans).
- If surgical treatment is undertaken, *the fracture is reduced by use of various direct/indirect techniques* to achieve acceptable reduction, and the reduction is held in place until fracture unites using internal/external implants.
- *The fractures are fixed in order to achieve stability,* which may be *absolute,* as in case of articular fractures, allowing no motion at the fracture site, aiming at primary healing or *relative* as in case of stable diaphyseal fractures, which allows micromotion at fracture site stimulating callus formation and healing by secondary intention.

13.3 Techniques for Fracture Reduction

13.3.1 Direct Techniques

When we open the fracture site to visualise the fracture anatomy and reduce the fracture under direct vision, we use direct techniques.

The advantages of direct reduction are: (1) It is done under vision, so there is minimal chance of neurovascular injuries during the process. (2) We can achieve perfect reduction by aligning the fracture fragments as per anatomy. It is advised in articular fractures. (3) It is easier to put in implants onto the fracture under vision. (4) Healing occurs by primary intention due to direct bone-to-bone contact.

Disadvantages of direct reduction are: (1) There is a lot of soft tissue injury involved during exposure of fracture site. (2) The soft tissue around the fracture is stripped, which decreases the blood supply to the fracture site. Hence, it is not advised in multifragmentary fractures. (3) The fracture haematoma is dislodged, which delays fracture healing. (4) Access to the fracture site may be difficult due to the presence of important neurovascular structures around.

13.3.2 Indirect Techniques

When we do not open the fracture site and rely upon indirect techniques like traction, ligamentotaxis, special instruments, etc., to achieve fracture reduction.

Advantages of indirect techniques are: (1) There is minimal soft tissue injury in the process of fracture reduction. It is the preferred method in multifragmentary fractures. (2) There is practically no soft tissue stripping around fracture site. (3) The fracture haematoma is not disturbed.

Disadvantages of indirect techniques are: (1) The reduction achieved may not be perfect in terms of end-to-end contact. Hence, not useful for articular fractures. (2) The techniques require specialised instruments and intraoperative imaging. There are radiation risks involved. (3) Excessive traction may cause neurovascular injuries.

The earliest implants used for fracture fixations were external fixators and stainless-steel wires. The fixators were used to span the length, while the wires were used to apply cerclage around the fracture fragment to keep it reduced.

With time, the implant designs and material used for implants have improved. The use of 'MRI-compatible stainless steel' and 'titanium' as implant material and the availability of 'locking plates', 'anatomical plates', 'bioabsorbable screws' have improved the outcomes of surgery.

Types of implants used in orthopaedic surgeries

1. Screws:

   They are used to hold bone fragments together and compress them when using interfragmentary screws or else to hold the plates with the bone surface in case of a plate screw construct.

   There are two types based on the type of bone they are used to hold.

   (i) Cortical screws—The screw has shallow, closely placed threads. They have larger core-to-thread ratio.
   (ii) Cancellous screws—These screws have widely placed threads and a smaller core-to-thread ratio. The deep threads allow better hold to cancellous bone.

   They may be non-cannulated with a solid core or cannulated with a hole in the core to pass guide wire through it. They may be fully or partially threaded.

There are three types based on the type of head.

(i) Locking screws—They have threads on their head, which allow them to lock onto the locking plates. This increases the pull-out strength of the plate screw construct.
(ii) Non-locking screws—These are traditional screws with no threaded head. They can be used for interfragmentary fixation or plate screw constructs.
(iii) Headless screws—These screws have cortical threads on one end and cancellous threads on the other end. They are cannulated. They are used for interfragmentary compression of articular fragments, as they can be buried into the bone.

Bio-absorbable screws have been used in arthroscopic surgeries of shoulder and knee and have benefit of not needing a second surgery for implant removal in future.
They are used to hold fracture reduction and are applied over the surface of the bone. They can be of different types.
Based on the morphology

(i) Reconstruction plates—They are low-profile, malleable plates used for holding reductions which are stable, preferably in paediatric cases or small bones.
(ii) 1/3rd tubular plates—They are thin, malleable plates used in bones that are subcutaneous.
(iii) Dynamic compression plates (DCP)—These are rigid plates and come with oval screw holes which allow sliding of screws inside the holes, causing compression of the fracture ends, if desired, by eccentric screw placement.

They may be locking if the screw holes have threads to lock the screw heads in them or non-locking, having no threads in the screw holes.

(i) Low contact DCP (LC DCP)—These are DCPs with minimal point contact between the plate bone interface which causes very little periosteum damage and allows better healing.

(ii) Angled blade plates—They are rigid plates with a predefined angle at one end. They are used for fixation of fracture of proximal or distal femur.

(iii) Anatomical plates—These are side-specific pre-contoured locking plates made to be used at specific anatomical sites.

Anatomical plates are very useful in stable fixation of peri-articular fracture patterns and allow early mobilisation.

2. Nails

These are intramedullary devices used for fixation of fractures of the shafts of long bones. They can be either locking nails, having option for bolt insertion through the nail to provide rotational stability to the nail-bone construct, or non-locking nails with no slots for bolt insertion, thus having no rotational stability. E.g.

(a) Non-locking nails—K nails, V nails, square nails

(b) Locking nails—Gamma nail, proximal femoral nails, etc.

3. K (Kirshner) wires—They have a sharp tip and are driven across the fracture fragments. They are used for temporary stabilisation of fracture fragments while reducing the fractures or can be used as a definitive means of fixation too in certain cases.
4. SS (stainless steel) wires—They are used to tie up the fracture. They are mostly used in combination with the K wire to do tension band wiring.
5. External Fixators—They are used to align and stabilise the limbs in cases of open fractures or extremely comminuted fractures not amenable to internal fixation. They can be of two types:

(a) Rod Clamp type of External fixators—They comprise a set of rods held with clamps over pins driven through the bone parallel to the limb to be stabilised. E.g. AO type of fixators, rail fixators.

(b) Circular fixators—They comprise circular rings held around the limb over wires and pins driven through the bone. They are inherently more stable, as they provide 360° support to the limb. E.g. Ilizarov ring fixators, Orthofix ring fixators.

6. Spinal implants: Special implants like pedicle screws, mesh, cages, connecting rods, etc. are used for instrumentation of the vertebral column during spine surgeries.
7. Prosthesis—Joint replacement surgeries (arthroplasty) use various prostheses for replacement of the shoulder, elbow, hip, knee and ankle joints.

The concept of fracture fixation has also seen a shift from initial 'rigid fixation' and 'trying to fix every fragment' to 'relative stability' and 'biological fixation with minimal soft tissue insult', which has further improved the outcomes in terms of fracture healing.

13.4 Recent Updates

For cast application: Fibreglass material is being used increasingly for cast application, especially for lower limbs, as they are harder and lighter than traditional POP. These casts are strong and durable and ideal for walking casts in lower limbs.

The advent of newer anaesthetic agents and modalities has made it possible for high-risk patients with multiple comorbidities to undergo surgeries. This becomes important as the proportion of older patients is increasing in the general population with the increased life expectancy, and they are the ones who are prone to have a fall and suffer from fragility fractures. This is the group of patients who also suffer from an array of comorbidities and are usually a high-risk group for anaesthesia.

The availability of newer implants like

1. Anatomically contoured plates for juxta-articular fractures
2. LISS (less invasive stabilisation system) for biological fixation by indirect methods
3. Carbon frames for external fixation to make the construct lighter and radiolucent

4. LRS (Limb reconstruction system) for stronger fixation in cases needing external fixator application
5. Fenestrated bone screws for cement augmentation of fixation in osteoporotic bones
6. Bioabsorbale screws for arthroscopic surgeries
7. Expandable rods and nails for paediatric patients

have improved outcomes in various challenging fractures.

The recent research has shown the importance of providing adequate cellular and molecular environment for fracture healing after its adequate stabilisation. Various pharmacotherapy and gene therapy have been developed to target the deficiencies in the healing of fractures.

The availability of bone substitutes: (1) Ceramic-based—Hydroxyapatite, Tricalcium phosphates, and (2) Growth factors like Bone morphogenetic proteins (BMP), Demineralised Bone matrix (DBM), Platelet-rich Plasma (PRP) (3) Composite of collagen and hydroxyapatite has also improved outcomes in complex fractures and bone loss situations.

Newer imaging modalities for preoperative imaging like C-arm, O-arm, have been developed.

The use of navigation tools and robotics in spine and arthroplasty surgeries has led to improvement in surgical precision.

The availability of prosthetics made of various materials like ceramics, titanium, porous-coated.

The use of microscopes and endoscopes along with better illumination has led to improvement in the field of minimally invasive surgeries of spine and joints.

Advancements in 3D printing technology have been used extensively in the planning of difficult surgeries (acetabular fractures, deformity correction) and development of implants and tools for complex bones (pelvis, acetabulum, cervical spine) and production of customised prostheses and implants to suit the specific needs of tumour surgery, deformity correction, etc.

Multiple Choice Questions

1. PTB is used for functional bracing of
   (a) Tibia fracture
   (b) Humerus fracture
   (c) Femur fracture
   (d) Forearm fracture
2. The circular external fixators are called
   (a) LRS
   (b) LISS
   (c) Ilizarov fixator
   (d) AO fixator
3. Pedcile screws are used for
   (a) Tibia fracture
   (b) Radius fracture
   (c) Spine surgery
   (d) Femur fracture
4. Bone graft substitutes include
   (a) Hydroxy apatite
   (b) Tricalcium phosphates
   (c) Both of them
   (d) None of them
5. The AO has its headquarters at
   (a) London
   (b) Dublin
   (c) Brussels
   (d) Davos

Answers: 1. (a), 2. (c), 3. (c), 4. (c), 5. (d)

Further Reading

Bartoníček J. Early history of operative treatment of fractures. Arch Orthop Trauma Surg. 2010;130(11):1385–96. https://doi.org/10.1007/s00402-010-1082-7.

Hernigou P. History of external fixation for treatment of fractures. Int Orthop. 2017;41(4):845–53. https://doi.org/10.1007/s00264-016-3324-y.

Broos PL, Sermon A. From unstable internal fixation to biological osteosynthesis. A historical overview of operative fracture treatment. Acta Chir Belg. 2004;104(4):396–400.

Kulkarni PG, Paudel N, Magar S, et al. Overcoming challenges and innovations in orthopedic prosthesis design: an interdisciplinary perspective. Biomed Mater Devices. 2023; https://doi.org/10.1007/s44174-023-00087-8.

Chao EY, Hein TJ. Mechanical performance of the standard Orthofix external fixator. Orthopedics. 1988;11(7):1057–69. https://doi.org/10.3928/0147-7447-19880701-09.

14 Complications of Fractures

Vikash Raj and Rajeev Anand

Fractures may be associated with many complications. They may be classified into

Immediate—occurring at the time of fracture

Early—occurring within a few of fracture

Late—occurs days to weeks after the fracture

based on time of occurrence (Table 14.1)

Table 14.1 Complications of fracture

Immediate	Early	Late
Local: 1. Injury to blood vessels 2. Injury to nerves 3. Injury to muscles and tendons 4. Injury to joint 5. Injury to viscera	Local: 1. Infection 2. Compartment syndrome	1. Delayed union 2. Non-union 3. Malunion 4. Cross union 5. AVN (avascular necrosis) 6. Joint stiffness 7. CRPS (complex regional pain syndrome) 8. Osteomyelitis 9. Myositis Ossificans 10. Osteoarthritis
Systemic: 1. Hypovolemic shock	Systemic: 1. Hypovolemic shock 2. Fat embolism 3. ARDS (acute respiratory distress syndrome) 4. DVT (deep vein thrombosis) 5. Septicaemia 6. Crush syndrome	

V. Raj (✉)
Department of Orthopedics, All India Institute of Medical Sciences, Deoghar, Jharkhand, India

R. Anand
Patna Medical College & Hospital, Patna, Bihar, India

V. Kumar et al. (eds.), *A Quick Guide to Essential Orthopedics*,
https://doi.org/10.1007/978-981-95-2676-5_14

14.1 Hypovolemic Shock

Shock is a state of global hypo-perfusion at cellular level causing hypoxia and dysfunction.

It is of four types based on the etiology:

1. *Distributive shock*—It occurs due to peripheral vasodilation, usually seen in cases of septic shock or cervical spine injury causing sympathetic failure
2. *Hypovolemic shock*
3. *Obstructive shock*—It occurs usually in cases of cardiac tamponade or obstructive pneumothorax leading to constriction of heart itself
4. *Cardiogenic shock*—It results due to failure of heart due to cardiac injuries or any other cause.

Hypovolemic shock is a potentially life-threatening condition. The successful outcome in this situation depends on early diagnosis and intervention.

Definition—It results due to failure of circulation caused by effective loss of volume of blood/body fluid circulating. This results in tissue hypoperfusion and hypoxia. If left untreated, it leads to failure of vital organs due to ischaemia and ultimately death because of multi organ failure.

Hypovolemic shock can be of two types—(1) Haemorrhagic and (2) Non-haemorrhagic.

Haemorrhagic shock occurs due to bleeding by blood vessel injuries and is commonly seen in trauma scenario.

Non-haemorrhagic blood loss occurs due to loss of body fluids as seen in cases of intractable diarrhoea, continuous vomiting, GI fistulas, intestinal obstructions, nephropathies, burn.

Whenever the body fluid or blood volume decreases due to any cause, the compensatory mechanism of our body kicks in and there is sympathetic overactivity which leads to increase in heart rate, increased cardiac contractility and peripheral vasoconstriction. This result in increase in net effective diastolic blood pressure and narrowed pulse pressure.

But, if there is massive loss of blood or body fluid leading to shrinkage of the total volume by around 30% the compensatory mechanism starts to fail and now the patient had tachycardia, drop in blood pressure and oligouria. The sympathetic overdrive results in diversion of all the blood from peripheral circulation to central part to maintain the supply to brain and heart. This results in decrease in the oxygen supply to the tissues and they switch to anaerobic metabolism from aerobic one to meet their energy demands. There is deposition of lactic acid in the tissues causing acidosis. There is ischaemia of vital organs including heart and patient develops multi organ failure.

14.1.1 Clinical Features

- History of trauma with evident bleeding
- Patient complains of thirst, cramps
- Dry mouth, lips
- Orthostatic hypotension
- Weak pulses
- Cold, clammy skin
- Lethargic, confused and agitated patient in severe cases

14.1.2 Investigation

- CBC—Low haemoglobin in case of haemorrhagic causes
- RFT—

Electrolyte (Na, K, PO_4) imbalanceHigh Serum creatinine, BUN (blood urea nitrogen) } Pre Renal failure

- Low pH: Acidosis
- Central venous pressure—decreased

14.1.3 Treatment

- Early and prompt diagnosis
- Control of bleeding
- Intravenous fluid therapy: Crystalloid are preferred over colloids in non-haemorrhagic causes
- Blood transfusion, if haemoglobin falls below 10 g%
- Better results are seen with balanced transfusion of 1:1:1 Plasma to Platelets to Packed RBC

Successful treatment results in restoration of fluid volume leading to normalisation of blood pressure, pH and urine output. Circulatory overload must be prevented as it may again cause complications.

14.2 Compartment Syndrome

It was first described by Volkman in the nineteenth century in patients having long bone fractures.

Definition—An increase in the intra compartmental pressure of a closed osteo fascial compartment causing impairment of the local circulation, ischaemia and eventually necrosis is termed 'compartment syndrome.'

The threshold is >30 mm of Hg rise in the intra compartmental pressure but it is not always necessary. The muscles in the limbs are enclosed in thin fascia which does not allow for rapid expansion of the compartments. The common sites for compartment syndrome are leg, forearm, hand, thigh, buttock, and foot. It is also common in open fractures.

Common causes for acute onset compartment syndrome are fractures of the forearm or leg, burns, vascular injuries, crush injuries, thrombosis, DVT, infections, cellulitis, reperfusion injuries, very tight cast/splints, circumferential bandages, improper limb positioning during surgery, penetrating appearance, etc.

A chronic form of compartment syndrome has been described in case of overexertion of muscles by excessive exercise, marching drills, long distance running, football players, etc.

Tibial fractures in adults and Supracondylar humerus fractures in children are the most common causes of compartment syndrome.

Normally, there is an equilibrium in the amount of fluid inside the osteo fascial compartment and the arterial inflow is matched by the venous outflow. If the arterial inflow increases or the venous outflow decreases, the fluid content inside the compartment increases. It leads to increase in the pressure inside the compartment. If the compartment pressure rises above the capillary pressure, it causes compression of the capillaries which decreases the flow into the compartment and ischaemia sets in. The normal capillary pressure is ≤10 mm of Hg and if it rises above 30 mm of Hg then acute compartment syndrome arises.

It may occur immediately after trauma and may be set in up to 48 h after initial trauma.

Clinical signs and symptoms

14.2.1 5 "P"S: Pain, Paraesthesia, Paralysis, Pallor and Pulseness

- Pain out of proportion, not relieved by rest and medication
- Pain on passive stretching
- Tense, shiny skin
- Poor two-point discrimination
- Altered or decreased sensation
- Cold periphery
- Decreased or absent pulses, rarely

14.2.2 Investigation

- X-ray of the limb
- Measurement of compartment pressure (Normal value 20–30 mm of Hg)
- Compartment pressure post-exercise for chronic compartment syndrome (values >30 mm of Hg post 1 min exercise & 20 mm of Hg post 5 min exercise)
- USG of the limb to look for thrombus.

- Creatinine phosphokinase (CPK) levels; it is increased in ischaemia or rhabdomyolysis
- Renal function test
- Urinary myoglobulin levels

14.2.3 Treatment

- Removal of tight cast/circumferential bandages
- Elevate the limb to heart level
- Prevent hypotension
- O2 support
- Immediate fasciotomy if above measures fail to relieve symptoms or the compartment pressure is above 30 mm of Hg

14.2.4 Complications

- Gangrene
- Volkmann's Contractures

Ideally, fasciotomy should be planned within 6 h of injury. Fasciotomy is not useful if done 36 h after injury as tissue necrosis already sets in. Amputation may be needed if there are massive necrosis and gangrene in the limb.

14.3 Fat Embolism

'Fat embolism Syndrome' results from dissemination of fat emboli into systemic circulation. It causes micro vascular damage and develops systemic inflammatory response syndrome in the patient. The end organ damage may express as (1) Skin changes (2) CNS involvement (3) Respiratory system involvement (4) Retinal changes.

Fat embolism is most common in orthopaedic fractures. Other causes are Pancreatitis, Liposuction, Bone marrow transplantation, fatty liver, hemoglobinopathies, Sickle cell disease, severe burn injuries, etc.

Risk factors for fat embolism: Young age, Multiple fractures, and vigorous reaming of long bones.

The fat globules released into the circulation due the fracture reaches the end organs like brain, lungs, retina or skin and gets deposited in the micro capillaries. These droplets block the capillaries causing decreased perfusion and ischaemia. The inflammatory cascade is also induced releasing acute phase reactants.

The patients present with

- Long bone fractures
- May experiences weakness, nausea, headache, respiratory difficulty
- The patients with pulmonary fat embolism also have Tachycardia, Tachypnoea, Diaphoresis
- The patients with Central Nervous involvement will have Agitation, Confusion, Seizures, Coma
- Retinal involvement causes retinal haemorrhages
- The skin may show multiple petechial rashes

Gurd's criteria for diagnosing fat embolism

Major criteria	Minor criteria
Petechial rash Respiratory insufficiency Cerebral involvement in non-head injury patient	Fever greater than 38.5 C Tachycardia heart rate greater than 110 beats per minutes Retinal involvement Jaundice Renal signs Anaemia Thrombocytopenia High erythrocyte sedimentation rate Fat macroglobulinemia

*Fat embolism is diagnosed when two major criteria or at least one major and four minor criteria are present

14.3.1 Investigations

- CBC—anaemia, thrombocytopenia
- pH—metabolic acidosis
- RFT—increased creatinine and blood urea nitrogen levels
- Increased alveolar arterial gradient (normal range 0–25 mm of Hg)
- Lipid inclusions in macrophages from bronchoalveolar lavage
- Fat globules in sputum, urine, blood

- 'Snow storm' appearance in chest X ray
- CT chest shows pulmonary edema and vascular congestion
- MRI brain

14.3.2 Treatment

- Supportive care
  - O2 supplementation
  - Adequate ventilation
  - Adequate hydration and nutrition
  - Blood pressure monitoring and maintenance
- IV Albumin to maintain blood volume
- IV Mannitol to reduce cerebral edema

Most patients recover by supportive care and further episodes are prevented by early fracture fixation. Mortality is seen in patients developing ARDS or cerebral edema.

14.4 ARDS (Acute Respiratory Distress Syndrome)

Definition—It is acute onset diffuse inflammatory infiltration of pulmonary tissue leading to poor oxygenation of the blood. It is usually seen in seriously ill patients and is often life-threatening condition. It usually manifests within 72 h of injury.

The condition is defined by a fall in the ratio of oxygenation of arterial blood (PaO2) with the amount of oxygen in inhaled air (FiO2) because of the decrease in the available alveolar surface for gaseous exchange to occur. It is characterised by absence of any cardiogenic pulmonary edema.

Risk factors—Advanced age, Female gender, Smoking, Alcohol use, Aortic vascular surgery, Cardiovascular surgery, Traumatic brain injury, Pancreatitis, Pulmonary contusion, Infectious pneumonia, Drugs (radiation, chemotherapeutic agents, amiodarone).

Pathology—The disease starts with alveolar capillary injury due to inflammatory agents leading to alveolae edema which reduces the gaseous exchange causing hypoxaemia. As the acute phase is over the lung tissue heals with fibrosis causing lung tissue elasticity to decrease leading to pulmonary hypertension.

Clinical features—The patients complain of progressively worsening dyspnoea developing over a few hours with signs of hypoxia.

Patient has dyspnoea, tachypnoea, altered mental status. Chest auscultation reveals basal rales.

14.4.1 Investigation

- Routine hemogram to look for signs of sepsis, renal impairment, and pH imbalance, electrolyte imbalance
- X ray chest—Bilateral lung infiltration
- CT scan of chest is done to look other pulmonary causes like pneumothorax, pleural effusion, mediastinal mass, etc.
- PaO2/ FiO2 < 300 mm of Hg
- 2D Echo to rule out cardiac causes

14.4.2 Treatment

It is directed towards increasing oxygen delivery and reducing further insult to pulmonary tissue

- Mechanical ventilation
- Measured fluid replacement to avoid cardiac overload
- Diuretics to wash out excess fluid
- Parenteral nutritional supplements
- Antibiotics to avoid secondary infections
- Treatment of underlying causes

Differential Diagnosis: Cardiogenic edema, Exacerbation of interstitial lung disease, Acute interstitial pneumonia, Diffuse alveolar haemorrhage, Acute eosinophilic lung disease, Organising pneumonia, Bilateral pneumonia, Pulmonary vasculitis, Cryptogenic organizing pneumonia, Disseminated malignancy

Complications: Barotrauma from high pressure ventilation, Tracheostomy due to prolonged ventilation, Laryngeal edema, Subglottic stenosis, hospital acquired infections, Pneumonia, UTI, DVT, Renal failure, Bed sores

14.5 Deep Vein Thrombosis (DVT)

Definition—The formation of blood clots in the deep veins of the body due to hinderance to blood flow. It usually occurs in the leg but can occur in upper limb, mesentery or the brain.

It is a source of emboli to the brain, heart and pulmonary tissue which causes obstruction of blood supply to these vital organs and ischaemia results.

14.5.1 Risk Factors

- Immobility due prolonged bed rest, anaesthesia, stroke, long flights, fractures, etc
- Increase in the resistance to venous flow due to mechanical compression (tight bandages, splints), pregnancy, stenosis, etc.
- Injury to the veins
- Increase in the blood viscosity due to polycythemia, thrombocytosis, dehydration
- Increase in the coagulation activity of blood due to genetic defects like Protein C or S deficiency, Factor V mutation
- Malignancy
- Heart failure
- Vasculitis
- Smoking
- Chronic diseases like diabetes, hypertension
- Inflammatory diseases like SLE, IBD
- Obesity
- Old age

14.5.2 Pathophysiology

The Virchow's triad (Fig. 14.1) is responsible for DVT.

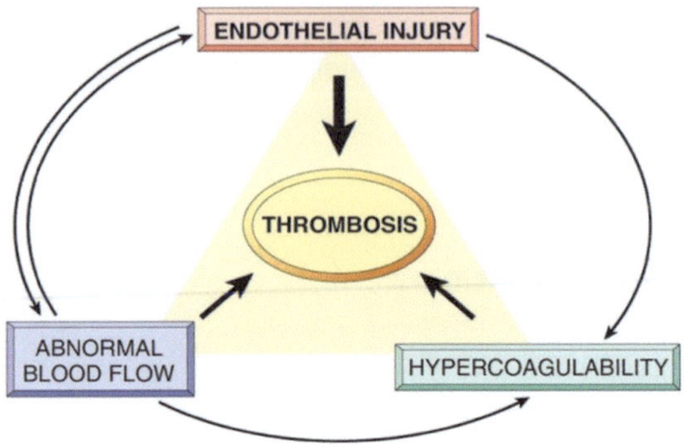

Fig. 14.1 Virchow's triad

14.5.3 Clinical Features

No specific set of signs and symptoms are there but usually patients present with

- Pain and swelling of involved limb
- Tenderness
- Erythema
- Local rise of temperature
- Calf squeeze (Homan's sign) is painful
- Peripheral cyanosis
- Gangrene in advanced stages

14.5.4 Investigations

- Venous Doppler of affected limb
- Coagulation profile
- D dimer levels
- CT angiograms can be done when in doubt

14.5.5 Treatment

- Anticoagulation therapy—Low molecular weight Heparin along with Factor Xa inhibitors is used for 5–6 days
- Vitamin K antagonists are given for 3 months or more
- Thrombolysis can be done for acute cases

14.5.6 Prevention

- Use of DVT garments in cases needing prolonged immobilisation
- Prophylaxis with Factor Xa inhibitors in high-risk patients with hypercoaguable state.
- Use of venous foot pumps
- Quit smoking

Differential Diagnosis: Cellulitis, Ruptured Baker cyst, Trauma, Superficial thrombophlebitis, Venous or lymphatic obstruction, Vasculitis, Peripheral edema, heart failure, cirrhosis, nephrotic syndrome

14.6 Crush Syndrome

Definition—It is defined as the systemic manifestation of crush injury which can cause multiple organ dysfunction especially acute renal failure and lead to death of patient.

14.6.1 Causes

Crush injury to limbs or body parts in case of

- Road traffic accidents
- Machine injury
- Burns and electrical injury
- Industrial and Construction site Injuries
- Disasters like earthquakes, floods
- Stampedes, etc

14.6.2 Pathophysiology

Crushing of muscle cells release myoglobin into circulation, minerals like sodium, potassium, calcium, phosphates, and enzymes like lactate dehydrogenase (LDH), creatinine phosphokinase (CPK) in large amounts. These have toxic effects. The myoglobulin blocks the renal microvasculature and causes renal vasoconstriction leading to acute renal injury (AKI). The excess potassium and calcium in circulation causes involuntary muscle contractions causing cramps and cardiac arrythmias. The excess lactic acid causes metabolic acidosis.

14.6.3 Clinical Features

- H/O of crush injury
- Oligouria
- Dark coloured urine
- Nausea
- Vomiting
- Delirium
- Cardiac arrythmia

14.6.4 Investigations

- Blood investigation:
  - Elevated CPK levels (>1000 IU/L)
  - Increased levels of Serum aldolase, Serum myoglobin, Serum Lactic acid, Serum LDH, Serum AST, Serum ALT, Serum urea, Serum creatinine, Serum potassium
  - Hypocalcaemia
  - Stress induced hyperglycaemia
  - Myoglobinuria
- ECG—may show arrythmia in case of hyperkalaemia
- Arterial blood gas analysis—reveals metabolic acidosis

14.6.5 Treatment

- Initial resuscitation at site of injury as per BLS/ATLS protocol: securing airway, ensure patient is breathing and the circulation is maintained by giving compression to control bleeding.
- The patient should be given adequate fluid replacement at the earliest to avoid hypovolemia. The type and amount of fluid given depends upon the electrolyte imbalance as evident on ABG and the central venous pressure (CVP) of the patient.
- Diuretics may be prescribed to maintain the urinary output above 300 ml/hr. along with fluid replacement.

- Dialysis should be started if the urinary output is low and patient has fluid overload with increase in serum creatinine levels, BUN and bicarbonate levels or there is hyperkalaemia.
- Hyperbaric oxygen therapy has been shown effective in promoting wound healing and prevent anaerobic infections.
- Prophylactic broad-spectrum antibiotics to prevent bacterial infections.
- Emergency Surgery in the form of laparotomy, thoracotomy, fracture treatment, fasciotomy or amputation may be needed.
- Aggressive debridement of dead and necrotic tissues is required.
- Rehabilitation of patient is done after primary treatment.

14.7 Delayed Union and Non-union

Bone is a unique tissue as it heals by formation of new bone tissue similar to the original bone and not scar tissue as in case of other tissues being injured. Fracture healing involves four stages:

(i) Stage of hematoma formation:
This stage is characterised by bleeding at the fracture site due to injury to the blood vessels immediately after the injury. The bleeding is controlled by local vasocontriction within a few hours.
The hematoma is rich in polymorphonuclear leucocytes and lymphocytes. These are replaced by macrophages in 24–48 h. These cells secrete inflammatory cytokines like interleukins (IL-1, IL-6) and tumour necrosis factor (TNF-α) as well as growth factors like platelet derived growth factor (PGDF), transforming growth factor (TGF-β), bone morphogenic proteins (BMP).

(ii) Stage of soft callus formation:
The bone periosteum forms the callus at fracture site. The osteoprogenitor cells of the periosteum form cartilaginous matrix in the central part under the influence of the growth factors.
The process starts in the first week of injury and requires stability around fracture site which will allow the hematoma to consolidate into fibrin meshwork to bridge the fracture gap and angiogenesis to regenerate the injured blood vessels.

(iii) Stage of hard callus (modelling phase)
The cambium layer of periosteum forms osteoblasts which produces inorganic matrix composed of collagen and it eventually mineralises to form woven bone tissue.
The cartilaginous callus matures by mineralisation.
This takes around 4 weeks time. It is clinically evident by loss of movement across fracture site, decreased pain and increased mobility in the injured limb. X ray done shows reduced fracture gap and callus formation.

(iv) Stage of remodelling
The woven bone across the fracture site is gradually replaced by lamellar bone over years. The process is faster in children and young while very slow in elderly. The process of remodelling occurs due to the balanced action of osteoclast bone resorption and osteoblast bone formation. The extracellular matrix is progressively mineralised.

The fracture healing occurs histologically through three routes

(i) Inter cortical bridging (early endosteal callus)—healing occurs through normal cortical remodelling when the fracture gap is obliterated and stabilised. This type of healing requires intact endosteal blood supply. It is also called primary bone healing. No external callus is seen.
(ii) External bridging callus (periosteal callus)—it is seen when fracture site has some amount of mobility (micromotion). An external callus is seen.
(iii) Intramedullary bridging callus (late Endosteal callus)—healing by this method is seen in cases of delayed union when primary periosteal bridging callus has failed to achieve union.

Fracture healing is determined by the degree of stabilisation at fracture site, amount of blood supply to fracture site and the biomechanical environment of the fracture site.

The stability at fracture site is important for a stable hematoma formation and angiogenesis to take place. The amount of callus formed is governed by the grade of apposition and mobility permitted across the fracture, good apposition with no mobility allows healing by primary intention where no external callus forms and bone heals primarily by cortical bridging while micromotion at fracture site causes external callus to form and healing occurs by external bridging callus.

The blood supply of the fracture site is responsible for hematoma formation and delivers inflammatory cells to the fracture site which bring about necessary biological agents required for bone healing.

The conducive nature biomechanical environment of the fracture site is very important as in cases with high energy trauma or open wounds or in patients with compromised immunity or comorbidity, bone healing is either delayed or fails to occur in spite of good reduction and stability across fracture site. The lack of blood supply, adequate inflammatory response and presence of progenitor cells at the fracture site will hamper fracture healing.

The 'diamond concept' of fracture healing (Fig. 14.2):

It gives equal importance to mechanical stability and biological environment for aiding in fracture healing. The vascularity of bone and the physiological state of patient are deemed important for initiation of healing as they supply the osteoinductive cells and mediators to the fracture site. The osteoblastic activity starts once the osteoconductive matrix has been laid down and there is mechanical stability with only micromotion at the fracture site.

Delayed union—It is defined as a delay in the fracture healing i.e. a particular bone with a particular fracture pattern requiring more than the usual time for adequate healing.

The fracture shows signs of union like callus formation, obliteration of fracture margins on X rays and decreased mobility across fracture with

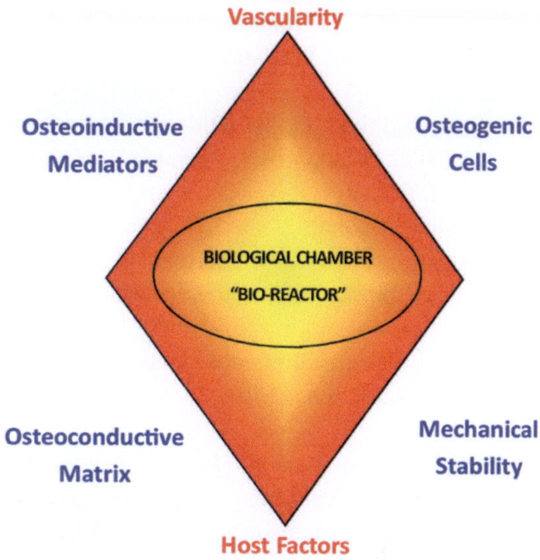

Fig. 14.2 Diamond concept of fracture healing. (Sourced from: Giannoudis PV, Einhorn TA, Marsh D. Fracture healing: the diamond concept. Injury. 2007 Sep 1;38:S3–6.)

decrease in pain on clinical but these changes take more than the usual time. The time frame for stamping a fracture going into delayed union is kept at 4–6 months.

Non-union—It is defined as a condition where in the fracture fails to unite. The fracture site shows no progression in the signs of union on successive follow-up. The x-rays show persistent gap at fracture site, sclerosis and rounding off of fracture ends and resorption of the callus. The fracture site may have mobility, but it may be absent if there is fibrous union. The time frame taken is 9–12 months.

As per FDA, if a fracture fails to unite at 9 months and does not show signs of healing in 3 consecutive months, then it is said to be in non-union.

14.7.1 Causes

- Unstable fracture pattern: long spiral pattern, multi-fragmentary fracture pattern
- Excessive movement across fracture site: poor mechanical stability, lack of splinting
- Inadequate fracture apposition: interposed soft tissue, bone loss
- Open fractures

- Precarious blood supply—Scaphoid #, Neck of femur #, Talus #, Distal tibia #
- Infection
- Co morbid conditions: Old age, Anaemia, DM, HIV, Osteoporosis, Peripheral vascular disease, Obesity
- Smoking, Alcohol
- Medications: NSAIDs, Steroids, Anticoagulants, Antibiotics, Chemotherapeutics, Insulin

Non-union is classified into two broad categories (Weber and Cech, 1976):

A. Hypertrophic non-union—It is characterised by the presence of exuberant callus across fracture site, but the fracture lines are not obliterated. These fractures have viable biology and good blood supply. Inadequate fracture stability or excess strain at fracture site hampers fracture healing. Based on the callus morphology on X-ray, it can be of following types (Fig. 14.3).

The treatment of hypertrophic non-union is done by improving mechanical stability using reamed locked intramedullary nails of adequate diameter, compression plating or ilizarov/ LRS external fixator system. There is no need for bone grafting.

B. Atrophic non-union—It is characterised by lack of callus at fracture site and the fracture ends are sclerosed with a persistent fracture gap. This results due to poor biology, infection, interposition of soft tissues or loss of bone fragments at the fracture site which hampers the healing process.

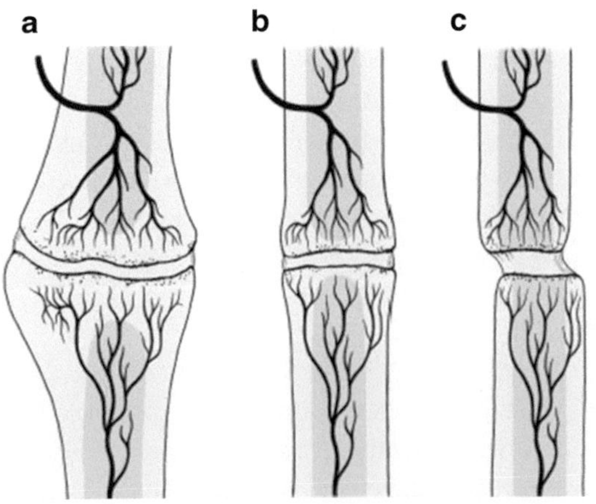

Fig. 14.3 It shows different types of Hypertrophic Non Union (**a**) Elephant foot type. (**b**) Horse hoof type. (**c**) Oligotrophic type

It can be of the following types based on the etiology (Fig. 14.4)

A. Dystrophic non-union: The intermediate fragment heals with one of the main segments but not the other
B. Necrotic non-union: The fractured bone fragment is avascular and fails to heal
C. Gap non-union: There is a bone loss creating a gap at fracture site
D. Atrophic non-union: The fracture site is filled with soft tissue which hinders fracture healing

14.7.2 Investigations

- X-ray
- Routine blood investigation: CBC, ESR, CRP, LFT, RFT
- DEXA Scan for osteoporosis
- Pus C&S

14.7.3 Treatment

- Hypertrophic non-union has intact biology and needs mechanical stability for fracture healing. The X-ray shows exuberant callus formation. Local infection should be ruled out. It is treated by stabilising the fracture either by POP cast for stable fracture pattern with no or minimal mobility or else operative fixation of fracture by compression plating or thick reamed intramedullary nail after freeing up the fracture site of excess callus and proper alignment of fracture ends.
- Atrophic non-union results due to lack of biological activity at fracture site. The fracture site has no callus; instead, fibrous tissue is formed around the fracture ends, which tries to stabilise the fracture. We should look for the

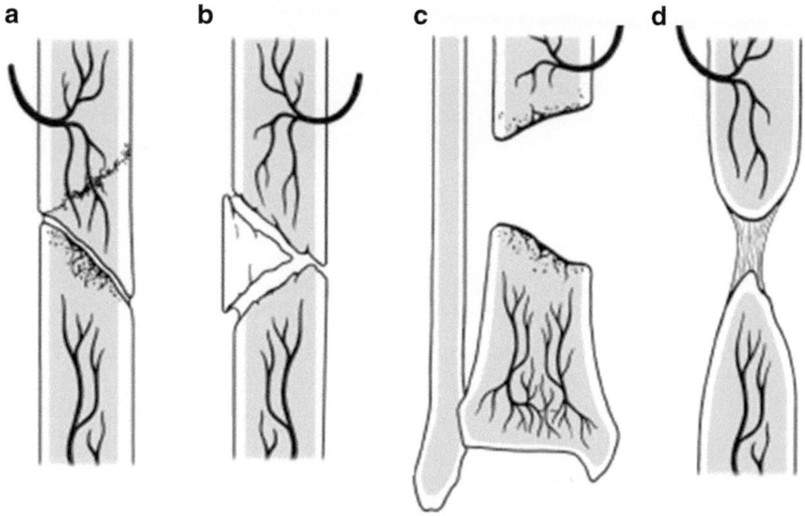

Fig. 14.4 It shows varoius types of Atrophic Non Union (**a**) Dystrophic type. (**b**) Nicrotic type. (**c**) Defect type. (**d**) Atrophic type

risk factors for non-union and treat the patient accordingly.

Any local infection is treated by aggressive debridement, and the fracture is stabilised temporarily by external fixators or splints. After infection is controlled, then definitive fixation is planned with an external fixation device, plates or intramedullary rods along with bone grafting to boost fracture healing. We can use osteoinductive molecules in place of bone grafting too.

14.7.4 Complications

- Persistent infection
- Joint stiffness
- Implant failure
- Recurrence of fracture

14.8 Malunion

The treatment of fracture is aimed at reducing the displaced fracture and maintain an anatomically acceptable length, alignment and rotation so that the patient's functions are not hampered. Any deviation in the length, alignment and rotation is termed as malunion (Fig. 14.5).

Cross Union—It is a malunion between the two forearm/leg bones in cases of both bone fracture. It results in restriction of pronation and supination movements in the forearm (Fig. 14.6).

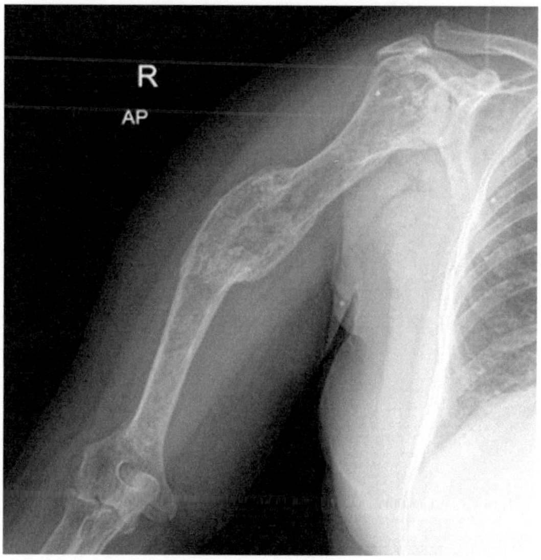

Fig. 14.5 Malunion of midshaft humerus fracture

14.8.1 Causes of Malunion

- Lack of treatment for the fracture
- Inadequate immobilization of the conservatively treated fractures
- Unstable fracture fixation in case of surgical treatment

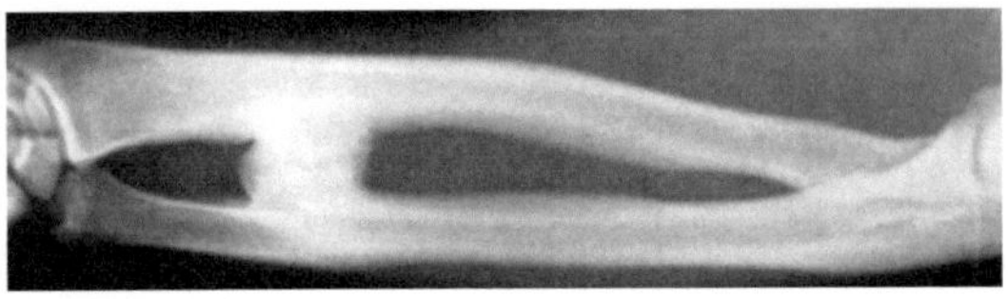

Fig. 14.6 Cross union of fracture radius and ulna

- Early mobilization and weight bearing before callus is strong enough
- Growth disturbances in growing children due to physeal arrest or overactivity

14.8.2 Malunion Can Lead to

- Restriction of joint mobility, especially in intra articular fractures
- Loss of function, due to loss of tension in muscles across the fracture
- Early arthritis, due to increased stress on adjacent joints
- Limp due to limb length discrepancy

14.8.3 Investigations

- X rays
- CT scans

14.8.4 Treatment

Surgical treatment is the only option. It is done by recreating the fracture line and fixation of fracture in correct length, alignment and rotation. It is done only if the patient is symptomatic and his activities are affected.

14.9 Avascular Necrosis of Bone (AVN)

It is a degenerative disease of bone characterised by cell death secondary to lack of bone supply to the bone. It is also called 'osteonecrosis', 'aseptic necrosis' and 'ischaemic bone necrosis'.

It is usually seen epiphysis of long bones and may lead to collapse of weight bearing bones.

14.9.1 Risk Factors

- Trauma: major joint dislocation, repetitive trauma
- Fracture Neck of femur, scaphoid, talar neck, proximal humerus
- Steroid therapy
- Smoking
- Alcohol
- Sickle cell disease
- Pregnancy
- Caisson disease
- Gaucher disease
- Anti phospholipid syndrome
- SLE
- Organ transplant
- Idiopathic

14.9.2 Clinical Features

AVN commonly affects the hip, knee, wrist and ankle joints. The AVN of femoral head is very common. The atraumatic cases may have a bilateral involvement. The osteonecrosis of the femoral head is classified based on the X-rays by 'Ficat and Arlet classification' and based on the MRI by 'Steinberg classification'. These classifications help the clinician to plan the management and give prognosis to the patients.

Although uncommon, spontaneous osteonecrosis of the knee is the most common type followed by the secondary type, which may occur due to any of the risk factors. The disease is common in older population. They are classified radiologically using the 'Koshino classification'.

The proximal humerus may develop AVN following fracture at the anatomical neck or a multifragmentary fracture. The 'Cruess classification' system is used for radiological classification.

AVN of talus results commonly after a displaced fracture at talar neck. It is classified using 'Hawkins classification'.

The osteonecrosis of lunate is also called 'Keinbock disease' and may result due to repeated trauma or any of the risk factors. The 'Lichtman staging system' is used for its classification.

The AVN of scaphoid, also called 'Preiser disease' may result due to any of the risk factors. It is common in fracture of scaphoid waist. The 'Herbert and Lanzetta classification' is used for it.

The presenting complains of the patients are

- Pain and stiffness of the involved joint
- Restricted ROM
- Shortening of involved limb

14.9.3 Investigation

- MRI, in early and doubtful cases
- Blood investigation—CBC, ESR, Coagulation profile, LFT, RFT to look for systemic causes

14.9.4 Treatment

- Non-operative treatment:
  - Bisphophonates therapy
  - Rest
  - Traction
- Operative treatment
  - Core decompression in early cases with no bony deformity
  - Osteotomy to divert the weight bearing surface away from the lesion
  - Joint replacement/arthroplasty for advanced cases with joint restriction

14.9.5 Complications

- Arthritis

14.10 Complex Regional Pain Syndrome (CRPS)

It is a multifactorial neuropathic pain disorder characterised by excessive pain disproportionate to the amount of injury and persists for a long time beyond the usual duration of healing of the tissue injury.

14.10.1 Causes

- Fractures: most common after wrist, shoulder, ankle, metacarpal fractures
- Surgery: common in patients undergoing foot and ankle surgeries, distal radius surgeries
- Genetical predisposition

14.10.2 Clinical Features

- History of trauma, fracture, surgery, burn, etc.
- Excessive pain involving the nearby joints with no fixed distribution pattern
- Skin changes—tense, shiny, red skin with loss of wrinkle lines
- Excessive sweating
- Hyperalgesia
- Allodynia
- Wasting of muscles
- Restriction of movement

The pain and swelling in CRPS are said to be a result of hyperactivity of the inflammatory and immunological cascade, while the neural sensitisation causes the symptoms like hyperalgesia and allodynia. The patient has a regional involvement for e.g. forearm, wrist and fingers are involved in CRPS secondary to Colle's fracture. The local skin temperature may rise in cases where there is sympathetic overactivity. The patients are disabled by the condition as it adversely affects their daily activities.

It is of two types (based on the injury)

1. Type I, also called 'Reflex sympathetic dystrophy (RSD)'.
2. Type II, also called 'Causlagia'

Causalgia results in cases with nerve injuries while RSD is seen in patients with no nerve injury.

It is classified into three types (based on the disease activity and duration)

1. Acute—It may last up to 3 months. It is characterised by severe pain, swelling with warm, shiny and tense skin. The joint mobility is restricted.
2. Dystrophic—It can last up to 12 months after the acute phase. It is characterised by weakening of muscles, stiffness of joints, loss of skin wrinkles, hyperalgesia, cool skin and brittle nails.
3. Atrophic—It follows the dystrophic phase. The affected area develops contractures, and the skin looks pale and shiny.

14.10.3 Investigation

1. X-ray: to look for bony injuries. It may show rarefaction of bones of the involved body part
2. Routine blood test: to rule out any other causes, infections

14.10.4 Treatment

- The disease has a self-limiting course. The symptoms improve with the passage of time.
- Non-interventional therapy
  - Physical therapy: local ultrasound therapy, TENS (transcutaneous electrical nerve stimulation), ROM excercises
  - Medications: Anti-inflammatory—NSAIDs, Anti-depressants—Gabapentin, Amytryptiline, NMDA antagonist—Ketamine
- Interventional therapy
  - Sympathetic blocks
  - Dorsal root ganglion stimulation

14.11 Myositis Ossificans

It is defined as the of formation of mature bone in the extra skeletal soft tissue. It is also called 'Heterotopic ossification'.

14.11.1 Causes

- Traumatic:
  - Head injury
  - Fractures, dislocation
  - Burn injury
  - Arthroplasty
- Neurogenic:
  - Stroke
  - Brain tumours
  - Spinal cord injury

14.11.2 Risk Factors

- Old age
- DVT
- Long bone fractures
- Repetitive trauma
- Coma patients
- Brain injury
- Ankylosing spondylitis
- Paget's disease
- DISH (diffuse idiopathic hyperostosis)
- Tracheostomy

The heterotopic tissue has mature woven bone in periphery and immature osteoblasts in central part.

14.11.3 Clinical Features

- Swelling: firm to hard
- Stiffness
- Pain

Symptoms start by second week after trauma and gradually progress.

14.11.4 Investigations

- X ray: it shows bony mass in the soft tissue
- CT scan
- Blood investigation: raised ESR, CRP, ALP, CK

14.11.5 Treatment

- Prophylaxis in high-risk patients for DVT, hypoxia
- Early ROM exercises

- Medications: Indomethacin, selective COX 2 inhibitors (celecoxib, rofecoxib), bisphonate (Etidronate)
- Local irradiation
- Surgical resection of an organised ossification can be planned, to increase ROM, once the bone has matured

Multiple Choice Questions

1. Keinbock disease affects
   (a) Scaphoid
   (b) Lunate
   (c) Capitate
   (d) Hamate
2. AVN of Femur head is classified using
   (a) Koshino classification
   (b) Herbert and Lanzetta classification
   (c) Cruess classification
   (d) Ficat and Arlet classification
3. Which is not a type of hypertrophic non union
   (a) Elephant foot
   (b) Horse hoof
   (c) Oligotrophic
   (d) Atrophic
4. Virchow's triad does not consist of
   (a) Damage to endothelium
   (b) Damage to nerves
   (c) Turbulence in blood flow
   (d) Hypercoagulability
5. Not a major criteria as per Gurd's criteria for diagnosis of fat embolism
   (a) Petechial rash
   (b) Respiratory insufficiency
   (c) Tachycardia
   (d) Confusion

Answers: 1. (b), 2. (d), 3. (d), 4. (b), 5. (d)

References for Further Reading

1. Hooper N, Armstrong TJ. Hemorrhagic shock. In: StatPearls. Treasure Island (FL): StatPearls Publishing; 2022.
2. Gitz Holler J, Jensen HK, Henriksen DP, et al. Etiology of shock in the emergency department: a 12-year population-based cohort study. Shock. 2019;51(1):60–7. https://doi.org/10.1097/SHK.0000000000000816.
3. Oczkowski S, Alshamsi F, Belley-Cote E, et al. Surviving Sepsis Campaign Guidelines 2021: highlights for the practicing clinician. Pol Arch Intern Me. 2022;132(7-8):16290. https://doi.org/10.20452/pamw.16290.
4. Elliott KG, Johnstone AJ. Diagnosing acute compartment syndrome. J Bone Joint Surg Br. 2003;85(5):625–32.
5. Schmidt AH. Acute compartment syndrome. Injury. 2017;48(Suppl 1):S22–5. https://doi.org/10.1016/j.injury.2017.04.024.
6. Osborn CPM, Schmidt AH. Management of acute compartment syndrome. J Am Acad Orthop Surg. 2020;28(3):e108–14. https://doi.org/10.5435/JAAOS-D-19-00270.
7. Liu B, Barrazueta G, Ruchelsman DE. Chronic exertional compartment syndrome in athletes. J Hand Surg Am. 2017;42(11):917–23. https://doi.org/10.1016/j.jhsa.2017.09.009.
8. Misra I, Glasgow J, Moosavy F. Fat emboli syndrome. Del Med J. 2017;89(5):148–50.
9. Guerado E, Bertrand ML, Cano JR, Cerván AM, Galán A. Damage control orthopaedics: State of the art. World J Orthop. 2019;10(1):1–13. Published 2019 Jan 18. https://doi.org/10.5312/wjo.v10.i1.1.
10. Rawal G, Yadav S, Kumar R. Acute respiratory distress syndrome: an update and review. J Transl Int Med. 2018;6(2):74–7. Published 2018 Jun 26. https://doi.org/10.1515/jtim-2016-0012.
11. Fan E, Brodie D, Slutsky AS. Acute respiratory distress syndrome: advances in diagnosis and treatment. JAMA. 2018;319(7):698–710. https://doi.org/10.1001/jama.2017.21907.
12. Stubbs MJ, Mouyis M, Thomas M. Deep vein thrombosis [published correction appears in BMJ. 2018 Mar 21;360:k1335]. BMJ. 2018;360:k351. Published 2018 Feb 22. https://doi.org/10.1136/bmj.k351.
13. Ruskin KJ. Deep vein thrombosis and venous thromboembolism in trauma. Curr Opin Anaesthesiol. 2018;31(2):215–8. https://doi.org/10.1097/ACO.0000000000000567.
14. Rahaghi FN, Minhas JK, Heresi GA. Diagnosis of deep venous thrombosis and pulmonary embolism: new imaging tools and modalities. Clin Chest Med. 2018;39(3):493–504. https://doi.org/10.1016/j.ccm.2018.04.003.
15. Rajagopalan S. Crush injuries and the crush syndrome. Med J Armed Forces India. 2010;66(4):317–20. https://doi.org/10.1016/S0377-1237(10)80007-3. Epub 2011 Jul 21. PMID: 27365733; PMCID: PMC4919827
16. Malinoski DJ, Slater MS, Mullins RJ. Crush injury and rhabdomyolysis. Crit Care Clin. 2004;20(1):171–92. https://doi.org/10.1016/s0749-0704(03)00091-5.
17. Thomas JD, Kehoe JL. Bone nonunion. [Updated 2023 Mar 6]. In: StatPearls [Internet]. Treasure Island (FL): StatPearls Publishing; 2023.

18. Fong K, Truong V, Foote CJ, et al. Predictors of nonunion and reoperation in patients with fractures of the tibia: an observational study. BMC Musculoskelet Disord. 2013;14:103. Published 2013 Mar 22. https://doi.org/10.1186/1471-2474-14-103.
19. Calori GM, Giannoudis PV. Enhancement of fracture healing with the diamond concept: the role of the biological chamber. Injury. 2011;42(11):1191–3. https://doi.org/10.1016/j.injury.2011.04.016.
20. Sheen JR, Mabrouk A, Garla VV. Fracture healing overview. [Updated 2023 Apr 8]. In: StatPearls [Internet]. Treasure Island (FL): StatPearls Publishing; 2023.
21. Matthews AH, Davis DD, Fish MJ, et al. Avascular necrosis. [Updated 2022 Nov 14]. In: StatPearls [Internet]. Treasure Island (FL): StatPearls Publishing; 2023.
22. Castillo-Guzmán TA, Nava-Obregón D, Palacios-Ríos JÁ, Estrada-Cortinas MC, González-García JF, Mendez-Guerra OG-S. Complex regional pain syndrome (CRPS), a review. Med Univ. 2015;17(67):114–21.
23. Vanden Bossche L, Vanderstraeten G. Heterotopic ossification: a review. J Rehabil Med. 2005;37(3):129–36. https://doi.org/10.1080/16501970510027628.
24. Sun E, Hanyu-Deutmeyer AA. Heterotopic ossification. In: StatPearls. Treasure Island (FL): StatPearls Publishing; 2022.

Fractures in Children 15

Ritesh Runu and Vishal Kumar

15.1 Paediatric Bone

- The bones are mostly cartilaginous, soft, pliable and vascular.
- They are covered with thick vascular periosteum, which provides support and good healing potential to the bones. It has growth plates at ends of bone, secondary ossification centres and abundant blood supply.
- It is divided into diaphysis, metaphysis, physis and epiphysis regions.
- The diaphysis region is a slender, tubular, hard cortical bone which provides length and strength to the bone. It is covered by thick periosteum.
- The metaphysis is a wide, flared area near the joint composed of cancellous bone. It has very high vascularity. Periosteal covering is thin.
- The physeal area is the growth plate area which provides growth to the bones, and any injury to this region may cause growth disturbances.
- The epiphysis is the broad rounded end of the bones which forms the joint and is covered with the articular cartilage.
- Shaft fractures are commonly undisplaced (due to periosteal tube) compared to periarticular and articular fractures where no periosteal covering is present.
- On histology, the bones have small units of osteons. It has osteoblasts, osteoclasts and matrix containing organic and inorganic materials. The osteoblasts form the bones by producing type 1 collagen rich in Extra Cellular Matrix (ECM), which mineralises later. These cells arise from the pluripotent cells. The ECM is removed by osteoclasts. These cells arise from the phagocytic macrophage series. The osteocytes are the bone cells which lay down new bones and provide strength to the body part.
- The rhythmic activity of osteoblasts and osteoclasts helps the bone to remain viable and elastic. This cycle of replacement of old bone by new bone is known as bone remodelling cycle.

15.2 The Development of Human Skeleton

- Starts at 7th week of intrauterine life. Most of the endoskeleton develops by 12th week. These bones have primary ossification centre.
- The formation of bone occurs by two processes. First is *intramembranous ossification* where mesenchymal tissue is directly con-

R. Runu (✉)
IGIMS, Patna, Bihar, India

V. Kumar
Department of Orthopaedics, PGIMER, Chandigarh, Chandigarh, India

V. Kumar et al. (eds.), *A Quick Guide to Essential Orthopedics*,
https://doi.org/10.1007/978-981-95-2676-5_15

verted to the bony tissue. The skull bones, and other flat bones are formed by this process.

- Another process is *endochondral ossification*. Here the mesenchymal cell differentiates into cartilaginous tissue and then ossifies to form the skeleton.
- These bones have a *primary ossification centre* which appears during intrauterine growth. The calcification of bone occurs from centre to periphery. The cartilaginous cells are pushed to periphery which later becomes growth plate. Later the end of bones calcifies through ossification centres at the periphery of bones known as *secondary ossification centres*. These appear after birth.
- The growth plate is used for age determination and for bone dysplasia diagnosis. At birth the secondary growth centres present and seen on x-ray are distal end of femur and proximal end of tibia.
- Later the growth of the skeleton occurs from the growth plate. This growth adds length to the bone while growth occurring from the periosteum is called *appositional growth*. It adds width or the circumference to the bones.
- Growth occurring from the ends of the bones but not adding length to the bones is called *apophyseal growth*. For example, trochanteric growth of femur. In the long bones, the proximal end of humerus and distal end of radius are the growing ends while in femur and tibia, the physis close to knee joints are the growing ends.
- The physis of metacarpals and metatarsals are distally placed except the first metacarpal where it is placed proximally.
- The *growth plate* has several layers.
  - From epiphysis the first layer is the zone of resting cells.
  - Second is zone of proliferation.
  - Third is zone of hypertrophy.
  - Fourth is zone of provisional calcification. It is the weakest layer because it lies between calcified and noncalcified areas (Salter and Harris). Most of the transverse physeal injuries occur through this zone.
  - Fifth is zone of enchondral ossification.
- Vertical compression forces and angular forces cause variable compression of physis leading to un-displaced or displaced fractures.
- The blood supply of physis is from both the metaphyseal and epiphyseal side, hence the risk of avascular changes in physis remains less.
- After trauma, in a few cases, a bridge of bone is formed which is known as a physeal bar. It can cause growth disturbances and deformities depending on its location. Central physeal bar may cause shortening while peripheral bars may cause angular deformities as well.

15.3 Types of Fractures

- Paediatric bones are soft and pliable. It is mostly cartilaginous and covered by thick periosteum in the diaphyseal area.
- Fractures of bone may occur due to trauma or diseases (pathological).
- Most common fracture in children are distal radius and ulna. Second most common are clavicle fractures.
- Paediatric fractures unite early, remodels well, may end up with overgrowth, may be associated with physeal injuries and may cause deformities.
- Post traumatic fractures (types)
  - Incomplete fractures
    - Plastic deformation of bones—due to compression and bending forces both the cortex bends but no fracture is noted. If angulation is more than 20° and age is more than 4 years then manipulation under anaesthesia is required. Example—plastic deformation of ulna.
    - Torus—when the bone gets compressed on one side without cortical break on other side in the metaphyseal area. Example: distal radius fractures, dorsal cortex compressed and distal tibial fractures, medial cortex compressed. It

usually presents late due to minimal pain and swelling. It remodels well.
    - Greenstick—when bending force breaks one cortex of bone and bends the other cortex. Most commonly seen in forearm bone fractures. Risk of refracture is high.
- Complete fractures
    - Undisplaced—when fracture fragments are in place due to thick periosteal tube. Mostly treated by plaster slab.
    - Displaced—when fracture fragments are displaced it requires reduction under anaesthesia and plaster immobilisation. The acceptable range of reduction in paediatric age groups depends remodelling capacity which depends on growth remaining, plane of deformity in relation to adjacent joint, proximity to growing physis, and the age of child. Remodelling is highest in sagittal plane, less in coronal plane and NIL in rotation. Wolff's law—bone remodelling depends on the stress working across the fracture site.
    - Displaced fractures are managed by bandages (clavicle fracture—figure of eight bandage and collar and cuff sling), manipulation under anaesthesia and plaster splinting (forearm bone fractures), Dunlop's traction (unreduced supracondylar fracture of humerus), Gallow's traction (femoral shaft fractures in infants), Thomas splinting (femoral shaft fractures in children), Krammer wire splinting.
    - Operative intervention is needed for irreducible fractures, neurovascular involvement with fracture, intraarticular fractures, multiple fractures, polytrauma, compound fractures and avulsion fractures.

15.4 Physeal Injuries and Classification

- Physis/Growth plate can be injured due to direct hit over the metaphyseal area or due to bending force, vertical compression or angular force creating side compression.
- The classifications for physeal injury were given by Salter and Harris (1963), Peterson, Rang, Ogden, Aitken, Poland, etc.
- Epiphyseal plate has secondary ossification centre. It ossifies and fuses with the metaphysis at maturity.
- After injury to the growth plate, temporary growth arrest occurs which is radiologically seen as transverse dense (sclerotic) line parallel to the physis, known as a Harris growth arrest line or Park's line.

15.4.1 Salter and Harris Classification

- Type 1—the whole of epiphysis is displaced from the physeal layer (zone of provisional calcification) without any fracture of epiphysis and metaphysis. Good prognosis.
- Type 2—the epiphysis is displaced with the triangular piece of metaphysis (Thurston Holland Fragment). Example—distal radial fracture.
- Type 3—the epiphysis is fractured without any displacement. It is an intraarticular fracture without any effect on growth of bones Example—distal tibial physeal injury.
- Type 4—the intraarticular fracture of epiphysis is displaced along with triangular piece of metaphysis. An unstable fracture requires accurate reduction and fixation. For example—lateral condyle fracture of distal humerus. The triangular metaphyseal bony fragment is known as Holland Thurston fragment.
- Type 5—this is the compression type of physeal injury where, the periphery of the growth

plate is injured but not seen on x-rays immediately. The effect of physeal injury is visible later with deformity. Example distal radial growth arrest.
- Type 6—added by Rang. Perichondral ring injury. Affects the physeal growth.
- Peterson reclassified the Salter Harris classification.

15.5 Management of Physeal Injuries

- Undisplaced fractures and physeal injuries are managed by plaster splint for 3–6 weeks.
- Undisplaced physeal injuries type II, III and IV requires closed/ open reduction and fixation with smooth pins and wires. Plaster splint for 3–6 weeks. Pins across physis are avoided due to risk of physeal injury.
- Displaced injuries of physis type II, III and IV requires anatomical reduction and fixation. Pins across physis are avoided. If required, smooth pins are applied. Type 4 physeal injuries are very unstable fractures. They need anatomical reduction and fixation.
- Type 5 fractures are usually identified later. The complications like deformity and shortening are managed later.

15.6 Complications of Fractures

- *Growth Disturbances*: Injury to physis may cause formation of calcified bars across it. If the physeal bar is in the central area of the growth plate then it affects the overall growth of bone leading to shortening of limb. Physeal bars are diagnosed by X-rays, CT scan and MRI.
- *Angular Deformities*: Formation of physeal bar in the peripheral area of the physis, may cause angular deformities. The location and size of the physeal bar is determined by MRI or CT scan. The physeal bars can be resected to regain the growth and to prevent further angular deformity to progress. Temporary epiphysiodesis is done to prevent progression of angular deformity. For non-progressive deformity, corrective osteotomy and bone lengthening is done.
- *Nonunion*: Displaced physeal fragment, inadequately fixed fracture may end up with nonunion. It may lead to joint stiffness, angular deformities and neurovascular problems. It is managed by early reduction, fixation and bone grafting.
- *Joint Stiffness*: Intra-articular and periarticular injuries, after prolonged immobilisation, excessive massage over the joint area can cause joint stiffness. Anatomical reduction and fixation of intraarticular fractures and early mobilisation can prevent stiffness. In severe cases, arthrolysis (debridement of joint) and manipulations are needed.
- *Arthritis*—It is a late complication of intra articular injuries. During early adulthood the patient may present with arthritis and stiffness.
- *Compartment syndrome*—This is acute complication of fractures in forearm and leg commonly. Muscles around the bone along with vessels and nerves surrounded by fascial sheath is known as a compartment. In forearm, the groups of muscles are arranged in superficial flexor compartment, deep flexor compartment and extensor compartment. In leg, the compartments enclosed by fascial sheath are anterior, lateral, superficial posterior and deep posterior compartment.
  Due to direct trauma to muscles or due to ischaemia or due to fluid extravasation, the compartment pressure rises causing severe pain. To accommodate the swollen muscle, fascial sheath expands to a limit, after which the arteries are compressed causing ishaemia to muscles and nerves. This causes pallor and paraesthesia. The ischaemic muscles break down creating a vicious cycle of increased pressure, ischaemia, muscle injury and nerve injury. As late signs, pulselessness and paralysis are observed.
  Clinically, tense tender compartment in limbs following trauma causing excruciating pain on toes or finger movement with raised compartment pressure is diagnosed as compart-

ment syndrome until proved otherwise. It is managed by splinting and elevation of limb, ice fomentation, analgesics and continuous monitoring. If resolution doesn't occur then, immediate bandages are removed, fasciotomy is done and limb is kept under observation.

The muscles in the compartment are replaced by fibrous tissue which is non contractile causing flexion deformity in fingers and wrist known as Volkmann's ischaemic contracture. On flexion of wrist, the fingers can extend at interphalangeal joints and metacarpophalangeal joints while reverse occurs with wrist extension. This phenomenon is called Volkmann's sign. Similar deformity with sensory deficit, it is confused with ulnar nerve palsy.

- *Vascular injury*—Due to close proximity of vessels to the bone, vascular injury can occur. Example—elbow joint injuries may cause brachial artery injury, distal femur or proximal tibial injuries may cause popliteal artery injury.

  The degree of injury may be either intimal injury or full thickness arterial wall injury or complete arterial disruption or direct extrinsic compression or indirect compression. The diagnosis of injury can be done by immediate arterial colour doppler, angiography or CT angiography. Any compression or thrombosis needs urgent intervention for resumption of blood supply distal to the block. Delay in intervention may lead to ischaemic necrosis of the part, Gangrene.
- *Plaster related complications*—Paediatric fractures are mostly managed by plaster slab or cast immobilization. It can cause skin lesion and joint stiffness also known as *plaster disease*. To prevent, plaster is applied for the minimum duration required and early mobilization is done.

  Tight plaster may cause neurocirculatory problems. *Compression of the superficial nerves* like common peroneal nerve over the fibular neck may cause foot drop. To prevent it, extra padding is done over the bony prominences and superficial nerves area. Tight plaster may also cause *compartment syndrome like features*. Hence, post plaster elevation of the limb, regular finger and toe movement and continuous monitoring for signs of compartment syndrome is done. Any sign of complication warrants removal of plaster immediately. While application of plaster, the edge of plaster over the cubital fossa and popliteal fossa may compress the artery causing compartment syndrome. To prevent, plaster application is done with care and bridging of plaster is done over the popliteal and cubital area.

  Inadequate length of cast may cause loosening and loss of reduction of fracture.
- *Traction related complications*—in children, skin traction is frequently applied. Tight bandaging of skin traction may compress the superficial nerves causing palsy, may compress the arteries causing vascular problems, may compress the muscles of leg or thigh causing the compartment syndrome. To prevent it, a finger is insinuated after bandage application to check the tightness of bandaging. Post procedure monitoring is done to check for any problems.

  Skeletal pin application may damage the physis causing growth disturbances and limb length disturbances.

15.7 Pathological Fractures

- A compromised bone (strength and structure) due to local or systemic conditions may fracture with minimal trauma.

15.7.1 Causes of Pathological Fractures in Children

- Tumours—benign and malignant.
- Bone marrow disorders—Leukaemia.
- Neuromuscular disorders—Cerebral Palsy, Myelomeningocele, Muscular Dystrophy, Arthrogryposis.

- Congenital and hereditary conditions—Osteogenesis imperfecta, Osteopetrosis, Sickle cell disease, Haemophilia (factor VIII and IX deficiency).
- Metabolic disorders—Rickets, Scurvy, Copper deficiency, hyperparathyroidism (primary and secondary), Cushings syndrome, Gaucher's disease and Renal failure.
- Medications causing osteoporosis—Steroids, Phenytoin, Aspirin, Ifosphamide, cancer therapy.
- Disuse osteopenia—Prolonged illness.
- Infections—Chronic osteomyelitis.
- Juvenile idiopathic osteoporosis.

15.7.2 Investigation

- X-rays are the first and most informative investigative tool. Osteoporosis is evident on x-ray after loss of 30% of bone mass. It shows the pattern of bone loss, periosteal reaction, metaphyseal bone loss, cortical thickness and medullary status.
- Quantitative CT scan measures the bone density, and the risk of fracture can be predicted.
- MRI is suggested in cases of soft tissue lesions like inflammation in osteomyelitis and soft tissue extension of tumours.
- Bone Scan—shows the extent of osseous involvement due to tumourous or infective lesions. It also shows any metastatic lesions.
- Hemogram, Peripheral blood smear, Liver function test, Kidney function test, Calcium, Phosphorus, Alkaline phosphatase, Hormonal assay, serum creatine kinase, Vit D level, Serum parathyroid level, serum hydroxyproline level, serum ascorbic acid level and relevant investigation are done.
- Bone marrow biopsy.

15.7.3 Management

- Pathological fractures are immediately immobilised to reduce pain and further displacement.
- Apart from fracture management, the primary condition is also managed simultaneously.
- Most of these fractures can be managed conservatively by plaster immobilisation. Few cases may require operative intervention, like osteogenesis imperfecta, chronic osteomyelitis, femoral neck fractures due to cystic lesion.
- Bisphosphonates are used in conditions with severe osteoporosis to increase the bone mass and to prevent further fractures especially in osteogenesis imperfecta.
- Calcium, vitamin D and other nutritional supplements are advised in high doses for deficiency conditions.
- Early mobilisation is suggested to reduce the risk of further osteoporosis due to immobilisation.

1. Child abuse (Non-accidental injury)
    - Fractures in children (age less than 18 years) may occur due to abuse which is common in premature, single child with care givers or step parents. Poor parents with low level of literacy and frustration increases the risk of child abuse.
    - It may be associated with emotional, sexual abuse and neglect.
    - Usually, these infants are brought to hospital by the care givers.
    - The history is inconsistent, clinical findings are confusing and multiple injuries are usually found. Areas of large ecchymosis along with fracture are consistent with NAI.
    - Most common bones fractured humerus, femur, tibia, skull, forearm, distal radius. Fibula is the least affected bone.
    - On skeletal survey, essential in kids less than 2 years, all long bones, skull and spine are screened. Corner fractures at epiphysiometaphyseal junction are usually pathognomonic.
    - Fractures at various stages of healing is seen. Most common differential is osteogenesis imperfecta.
    - Spinal injuries do not show any bony injury on X-ray. SCIWORA—spinal cord injury without radiological abnormality.

- Apart from the treatment of fractures, its reporting to child care authorities is essential.

Multiple Choice Questions

1. Growth plate is located in
   (a) centre of bone
   (b) one of the bone ends
   (c) both ends of bone
   (d) none
2. Bone remodelling unit comprises
   (a) osteoblasts,
   (b) osteoclasts
   (c) both
   (d) none
3. Longitudinal growth of bone occurs by
   (a) endochondral ossification
   (b) intramembranous ossification
   (c) appositional ossification
   (d) apophyseal ossification
4. Weakest layer of growth plate is
   (a) zone of proliferation
   (b) zone of hypertrophy
   (c) zone of provisional calcification
   (d) zone of endochondral ossification
5. Physeal bars are
   (a) normal physeal structures
   (b) post traumatic features
   (c) post infective features
   (d) post ischaemic features
6. Plastic deformation of bone is seen in
   (a) rickets
   (b) osteomyelitis
   (c) trauma
   (d) tumour
7. Torus fracture is commonly seen in
   (a) adults
   (b) children
   (c) infants
   (d) geriatric
8. Greenstick fractures are
   (a) Complete fractures
   (b) incomplete fractures
   (c) pathological fractures
   (d) All
9. Gallow's traction is applied for
   (a) fracture Clavicle
   (b) Fracture Femur
   (c) fracture tibia
   (d) fracture spine
10. Salter Harris classification is used for
    (a) paediatric fractures
    (b) adult fractures
    (c) geriatric fractures
    (d) pathological fractures
11. Thurston Holland sign is seen in Salter Harris type
    (a) one
    (b) two
    (c) three
    (d) four
12. Volkmann Ischaemic Contracture is due to
    (a) Ischaemia
    (b) ischaemia and neurological injury
    (c) ischaemia and muscle damage
    (d) All
13. Compartment syndrome is due to
    (a) ischaemia
    (b) muscle damage
    (c) tight compartment
    (d) All
14. Investigation of choice for ligament injury
    (a) X-ray
    (b) ultrasound assessment
    (c) Computed Tomography scanning
    (d) MRI
15. Pathological dislocation of joints may occur due to
    (a) Ligament laxity
    (b) Infection
    (c) Dysplasia of joints
    (d) All

Answers: 1. (c), 2. (c), 3. (a), 4. (b), 5. (b), 6. (c), 7. (b), 8. (b), 9. (b), 10. (a), 11. (b), 12. (d), 13. (d) 14. (d) 15. (d),

Suggested Readings

1. Solomon L, Warwick D, Nayagam S. Apley's system of orthopaedics and fractures. 9th ed. UK: Hodder Arnold; 2010.
2. Flynn JM, Skaggs DL, Waters PM. Rockwood and Wilkins' fractures in children. 8th ed. USA: Wolter Kluwer; 2015.

Approach to a Patient with Limb Injury

16

Shivji Prajapati

RTA is one of the most common causes of polytrauma, other than natural calamities, train accidents, flight crashes, etc. These may result in head injury, chest injury, abdominal injury, pelvis injury, spine injury and limb trauma.

Management of polytrauma can be divided in two major parts: As given below in Table 16.1.

Basic survey at site is done by clinician or expert person to identify the level of trauma and casualities that have happened so he can call for support from an expert team at site with equipment.

First aid is the initial care of the injured at the place of accident.

Table 16.1 Management of polytrauma patient on basis of treatment site

1. Action at the site of injury	2. Management at hospital
Basic survey First aid Triage ATLS, immediate resuscitation GCSShifting the patient to hospital	Detailed clinical examination/ vitals Resuscitation / monitoring/ reevaluation Wound inspection & classification ETO vs. DCO Fracture management

16.1 Goals of First Aid Treatment

Three Ps aptly describe goals of first aid treatment:

- *P*reserve life by carrying out appropriate resuscitative measures.
- *P*revent further injuries by careful handling.
- *P*romote recovery.

16.1.1 Glasgow Coma Scale (GCS)

Total Glasgow Coma Scale (tGCS) scores range from 3 to 15, with lower scores for lower levels of consciousness, generally correlating with more severe injury requiring more intensive care. Components and scoring are given below (Table 16.2).

Scores of 3–8 are considered to denote severe head injury, 9–12 moderate and 13–15 mild.

S. Prajapati (✉)
Popular Hospital, Varanasi, Uttar Pradesh, India

V. Kumar et al. (eds.), *A Quick Guide to Essential Orthopedics*,
https://doi.org/10.1007/978-981-95-2676-5_16

Table 16.2 Glasgow coma scale

Eye opening	
Does not open eyes	1
Opens eyes in response to pain	2
Opens eyes in response to voice	3
Opens eyes spontaneously	4
Verbal	
Makes no sounds	1
Incomprehensible sounds	2
Inappropriate words	3
Confused and disoriented, but able to answer questions	4
Oriented to time, person, and place, converses normally	5
Motor	
Makes no movements	1
Abnormal extension (decerebrate posture)	2
Abnormal flexion (decorticate posture)	3
Flexion / Withdrawal from painful stimuli	4
Moves to localise pain	5
Obeys commands	6
Total	15

16.2 Triage

It includes preliminary assessment of patients in order to determine the *urgency* of their need for treatment and the nature of treatment required. Classified in *four* categories with colour code *red, yellow, green, white/black* are given below as per (Table 16.3).

Table 16.3 Triage system with colour code

Category 1: Immediate	RED	Life threatening illness/injury Need immediate resuscitation	Shock, pneumothorax, flail chest, burn 3rd degree.
Category 2: Urgent	YELLOW	Non ambulatory patient Can be delayed up to1 hour	Fracture tibia, femur, dislocation Respiratory distress and chest pain
Category 3: Delayed	GREEN	Ambulatory patient Can be delayed up to 3 hours	Laceration, abrasion, fracture of non wt. bearing bone.
Category 4: Deceased /Expectant	Black / White	Dead and morbid pt.	No care needed.

16.3 Principal of Management: Four Stages

1. Immediate care—ATLS Protocol
2. Acute care—life saving procedure to control haemorrhage, respiratory and circulatory support; DCO begins
3. Intermediate care—skeletal stabilization—DCO
   Nutritional support and pain control
4. Definitive care—Comprehensive management of injury and rehabs

16.3.1 ATLS Protocol

(Mnemonic—ABCDE)

1. *Airway*: Listen air movement, look for intercostal movement, check for foreign body and remove it.
   Achieve 3 *P*
   - Achieve *p*atency
   - *P*rotect aspiration
   - *P*ositive pressure ventilation.
2. *Breathing*: Observe respiratory rate and depth of breathing.
   Check for tension pneumothorax, flail chest, massive pneumothorax and manage it.
3. *Circulation*: Examine the radial pulse and the carotid pulse for the function of cardia. If the pulse is absent, initiate cardiac resuscitation with CPR. Monitor BP, Pulse, urine input and output. It is advisable to arrest the bleeding by elevation or direct application of pressure over the bleeding points and prevent shock (Fig. 16.1).
4. *Disability*: Neurological Examination (AVPU Scale) & GCS Score
   *A*lert
   *V*ocal response
   *P*ain response
   *U*nresponsive to all stimuli
   Prevent further injury to brain by proper oxygenation and perfusion by maintaining blood pressure.
5. *Exposure*: Remove all clothes to examine other site of injury, prevent hypothermia and logroll to shift the patient (Fig. 16.2).

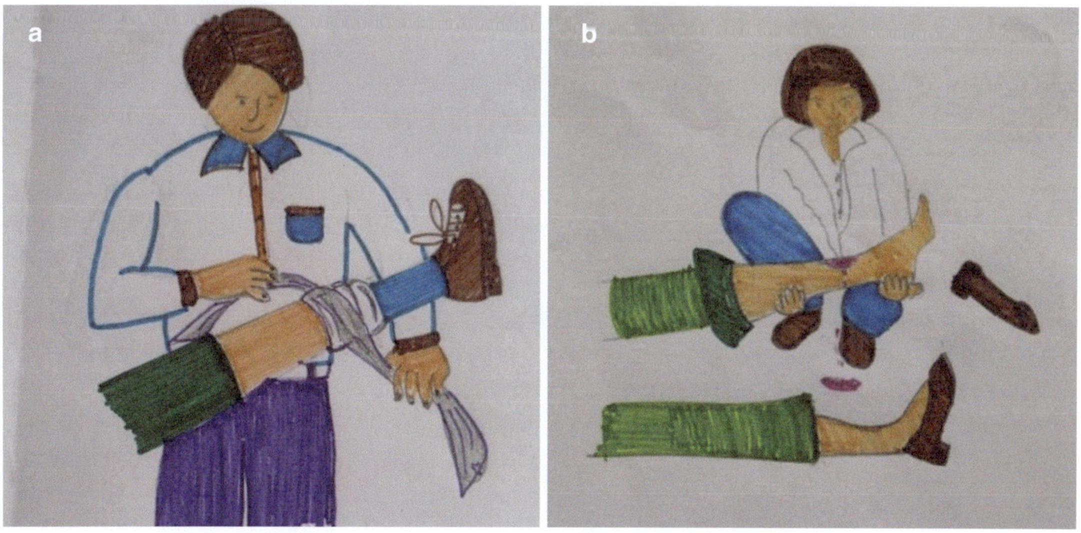

Fig. 16.1 Methods to control bleeding. (**a**) Firm pressure and bandaging (**b**) Limb elevation

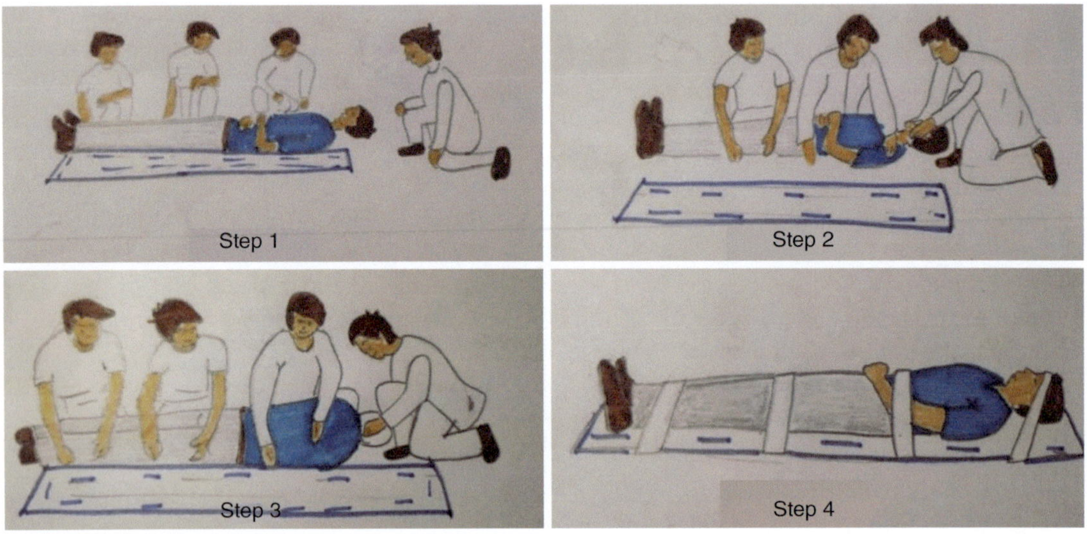

Fig. 16.2 Logroll technique

16.3.2 Management at Hospital

A to F management guidelines at hospital.

- Airway management
- Blood and fluid replacement
- Central nervous system management
- Digestive system management
- Excretory system management
- Fracture management

Secondary Survey Performed only after primary survey and resuscitation once patient clinically stable include head to toe examination and history.

16.4 Sample History

*S*ymptoms—pain, breathlessness, dizziness
*A*llergy—any specific drug/substance
*M*edication—regular/before event
*P*ast history—any medicine/surgery
*L*ast—meal timing
*E*vent—responsible for trauma

More severe injury should address first-head injury, pelvis injury, abdominal trauma, bladder injury, closed fracture

16.5 Wound Classification and Management

Open fracture needs wound care as well as fracture management.

On the basis of severity of wound, Gustilo & Anderson classified wound in three grades (Table 16.4). Sequence of management includes

Copious irrigation of wound—debridement—prophylactic antibiotics—splitting with external fixator/LRS, Illizarov—healed wound—definitive fixation.

16.5.1 ETO vs. DCO

Early total care: Earlier, it was considered to treat ortho injury by definitive fixation of all fracture in one trip to operation theatre. It involves definitive surgical stabilization of all long bone fracture during early phase of treatment (24 h).

Damage control orthopaedics is an approach which stabilizes orthopaedics injury so that patient's overall physiology can be improved.

Table 16.4 Gastelo & Anderson Classification of open wound

Gustilo and Anderson classification	
Grade I	Clean skin opening of <1 cm, usually from inside to outside; minimal muscle contusion; simple transverse or short oblique fractures
Grade II	Laceration >1 cm long, with extensive soft tissue damage; minimal to moderate crushing component; simple transverse or short oblique fractures with minimal communication.
Grade III	Extensive soft tissue damage, including muscles, skin and neurovascular structures: often a high energy injury with severe crushing component.
Grade IIIA	Extensive soft tissue laceration, adequate bone coverage; segmental fractures, gunshot injuries, minimal periosteal stripping.
Grade IIIB	Extensive soft tissue injury with periosteal stripping and bone exposure requiring soft tissue flap closure; usually associated with massive contamination
Grade IIIC	Vascular injury requiring repair.

Goal of DCO

- To avoid "second hit" phenomenon of major surgery during the acute systemic inflammatory response to trauma.
- Control to haemorrhage and manage soft tissue injuries (Fig. 16.1)
- Achievement of provisional fixation.

16.5.2 Fracture Management

Fracture is not an emergency but dislocation is emergency and need reduction as soon as possible. Fracture needs to be splinted with whatever material is available at the scene of accident (Fig. 16.3). Most of them can be managed electively later.

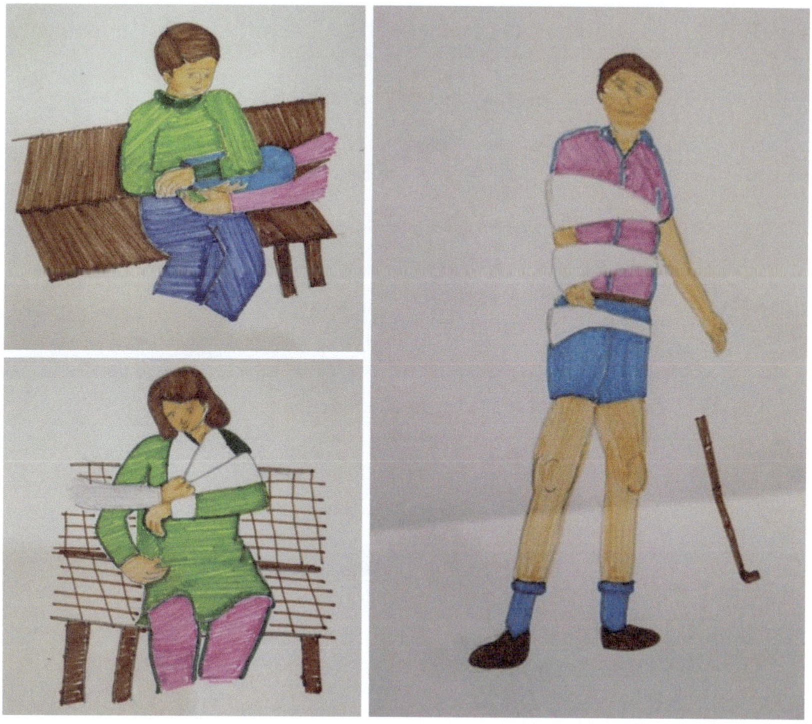

Fig 16.3 Various methods of splinting with cloths, sling and body bandage, own body part

POLYTRAUMA

Primary survey (ATLS)

- Assessment of vital functions and resuscitation
- ABCDE
- Focused Assessment with Sonography for Trauma(FAST) USG / AP chest and pelvic X-rays

Stable

AMPLE history
(Secondary survey)
- "Head-to-toe" Examination
- CT scan, X-ray spine & extremities, ECG, Echo

Reassessment (ATLS)

Stable

Delayed primary surgery
- Surgical management of non-immediately life-threatening injuries.
- Soft-tissue Debridement. External fixation of fractures, LRS.
- Definitive fixation of fracture.

Unstable

Damage control
- Life-saving surgery
- Prevent MODS/ARDS ,2 HIT

Unstable

Intensive care

- Restoration of the physiological "endpoints of resuscitation"

Which of the following is the most common cause of bleeding in Polytrauma Patient
A. Pelvis and Femur Fracture
B. Brain Haemorrhage
C. Rupture of Aorta
D. None of the above

Multiple Choice Questions

1. Which of the following is the most common cause of bleeding in Polytrauma Patient
   (a) Pelvis and Femur Fracture
   (b) Brain Haemorrhage
   (c) Rupture of Aorta
   (d) None of the above
2. If there is an incident of polytrauma in your locality, then which of the technique should you consider while transporting patient from trauma site to hospital to avoid progression of injury ?
   (a) Logroll technique
   (b) Slide board transfer
   (c) Rolling over technique
   (d) All of these
3. You are an Intern posted in Orthopaedic department and suddenly a Patient presents with Injury to the lower limb associated with severe pain and restriction in the range of motion, you made a diagnosis of Open fracture resulting from trauma to lower limb. Which of the following is true about an open fracture?
   1. Tibia and phalanges are most involved.
   2. Usually, no co-existing injuries.
   3. Compartment syndrome does not occur in open fractures.
   4. Early debridement should be done.
      (a) 1 and 4.
      (b) 1 and 2.
      (c) 2 and 4.
      (d) 2 and 3.
4. There is an incidence of mass casuality in your nearby area. You are posted in ED and a patient was brought to you with a suspected Head Injury. What should be the correct order of priorities which you should follow for the initial management of this patient?
   (a) Airway, breathing, circulation treatment of extracranial injuries.
   (b) Treatment of extracranial injuries, Airway, breathing, circulation.
   (c) Circulation, Airway, breathing, treatment of extracranial injuries.
   (d) Airway, circulation, breathing treatment of extracranial injuries.
5. In an unconscious severely injured patient of multiple fractures and an open bleeding wound on the right thigh, the first thing to be done is?
   (a) Secure airway.
   (b) Blood transfusion and treat shock.
   (c) Tourniquet and splinting.
   (d) GCS scoring.
6. Vascular repair is warranted in which type of Gustilo Anderson injury?
   (a) A.III c
   (b) B.I
   (c) C.II
   (d) D.III B
7. Which one is correct sequence of ATLS protocol?
   (a) Airway, breathing, circulation, disability, exposure
   (b) Breathing, Circulation, Airway, Exposure, Disability
   (c) Circulation, Airway, Breathing, Disability, Exposure
   (d) Breathing, Airway, Circulation, Disability, Exposure
8. What is maximum and minimum value of GCS score?
   (a) 15, 0
   (b) 15, 5
   (c) 15, 3
   (d) 12, 3
9. What is colour code for Triage patient who needs immediate response?
   (a) Blue
   (b) Green
   (c) Red
   (d) Yellow

Answers: 1. (a), 2. (d), 3. (a), 4. (a), 5. (a), 6. (a), 7. (a), 8. (c), 9. (c)

Introduction to Functional Bracing and Distraction Osteogenesis 17

Rama Priya Yasam

17.1 Functional Cast Bracing

17.1.1 Introduction

- The concept of functional cast bracing was described in the early eighteenth century.
- Sarmiento re-established the ideology in the late 60s as the Sarmiento principle: "In the closed system of the brace the dislocating forces are transformed into compression forces activated by the muscles."
- FCB is a type of bracing where the limb is allowed to do restricted functions with the brace in.

17.1.2 Definition

- Functional bracing is a therapeutic technique used for treating musculoskeletal injuries, which involves the use of specialized braces or orthoses to support and protect injured joints or body parts.
- The goal is to provide stability, promote healing, and facilitate the return to normal activity levels.

17.1.3 Purpose and Benefits

- Restricts specific movements that could further aggravate the injury.
- It allows controlled movement while protecting the injured area, unlike immobilization.
- Helps promote healing and prevent re-injury.
- It prevents muscle atrophy, joint stiffness, and other complications associated with prolonged immobilization.
- Provides support, reduces pain, and enhances the patient's sense of security.

17.1.4 Theoretical Basis

- FCB works on the concept of Pascals law, i.e., fluid is not compressible. The deep fascia surrounding the muscle compartments acts as a fluid mass. Fluid cannot be compressed, and fascia cannot be extended beyond the cast's boundaries. Because of this, pressure and load are communicated after a particular amount of displacement without additional distortion. As a result, the bone fragments are held in place more firmly (Fig. 17.1).
- In FCB, fracture healing is mostly accomplished by the creation of external bridging callus. It outperforms the medullary callus in terms of mechanical advantage. Intermittent loading of the fracture location by muscle activity and weight bearing stimulates local

R. P. Yasam (✉)
Department of, Orthopedics, Government Institute of Medical Sciences and Research Institute, Srinagar, Uttarakhand, India

V. Kumar et al. (eds.), *A Quick Guide to Essential Orthopedics*,
https://doi.org/10.1007/978-981-95-2676-5_17

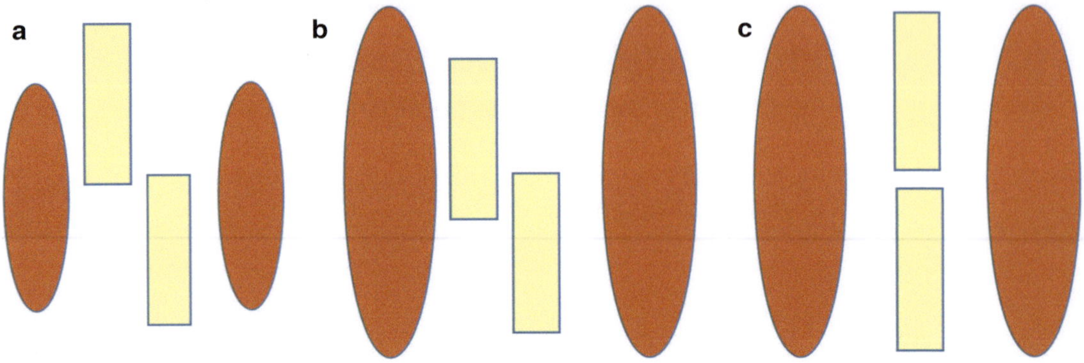

Fig. 17.1 Concept of pascals law in FCB (**a**) without muscle contraction (**b**) with muscle contraction (**c**) with muscle contraction and cast

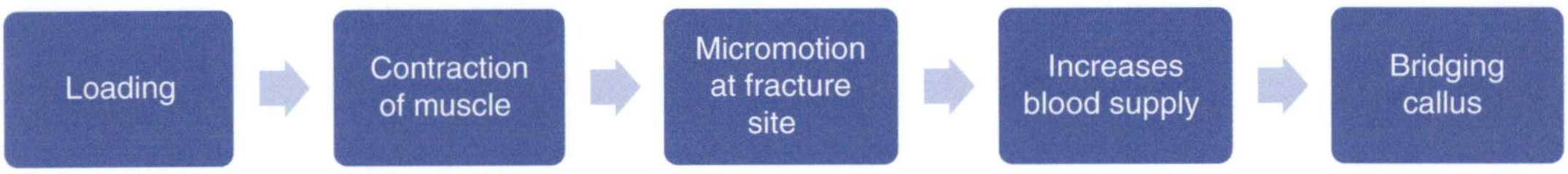

Fig. 17.2 Flowchart showing formation of bridging callus in DO

blood flow and the formation of electrical fields that aid in healing (Fig. 17.2).

17.1.5 Indications

- All middle third shaft fractures and lower third junction fractures in long bones.
- Ligament injuries, tendonitis, osteoarthritis, and fractures.
- Specific braces and designs are used based on the injury or condition being treated.

17.1.6 Time of Application

- Fracture ends sticky
- After pain and swelling subsides
- Minor movements at the fracture site should be pain-free
- Any deformity should disappear once deforming force removed
- Reasonable resistance to telescoping
- Shortening should not exceed 6 mm for the tibia and 1.25 cm for the femur
- For low-energy injuries bracing can be done in the first 2 weeks
- High energy injuries 3–4 weeks
- For humerus fractures, 7–10 days
- Median time for brace removal: tibia-18 weeks and humerus-10 weeks

17.1.7 Contraindications

- Intraarticular fractures
- Compound fractures
- Lack of cooperation by the patient
- Patient with spastic disorders
- Bedridden and mentally incompetent patients
- Deficient sensibility of the limb
- Fractures of both bones forearm when reduction is difficult

17.1.8 Not Used In

- Galeazzi fractures
- Monteggia fractures
- Proximal half of the shaft of the femur
- Isolated fractures of the tibia, fibula
- Tends to cause varus angulation and delay in the consolidation of fractures

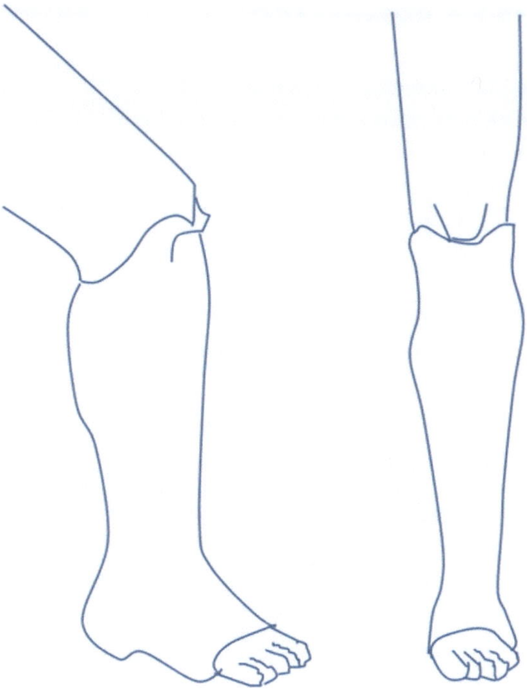

Fig. 17.3 PTB cast

17.1.9 Acceptable Reduction

- 50% cortical contact
- Less than 5–10° of varus or valgus angulation
- Less than 10–15° of anterior or posterior bowing
- Less than 5–7° of internal or external rotation
- Not more than 10–15 mm of shortening

17.1.10 Examples

- Patellar Tendon Bearing (PTB) Cast (Fig. 17.3)
- The functional cast of the humerus (Fig. 17.4)

17.1.11 Rehabilitation and Progressive Adjustment

- Functional bracing plays a crucial role in the rehabilitation process.
- It can be adjusted or modified over time to accommodate changes in the injury or the patient's healing progress.

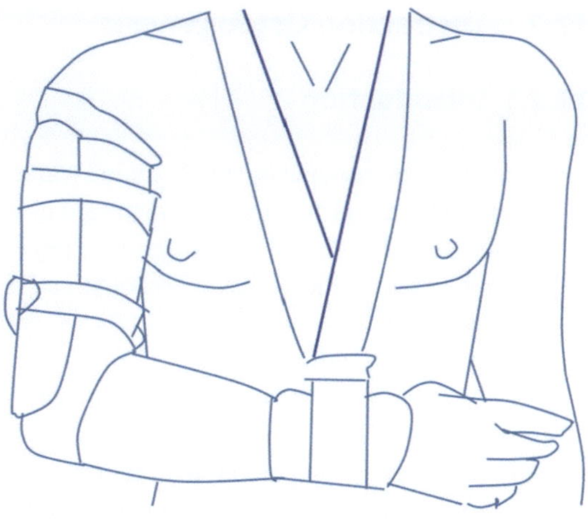

Fig. 17.4 FCB of humerus

- Gradual adjustments allow for an increased range of motion and functional activity as the injury improves.

17.1.12 Integration with Other Treatments

- Functional bracing is often combined with physical therapy, exercise programs, and pain management techniques.
- These complementary treatments enhance the overall rehabilitation process and optimize functional outcomes.

17.1.13 Conclusion

- Functional bracing offers advantages over immobilization by allowing controlled movement and promoting healing.
- It is effective in treating various musculoskeletal conditions and supporting the rehabilitation process.
- Proper implementation and supervision by healthcare professionals are essential for optimal outcomes.

17.2 Distraction Osteogenesis

17.2.1 Introduction

- Distraction osteogenesis (DO), called callus distraction, callotasis, and osteodistraction, is a process used in orthopedic surgery to repair skeletal deformities and reconstructive surgery.
- Developed by Ilizarov in 1956
- Mechanical induction of new bone that occurs between vascular bony surfaces that are gradually pulled apart by gradual distraction
- New bone formed bridges the gap and remodels to normal bone macrostructure
- Treatment stress effect on growth and genesis of tissues
- The procedure involves cutting and slowly separating bone, allowing the bone healing process to fill in the gap.
- Highly modular fixators allow the formation of new bone in almost any play as distraction osteogenesis follows the vector of applied force

17.2.2 Indications

- Non-union, LLD, deformity, bone defects secondary to complex trauma, infection, tumor.

17.2.3 Osteotomy

- osteotomy is performed at the metaphyseo diaphyseal junction which allows enough room for secure fixation of the cancellous fragment and yet still has good regenerate potential (good blood supply and large surface area).
- "Afghan type" of osteotomy involves percutaneous placement of a Gigli saw beneath the periosteum, which allows percutaneous osteotomy

17.2.4 Biology of DO

- Inflammatory response
- Callus formation
- Angiogenesis
- Osteogenesis
- Remodeling

17.2.5 Advantages of Osteotomy over Bone Grafting

- Reduces donor site morbidity.
- Autograph is limited.
- No fear of transmission of antigens, bacteria, viruses, or dead foreign bodies.
- In infected wounds.
- Risk of fracture in bone graft over an extended period.
- Bone graft will never incorporate into living bone.

17.2.6 Disadvantages

- Complete osteotomy disrupts medullary bone and its blood supply

17.2.7 Phases of DO

- Application of external fixator
- Corticotomy
- Latency period
- Distraction phase
- Consolidation phase

17.2.8 Corticotomy

- In this phase, the bone is cut either partially only through the hard exterior, or completely and a device is fitted which will be used in the next phases.

- Low energy osteotomy performed using an osteotome/corticotome to cut only the cortical surface thus preserving the medullary canal nutrient vessel, endosteum, and periosteum.
- Allows reliable tubular bone growth at 1 mm per day.
- As compared to osteotomy, corticotomy allows faster progression of new bone growth.
- The main difficulty with corticotomy is not knowing whether the corticotomy is complete or not.

17.2.9 Latency Period

- This is the second phase that lasts generally 7–10 days.
- Allows bone healing to progress through the acute inflammatory phase and enter into the reparative of bone healing and mobilization of bone progenitor cells.

17.2.10 Distraction Phase

- In this phase, the device mounted to the bone on each side of the cut gradually separates the two pieces, allowing new bone to form in the gap.
- Distraction of 1 mm per day (0.25 mm 6th hrly) yields the most optimal results
- Distraction less than 0.5 mm/day may result in premature consolidation, whereas more than 2 mm per day over-extends the bone regeneration process
- It is influenced by factors such as age, bone vascularity, etc.
- If the radiographic appearance of the regenerate contains central radiolucency greater than 8 mm then the distraction may be too fast and conversely, if the central radiolucency is less than 2 mm then the distraction may be proceeding too slowly
- Radiographs taken in the 4th postoperative week should reveal some callus formation
- If the callus is not seen, then distraction should be temporarily slowed or reversed
- If premature consolidation is present, then consider increasing distraction to 1.25 mm per day
- External fixation is then maintained until the callus becomes mature.

17.2.11 Consolidation Phase

- When the desired or possible length is reached, a consolidation phase follows in which the device keeps the bone stable to allow the bone to fully heal.
- It lasts twice as long as the distraction phase in children and three to four times as long as the distraction phase in adults.
- Plane X Rays are done on a monthly basis to know the condition of the Cortex and medullary canal in the osteogenic area
- After the consolidation phase, the device is removed in a second surgical procedure.

17.2.12 Healing Index

- Number of months of treatment per cm of new bone
- Adults: 1.8 months/cm
- Tibia
  - Children: 0.87 months per cm
  - Adults: 1.5 months per cm

17.2.13 Accordion Technique

- Mono-focal compression distraction technique for non-union treatment
- Alternate compression and distraction maneuver is used two to three times to stimulate bone neogenesis
- Local scar tissues are initially crushed to be transformed into tissues capable of neogenesis

17.2.14 Complications

- Pin tract infections
- Neurovascular injury
- Premature consolidation or delayed healing
- Hardware-related Problems
- Psychosocial Considerations

17.2.15 Conclusion

- Distraction osteogenesis is an innovative surgical technique that has transformed the way that different skeletal abnormalities and bone defects are treated.
- It offers customizable correction, preserves soft tissues, enhances bone regeneration, and expands treatment options.
- With careful patient selection, meticulous surgical technique, and appropriate postoperative management, it improves the quality of life for individuals with skeletal abnormalities.

Multiple Choice Questions—FCB

1. Functional cast bracing works on the principal of
   (a) Pascals law
   (b) Wolffs law
   (c) Hueter Volkmann law
   (d) Newtons law
2. Functional cast bracing can be combined with
   (a) physical therapy
   (b) exercise programs
   (c) pain management techniques
   (d) all of the above
3. Contraindications of FCB
   (a) diaphyseal fractures
   (b) closed fractures
   (c) Patient with spastic disorders
   (d) mentally competent patients
4. Time of application of FCB is
   (a) after the Fracture unites
   (b) after fracture ends become sticky
   (c) before pain and swelling subsides
   (d) immediately after fracture occurs
5. Benefits of FCB
   (a) prevents muscle atrophy
   (b) promote healing
   (c) prevents muscle atrophy
   (d) all the above

Answers: 1. (a), 2. (d), 3. (c), 4. (b), 5. (d)

Multiple Choice Questions—DO

1. Accordion technique involves
   (a) only compression
   (b) only distraction
   (c) compression and distraction
   (d) osteotomy and distraction
2. Complications of distraction osteogenesis
   (a) Pin tract infections
   (b) Neurovascular injury
   (c) Premature consolidation
   (d) All of the above
3. Correct order of phases of DO
   (a) Latency period, Distraction phase, Corticotomy, Consolidation phase
   (b) Corticotomy, Latency period, Distraction phase, Consolidation phase
   (c) Distraction phase, Corticotomy, Consolidation phase, Latency period
   (d) Consolidation phase, Corticotomy, Latency period, Distraction phase
4. Distraction of yields the most optimal results
   (a) 0.25 mm per day
   (b) 2 mm per day
   (c) 0.5 mm 6th hrly
   (d) 1 mm per day
5. Corticotomy in DO is done at
   (a) metaphysis
   (b) diaphysis
   (c) metaphyseo-diaphyseal junction
   (d) epiphysis

Answers: 1. (c), 2. (d), 3. (b), 4. (d), 5. (c)

References

1. Van den Berg C, Haak T, Weil NL, Hoogendoorn JM. Functional bracing treatment for stable type B ankle fractures. Injury. 2018;49(8):1607–11. https://doi.org/10.1016/j.injury.2018.06.009. Epub 2018 Jun 4.
2. Drakos MC, Murphy CI. Bracing versus casting in ankle fractures. Phys Sportsmed. 2014;42(4):60–70. https://doi.org/10.3810/psm.2014.11.2092.
3. Aktuglu K, Erol K, Vahabi A. Ilizarov bone transport and treatment of critical-sized tibial bone defects: a narrative review. J Orthop Traumatol. 2019;20(1):22. https://doi.org/10.1186/s10195-019-0527-1. PMID: 30993461; PMCID: PMC6468024.
4. Millonig K, Hutchinson B. Management of osseous defects in the Tibia: utilization of external fixation, distraction osteogenesis, and bone transport. Clin Podiatr Med Surg. 2021;38(1):111–6. https://doi.org/10.1016/j.cpm.2020.09.006.
5. Li Y, Pan Q, Xu J, He X, Li HA, Oldridge DA, Li G, Qin L. Overview of methods for enhancing bone regeneration in distraction osteogenesis: potential roles of biometals. J Orthop Translat. 2021;27:110–8. https://doi.org/10.1016/j.jot.2020.11.008. PMID: 33575164; PMCID: PMC7859169.

Part III

Regional Traumatology

Injuries Around the Shoulder

18

Kshitij Gupta and Sitanshu Barik

18.1 Introduction

The shoulder is one of the most freely moveable joints in the human body. It is because of the glenohumeral joint, which is a ball-and-socket type of joint and provides mobility in almost all directions. But it is complex joint formed by multiple articulations between clavicle, scapula, and proximal humerus. In this chapter, we'll cover all the injuries involving these bones and their multiple joints.

18.1.1 Anatomical Considerations

The functioning of the shoulder joint involves four joints:

1. Sternoclavicular joint (SC joint).
2. Acromioclavicular joint (AC joint).
3. Scapulothoracic joint.
4. Glenohumeral joint (GH joint).

The sternoclavicular joint is a synovial saddle joint. It is the only joint that transmits the load of upper limb to the axial skeleton. It is formed between the medial end of clavicle and manubrium sterni, stabilized by costoclavicular ligaments. The acromioclavicular joint is a plane synovial joint that connects the acromion process of the scapula to the lateral end of clavicle. It is stabilized primarily by the coracoclavicular ligament and secondarily by superior and inferior acromioclavicular ligaments. The scapulothoracic joint is not truly a joint. It is the name given to the gliding motion of scapula over the rib cage, assisted by various muscles.

As already mentioned, the glenohumeral joint is a ball-and-socket synovial joint that is stabilized by the rotator cuff muscles that attach to the joint capsule, as well as the tendons of the biceps and triceps brachii. The humeral head articulates with the glenoid fossa of the scapula. Glenoid forms a shallow socket and accommodates less than one-third of the humeral head. The fibro-cartilagenous labrum attaches to the outer rim of the glenoid fossa and provides additional depth and stability, securing the humeral head.

The stability of the glenohumeral joint is maintained by passive and active mechanisms which include:

Passive

- Joint conformity.
- Vacuum effect of limited joint volume and synovial fluid.
- Scapular inclination.

K. Gupta (✉)
Department of Orthopedics, All India Institute of Medical Sciences, Rishikesh, Uttarakhand, India

S. Barik
Department of Orthopaedics, AIIMS Nagpur, Nagpur, Maharashtra, India

V. Kumar et al. (eds.), *A Quick Guide to Essential Orthopedics*,
https://doi.org/10.1007/978-981-95-2676-5_18

- Ligaments and capsule—it includes the joint capsule, the coracohumeral ligament and the superior, middle and inferior glenohumeral ligament.
- Glenoid labrum.
- Bony restraints—acromion, coracoids and glenoid fossa.

Active

- Biceps long head.
- Rotator cuff.
- Scapula stabilizing muscles.

18.2 Fractures of Clavicle

The clavicle is the first bone to ossify (fifth week of gestation) and the last ossification center to fuse (sternal end) at 22–25 years of age. In children the clavicle fractures easily, but it almost invariably unites rapidly and without complications. In adults it accounts for 2.6–4% of all fractures. The most common site of fracture is middle third, on account of being devoid of muscular and ligamentous supports, followed by lateral third and medial third, respectively.

18.2.1 Mechanism of Injury

The most common mechanism of injury is fall onto the affected shoulder (85%). It is followed by direct impact on the clavicle and fall on outstretched hand in that order. It can be fractured by minimal trauma also in case of pathological changes. In case of midshaft fracture, the lateral fragment is pulled down by the weight of the arm and the medial half is held up by the sternocleidomastoid muscle. In fractures of the lateral end, if the ligaments are intact, there is little displacement. But if the coracoclavicular ligaments are torn, or if the fracture is medial to these ligaments, displacement may be more severe.

18.2.2 Clinical Features

Usually, the arm is clasped to the chest and supported by the opposite hand for immobilization. On examination, there might be palpable bulge or skin tenting in the lower neck. Tenderness and abnormal mobility at the fracture is also elicitable. It is wise the check the neurovascular status of the limb especially in case of medial third fracture in view of the neuro-vascular structures lying posterior to the clavicle.

18.2.3 Imaging

A clavicle fracture is usually apparent in an antero-posterior (AP) projection. An additional view in 30° of cephalic tilt may be taken to identify any occult fractures or assess for fracture—dislocation of the SC or the AC joint.

18.2.4 Classification

Clavicle fractures are usually classified on the basis of their location:

- Group I—middle-third fractures.
- Group II—lateral-third fractures.
- Group III—medial-third fractures.

Group II was further subclassified by Neer into three types:

- Type I—Fracture lateral to CC ligaments with CC ligaments intact and minimal displacement.
- Type II—Fracture medial to CC ligament of between the CC ligaments with ligaments intact or torn, associated with significant displacement.
- Type III—Fracture extending into the AC joint (Fig. 18.1).

18.2.5 Management

Nonoperative management—Most of the closed, undisplaced clavicle fractures with no neurovascular deficits can be managed nonoperatively. It can be managed using an arm sling or a figure of eight bandage. None of the techniques have shown any superiority over the

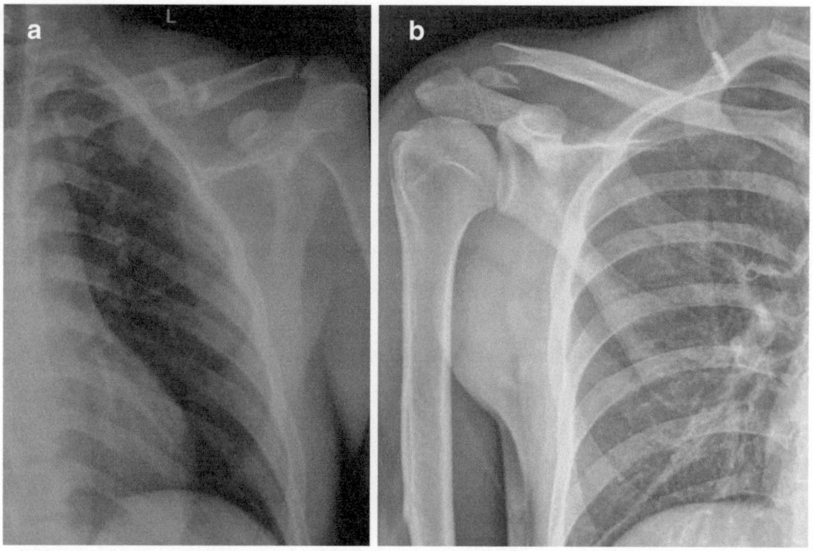

Fig. 18.1 (**a**) Middle third clavicle fracture, (**b**) Lateral third clavicle fracture

other. Though figure of eight strapping has been shown to cause more pain and has potential risk of pressure sores. Arm is kept in a sling for 2–3 weeks and gentle movements are started afterwards once pain subsides.

Operative fixation—Indications of operative fixation include:

- Open fractures.
- Displacement >2 cm.
- Fracture associated with skin tenting and future possibility of pressure sore or open injury.
- Vascular injury.

There are various options available for operative fixation of clavicle such as, anatomically contoured plates, hook plates as well as intramedullary devices and K-wires.

18.2.6 Complications

Early complications: Early complications as usually the associated injuries such as vascular injuries, brachial plexus injuries, rib fractures and occasional pneumothorax.

Late complications:

- Nonunion—Rate of nonunion in displaced clavicle fractures is 1–15%. The patients are usually asyptomatic. Symptomatic nonunions can be treated with fixation and bone grafting and mostly move onto union.
- Malunion—Most of the displaced fractures unite in a non-anatomical position with some shortening and/or angulation. It might be asymptomatic or can can periscapular pain. In cases of intractable pain, a corrective osteotomy and fixation can be attempted.

18.3 Fractures of Scapula

These are rare fractures usually caused by high energy trauma. The most commonly affected age group is 25–50 years. It can be associated with other injuries such as rib fractures, intra-thoracic injuries, shoulder dislocations, humerus, and clavicle fractures.

18.3.1 Mechanism of Injury

These are mostly the result of high energy trauma such as motor vehicle collisions (70%). It can also be caused by indirect trauma in case of fall on outstretched hand. Glenoid fossa and neck fractures can also occur in case of shoulder dislocations.

18.3.2 Clinical Features

Patient presents with a history of high energy trauma with diffuse pain around the affected shoulder. Because of energy required to damage scapula, it can also be associated with severe injuries to the chest, brachial plexus, spine, abdomen and head. There will be localized tenderness and abnormal shoulder contour, abrasions, or open wounds over the scapula. Careful neurological and vascular examinations are essential.

18.3.3 Imaging

Scapular fractures are difficult to assess on a plain x-ray owing to the surrounding soft tissue. A true AP of scapula, scapular Y view and axillary lateral views might be helpful. CT scan and 3D reconstruction are useful in demonstrating the morphology of the fracture (Fig. 18.2).

18.3.4 Classification

Scapula fractures are classified based on the anatomical location of the fracture into scapular body, glenoid neck, glenoid fossa, acromion and coracoids process.

18.3.5 Management

Body fractures: Usually managed conservatively. Patient wears a sling for support and pain relief and early mobilization after pain relief is promoted.

Glenoid neck fractures: The fractures are often displaced and further displacement is unlikely. They can be managed nonoperatively owing to their extra-articular nature.

Glenoid fossa fractures: These are intra-articular fractures and have to be treated as such. Smaller fracture fragments with humeral head centered over the glenoid with a stable shoulder need not be fixed and can be managed on a sling. If fracture involves more than 25% of the glenoid surface area with humeral head subluxation or an articular step-off of >5 mm, it needs to be fixed. Comminuted fracture of the glenoid fossa is likely to lead to osteoarthritis later on.

Acromion fractures: Undisplaced fractures are managed conservatively. Displaced fractures with reduced sub-acromial space needs operative intervention to restore anatomy.

Coracoid fractures: Fractures distal to the AC ligaments do not cause significant displacement while those proximal to it might cause acromio-clavicular separation and may require operative intervention.

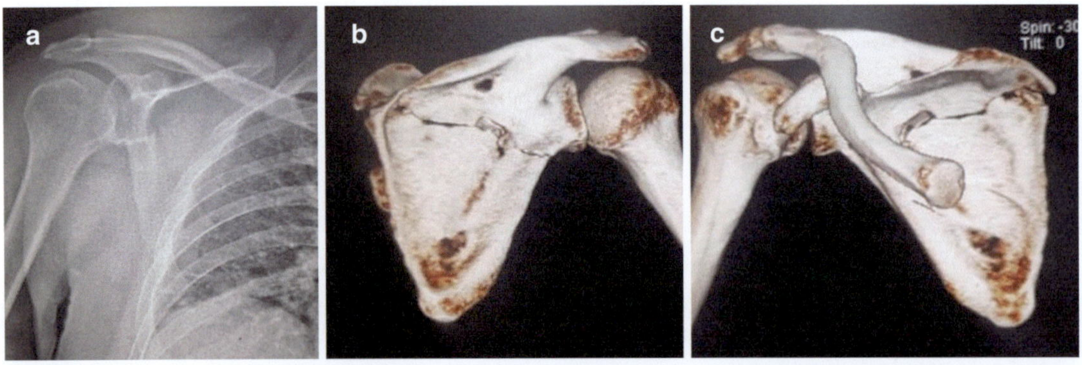

Fig. 18.2 (**a**) Scapular body fracture, (**b**) and (**c**) 3D reconstruction CT scan showing infraglenoid scapular body fracture

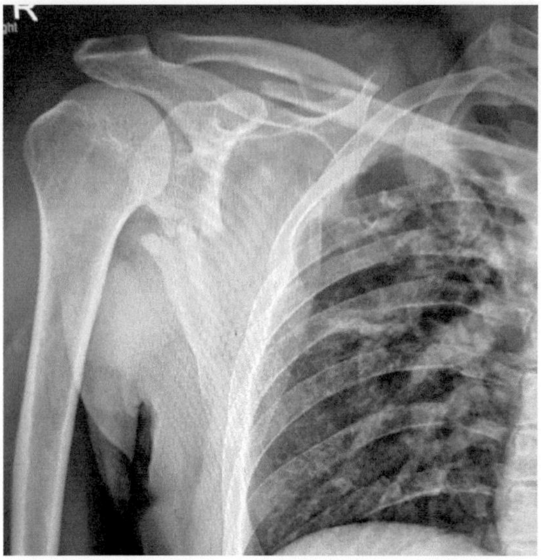

Fig. 18.3 Floating shoulder injury showing ipsilateral clavicle with glenoid neck fracture

18.3.6 NOTE: Floating Shoulder

Traditionally floating shoulder means ipsilateral glenoid neck fracture with clavicle fracture. But, recent evidence suggests that ligamentous disruption with glenoid neck fractures is a functional equivalent to this and has been included under this umbrella term. Minimally displaced fractures can be managed conservatively. But, individual indications for surgery for each fracture also warrant surgery for this injury. Even borderline cases might be taken up for surgery owing to the unstable pattern of this injury and one or both of the fractures might need to be fixed (Fig. 18.3).

18.4 Scapulothoracic Dissociation

Scapulothoracic Dissociation is a high-energy traumatic disruption of the scapulothoracic articulation often associated with severe neurovascular injuries, scapula, and clavicular fractures. It is usually caused by lateral traction injury to the shoulder girdle and involves significant trauma to heart, chest wall, and lungs. This injury caries a mortality rate of around 10%.

18.4.1 Clinical Features and Imaging

Patient presents with pain in the involved limb or a flail limb with sensory-motor deficits. There might be swelling and bruising around the shoulder. Neurovascular examination might reveal absent or decreased pulses and neurological deficits and is a critical part of the examination.

It is usually diagnosed by edge of scapula displaced >1 mm from spinous processes as compared to the contralateral side as seen on AP projection of the chest. It can also show associated clavicle, scapula fractures and SC joint, AC joint dislocations. A CT scan will show asymmetric distance between spinous process and medial edges of both scapulas. An angiogram may be required to assess injuries to subclavian and axillary artery.

18.4.2 Management

Management will include immobilization of affected limb with supportive care for patients without any significant vascular injury who are hemodynamically stable. An associated vascular injury might warrant an early visit to the OR for emergent management of vascular injury. Associated fractures and dislocations might be repaired at that time if patient hemodynamics allow. Functional outcome is dependent on neurological injury. If return of neurological function is unlikely, an early amputation will be beneficial to the patient.

18.5 Acromioclavicular Joint Injury

Acute injury of AC joint forms 12% of shoulder injuries. Chronic sprain of AC joint might be found in patients engaged in heavy lifting activities.

18.5.1 Mechanism of Injury

A direct fall on the shoulder may sprain or tear the AC ligaments and will lead to AC joint subluxation. A larger force might tear the CC ligaments, resulting in frank dislocation of the joint.

18.5.2 Clinical Features

The patient presents with pain at the site of AC joint. There might be no visible deformity but, joint might be tender on palpation in case of a sprain. While a dislocation may have a palpable and visible step superficially. Shoulder movements may also be limited.

18.5.3 Imaging

Imaging might include a standard AP view, 15° cephalic tilt view (Zanca view) and axillary view. In addition stress views with weight in the affected limb to increase the displacement might aid in diagnosis. A CT scan will show the exact morphology of the dislocation and might detect any fractures of distal clavicle or acromion which might have been missed on radiographs (Fig. 18.4).

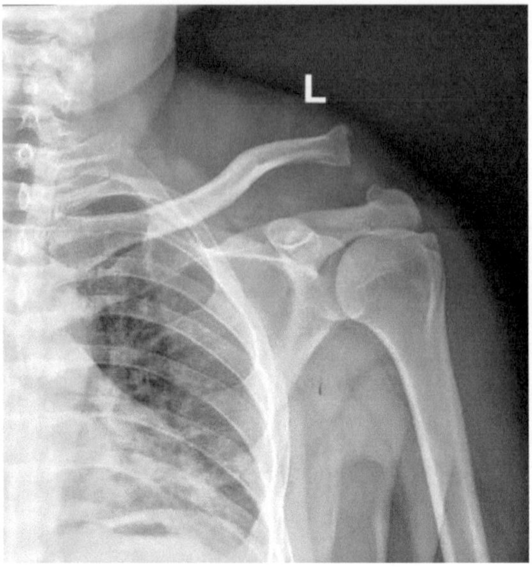

Fig. 18.4 Radiograph showing AC joint disruption

18.5.4 Classification (Table 18.1)

Table 18.1 Rockwood classification of AC joint injuries

Type	AC ligament	CC ligament	Radiograph	Treatment
Type I	Sprain	Normal	Normal	Sling
Type II	Torn	Sprain	AC joint disrupted, CC distance increased <25% of contralateral side	Sling
Type III	Torn	Torn	AC joint disrupted, CC distance increased 25–100% of contralateral side	Controversial
Type IV	Torn	Torn	Lateral clavicle displaced posteriorly through trapezius	Surgery
Type V	Torn	Torn	CC distance increased >100% of contralateral side	Surgery
Type VI	Torn	Torn	Inferior displacement of lateral clavicle	Surgery

18.5.5 Management

Ligament sprains can be managed with just a sling for pain relief and early shoulder mobilization once pain subsides. There is not enough evidence to show benefit of surgical management over conservative approach for type III injuries and management is controversial. Type IV, V and VI injuries require operative intervention with ORIF and/or ligament reconstruction. There are various techniques available to achieve it. Ligament stability can be achieved by either transferring existing ligaments (Coracoacromial ligaments or conjoined tendons) or by using a free graft (autogenous or synthetic). Fixation can be done with sutures, hook plates, CC screws, or K-wires. One procedure worth mentioning is the modified Weaver-Dunn procedure which includes resection of distal clavicle with transfer of coracoacromial ligament to distal clavicle to recreate CC ligament. Though none of the procedures has shown superiority to others.

18.5.6 Complications

- Rotator cuff problems—It can be either primary suffered during the time of injury of secondary to AC joint injury due to edema, inflammation, or arthritis. Treatment is anti-inflammatory medications and surgery in case of severely symptomatic tears.
- Residual dislocation and pain—Unreduced joint might have pain later on and may require surgical intervention. Residual pain is present in 30–50% cases.
- Secondary osteoarthritis of AC joint—It is a late complication, more common with operative intervention than with conservative management. It can be managed with pain relief with NSAIDs and physical therapy with surgery reserved for intractable cases.

18.6 Sternoclavicular Dislocation

Sternoclavicular Dislocations are uncommon injuries to the chest that consist of traumatic or atraumatic dislocations of the sternoclavicular joint. Anterior dislocation is more common but, posterior dislocation is more troublesome on account of placing mediastinal structures at risk. Usually caused by high energy injury such as motor vehicle collision, contact sports. Occasionally atraumatic subluxation may occur in young patients with overhead elevation of arm.

18.6.1 Clinical Features and Imaging

Anterior dislocation is visible as a bump in front of the SC joint. Posterior dislocation might be associated with dyspnea, dysphagia, tachypnea, and stridor. Closeness of neurovascular structures to the SC joint warrant a neurovascular examination.

It can be diagnosed of standard AP view of chest. Serendipity view (40° cephalic tilt) can show the direction of displacement—affected clavicle will be above/ below contralateral clavicle in anterior and posterior dislocation respectively. CT scan is the study of choice and can aid in assessing both the dislocation as well as associated injuries to mediastinal and neurovascular structures.

18.6.2 Management

Atraumatic subluxations and chronic anterior dislocations (>3 weeks) just require reassurance and local symptomatic treatment. Acute dislocations require a closed reduction either in emergency or under general anesthesia. Once reduction is achieved, shoulder can be braced in a figure of eight or velpeau bandage. Though the joint might redislocate, but, anterior dislocations are usually asymptomatic and patient gains good function. Failed closed reduction and posterior dislocations with symptoms of mediastinal structures compression and neurovascular deficit might require an open reduction. Great care needs to be taken not to injure mediastinal structures and a backup of cardio-thoracic surgeons might be needed.

18.7 Shoulder Dislocation

Shoulder joint is the most commonly dislocated joint among the large joints of the body. There is a high recurrence rate associated with shoulder dislocations, especially in younger population. Shoulder can dislocate in almost any direction including anterior, posterior, inferior with anterior being the most common direction. There are multiple factors responsible for this:

1. Shallow glenoid fossa.
2. Large multidirectional range of motion of the shoulder joint.
3. Underlying conditions such as ligamentous laxity, glenoid dysplasia.
4. Vulnerability of joint during stressful activities of upper limb.

We will deal with acute dislocations of the shoulder and their management in this chapter.

18.8 Anterior Shoulder Dislocation

18.8.1 Mechanism of Injury

It is mostly caused by a blow to the shoulder in an abducted, externally rotated, and extended extremity. It can also be caused by a fall on outstretched hand or a posterior impact on the shoulder.

18.8.2 Clinical Features

Patient presents with a history of trauma with affected limb abducted and externally rotated. Patient supports the affected limb with the contralateral hand for pain relief. There will an emptiness laterally while the humeral head may be palpated anteriorly below the clavicle. It is necessary to test and document the neurovascular status prereduction. One should check for the regimental badge sign to test for axillary nerve which is the most commonly affected nerve. There are a few named signs associated with shoulder dislocations such as,

Dugas test—When hand of the affected side is made to touch the opposite shoulder, the affected elbow cannot be touched to the chest which is diagnostic of a dislocated shoulder.

Hamilton ruler sign—It is considered positive when a straight ruler can be touched to both the acromion process and the lateral epicondyle when kept on the lateral aspect of the shoulder. Normally the shoulder contour prevents this from happening. The shoulder contour is lost in dislocation and hence the sign is positive.

18.8.3 Imaging

Normal plain anteroposterior radiographs will show the dislocation indicated by overlap of humeral head with displacement of humeral head medial to the glenoid fossa placed inferior to the coracoids process or clavicle. Axillary or lateral view can be used which will show the anterior dislocation of the humeral head compared to the glenoid. Occasionally a CT scan might be used to delineate fracture lines if, a fracture dislocation is suspected on radiographs (Fig. 18.5).

18.8.4 Management

Acute anterior shoulder dislocations require reduction. It can either be reduced in awake patient or might require sedation. Patient's pain is almost immediately decreased post reduction and can be used as a sign of reduction. There are multiple reduction techniques documented some of which currently carry only historical value. Some of these worth mentioning are:

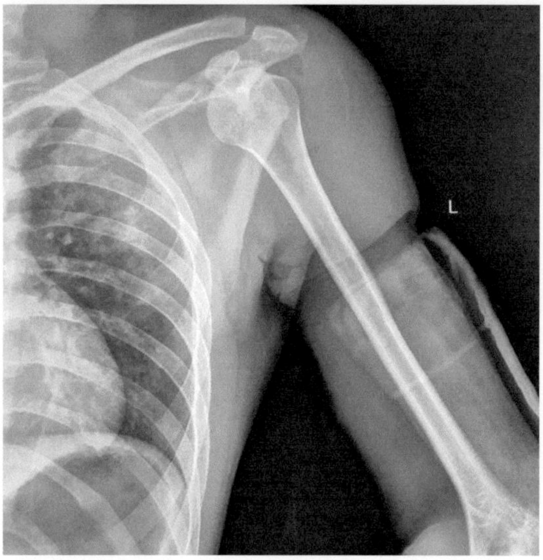

Fig. 18.5 Radiograph showing anterior shoulder dislocation

- *Stimson maneuver:* The patient lies in prone position with his arm hanging by the side of table. A downward traction to the arm is applied for 10–20 min by the practitioner or by attaching weights to the wrist of the patient. Then, the weights are released allowing the humerus to fall back into its position.
- *Milch technique:* The patient lies in a supine position. The practitioner holds the patient's arm at the wrist and the elbow externally rotating it to 90° followed by abduction to overhead position. Subsequently, the practitioner pushes the humeral head into a superior and lateral direction, reducing the shoulder.
- *Kocher maneuver (TEA-I):* The patient lies in supine position with his arm adducted to the thorax and his elbow flexed in 90°. The practitioner then provides a gentle traction and externally rotates the shoulder until resistance is felt. Then, the arm is adducted, retaining the external rotation in the shoulder. Finally, the arm is internally rotated and affected hand is placed on the contralateral shoulder completing the reduction maneuver.

Post reduction, the shoulder is immobilized in a sling or a shoulder immobilizer for 3 weeks period. Shoulder ROM is started after 3 weeks to allow the surrounding soft tissue to heal.

18.8.5 Complications

Early complications:

- Rotator cuff tears—This is particularly common in elderly patients. Associated with pain and weakness in movements of the affected shoulder based on the type and size of the tear. While it can be managed conservatively in low demand elderly patients, young patients with large tears will certainly require operative intervention.
- Neurovascular injury—Axillary nerve is the most commonly affected structure. It is associated with weakness of deltoid muscle (shoulder abduction) and regimental badge sign. Usually it is neuropraxia and recovers within a few weeks. If it does not recover, surgical exploration should be considered. It can also be associated with injury to the radial nerve, musculocutaneous nerve, and brachial plexus in general.
- Axillary artery is the most commonly affected vascular injury. Mostly affected in the elderly patients due to fragile vessels. It is also possible in overzealous reduction. It is necessary to check the vascular status both pre and postreduction.
- Fracture dislocations—Sometimes the dislocation might be associated with fracture of the proximal humerus. The first step still remains reduction of the joint. Once reduced the fracture can be managed based on the type and displacement of fragments postreduction like a proximal humerus fracture. A fracture dislocation might require an open reduction, if closed reduction fails.

Late complications:

- Shoulder stiffness—Prolonged immobilization post reduction is associated with shoulder stiffness, commonly inn patients >40 years of age. Active exercises should be started after 3 weeks of immobilization to loosen up the joint. Manipulation under anesthesia and arthroscopic repair can be undertaken in recalcitrant cases.

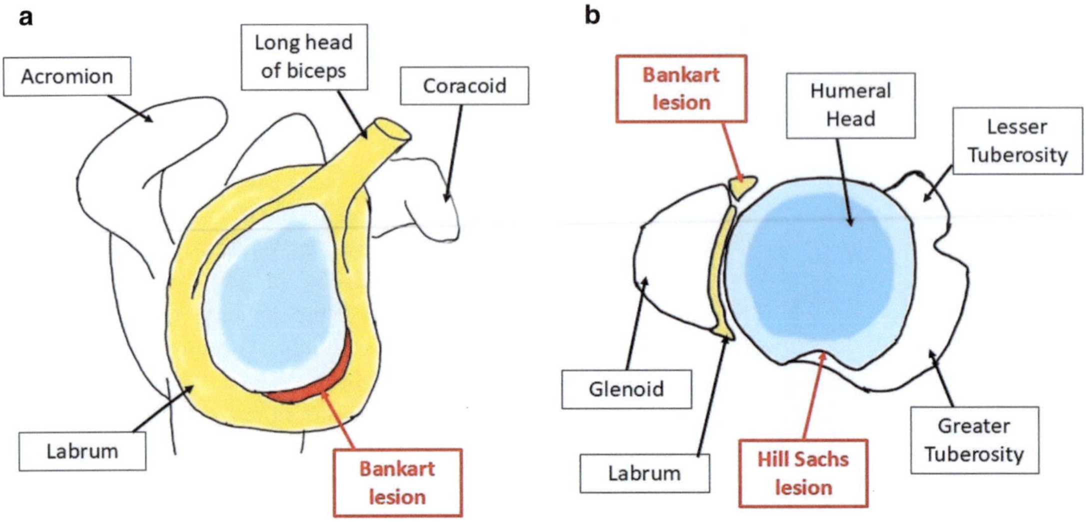

Fig. 18.6 Schematic diagrams showing (**a**) bankart lesion, (**b**) hill sach lesion

- Recurrent dislocation—Recurrence is quite common with shoulder dislocations. Usually occurs due to a tear in the glenoid labrum, making the joint unstable. Patient presents with history of multiple dislocation episodes with relatively trivial trauma and has apprehension test positive. Patient might be able to relocate the joint with subsequent dislocations. Usually requires an operative intervention based of the type of adjoining lesions.

18.8.6 NOTE

Bankart Lesion Bankart lesion represents an anterior and inferior labral detachment from the glenoid with an associated capsuloligamentous injury. It results in anterior shoulder instability. An associated bony fracture of the anteroinferior glenoid fossa is called a bony bankart lesion.

Hill Sach Lesion It is an osseous defect in the postero-supero-lateral aspect of humeral head caused by impaction of humeral head by anterior part of glenoid in case of anterior shoulder dislocations. Repeated dislocations can lead to a large lesion which can lock into the glenoid in dislocation and make relocation difficult.

Apprehension Test It is a test to assess patients with recurrent shoulder dislocations. Patient lies supine on the examination table. The affected shoulder is abducted, externally rotated and extended putting it in the vulnerable position for dislocation. Patient apprehension and not pain is considered positive test. Pain in the affected shoulder indicates an internal pathology such as impingement (Fig. 18.6).

18.9 Posterior Shoulder Dislocation

18.9.1 Mechanism of Injury

Large force resulting in marked internal rotation and adduction causes a posterior dislocation. It is mostly caused in cases of seizures and electric shock. It can also be possible in cases of direct anterior blow to the shoulder and fall on outstretched hand.

18.9.2 Clinical Features and Imaging

Patient presents with a history of trauma, seizure or electric shock with pain in the affected shoulder. The affected shoulder is held in adduction and internal rotation with restricted external rota-

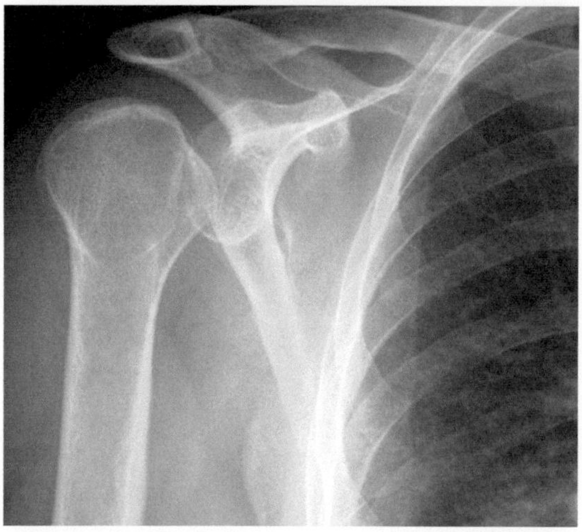

Fig. 18.7 Xray showing posterior shoulder dislocation showing light bulb sign

tion. Emptiness can be felt anteriorly and laterally with the round humeral head felt posteriorly.

A standard AP radiograph of the shoulder can be used for diagnosis. The humeral head is internally rotated, giving the typical light bulb sign. The humeral head also stays slightly away from the glenoid fossa, known as the empty glenoid sign. Lateral or axillary films can also be used which show posterior dislocation of the humeral head. CT scan might be taken in cases of suspected fracture (Fig. 18.7).

18.9.3 Management

The shoulder is reduced by applying traction to the arm in adducted and internally rotated position. Once the head is disengaged, another person can apply anterior and lateral force to the humeral head reducing it into the position. If reduction is stable, it can be immobilized in a sling or immobilizer. If unstable, it can be immobilized in an abducted and externally rotated position for 3–6 weeks. Shoulder movements can be started after 3–6 weeks once soft-tissues heal.

18.10 Inferior Shoulder Dislocation (Luxatio erecta)

It is a rare entity. It is caused by a severe hyperabduction force. Humeral head is levered out of the inferior end of glenoid with acromion acting as a fulcrum. Humeral head is displaced into inferior position with humeral head abducted into overhead position. Same features can be seen clinically and in radiographs. You should always look for neurovascular damage. Radiographs should also be inspected for associated fractures of the proximal humerus or glenoid. Inferior dislocation can usually be reduced by applying traction upwards in line with the abducted arm, with countertraction downwards over the top of the shoulder. If the humeral head is stuck in the soft tissues, open reduction is needed. It is important to examine for neurovascular injury. The arm is rested in a sling until pain subsides and movement is then allowed, but avoiding abduction for 3 weeks to allow the soft tissues to heal.

18.11 Proximal Humerus Fractures

Proximal humerus fracture forms 5–6% of adult fractures and is the most common humerus fracture. It mostly occurs in osteoporotic patients and is considered a fragility fracture. About 85% are undisplaced and can be managed conservatively. The remaining have considerable displacement of one or more fragments and can complications related to bone fragility, rotator cuff injuries and vascular insult to humeral head.

18.11.1 Anatomy

Proximal end of humerus includes a spheroid head which articulates with the socket of glenoid fossa of scapula to form the shoulder joint. The humeral head forms an angle of around

120–145° which is known as the humeral head inclination angle. Proximal humerus is also retroverted around 35–40° as compared to the distal humerus. The proximal humerus also includes 2 tuberosities known as the greater and the lesser tuberosity. These tuberosities provide attachment to the rotator cuff muscles with supraspinatus, infraspinatus and teres minor attaching to the greater tuberosity and subscapularis attaching on the lesser tuberosity. Long head of biceps passes between the tuberosities in the bicipital groove. The junction of the proximal humerus with the shaft is called as the surgical neck of humerus. The line along the physeal scar at the junction of head and tuberosities is known as the anatomical neck. Blood supply to the proximal humerus is provided by the combination of anterior circumflex humeral artery (36%) and posterior circumflex humeral artery (64%) (Fig. 18.8).

18.11.2 Mechanism of Injury

This fracture has a bimodal distribution with high energy trauma such as MVA forming the most common cause in young population. While in elderly, it is caused by a fall on outstretched hand, or fall from standing height and is considered a fragility fracture. It can occasionally be associated with a dislocation resulting in a fracture dislocation.

18.11.3 Clinical Features

Patient presents with pain and restricted mobility of shoulder. There may be presence of swelling, ecchymosis and bruising around the affected shoulder. A careful neurovascular examination is necessary considered the close proximity of brachial plexus and large vessels of the arm to the affected area.

18.11.4 Imaging

Standard antero-posterior radiographs of the affected shoulder are usually enough to identify the fracture. Additional views such as axillary lateral and scapular Y view need to be taken to rule out dislocation and identify the fracture mor-

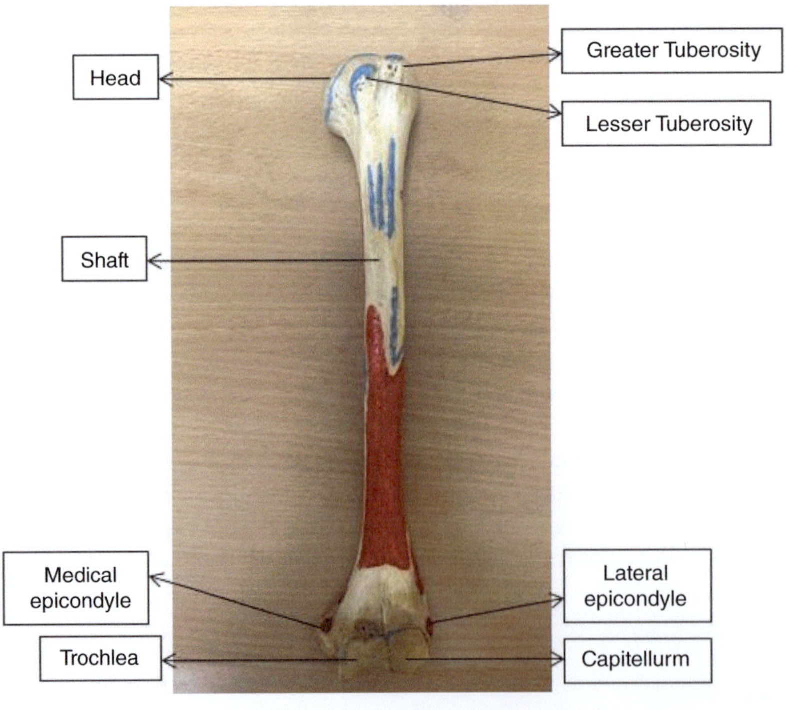

Fig. 18.8 Anatomy of humerus

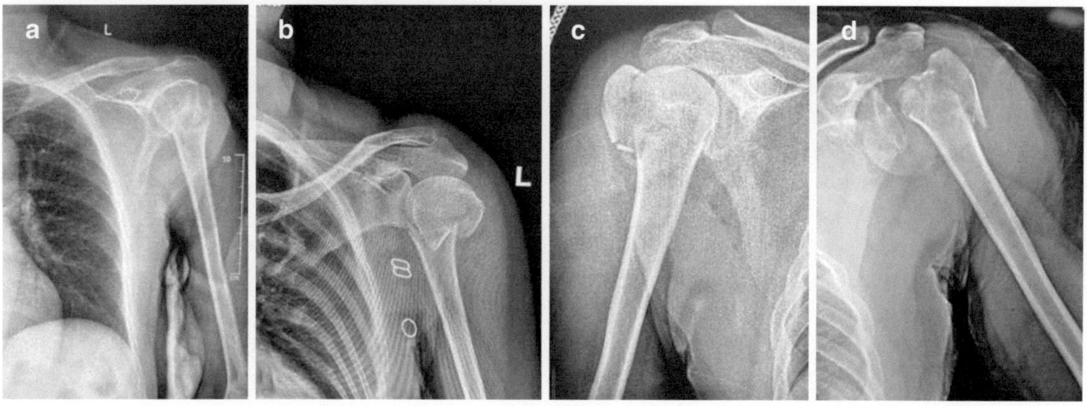

Fig. 18.9 Proximal humerus fractures, (**a**) one-part, (**b**) two-part, (**c**) three-part, (**d**) four part

phology. With the advent of 3D CT reconstruction, it is being increasingly used to characterize and classify proximal humerus fractures (Fig. 18.9).

18.11.5 Classification

The most widely accepted classification is the Neer's classification. Neer's classification is based on the displacement of the four major parts of proximal humerus namely head, greater tuberosity, lesser tuberosity and the shaft. Displacement according to Neer is defined as a translation>1 cm or angulation >45° between 2 fragments. Fracture can be classified into one, two, three or four part based on the number of fragments that are displaced. So, even if all of the four parts are fractured, if there is no displacement it is considered a one part fracture. Subsequently, if one part is displaced from others, it is a two part fracture. If, two parts are displaced, it is a three part fracture while a displacement of all the parts from each other is called a four part fracture. The classification was originally based on X-rays, but CT scan can also be used. Despite that, the classification has a very low inter and intra-observer reliability.

18.11.6 Management

18.11.7 Non-operative Management

Indications:

- Minimally displaced surgical and anatomic neck fractures.
- Greater tuberosity fracture displaced <5 mm.
- Elderly, low demand patients.

Minimally displaced proximal humerus fractures can be easily managed conservatively with a shoulder immobilizer or an arm sling and rest for 2–3 weeks. Passive exercises are started after this period while elbow, wrist and finger movements are encouraged throughout the rest period. Active exercises are started after 6 weeks once the fracture has united.

18.11.8 Operative Management

Indications:

- Displaced 2-part fracture.
- Greater tuberosity fracture displaced >5 mm.
- 3-,4-part fractures
- Head splitting fractures.
- Irreducible fracture dislocations.

There are multiple modalities available for operative management of proximal humerus fractures, which include:

- Closed reduction and percutaneous pinning.
- Open reduction and internal fixation with plate/screw.
- Intramedullary nailing.
- Arthroplasty—Hemiarthroplasty or reverse shoulder arthroplasty.

Each modality is indicated in a different scenario, which is also influenced by surgeon preference. Broad indications of each surgical modality have been enumerated in the Table 18.2 below.

Table 18.2 Indications for various surgical techniques for management of proximal humerus fracture

Technique	Indications
Closed reduction and percutaneous pinning	2-part surgical neck fractures 3-part and valgus-impacted 4-part fractures in patients with good bone quality, minimal metaphyseal comminution
ORIF with plating/ screw fixation	Greater tuberosity displaced >5 mm Displaced 2-part fractures 3-, and 4-part fractures in younger patients Head-splitting fractures in younger patients
Intramedullary nailing	Surgical neck fractures or 3-part greater tuberosity fractures in younger patients Combined proximal humerus and humeral shaft fractures
Hemiarthroplasty	Younger patients (40–65 years old) with complex fracture-dislocations that may fail fixation
Reverse shoulder arthroplasty (RSA)	low-demand elderly individuals with non-reconstructible tuberosities and poor bone stock

18.11.9 Complications

- Neurovascular injuries: Proper neurovascular examination both at the time of initial presentation and post-surgery is necessary. Axillary nerve is the most commonly injured nerve, both pre- and post-operatively.
- Avascular necrosis (AVN): The risk of avascular necrosis is around 10–30% in 3-part fractures and 10–50% in 4-part fractures. It is necessary to assess the risk for avascular necrosis, so that an early decision can be made if patient needs arthroplasty instead of fixation. Majority of the blood supply to humeral head comes from posterior circumflex humeral artery followed by anterior circumflex artery. Blood supply from both the sources can be disrupted in a severely displaced 3- or 4-part fracture and increases the risk of AVN.
- Malunion: Majority of conservatively managed fractures land up in some form of malunion. But, it leads to less problems to the patient and is usually well tolerated.
- Stiffness: Joint stiffness is essentially a dictum in upper limb fractures and shoulder is no different. It is more common in elderly population in which the limb has been immobilized for long. It can be prevented/reduced with early mobilization.

Multiple Choice Questions

1. A 31-year-old male sustains the injury shown in Fig. A. As compared to treatment with a simple sling, what is the primary advantage of treatment with a figure-of-eight brace?
   (a) Decreased sleep disturbance
   (b) Decreased rate of malunion
   (c) Improved long-term clinical outcomes
   (d) No advantage, equivalent results of both

2. A 20-year old male presents with history of road traffic accident with left shoulder pain and difficulty in moving. Radiographs of the patient are shown in the following figure. Which of the following techniques cannot be used for management of this patient?

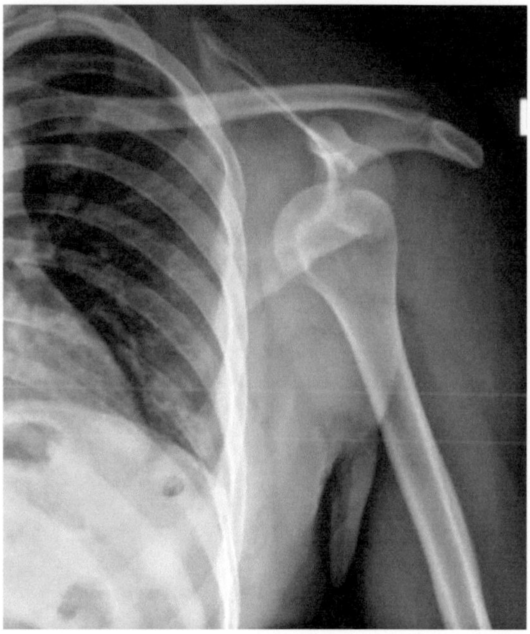

   (a) Stimson maneuver
   (b) Kocher maneuver
   (c) Hippocratic maneuver
   (d) Allis maneuver
3. Which of the following parts if not used for classification of proximal humerus fracture according to Neer's classification?
   (a) Head
   (b) Neck
   (c) Greater tuberosity
   (d) Shaft
4. Which of the following views are used for assessment of sternoclavicular (SC) joint and acromioclavicular (AC) joint respectively?
   (a) Serendipity view, Zanca view
   (b) Zanca view, Serendipity view
   (c) Grashey view, Stykernotch view
   (d) Strykernotch view, Grashey view
5. Which of the following is not an indication for operative management in proximal humerus fractures?
   (a) 3 part fracture
   (b) Fracture dislocation
   (c) Greater tuberosity fracture displaced >5 mm
   (d) Head split fractures

Answers: 1. (d), 2. (d), 3. (b), 4. (a), 5. (b)

References

1. Tornetta P III, Ricci WM, Ostrum RF, Mcqueen MM, McKee MD, Court-Brown CM. Rockwood and green's fractures in adults (9th edn). Philadelphia: Lippincott Williams & Wilkins (LWW); 2019.
2. Ropars M, Thomazeau H, Huten D. Clavicle fractures. Orthop Traumatol Surg Res. 2017;103(1S):S53–9.
3. Frank RM, Cotter EJ, Leroux TS, Romeo AA. Acromioclavicular joint injuries: evidence-based treatment. J Am Acad Orthop Surg. 2019;27(17):e775–88. https://doi.org/10.5435/JAAOS-D-17-00105.
4. Abrams R, Akbarnia H. Shoulder dislocations overview. [Updated 2022 Aug 8]. In: StatPearls [Internet]. Treasure Island (FL): StatPearls Publishing; 2023. Available from: https://www.ncbi.nlm.nih.gov/books/NBK459125/.
5. Pencle FJ, Varacallo M. Proximal humerus fracture. [Updated 2022 Sep 4]. In: StatPearls [Internet]. Treasure Island (FL): StatPearls Publishing; 2023. Available from: https://www.ncbi.nlm.nih.gov/books/NBK470346/.

19 Injuries of Arm

Kshitij Gupta

19.1 Shaft of Humerus Fracture

Shaft of humerus fractures constitute 3–5% of all adult fractures. It has a bimodal age distribution, caused by high energy trauma in young patients and low energy trauma in elderly osteoporotic bones. It is a diaphyseal fracture which can usually be managed conservatively with some impetus on maintaining alignment.

19.1.1 Anatomy

Humeral shaft is cylindrical in shape in the proximal part while the distal part is triangular in cross-section. Proximally, humeral head articulates with glenoid fossa of scapula to form the shoulder joint, while distal part articulates with forearm bones, radius, and ulna to form the elbow joint. Fracture displacement can be influenced by the muscle insertions. If fracture occurs proximal to deltoid insertion, it is adducted medially by the pectoralis major. While in fractures distal to deltoid insertion, the proximal fragment is abducted by deltoid muscle.

Humeral shaft is closely placed to radial nerve. Radial nerve courses posteriorly across the shaft in the spiral groove from medial side to lateral side. The nerve lies 14 cm proximally from the lateral epicondyle and 20 cm from the medial epicondyle.

19.1.2 Mechanism of Injury

The type of humeral fracture depends on the mechanism of injury resulting in different types of forces. A fall on outstretched hand results in twisting force and a resultant spiral fracture. While a fall on the elbow results in a bending force and causes an oblique or transverse fracture. A direct blow to the arm causes a comminuted or transverse fracture. Fractures in elderly might also be result of a pathological process such as metastasis or osteoporosis.

19.1.3 Clinical Features

Patient presents with pain history of/ trauma with pain in the affected arm. There might be visible deformity and bruising of the arm. There is tenderness and presence of abnormal mobility on palpation. It is necessary to do a radial nerve examination pre-reduction and post reduction given its close proximity to the bone. Any alteration in radial nerve function post reduction is an indication for surgery.

K. Gupta (✉)
Department of Orthopedics, All India Institute of Medical Sciences, Rishikesh, Uttarakhand, India

V. Kumar et al. (eds.), *A Quick Guide to Essential Orthopedics*,
https://doi.org/10.1007/978-981-95-2676-5_19

19.1.4 Imaging

Routine AP and lateral radiographs of humerus including the shoulder and elbow joints can show the fracture pattern. Radiographs can also aid in examining any pathological lesions (Fig. 19.1).

19.1.5 Classification

Fracture can be classified based on location into proximal, middle, and distal shaft. Type of fracture pattern like transverse, spiral, comminuted, etc. can also be used to define the fracture.

NOTE: Holstein-Lewis Fracture (Fig. 19.2) This fracture pattern is a simple spiral fracture of the distal third of humeral shaft with distal fragment displaced with its proximal end deviated radially. This fracture pattern is associated with higher incidence of radial nerve palsy (22% vs. 8%). Majority of these palsies are neuropraxias and require only expectant management. This fracture pattern is only a relative indication of operative fixation and decision lies solely on surgeon's discretion.

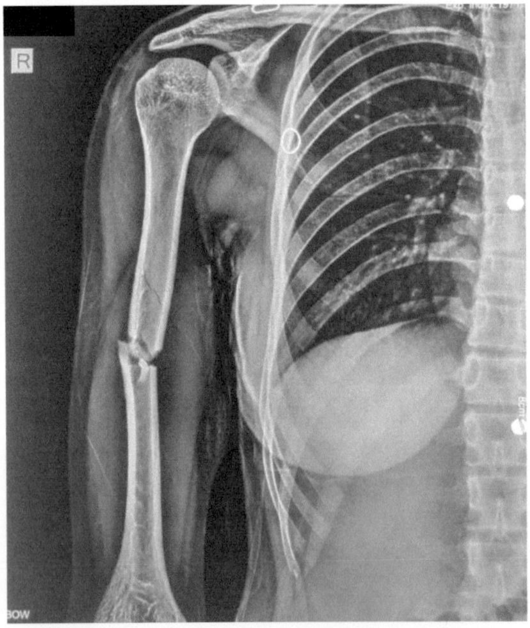

Fig. 19.1 Radiograph of shaft of humerus fracture

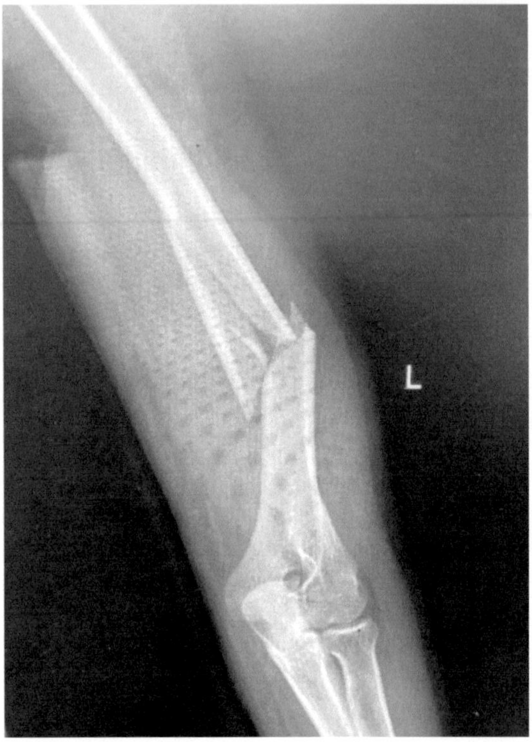

Fig. 19.2 Radiograph of Holstein Lewis fracture showing a radial side spike of distal fracture fragment

19.1.6 Management

19.1.6.1 Nonoperative Management

Most of the humeral shaft fractures can be managed conservatively using a U slab (Fig. 19.3), hanging cast, coaptation splint, functional brace, etc. Acceptable reduction is:

1. <20° anterior angulation
2. <30° varus/valgus angulation
3. <3 cm shortening.

The fracture is usually splinted after reduction in a U-slab in the acute stage. It is followed by a hanging cast after 3–5 days which uses gravity to keep the fracture fragments aligned. Once the fracture has become sticky after 3–4 weeks, patient can be given a functional cast or brace for further 6 weeks which immobilizes only the shaft and allows move-

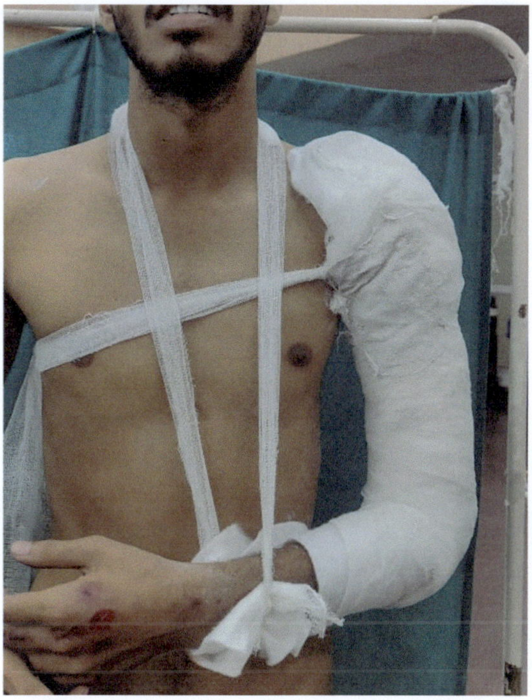

Fig. 19.3 U slab used for management of shaft of humerus fracture

ment of elbow and shoulder. Aim is to prevent stiffness of adjoining joints which is quite common in upper limb fractures. While a pre-reduction radial nerve palsy is not a contraindication for non-operative management, a post-reduction radial nerve deficit warrants a surgical exploration for the likely entrapped radial nerve.

19.1.6.2 Operative Management

Indications of operative management:

- Open fracture.
- Segmental fractures.
- Vascular injury requiring repair.
- Brachial plexus injury.
- Ipsilateral forearm fracture (floating elbow).
- Compartment syndrome.
- Radial nerve palsy after manipulation.
- Non-union.

Various options are available for operative management including plating, intramedullary fixation with elastic or interlocking nail or external fixator which is usually used for open fractures.

19.1.7 Complications

19.1.7.1 Early Complications

- Vascular injury—If there are signs of vascular insufficiency the affected limb, brachial artery damage must be suspected. It can be confirmed on an angiogram. This is an emergency and requires immediate repair. If brachial artery is being repaired, fracture fixation is also recommended.
- Radial nerve injury—As already mentioned, radial nerve lies in close proximity to humerus and hence it is important to look out for radial nerve palsy (wrist drop and finger drop) in shaft of humerus fractures (esp. Holstein Lewis fracture). Expectant management for 3 months is the usual policy for radial nerve palsy associated with humeral shaft fractures. If, nerve function does not return after 3 months, radial nerve exploration is warranted. Mostly a neurolysis is all that's needed but, nerve grafting can be done in case of discontinuity of nerve. If results are unsatisfactory, tendon transfers can be used to restore the lost functions. While a pre-reduction radial nerve palsy is not a contraindication for non-operative management, a post-reduction radial nerve deficit warrants a surgical exploration for the likely entrapped or transected radial nerve (Fig. 19.4).

19.1.7.2 Late Complications

- Joint stiffness—Joint stiffness is very common in majority upper limb fractures. It can be avoided by allowing early mobilization of adjoining joints whenever possible.
- Delayed union or non-union—Fractures which have been excessively distracted by a heavy hanging cast or which have been inadequately reduced in an operatively managed

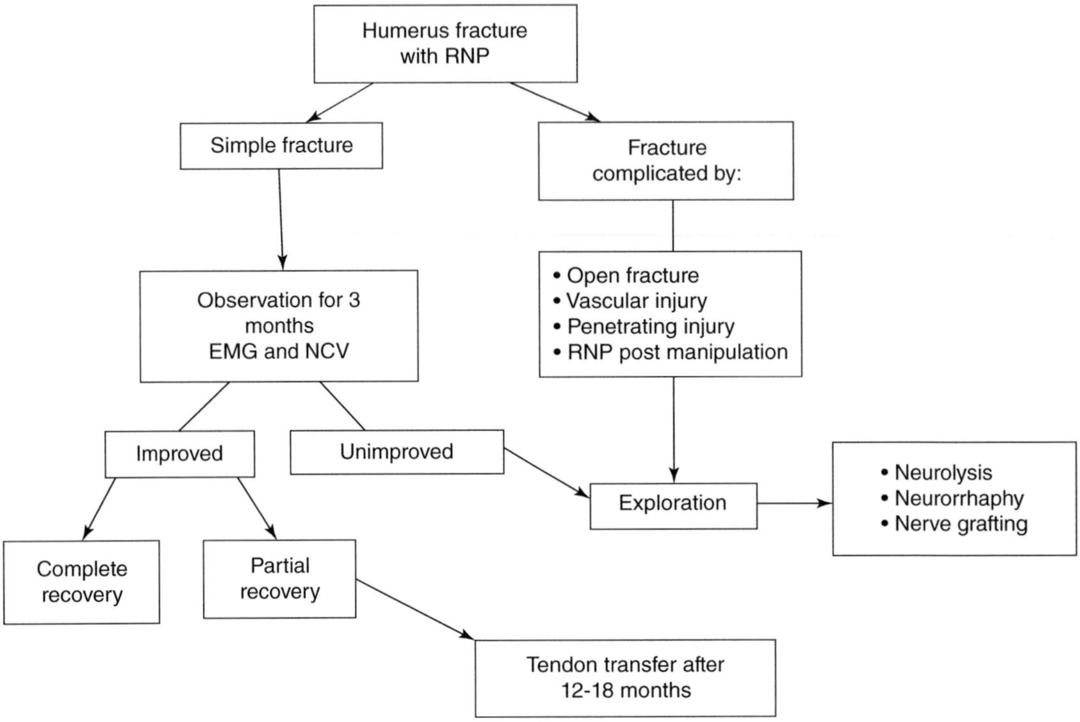

Fig. 19.4 Flowchart for management of radial nerve palsy (RNP) associated with humerus fracture

case tend to go into nonunion. As long as there are signs of callous formation, fracture can be expected to unite and requires minor tweaking in the technique. In cases of frank nonunion, operative management in terms of exchange nailing or plating with freshening of bone end and insertion of cancellous bone graft yields good results.

- Malunion—Conservatively managed fractures can malunite but rarely lead to any functional deficits with minimal cosmetic concerns. A malunited fracture not hampering the patient's functionality need not be operated.

19.2 Pediatric Humeral Shaft Fractures

It constitutes <10% of fractures in pediatric age groups. These are typically associated with trauma, but, a shaft humerus fracture in pediatric age group should raise a suspicion of child abuse and the child should be properly examined for additional injuries. Upto 5% of these fractures are associated with radial nerve palsy. Almost all of these fractures can be managed conservatively by a sling, cuff, coaptation splint or hanging arm cast owing to the high remodeling capacity of pediatric age group. Range of motion exercises can be initiated in 2–3 weeks once pain subsides. There are very few indications for operative management like open fractures, multiply injured patient, floating elbow, etc. It is usually undertaken by flexible intramedullary nail fixation.

19.3 Multiple Choice Questions

1. A 19-year-old girl presents with the fracture shown in the following fracture. Which of the following will be a contraindication to conservative management with cast application?

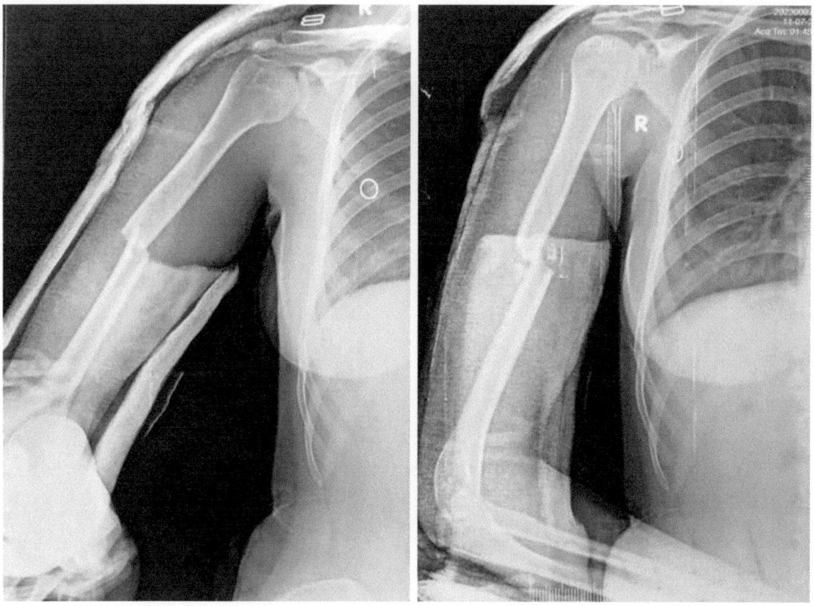

   (a) Radial nerve palsy
   (b) 1 cm shortening
   (c) 20° varus deformity
   (d) Brachial plexus injury
2. Radial nerve is closely related to humerus at what location?
   (a) Anatomical neck
   (b) Surgical neck
   (c) Radial groove
   (d) Medial epicondyle
3. A 35-year-old patient presents with the radiograph shown in Q1. Patient is able to extend the elbow but is unable to extend his wrist and fingers. Which of the following palsies has the patient developed?
   (a) Very high radial nerve palsy
   (b) High radial nerve palsy
   (c) Low radial nerve palsy
   (d) Ulnar nerve palsy
4. How will you manage radial nerve palsy in this patient?
   (a) Neurolysis
   (b) Neurorrhapy
   (c) Observation for 3 months
   (d) Tendon transfer
5. U slab is used for the management of which fracture?
   (a) Proximal humerus fracture
   (b) Shaft of humerus fracture
   (c) Distal humerus fracture
   (d) Forearm fracture

Answers: 1. (d), 2. (c), 3. (b), 4. (c), 5. (b)

References

1. Tornetta P III, Ricci WM, Ostrum RF, Mcqueen MM, McKee MD, Court-Brown CM. Rockwood and Green's fractures in adults (9th edition). Philadelphia: Lippincott Williams & Wilkins (LWW); 2019.
2. Bounds EJ, Frane N, Jajou L, et al. Humeral shaft fractures. [Updated 2023 Mar 1]. In: StatPearls [Internet]. Treasure Island (FL): StatPearls Publishing; 2023. Available from: https://www.ncbi.nlm.nih.gov/books/NBK448074/.
3. Rocchi M, Tarallo L, Mugnai R, Adani R. Humerus shaft fracture complicated by radial nerve palsy: is surgical exploration necessary? Musculoskelet Surg. 2016;100(Suppl 1):53–60. https://doi.org/10.1007/s12306-016-0414-3.
4. Nowak LL, Dehghan N, McKee MD, Schemitsch EH. Plate fixation for management of humerus fractures. Injury. 2018;49(Suppl 1):S33–8. https://doi.org/10.1016/S0020-1383(18)30300-0.

20 Injuries Around Elbow

Syed Ifthekar

20.1 Introduction

Elbow injuries need immediate attention and appropriate treatment to avoid complications. A basic understanding of the anatomy and radiology of the elbow is vital for optimal management of elbow injuries.

20.2 Anatomical Considerations

The elbow is a hinge joint that has three individual joints held together in a common synovial cavity (Fig. 20.1). The joints are formed by articulation of distal humerus with ulna (Ulno-humeral joint), distal humerus with radius (Humero-radial joint), and articulation between radius and ulna (radio-ulnar joints). The distal humerus is expanded Medio-laterally to form a medial trochlea and a lateral capitellum. The most prominent parts of the medial and lateral supracondylar ridges are termed medial and lateral epicondyles.

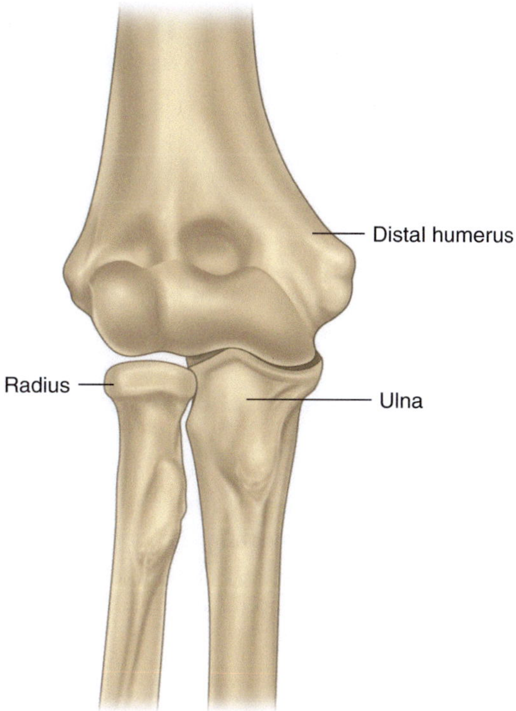

Fig. 20.1 Elbow joint showing articulation of distal humerus with ulna (Ulno-humeral joint), distal humerus with radius (Humero-radial joint), and articulation between radius and ulna (radio-ulnar joints)

S. Ifthekar (✉)
Department of Orthopedics, All India Institute of Medical Sciences, Bibinagar, Telangana, India

V. Kumar et al. (eds.), *A Quick Guide to Essential Orthopedics*,
https://doi.org/10.1007/978-981-95-2676-5_20

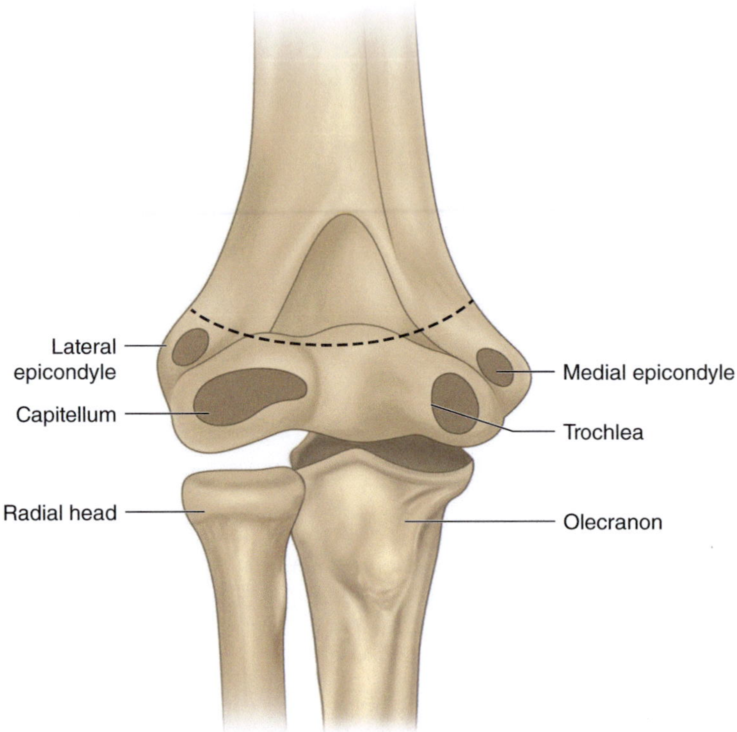

Fig. 20.2 The age of ossification for the various anatomical structures around elbow

20.2.1 Ossification of the Elbow

Having a knowledge of ossification of the elbow is important to diagnose the fractures around the elbow in pediatric population. The girls have an earlier ossification than boys. The age of ossification for the various anatomical structures around elbow are as below (Fig. 20.2).

20.3 Supracondylar Fractures of the Distal Humerus

These are one of the most common injuries seen in pediatric population. These fractures when not treated adequately result in mal-union and result in a typical "Gun-stock deformity".

20.4 Mechanism of Injury and Anatomy

These fractures usually occur as a result of fall on an outstretched hand. Based on the direction of displacement of the distal fragment, these are broadly divided into extension type and flexion type of fractures (Fig. 20.3). The extension type of supracondylar fracture is most common (97–99%) and is described in detail in this section.

When the child falls on an outstretched hand with elbow in hyperextension, the olecranon articulates with olecranon fossa and acts as a fulcrum to transmit an extension force across the distal humerus. The anterior capsule of the elbow joint is thick. These capsule fibers become tense

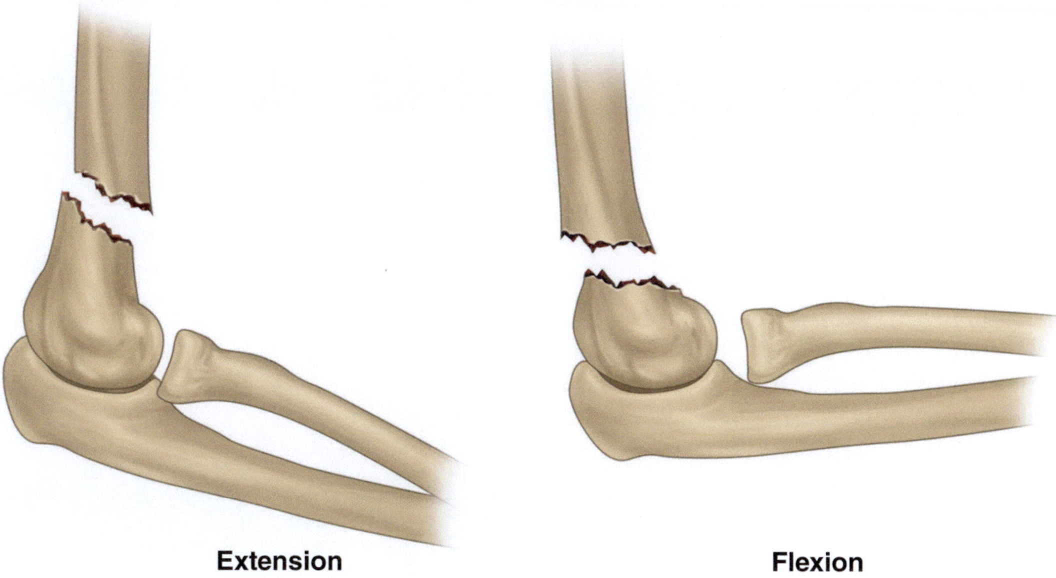

Fig. 20.3 Extension type and flexion type of supracondylar fractures

with hyper-extension of elbow and propagate a firm force between ulna and distal humerus. The fulcrum of rotation is then transmitted to the tip of olecranon in the supracondylar area, resulting in a supracondylar fracture.

The anterior periosteum is usually torn in the extension type supracondylar fractures. But the posterior periosteum may be intact which provides vital periosteal hinge to reduce and stabilize the fracture.

The common displacements of the distal fragment in a supracondylar fracture are:

(i) Posterior tilt
(ii) Posterior shift
(iii) Apposition or proximal shift
(iv) Medial shift
(v) Medial tilt
(vi) Internal rotation

Based on the medial or lateral displacements of the distal fragment, the extension type supracondylar fractures are classified as posteromedial and posterolateral type of supracondylar fractures. The Posteromedial supracondylar fractures are more common than the posterolateral type of supracondylar fractures. The displacement and nomenclature are important because they determine the vital structures at risk following the fractures. The posteromedial type of fracture has an increased risk for the radial nerve injury, and posterolateral type of fractures has an increased risk for median nerve injury and brachial artery.

Further based on the degree of displacements of the distal fragment, the supracondylar fracture is classified into four different types. The most common classification system in use is modified Gartland classification.

Type I	Undisplaced	Swollen fat pad
Type II	Hinged posteriorly	Anterior humeral line Anterior to capitellum
Type III	Displaced	Loss of complete cortical continuity
Type IV	Displaces into extension and flexion	Diagnosed with manipulation under C-arm.

20.5 Clinical Features

20.5.1 History

A child is usually brought to hospital with complaints of fall during play and inability to use his upper limb following fall. There may be com-

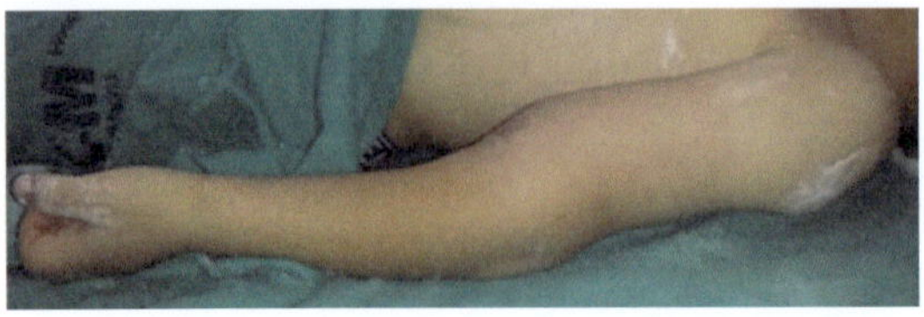

Fig. 20.4 S shaped deformity of the involve limb following supracondylar fracture of left elbow

plaints of severe swelling around the elbow joint and inability to move fingers or loss of sensations in the forearm or hand. An attempt should be made to identify blebs or color changes of the upper limb if the presentation is late to diagnose compartment syndrome.

20.5.2 Clinical Examination

A child with supracondylar fracture may typically present with an S shaped deformity of the involved limb (Fig. 20.4). The elbow will be grossly swollen, and the movements are painful. Examination of the elbow may be restricted due to tenderness. There may be puckering of the skin on the anterior aspect of the elbow due to penetration of the proximal bony fragment through brachialis and fascia. A complete neural and vascular examination should be done to diagnose the vascular or nerve injuries. Vascular status may be confirmed by examining the pulse, local warmth of fingers or a pulse oximeter may be used to objectively diagnose vascular compromise.

20.6 Investigations

Good quality anteroposterior and lateral view X-rays of the involved elbow should be done to diagnose supracondylar fractures of humerus (Fig. 20.5).

In very young children or in rare cases, comparative X-rays of the normal limb may be required for the diagnosis-rays should be examined with a high index of suspicion if no obvious fracture is seen. A posterior fat pad sign may be the only positive finding in few patients.

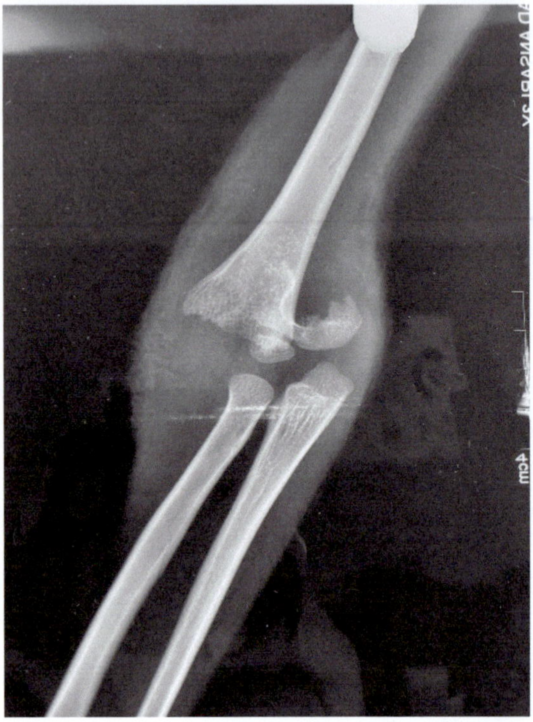

Fig. 20.5 X-rays of the elbow showing supracondylar fracture

A normal elbow of the child should have the anterior humeral line crossing the capitellum through the middle third on a true lateral x-ray of the elbow. If the anterior humeral line crosses anterior to the capitellum, then there is an extension type of supracondylar fracture.

20.7 Differential Diagnosis

Nursemaid's elbow/Pulled elbow
Epiphyseal separation
Posterior dislocation of elbow
Fracture Lateral condyle of Humerus
Fracture Medial condyle of Humerus

20.7.1 Treatment

Casting in-situ This treatment method is good for Type 1 fractures. This cannot be used for displaced fractures.

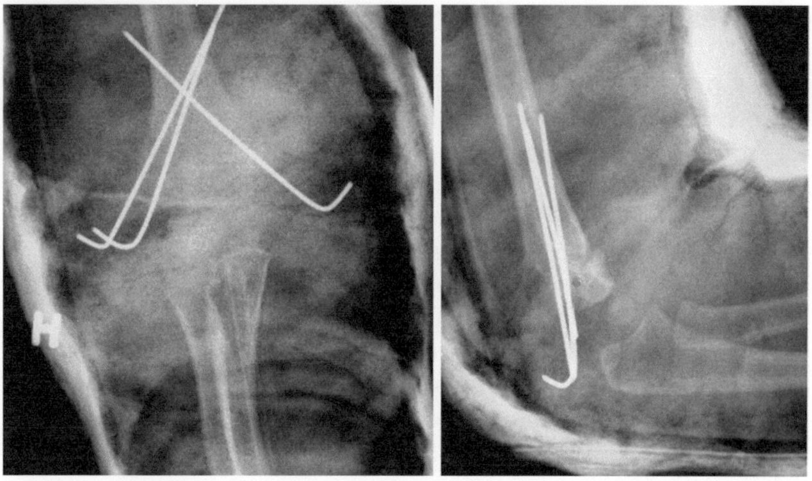

Fig. 20.6 Satisfactory reduction in both AP and lateral views

20.7.1.1 Closed Reduction and Casting

This treatment can be used for partially displaced fractures with intact periosteal hinge. The elbow is reduced in flexion. There may be a risk of compartment syndrome due to excessive flexion. Pulse should be palpated while flexing the elbow and the flexion should be reduced if the pulse is not palpable. If the pulse is palpable in full flexion of the elbow, then the elbow should be immobilized in full flexion.

20.7.1.2 Closed Reduction and Percutaneous Pinning

This technique can be used in grossly displaced fractures. This technique has a good and predict able outcome.

20.7.1.3 Open Reduction and Pinning

This is rarely required. The indications for open reduction are:

A. Associated vascular or neural injuries
B. Type 3 or Type 4 fractures which are irreducible by closed methods
C. After fasciotomy in fractures with compartment syndrome

and this technique is mostly used when there are associated vascular or neural injuries.

20.7.1.4 Technique of Closed Reduction and Percutaneous K-wire Fixation

This procedure can be done under general anesthesia or adequate sedation. This technique requires expertise to achieve a good reduction in minimal time. Traction counter-traction method is used to dislodge the fractured fragments. Correction in medio-lateral plane or rotation should be done. This is followed by gradual reduction of the distal fragment by putting a pressure over the tip of olecranon and simultaneously flexing the elbow. The radial pulse should be felt at each stage of reduction and flexion should be reduced as soon as radial pulse disappears or becomes feeble. The reduction at each step should be monitored under c-arm to check for the acceptability. The reduction should be deemed satisfactory only if it is acceptable in both AP and lateral views (Fig. 20.6). A tear drop view on lateral view and restoration of Baumann's angle on AP view suggest acceptable reduction.

20.8 Complications

The complications of supracondylar fractures can be divided into

1. Early complications
2. Late complications

20.8.1 Early Complications

20.8.1.1 Vascular Injury

Brachial artery may be injured by the sharp bony edge of the proximal fragment. There is good collateral network of vessels around the elbow and the perfusion may be maintained by these collaterals even after injury to brachial artery. The arterial occlusion may also be due to the pressure on the brachial artery by the displaced fragment and mere reduction may allow reperfusion of the limb. So, time shouldn't be wasted in investigating studies like angiograms and priority should be given to reduction of the fracture.

20.8.1.2 Injury to Nerves

The radial nerve, median nerve especially the anterior interosseous branch of median nerve and ulnar nerve may be involved in the supracondylar fracture. Formal tests should be done for each nerve following the injury. Spontaneous recovery occurs in majority of the cases once the fracture is reduced and treated. If the nerve injury occurs after reduction of the fracture, it is mainly due to the entrapment during reduction and the fracture should be explored to release entrapment.

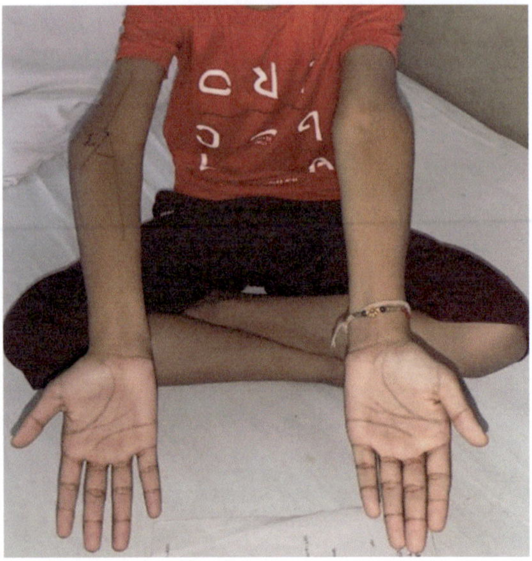

Fig. 20.7 Mal-union of a supracondylar fracture Humerus with a gunstock deformity

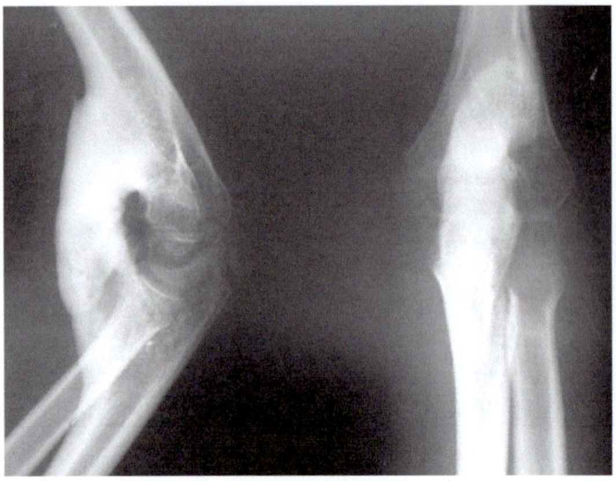

Fig. 20.8 X ray showing Myositis ossificans around elbow

20.8.2 Late Complications

20.8.2.1 Mal-union

Since the fracture involves the metaphyseal area, non-union is very rare and most of the untreated fractures end up in mal-union. The most common deformity seen as a result of mal-union is cubitus varus deformity (Gun-stock deformity) (Fig. 20.7). The deformity does not lead to functional disability. The main concern of the mal-union is cosmetic deformity. This can be addressed by osteotomy (French/step-cut/modified French) y. There may be tardy ulnar nerve palsy in long standing cubitus varus deformity and the treatment should be focused towards treating nerve injury and rehabilitation.

20.8.2.2 Myositis Ossificans

When aggressive massaging is done after injury, ectopic new bone may be formed around the elbow. This new bone is called myositis ossificans (Fig. 20.8). This may also lead to stiffness of the elbow.

20.8.2.3 Volkmann's Ischemic Contracture

This is a serious long-term complication if compartment syndrome is not diagnosed and treated early in the course of treatment. Due to compartment syndrome, there is a compromise in the blood supply to the muscles and nerves, espe-

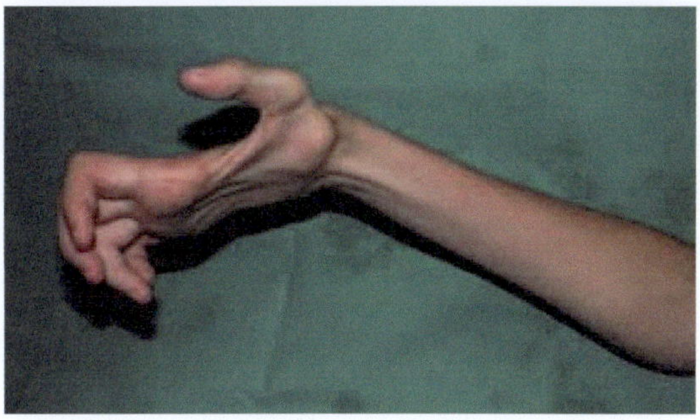

Fig. 20.9 Typical deformity of the hand in Volkmann's Ischemic contracture (VIC)

cially to the deep flexor compartment of the forearm. The most commonly affected muscle is flexor digitorum profundus. The muscle tissue is converted into fibrotic tissue and a typical deformity of the hand ensues as the disease progresses (Fig. 20.9).

20.8.2.4 Volkmann's Sign

The ability to passively extend fingers when the wrist is flexed which is not possible if the wrist is extended is known as Volkmann's sign. This occurs due to fixed length phenomenon.

20.9 Flexion-Type Supracondylar Fractures

Flexion-type supracondylar humeral fractures are very rare and account only for about 2% of humeral fractures. It may be difficult to identify the flexion pattern until reduction is attempted because initial radiographs are inadequate. A key to recognizing a flexion-type supracondylar fracture is that it is unstable in flexion, whereas extension-type fractures generally are stable in hyperflexion. A laterally displaced supracondylar fracture may actually be a flexion-type injury.

The clinical signs and investigations are similar to that of the extension type fractures. Treatment includes casting with elbow in extension or if pinning is required then the elbow can be immobilized in flexion.

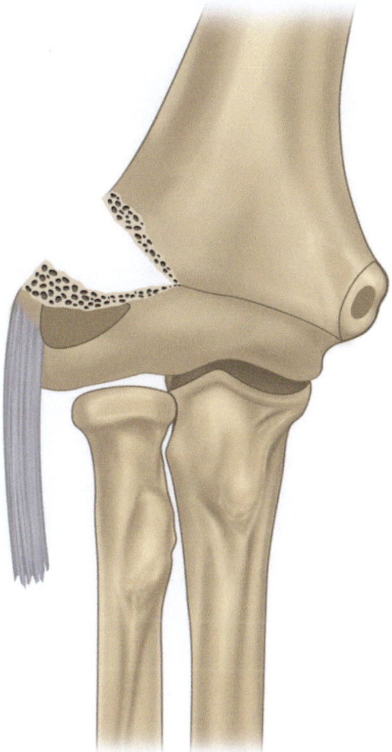

Fig. 20.10 Pull-off mechanism leading to lateral condyle fracture of humerus

20.10 Fractures of the Lateral Condyle

20.10.1 Mechanism of Injury

The fractures of lateral condyle also occur in pediatric population who fall on an outstretched hand. When the child falls on an extended elbow and when the elbow is forced into varus, lateral condyle is avulsed by the extensors of the wrist. This mechanism is known as pull-off mechanism (Fig. 20.10). Sometimes there may be direct compression of the lateral condyle rather than the avulsion pattern. This mechanism is known as push-off mechanism. The fracture line runs along the physis and extends into the trochlea. Rarely the fracture line may continue through the medial epiphysis and exits through the capitello-trochlear groove. When the injury is severe there may be associated dislocations of the elbow. The exten-

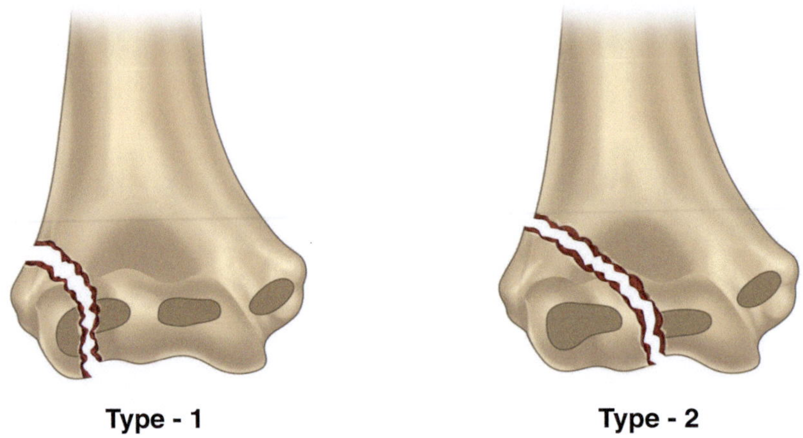

Fig. 20.11 Milch classification of Lateral Condyle fractures

sor carpi radialis longus and brevis muscles remain attached to the free distal fragment, along with the lateral collateral ligaments of the elbow.

Displacement is common and occurs due to the 'pull' of the common extensor muscles which take origin from the lateral epicondyle. The fragment is rotated outwards along its vertical and horizontal axis sometimes even as much as 90°.

20.10.2 Classification

Milch classified these fractures into two types (Fig. 20.11)

20.10.2.1 Type 1

The fracture running through the lateral condyle into the capitello trochlear groove. These are uncommon injuries but have a large potential to cause growth disturbances. These are classified according to salter Harris classification as Type 4 injuries.

20.10.2.2 Type 2

The fracture running through the trochlea. This type of fracture is common. These injuries are classified according to salter Harris classification as Type 4 injuries.

20.11 Clinical Features

20.11.1 History

A child is usually brought to hospital with complaints of fall during play and inability to use his upper limb following fall. There may be complains of swelling of elbow.

20.11.2 Clinical Examination

Compared with the marked distortion of the elbow that occurs with displaced supracondylar fractures, little distortion of the elbow, other than that produced by the fracture hematoma, may be present with lateral condylar fractures. The key to the clinical evaluation of this fracture is the location of soft tissue swelling concentrated over the lateral aspect of the distal humerus. The movements are painful. Passive flexion of the wrist may elicit tenderness due to the pull of extensors.

20.11.3 Investigations

X rays of the involved elbow in AP and Lateral views (Fig. 20.12) are needed to diagnose frac-

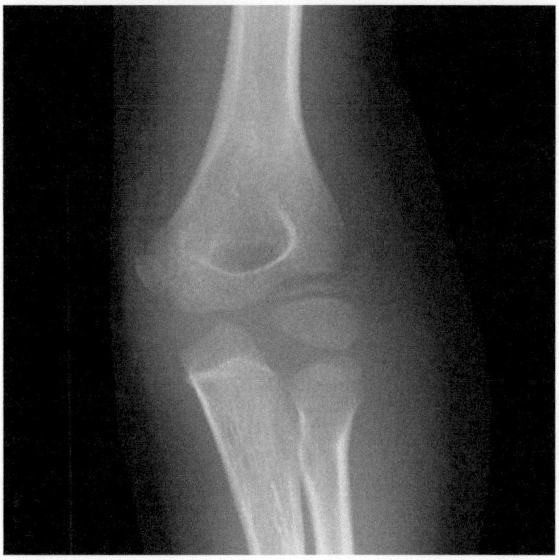

Fig. 20.12 X ray showing lateral condyle fracture of humerus

ture lateral condyle. The x rays may not be able to diagnose the fracture and few modified views may be necessary.

An internal oblique view helps in better diagnosis of the fracture and also in quantifying the displacement of the fracture. A major diagnostic difficulty lies in differentiating this fracture from a fracture of the entire distal humeral physis. In a young child in whom the condyle is unossified, an arthrogram or MRI may be helpful. The condylar epiphysis is mostly cartilaginous, so the bony fragment may look very small on an x-ray. In addition, any displacement of the proximal radius and ulna is more likely to be lateral due to the loss of stability provided by the lateral crista of the distal humerus.

20.11.4 Treatment

20.11.4.1 Un-displaced Fractures

Forty percent (40%) of lateral condylar physeal fractures are sufficiently undisplaced so that they can be treated by simple immobilization without surgical intervention. Undisplaced fractures can be immobilized in a posterior slab with the elbow flexed 90°, the forearm in neutral position and the wrist extended (this position relaxes the extensor mechanism which attaches to the fragment). The x-rays should be repeated after 5 days to make sure that the fracture has not displaced. If displaced, open reduction and fixation is the treatment of choice.

20.11.5 Closed Reduction and Percutaneous K-wire

Minimally displaced fractures (2–4 mm) with a congruent articular surface which are stable and have considerable intrinsic soft tissue attachments that prevent displacement of the distal fragment can be treated with closed reduction and percutaneous k-wires. Reduction is best achieved with the forearm supinated and the elbow extended. Placing a varus stress on the extended elbow allows further room for manipulation of the fragment.

20.11.6 Open Reduction

Open reduction of Lateral condyle fractures is done when the reduction is not acceptable. Since these fractures are intra-articular fractures, anatomical reduction and fixation is required for the optimal outcome. If there is any loss of reduction during conservative or closed reduction, open reduction should be employed.

20.11.7 Complications

1. Non-union: If unreduced, the fracture goes into non-union (Fig. 20.13). The causes are wide displacement of the fragment or a constant ‘pulling.
2. Cubitus valgus deformity: Diminished growth at the lateral side of distal humerus epiphysis results in a cubitus valgus deformity. This may result in tardy ulnar nerve palsy because of friction neuritis of the ulnar nerve as it moves over the medial epicondyle, every time the elbow is flexed and extended.

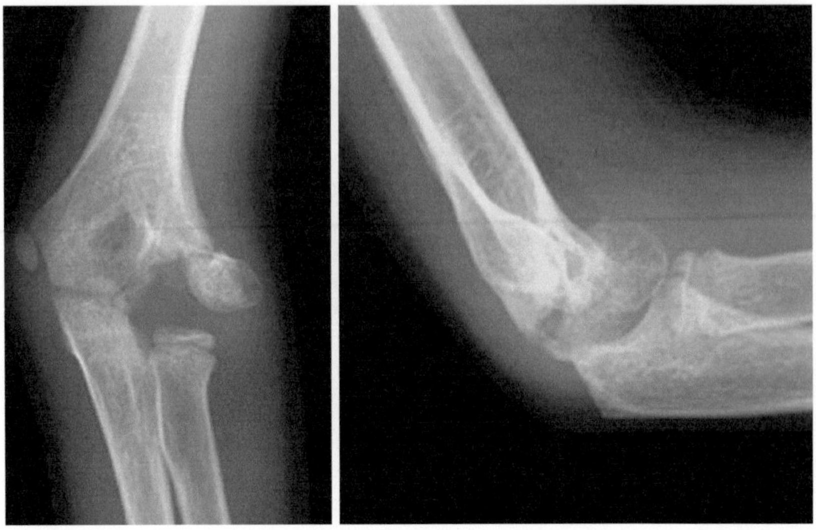

Fig. 20.13 X ray showing non-union of lateral condyle fracture Humerus

3. Cubitus varus: Lateral condylar fractures may heal with some residual cubitus varus angulation.
4. Recurrent dislocation: Occasionally recurrent posterolateral dislocation of the elbow may follow fracture lateral condyle.

20.12 Fracture of the Medial Condyle

This is rare when compared to lateral condylar fractures.

20.12.1 Mechanism of Injury

The injury is caused by a fall on an outstretched hand with the elbow forced into valgus. There would be an avulsion mechanism in this case. This may also occur due to direct blow to the point of the elbow. The fracture fragment may be displaced by the pull of the flexor muscle group.

20.12.2 Clinical Features

This is an intra-articular fracture. There may be considerable pain and swelling. The examination may be restricted due to pain. The tenderness may be localized on the medial aspect of the elbow.

20.12.3 Investigations

X rays of elbow in AP and Lateral view should form the standard diagnostic panel of examination. In older children the metaphyseal component is easily visualized on x-ray. In young children medial condylar epiphysis is cartilaginous and therefore not visible on x-ray.

20.12.4 Treatment

Un-displaced fractures are treated by Cast.

Displaced fractures are treated by either closed reduction (sometimes with percutaneous pinning) or by open reduction and fixation with pins.

Postoperative management is similar to that of lateral condyle fractures.

20.13 Separation of the Medial Epicondyle

20.13.1 Mechanism of Injury and Pathology

The medial epicondyle begins to ossify at the age of about 5 years and fuses to the shaft at about 16 years of age; a severe muscle or ligament strain may lead to avulsion between these ages (Fig. 20.14). A fall on the outstretched hand with

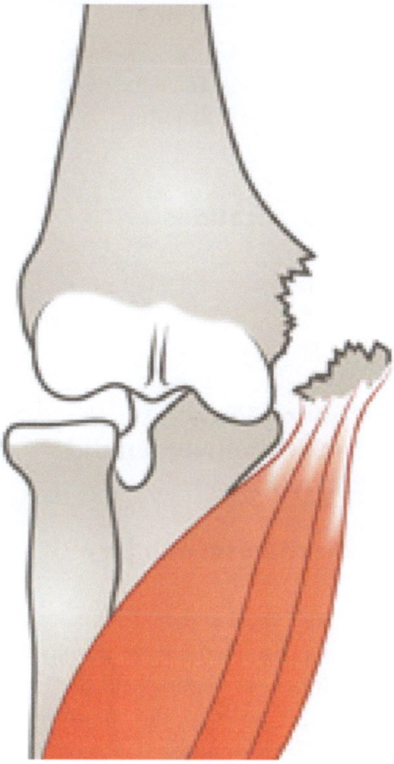

Fig. 20.14 Avulsion mechanism of medial epicondyle

the wrist and elbow extended and the elbow in valgus leads to separation of epicondyle. The unfused epicondylar apophysis is avulsed by tension on either the wrist flexor muscles or the medial ligament of the elbow. If the elbow subluxates (even momentarily), the small apophyseal fragment may be dragged into the joint. With more severe injuries the joint dislocates laterally.

20.13.2 Clinical Features

Pain, swelling and bruising on the medial side of the elbow following a fall. Deformity is obvious If the joint is dislocated. Ulnar nerve should be examined.

20.13.3 Investigations

X-ray in the anteroposterior view and lateral view should help in the diagnosis of medial epicondylar separation. The medial epicondylar epiphysis may be tilted or shifted downwards. The dislocation if present is obvious. The epicondyle may look like a loose body in the joint. If in any doubt, the normal side should be x-rayed for comparison.

20.13.4 Treatment

Minor displacement may be treated conservatively.

If the epicondyle is trapped in the joint (incarcerated fragment) it must be freed. Manipulation with the elbow in valgus and the wrist hyperextended may be successful. The joint must be opened if the maneuver fails.

Reduction and K-wire: If there is valgus instability (because of the attachment of the medial collateral ligament complex). A direct medial approach to the fracture site is used and an incision is given anterior to the medial epicondyle. The periosteum is cleared from the fracture site and the fracture reduced with the elbow in flexion and pronation. Then, the reduction is stabilized by either k-wires or screws depending on the size of the fragment.

20.13.5 Complications

Ulnar nerve damage is not uncommon. But it may recover spontaneously.

20.14 Fracture of Neck of the Radius

This is caused by a valgus injury of the elbow. It occurs commonly in children.

20.14.1 Clinical Features

There may be pain in the elbow following fall. Localized tenderness over the radial head and pain on rotating the forearm may be the findings on examination.

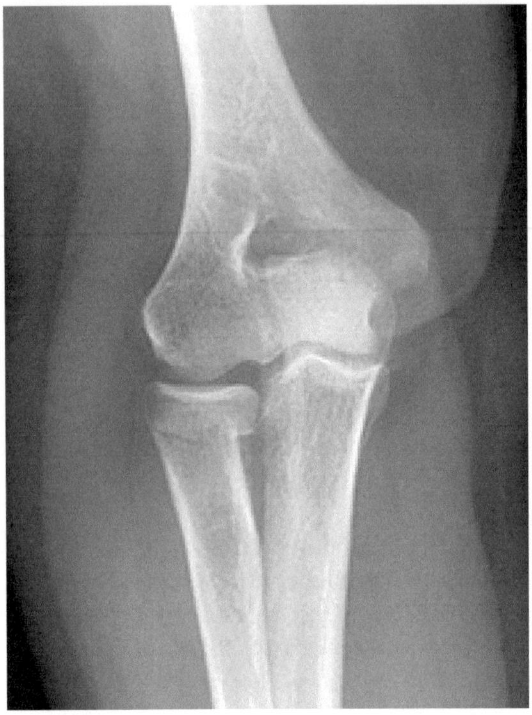

Fig. 20.15 X ray showing fracture of radial head

20.14.2 Investigations

X rays of the Elbow in AP and lateral view show mild displacements usually (Fig. 20.15). The proximal fragment is tilted distally, forwards and outwards. Sometimes the upper end of the ulna is also fractured or there may be a posterior dislocation of the elbow.

20.14.3 Treatment

20.14.3.1 Cast Immobilization

Undisplaced or minimally displaced fracture can be treated in an above-elbow plaster slab for 2–3 weeks. 30 Degrees of angulation and 3 mm of transverse displacement is acceptable.

20.14.3.2 Closed Reduction

30–60 degrees of angulation may require closed manipulation.

20.14.3.3 Open Reduction

Preformed occasionally in severe cases of angulation or displacement (usually more than 60°), fixation with K-wire is required.

20.14.4 Complications

Cubitus valgus deformity may occur in a malunited fracture.

20.15 Pulled Elbow Syndrome(Nursemaid's Elbow)

20.15.1 Mechanism of Injury

Usual mechanism of injury is the longitudinal traction on the extended elbow. Displacement of the annular ligament occurs with the forearm in pronation. In this position, the lateral edge of the radial head, which opposes the main portion of the annular ligament, is narrow and round at its margin. In supination, the lateral edge of the radial head is wider and more square at its margin, thereby restricting slippage of the annular ligament. Presumably, the annular ligament displaces proximally, partially over the radial head in this condition. After 5 years of age, the distal attachments of the sub-annular membrane and annular ligament to the neck of the radius have strengthened sufficiently to prevent its tearing and subsequent displacement.

Thus, the most widely accepted mechanism is that the injury occurs when the forearm is pronated, the elbow extended, and longitudinal traction is applied to the patient's wrist or hand.

20.15.2 Signs and Symptoms

The history is that of an episode of a longitudinal pull on the elbow of the young child. The initial pain usually subsides rapidly, and the child does not appear to be in distress except that he or she is reluctant to use the involved extremity. The upper extremity is typically held at the side with the forearm pronated. Any attempt to supinate the forearm produces pain. Local tenderness may be present over the radial head and annular ligament.

20.15.3 Imaging

X-rays—Anteroposterior and lateral x-rays usually are normal.

Ultrasonography may be helpful.

20.15.4 Treatment

Closed Reduction—By forceful supination and flexion of the involved elbow.

20.16 Injuries Around the Elbow in Adults

20.16.1 Fractures of Distal Humerus

The fractures occurring in adults around the distal humerus are often high-energy injuries which are associated with vascular and nerve damage. These fractures tend to be associated with stiffness of the elbow. The restoration of anatomical congruity and early mobilization to prevent stiffness should be of paramount importance in these patients.

The AO-ASIF Group have defined three types of distal humeral fracture (Fig. 20.16).

Type A—an extra-articular supracondylar fracture.

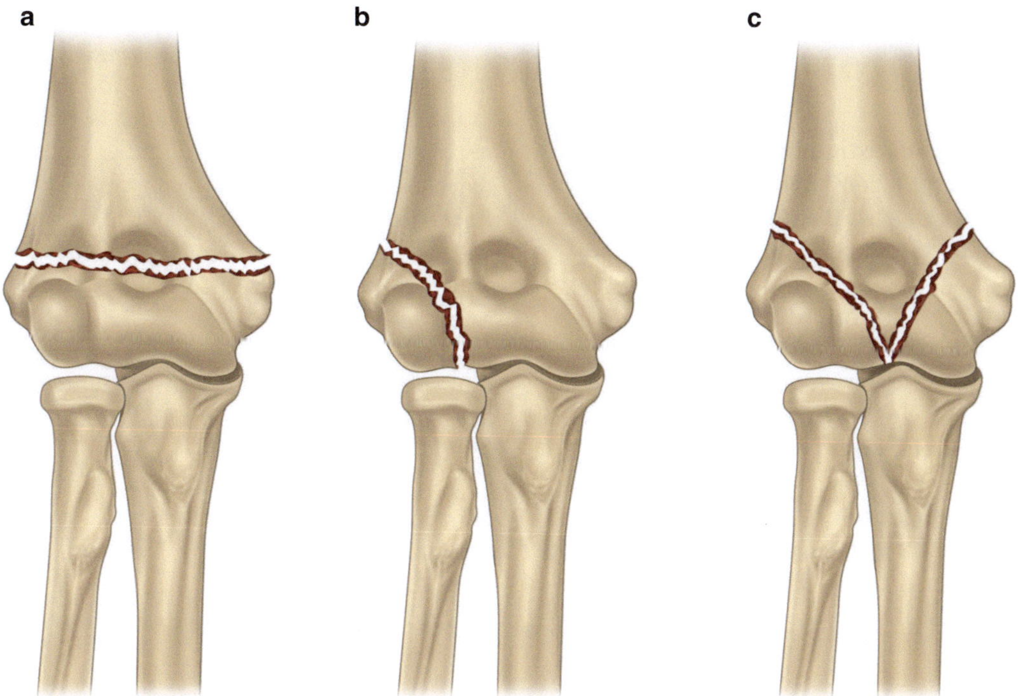

Fig. 20.16 AO-ASIF classification of fractures of distal humeral fracture

Type B—an intra-articular unicondylar fracture (one condyle sheared off).

Type C—bicondylar (Intercondylar) fractures with varying degrees of comminution.

20.16.2 Type A—Supracondylar Fractures

These are rare extra-articular fractures in adults. As there is no tough periosteum to tether the fragments, they are usually displaced and unstable. In high-energy injuries there may be comminution of the distal humerus.

20.16.2.1 Clinical Examination

The patient presents with high energy injury to the elbow and inability to use the upper limb following injury. On examination there may be swelling and severe tenderness over the injured elbow. Crepitus may be felt accidentally while examining the elbow. The distal neurovascular status needs to be examined as there may be neurovascular deficits.

20.16.2.2 Investigations

X rays of the elbow joint in AP and lateral views would be enough to diagnose most of the times. In case of uncertainty CT scans help in diagnosis.

20.16.2.3 Treatment

Closed Reduction

It is unlikely to be stable and K-wire fixation is not strong enough to permit early mobilization.

Open Reduction and Internal Fixation

This is the treatment of choice. The articular congruity should be restored and fracture secured with plates and screws.

20.16.3 Types B and C—Intra-articular Fractures

These are also called as intercondylar fractures. These are usually high energy injuries with severe soft tissue damage.

20.16.3.1 Mechanism of Injury

A severe blow on the point of the elbow drives the olecranon process upwards, splitting the condyles apart.

20.16.3.2 Clinical Examination

The patient presents with high energy injury to the elbow and inability to use the upper limb following injury. On examination there may be severe swelling and tenderness over the injured elbow. Crepitus may be felt accidentally while examining the elbow. The distal neurovascular status needs to be examined as there may be neurovascular deficits.

20.16.3.3 Investigations

X rays of the elbow joint in AP and Lateral views would be helpful to diagnose these fractures. CT scans can be helpful in diagnosing and planning the fixation for the fracture.

20.16.3.4 Treatment

Most of the times, Open reduction and internal fixation is the treatment of choice for these fractures. Good exposure of the joint is needed, if necessary, by performing an intra-articular olecranon osteotomy. The ulnar nerve should be identified and protected throughout. The articular congruity should be restored and fracture secured with two plates on two columns with locking screws.

Post-operatively, elbow is held at 90° with the arm supported in a sling. Movement is encouraged but should never be forced. Fracture healing usually occurs by 12 weeks.

20.16.3.5 Complications

Vascular injury
Nerve injury
Elbow stiffness
Heterotopic Ossification

20.16.4 Fracture Capitellum

20.16.4.1 Mechanism of Injury

This is an uncommon fracture, seen in adults. The patient falls on the hand, usually with the elbow straight. The anterior part of the capitellum is sheared off and displaced proximally. The chipped off capitellum may get displaced into the joint.

20.16.4.2 Clinical Features

The patient gives history of fullness in front of the elbow. Difficulty in using the arm is another symptom but the disability is not severe. The lateral side of the elbow is tender and flexion is grossly restricted.

20.16.4.3 Investigations

X-rays of the elbow in AP and lateral view should be taken (Fig. 20.17). The lateral view may show the fractured part in front of the lower humerus. Due to overlap of bones, the fracture fragment may go unnoticed on X-rays. CT scans can be helpful in clarifying the diagnosis.

20.16.4.4 Treatment

Conservative Un-displaced fractures can be treated by simple splintage.

Operative Treatment

If the fragment is small or comminuted, excision is carried out. If it is a big fragment, open reduction and internal fixation should be performed. Headless bone screws are ideally passed from front to back; alternatively, if the fragment is large enough, lag screws can be passed from back to front.

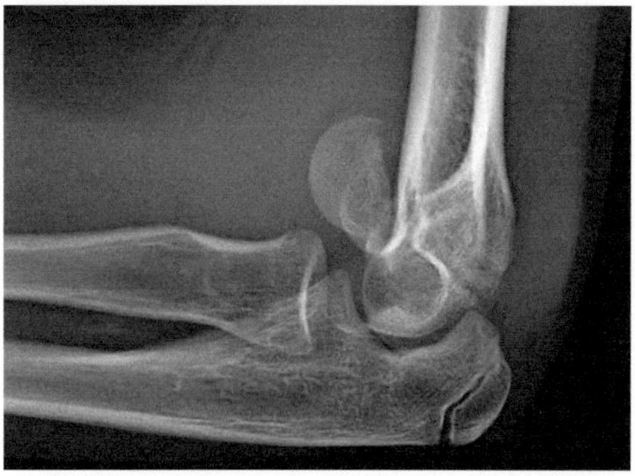

Fig. 20.17 X-rays of the elbow showing fracture of capitellum

20.16.5 Fracture Head of Radius

20.16.5.1 Mechanism of Injury

The common mechanism is fall on the outstretched hand with the elbow in extension and the forearm in pronation. This causes impaction of the radial head against the capitellum. The radial head may be split or broken. In addition, the articular cartilage of the capitellum may be bruised or chipped.

20.16.5.2 Clinical Features

There is history of fall on the ground from standing height. There may be mild to moderate pain along with difficulty in pronation and supination. Tenderness on pressure over the radial head may help clinch the diagnosis.

20.16.5.3 Investigations

X ray of the elbow joint AP and lateral views should be helpful in diagnosing the fracture. (Fig. 20.18). Associated fractures of capitellum should be looked for.

Mason classified these fractures into three types (Fig. 20.19)

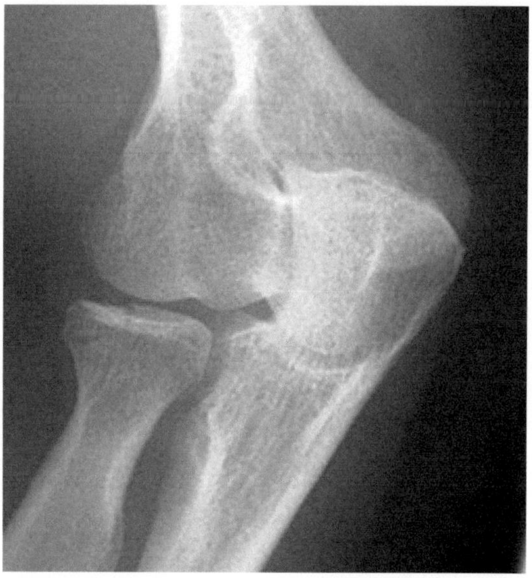

Fig. 20.18 X-rays of the elbow showing fracture of radial head

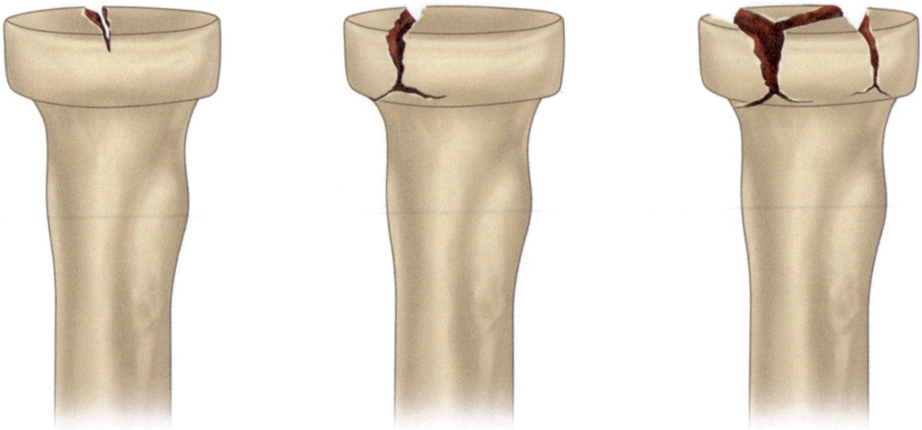

Fig. 20.19 Mason classification of fracture head of radius

Type 1—An un-displaced vertical split in the radial head.
Type 2—A displaced single fragment of the head.
Type 3—The head broken into several fragments (comminuted).

20.16.5.4 Treatment

Conservative

Type 1 fractures can be treated by immobilization for 3 weeks.

Operative Management

Open reduction and fixation should be done in Type 2 fractures. Headless screws can be used to hold the fractured fragments.

Type 3 fractures may have associated soft tissue injuries medial collateral ligament and interosseous membrane.

If the soft tissue is injured, excision of the radial head in type 3 is contraindicated.

If the soft tissue is intact, excision of radial head gives good results.

20.16.5.5 Essex Lopresti Lesion

Rupture of the interosseous membrane with fracture radial head.

20.16.5.6 Terrible Triad of Elbow

Combined fractures of the radial head and coronoid process plus dislocation of the elbow.

Complications

1. Joint stiffness.
2. Myositis ossificans.
3. Recurrent instability.

20.16.6 Fracture Olecranon

20.16.6.1 Mechanism of Injury

Fractures of the olecranon in adults occur due to two mechanisms. An indirect injury where there is avulsion of olecranon due to sudden contraction of triceps and a direct injury, which is due to direct blow on the olecranon. These fractures are intra-articular and should be treated according to the principles of intra-articular fractures.

20.16.6.2 Clinical Features

The patient gives history of either direct injury or a fall with sudden flexion of elbow. There may be bruises over the elbow in case of direct injury. The active extension of the elbow should be examined as this decides the continuity of exten-

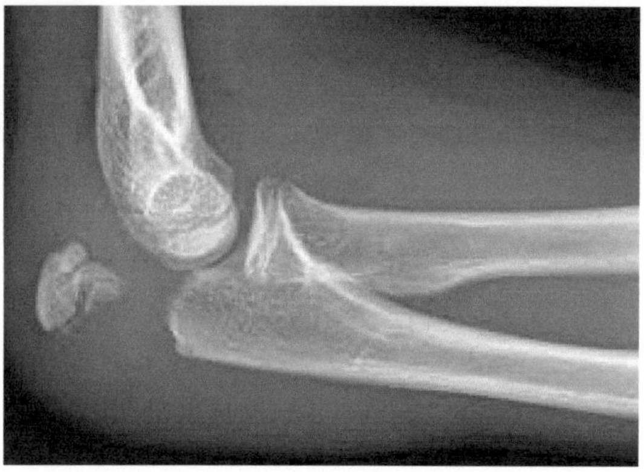

Fig. 20.20 X ray showing fracture of olecranon

sor mechanism and in turn decides the treatment. There may be a palpable gap over the olecranon.

20.16.6.3 Investigations

X rays of the elbow joint in AP and lateral view should be done. The lateral view gives the description of the fracture (Fig. 20.20).

20.16.6.4 Treatment

Conservative

This treatment option is considered for patients who have an un-displaced fracture which does not open up when the elbow is flexed. The elbow is immobilized in 60° of flexion for 3 weeks.

Operative

All displaced fractures require reduction and fixation for optimum outcomes. The fracture can be held with k-wires and a stainless-steel wire using tension band principle or tension band plates can be used to hold the reduced fracture.

20.17 Dislocations of the Elbow

20.17.1 Introduction

Dislocation of the elbow joint is more common in adults when compared to children. Ulno-humeral joint is usually involved in dislocation of elbow, but the soft tissue injuries may be extensive. The nomenclature of dislocation is based on the direction of displacement of proximal radio-ulnar complex.

20.17.2 Surgical and Applied Anatomy

The elbow is a constrained hinge joint and stabilized by dynamic and static stabilizers.

The surrounding elbow musculature provide dynamic stabilization to the elbow. The dynamic stabilizers of elbow are not as strong as shoulder and provide only a minimum role in stability.

The static stabilizers are again classified into ligamentous and bony stabilizers.

20.17.3 Bony Stabilizers

The coronoid and olecranon articulate with trochlea and olecranon fossa to provide stability. The concave surface of the radial head articulates with the convex capitellum to provide stability to the lateral aspect of the elbow joint.

20.17.4 Ligamentous Stabilizers

Annular ligament encircles radial head and neck, but inserts on ulna. Radial collateral ligaments originate from lateral epicondyle but insert into lateral aspect of ulna. The ulnar collateral ligament provides stability against valgus stress.

20.17.5 Classification

Elbow dislocations are classified according to the direction of displacement of the proximal radio-ulnar complex. In majority of the patients, radio-ulnar complex is displaced posteriorly or postero-laterally making posterior and postero-lateral dislocations as the commonest (Fig. 20.21).

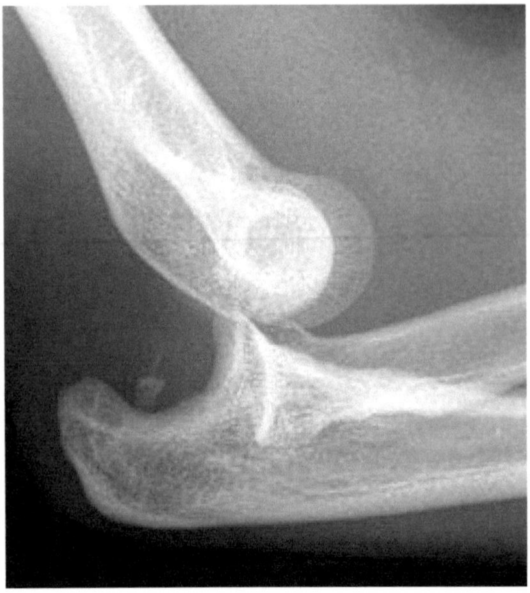

Fig. 20.21 X ray showing posterior dislocation of elbow joint

20.17.6 Mechanism of Injury

The posterior dislocation occurs in an adult due to fall on the outstretched hand. The disruption of the ulnar collateral ligaments is the first stage in a posterior or posterolateral dislocation. There is subsequent valgus instability. The biceps tendon is intact and acts as the center of rotation for the, thereby displacing the proximal radius and ulna.

The extensive ligamentous injury and bony fractures render the elbow unstable and reductions may tend to redislocate.

20.17.7 Clinical Features

The patient attends the emergency following fall on the outstretched hand and injury to elbow. The patient walks with supporting his forearm with the elbow in slight flexion. Swelling may be extensive, in some cases if the swelling is not severe, the bony landmarks (olecranon and epicondyles) may be palpable and can be detected at abnormal positions. The tip of the olecranon is displaced posteriorly and proximally. There may be puckering of skin over olecranon fossa.

A complete and thorough examination for neural and vascular injuries should be done as elbow dislocations may be associated with neurovascular injuries. There may be associated Fractures of medial epicondyle, radial head and neck, and coronoid process.

20.17.8 Investigations

X-ray of elbow joint in anteroposterior and lateral planes are usually diagnostic of an elbow dislocation.

CT scans may be necessary in the presence of extensive associated fractures to diagnose and plan the management.

20.17.9 Treatment

20.17.9.1 Closed Reduction

All the elbow dislocations should be attempted for close reduction as soon as possible. The dislocations reduced soon after the injury have better outcomes than those in which reduction is delayed.

20.17.9.2 Closed Reduction Maneuver

Under adequate anesthesia, the surgeon gives traction on the fore-arm with elbow in flexion. Sideways displacement is manipulated followed by pressure on olecranon and further flexion. Full flexion of the elbow indicates that the elbow is reduced. The elbow should be immobilized in arm pouch for 1 week followed by supervised physiotherapy.

The elbow should be examined for stability by performing flexion and extension maneuvers. Any instability is due to associated fractures or soft tissue injuries. These should be diagnosed and treated accordingly.

20.18 Surgical Treatment

20.18.1 Indications for Surgery

Inability to obtain a concentric closed reduction.
An open dislocation.
Displaced osteochondral fracture.

The associated fractures should be diagnosed and treated accordingly before the elbow is reduced in a surgery. Primary ligamentous repair is not routinely indicated.

20.18.2 Complications

20.18.2.1 Early Complications

Vascular Injuries
Brachial artery injury is one of the dreaded complications. If diagnosed, it should be treated as emergency.

Neurologic Injuries
Ulnar nerve is the most common nerve involved. The second most common is median nerve. The nerve injuries spontaneously recover in 6–8 weeks if the reduction is performed promptly and there are no associated injuries.

20.18.2.2 Late Complications

Elbow Stiffness
Stiffness is the most common complication following dislocation. Even with timely treatment, there may be 20–30 degrees of loss of extension. The most common cause of stiffness is prolonged immobilization.

Myositis Ossificans
It is the abnormal bone formation in the damaged tissues. The reason for this is not known but it is closely associated with massage. X-rays are not helpful in the initial phase because soft-tissue ossification is visible only after 4–6 weeks of injury. If the condition is suspected, exercises are stopped and the elbow is splinted in comfortable flexion until pain subsides. Gentle active physiotherapy is resumed later. Excision of the bone mass which markedly restricts movement and elbow function is the treatment of choice.

Recurrent Dislocations
Recurrent dislocation is one of the complication that has to be watched for in the future.

Osteoarthritis
Osteoarthritis can be a sequelae of dislocations of elbow.

Multiple Choice Questions

1. The last bone to ossify around elbow is
   (a) Lateral epicondyle
   (b) Trochlea
   (c) Olecranon
   (d) Radial head
2. Which artery should be felt during close reduction of supracondylar fracture of humerus?
   (a) Radial artery
   (b) Ulnar artery
   (c) Brachial artery
   (d) Anterior interosseus artery
3. Which angle is used in Anteroposterior view to assess adequate reduction of supracondylar fracture?
   (a) Baumann angle
   (b) wiberg angle
   (c) perkins angle
   (d) Radial angle
4. Type 1 Milch fractures of lateral condyle of humerus belong to which salter harris classification?
   (a) Type 1
   (b) Type 3
   (c) Type 2
   (d) Type 4
5. The most common deformity following untreated lateral condyle fracture is
   (a) Cubitus Valgus
   (b) Cubitus varus
   (c) Cubitus rectus
   (d) None of the above

Answers: 1. (a), 2. (a), 3. (a), 4. (d), 5. (a)

Injuries of the Forearm

21

Syed Ifthekar and Vishal Kumar

21.1 Fracture of Radius and Ulna

The fracture of both bones of the forearm is quite common. The forearm bones act as a ring and fracture of either bone disrupts the ring, leading to fracture or dislocation of other forearm bone at the proximal or distal radioulnar joint.

21.2 Anatomical Considerations

The location of the fracture in these two bones dictates the deforming forces and thereby gives an idea of immobilisation if treated conservatively.

The proximal part of radius gets the insertion of supinator and biceps brachii which are supinators of the forearm. The distal part of the radius gets the insertion of pronator quadratus which is the main pronator.

Now, if the fracture is distal to supinator muscle insertion but proximal to pronator teres muscle, the proximal fragment goes into supination and distal fragment is in pronation.

The fractures distal to supinator and pronator teres insertion leads to neutral alignment of the proximal fragment but pronation of the distal fragment due to pronator quadratus muscle.

21.2.1 Mechanism of Injury

The fractures of both bone forearm are mainly due to high velocity accidents. The fractures can also be caused due to direct trauma during fall or while protecting self from external blow.

21.3 Clinical Features

The patient presents with history of injury to forearm after fall, motor vehicle accident or direct injury during protection followed by gross deformity, swelling and inability to use the forearm.

On clinical examination, a careful examination with a keen eye on neurovascular status should be done as these injuries can lead to severe swelling and compartment syndrome. In the presence of compartment syndrome, an urgent fasciotomy to decrease the compartment pressure should be undertaken.

S. Ifthekar (✉)
Department of Orthopedics, All India Institute of Medical Sciences, Bibinagar, Telangana, India

V. Kumar
Department of Orthopaedics, PGIMER, Chandigarh, Chandigarh, India

V. Kumar et al. (eds.), *A Quick Guide to Essential Orthopedics*,
https://doi.org/10.1007/978-981-95-2676-5_21

21.4 Investigations

X-rays of forearm in anteroposterior and lateral views should reveal the diagnosis in majority of the cases. The x rays should include the proximal and distal radioulnar joints to assess the associated dislocations or fractures.

21.5 Treatment

21.5.1 Non-operative

In rare cases where the fractures of radius and ulna are undisplaced can be treated by above elbow cast in 90°. The patients should be examined radiologically every week for the possible loss of fracture reduction.

In children, plastic deformation of the bones (Green stick fractures) is common due to thick periosteum. These are incomplete fractures and should be completed to correct the deformity. These are stable fractures and can be treated conservatively.

The deforming forces at different levels of fractures dictate the forearm position during immobilisation.

Proximal third fractures: supination
Middle third fractures: neutral
Distal third fractures: pronation.

Th extremes of supination or pronation should be avoided.

21.5.2 Acceptable Deformity in Children

The angulation and bayonet apposition will correct in children as they grow but the rotational deformities seldom correct. The acceptable deformity is age and fracture dependent. Up to 15° of angulation can get corrected in children <10 years old at wrist. Bayonet apposition of 1 cm is acceptable in <10 year old children.

In children >10 years old, no deformity should be accepted.

21.6 Operative Treatment

In adults and older children, completely displaced fractures should be anatomically reduced and fixed with dynamic compression plates.

21.6.1 Principles of Plate Fixation

(a) To correct rotational alignment
(b) To restore radial bow
(c) To restore radial and ulnar length

Occasionally, intramedullary nail can be used in teenagers where plates cannot be used.

21.6.2 Complications

Non-union and malunion

Non-union is uncommon, but can be seen in patients treated with wrong surgical techniques.

Neurovascular injury

Nerve palsies can occur following forearm fractures.

Compartment syndrome

10% of forearm fractures are reported to develop compartment syndrome usually in the fractures of the proximal third of the forearm.

Volkmann contracture
Radioulnar synostosis
Fracture of Ulna shaft

Isolated ulnar fractures can be nightstick fractures or monteggia fracture dislocations.

21.7 Monteggia Fracture Dislocations

Monteggia fractures are the fractures of proximal ulna associated with radial head dislocation.

21.7.1 Classification of Monteggia Fractures

Monteggia fractures are classified into four types according to Bado classification:

Type 1: Anterior dislocation of radial head with anteriorly angulated fracture of ulna

Type 2: Posterior dislocation of radial head with posteriorly angulated fracture of ulna

Type 3: A lateral or anterolateral dislocation of radial head with a fracture of ulnar metaphysis

Type 4: Anterior dislocation of radial head with fracture of radius and ulna

21.7.2 Mechanism of Injury

Type 1: Forced pronation of the forearm

Type 2: Axial loading of the forearm with flexed elbow

Type 3: Forced abduction of the elbow

Type 4: Type 1 mechanism with additional failure of radius

21.7.3 Clinical Features

Patients with monteggia fracture have elbow swelling, pain and restricted movements along with pain and swelling over ulna. Rarely posterior interosseous nerve may be injured in this fracture.

21.7.4 Investigations

Anteroposterior and lateral views of the forearm with the elbow should be enough to make the diagnosis of the monteggia fracture.

A line drawn through the radial shaft and head should cut the capitellum in any position of elbow. This would help in the diagnosis of subtle radial head subluxation.

21.8 Treatment

21.8.1 Non-operative Treatment

Should be considered only in pediatric population.

Ten degrees of angulation of ulna in <10-year-old children are acceptable if the radial head is reduced.

21.8.2 Operative Treatment

Monteggia fractures in adults require surgical treatment to fix the ulnar fracture. Reduction of the fracture and stabilisation would lead to spontaneous reduction of radial head in majority of the cases.

If the radial head doesn't reduce spontaneously, open reductio should be done.

Usual causes for irreducibility of radial head are inaccurate reduction of ulna or interposed annular ligament.

Following surgery, patients forearm should be immobilised for a week.

21.8.3 Complications

Non-union- Seen in Bado type 2 fractures.

Nerve injury

Radial or Median nerves with posterior interosseous nerve or anterior interosseous nerve can be involved especially in type 2 and type 3 Bado injuries.

Recurrent radial head dislocation

21.9 Fractures of Radial Shaft

The radial shaft may be fractured at different positions throughout its length. The proximal shaft fractures may be isolated but the distal third fractures of shaft of radius are usually associated with distal radio ulnar joint subluxations.

21.9.1 Mechanism of Injury

Fall on an outstretched hand with a component of rotational force.

21.9.2 Clinical Features

The patient would have swelling, deformity and tenderness of the affected forearm with difficulty in rotation movements of forearm.

21.9.3 Investigations

Anteroposterior and lateral ray of the involved forearm with wrist and elbow should be requested for the diagnosis. The distal radioulnar joint is very commonly affected.

The signs of involvement of distal radioulnar joint are:

(a) Fracture at the base of ulnar styloid
(b) Widened distal radioulnar joint on AP x ray
(c) Subluxed ulna on lateral x-ray
(d) >5 mm radial shortening

21.9.4 Treatment

Open reduction and internal fixation are the treatment of choice for all galeazzi fracture dislocations.

The distal radioulnar joint may be reduced by k-wire and the k wires ca be removed at 6 weeks.

21.9.5 Complications

Malunion:
Instability of distal radioulnar joint:
Superficial radial nerve injury-rare.

Multiple Choice Questions

1. Both bone fractures if fractured in proximal one-third, should be immobilized in which position?
   (a) Supination
   (b) Pronation
   (c) mid-prone
   (d) None of the above
2. The acceptable angulation of forearm fractures in children less than 10 years is
   (a) 5 Degrees
   (b) 10 Degrees
   (c) 15 Degrees
   (d) 20 Degrees
3. The acceptable bayonet apposition of forearm fractures in children less than 10 years is
   (a) 1 cm
   (b) 2 cm
   (c) 3 cm
   (d) 4 cm
4. The mechanism of injury in type 1 Monteggia fracture is
   (a) Forced pronation of the forearm
   (b) Axial loading of the forearm with flexed elbow
   (c) Forced abduction of the elbow
   (d) Type 1 mechanism with additional failure of radius
5. Which of the following is not a sign of distal radioulnar joint injury?
   (a) Fracture at the base of ulnar styloid
   (b) Widened distal radioulnar joint on AP x ray
   (c) Subluxed ulna on lateral x-ray
   (d) 3 mm radial shortening

Answers: 1. (a), 2. (b), 3. (a), 4. (a), 5. (d)

22 Injuries of the Wrist

Sanny Kumar Singh and Rajeev Anand

22.1 Radiocarpal Fracture-Dislocation

Definition: Radiocarpal fracture-dislocation involves complete separation between the carpal bones and the distal radius, typically resulting from high-energy trauma.

Epidemiology: These injuries are rare, constituting about 0.2% of all wrist traumas annually, and are more prevalent in males. Most dislocations are dorsal rather than volar.

Mechanism: Commonly occurs in high-impact scenarios such as vehicular accidents or falls from height. The usual force involves hyperextension and pronation of the wrist with rotational or shearing forces.

Associated Injuries. These may include

- Distal radius fractures (especially volar marginal fragments)
- Radial/ulnar styloid fractures
- Injuries to key ligaments (radioscaphocapitate, short radiolunate)
- Carpal bone fractures (e.g., scaphoid, lunate)
- Median nerve neuropathy

Presentation: Pain, swelling, deformity (usually dorsal), bruising, and possible neurovascular compromise (cold or pale hand). Numbness is often present due to nerve involvement.

Examination: Check for range of motion (flexion/extension, rotation), crepitus, and neurovascular integrity. Evaluate median and ulnar nerves and radial/ulnar pulses.

22.1.1 Imaging

- PA View Assess Gilula lines and carpal alignment
- Lateral View Determines dislocation direction
- Teardrop View Reveals lunate facet involvement
- CT Evaluates comminuted fractures and articular involvement
- MRI Assesses ligamentous injuries (scapholunate, lunotriquetral)

22.1.2 Treatment

- Conservative Closed reduction and immobilization for stable injuries
- Surgical Open reduction, internal fixation, and ligament repair if unstable or irreducible

S. K. Singh (✉)
Department of Orthopaedics, Post Graduate Institute of Medical Education & Research, Chandigarh, India

R. Anand
Patna Medical College & Hospital, Patna, Bihar, India

V. Kumar et al. (eds.), *A Quick Guide to Essential Orthopedics*,
https://doi.org/10.1007/978-981-95-2676-5_22

Complications Potential for carpal tunnel syndrome, stiffness, arthritis, instability, and late intercarpal dissociation.

Outcome Early intervention generally yields favorable outcomes.

22.1.3 Scaphoid Fracture

Scaphoid fractures are the most frequently encountered carpal bone fractures, and they commonly result from a fall on an outstretched hand (FOOSH).

22.1.3.1 Incidence & Demographics

They represent approximately 15% of all acute wrist injuries and account for 60% of carpal fractures. The incidence is about 8 per 100,000 females and 38 per 100,000 males, with a 21 male predominance. These injuries are most frequent in individuals in their third decade of life.

22.1.3.2 Fracture Distribution

- Waist fractures ~65%
- Proximal third ~25%
- Distal third ~10%. In children, distal pole fractures were historically more prevalent due to the sequence of ossification, though waist fractures are now increasingly common.

Mechanism of Injury

Typically occurs due to an axial force on a wrist that is hyperextended, pronated, and ulnarly deviated, as seen in contact sports. Transverse fractures tend to be more stable than vertical or oblique patterns.

Associated Conditions

A major complication includes Scaphoid Nonunion Advanced Collapse (SNAC wrist).

22.1.3.3 Clinical Features

History

Often involves a fall onto an outstretched hand, with variable trauma intensity.

Symptoms

Pain localized to the wrist, particularly in the anatomical snuffbox.

Physical Findings

- Swelling is present, though ecchymosis and deformity are rare.
- Pain exacerbated by wrist circumduction and resisted pronation.

Provocative Tests

- Snuffbox tenderness (dorsal)
- Scaphoid tubercle tenderness (volar)
- Scaphoid compression test Pain with axial pressure through the thumb (sensitivity 87–100%, specificity ~74% if all three signs present within 24 h)

22.1.3.4 Imaging

- Radiographs Include PA (neutral), lateral, 45° oblique, and scaphoid views (30° wrist extension, 20° ulnar deviation). Waist fractures are best seen in these views.
- If initial X-rays are negative (in ~27% of cases), but clinical suspicion is high, repeat after 14–21 days.
- Bone Scintigraphy Useful in early detection of occult fractures.
- MRI Most sensitive within the first 24 h, also assesses ligamentous damage and proximal pole vascularity (especially on T1-weighted images).
- CT Scan Best for evaluating fracture orientation, angulation, displacement, and size, and for monitoring healing post-operatively. It's less sensitive than MRI for early fracture detection.

22.1.4 Management

22.1.4.1 Non-operative (Casting)

- Indicated for stable, non-displaced fractures, which make up the majority.
- If X-rays are normal but suspicion remains, immobilize in a thumb spica cast and re-evaluate in 2–3 weeks.
- Fractures with <1 mm displacement have a 90% union rate with conservative treatment.

22.1.4.2 Operative Management

- Percutaneous Screw Fixation Used for unstable or proximal pole fractures displaced >1 mm, or for stable waist fractures in active patients (for earlier return to activities). Union rate 90–95%.
- Open Reduction and Internal Fixation (ORIF) Indicated for
  - Significantly displaced fractures
  - Humpback deformity >15°
  - Radiolunate angle >15° (DISI pattern)
  - Intrascaphoid angle >35°
  - Fractures with perilunate dislocation, comminution, or unstable oblique/vertical lines
  - Precise reduction correlates with improved healing outcomes

22.1.5 Complications

- Nonunion Occurs in 5–10% of immobilized cases, with proximal fractures at greater risk. Factors include displacement >1 mm, vertical obliquity, age, and nicotine use.
- Avascular Necrosis (AVN) Seen in 13–50%, especially in fractures of the proximal fifth.
- Malunion Results in a humpback deformity, with flexion of the distal and extension of the proximal fragment due to pull from the scapholunate ligament.
- SNAC Wrist AVN risk increases with proximity to the proximal pole — 100% in proximal fifth, 33% in proximal third without treatment.

22.1.6 Lunate Dislocation/Perilunate Dissociation

Lunate and perilunate dislocations represent high-energy wrist injuries, often associated with median nerve involvement, and carry a risk of poor long-term function if missed or untreated.

22.1.6.1 Epidemiology

These injuries are rare, occurring in fewer than 1 per 100,000 annually. They are frequently overlooked, with up to 25% of cases not diagnosed at the initial presentation.

22.1.6.2 Mechanism of Injury

These injuries typically result from trauma, such as a fall or vehicular accident, with the wrist in an extended and ulnarly deviated position. This leads to intercarpal supination and progressive disruption of the carpal ligaments, starting with the scapholunate ligament.

22.1.6.3 Clinical Presentation

- Acute wrist swelling and intense pain
- Possible median nerve compression symptoms (e.g., numbness, tingling, or weakness), occurring in approximately 25% of cases, particularly when the lunate herniates into the carpal tunnel

22.1.6.4 Imaging Features

X-rays (PA and Lateral Views)

- PA View
  - Disruption of Gilula's arcs
  - Overlapping of the lunate and capitate
  - "Piece-of-pie sign" Triangular configuration of the lunate due to its palmar rotation
- Lateral View
  - Loss of normal alignment between the radius, lunate, and capitate
  - Scapholunate angle >70°
  - "Spilled teacup sign" Volar tilt of the lunate, appearing as if tipped over

MRI

- Generally not necessary for diagnosis, unless ligamentous or soft tissue detail is needed preoperatively.

22.1.6.5 Management

Non-operative (Rare)

- May be considered only in select acute, stable cases, involving closed reduction and casting

Operative

- Most cases require urgent closed reduction followed by
  - Open reduction
  - Repair of torn ligaments
  - Internal fixation
  - Carpal tunnel decompression, if median nerve compression is present

22.1.6.6 Complications

- Transient Lunate Ischemia
  - Seen in up to 12.5% of cases
  - Appears as increased bone density on X-rays, usually identified 1–4 months post-injury
  - Typically benign and self-resolving, requiring only observation

22.1.7 Triquetrum Fracture

Triquetrum fractures are among the most frequent carpal bone injuries and are often accompanied by other wrist trauma, particularly ligamentous or osseous injuries.

22.1.7.1 Incidence

- These fractures are the second most common of the carpal bones
- They account for approximately 15% of all carpal fractures

22.1.7.2 Commonly Associated Injuries

- Perilunate dislocations (found in 12–25% of cases)
- Distal radius or ulna fractures

22.1.7.3 Clinical Presentation

- Swelling and possible deformity localized to the ulnar side of the wrist
- Direct tenderness over the triquetrum on palpation
- Pain during wrist flexion and extension, especially in dorsal cortical fractures

22.1.7.4 Imaging Studies

Radiographs

- Standard PA and lateral views
- Special views such as internal rotation oblique and radial deviation views help detect dorsal fractures more clearly

CT Scan

- Recommended when there is a high index of suspicion and plain films are inconclusive

MRI

- Particularly useful for palmar cortical fractures due to the risk of carpal instability
- Also indicated when assessing for intercarpal ligament injury or occult fractures

22.1.7.5 Treatment Options

Nonoperative

- Suitable for
  - Dorsal cortical fractures with no instability
  - Nondisplaced fractures of the triquetral body
  - Palmar cortical fractures without signs of instability
- Managed with immobilization for 4–6 weeks, typically in a wrist splint or cast

Operative

- Required for
  - Dorsal cortical fractures showing signs of instability
  - Displaced body fractures
  - Palmar cortical fractures with demonstrated instability
- Managed with open reduction and internal fixation (ORIF)

22.1.8 Trapezium Fracture

Fractures of the trapezium, though relatively rare, can result from axial loading injuries and are often associated with thumb trauma or complex wrist injuries.

22.1.8.1 Epidemiology

- These fractures are uncommon, comprising less than 1% of all fractures.
- Among carpal bone fractures, trapezial fractures rank third, making up 1–5% of cases.

22.1.8.2 Etiology & Mechanism

- Usually caused by direct trauma, particularly from axial loading through the thumb.
- Often seen in association with Bennett fractures (fracture-dislocation at the base of the first metacarpal).
- Other possible concurrent injuries include fractures of the scaphoid, trapezoid, capitate, neighboring metacarpals, and distal radius—especially in high-energy trauma or fracture-dislocations.

22.1.8.3 Clinical Presentation

- Patients report a history of thumb trauma with sudden pain and swelling over the base of the thumb.
- Point tenderness is localized to the trapezium; ecchymosis may be present.
- Trapezial ridge fractures can present more subtly, often as dull, persistent pain over the volar base of the thumb.

22.1.8.4 Imaging Evaluation

22.1.9 X-rays

- Include PA, pronated AP, lateral, Bett's view, and carpal tunnel view (especially for ridge fractures).

22.1.9.1 CT Scan

- Indicated when X-rays are inconclusive despite clinical suspicion.
- Helps define fragment size, displacement, and involvement of the joint surface.

22.1.9.2 MRI

- Not routinely required, but can detect occult fractures or ligament injuries when needed.

22.1.9.3 Management

22.1.9.4 Nonoperative Treatment

- Thumb spica cast immobilization for 4–6 weeks is appropriate for
  - Non-displaced body fractures
  - Acute ridge fractures with stable first CMC joint

22.1.9.5 Operative Management

- Open reduction and internal fixation (ORIF) For displaced body fractures, especially in physically active patients
- Primary arthrodesis Reserved for severely comminuted fractures in high-demand individuals
- External fixation Considered for comminuted fractures with preserved joint congruity

22.1.9.6 Complications

- Non union
- Instability of the first carpometacarpal (CMC) joint
- Post-traumatic osteoarthritis

22.2 Hamate Fractures

22.2.1 Hook of Hamate Fracture

Hook of hamate fractures are uncommon and frequently missed injuries, most often seen in athletes involved in grip-heavy sports such as golf, baseball, and hockey. These injuries result from direct trauma to the volar-ulnar aspect of the wrist.

22.2.2 Epidemiology

- Represent 2–4% of all carpal bone fractures
- Occur more commonly in males, with a 21 male-to-female ratio

22.2.3 Risk Factors & Mechanism

- Repetitive or acute impact on the palm, particularly during actions such as
  - Striking the ground with a golf club
  - Batting in baseball
  - Falling on an outstretched hand
- Sports requiring tight gripping are a significant risk factor

22.2.4 Associated Injuries

- Ulnar nerve compression in Guyon's canal
- Bipartite hamate (an anatomical variant that may mimic or predispose to fracture)

22.2.5 Clinical Presentation

- Diagnosis is often delayed, with an average detection time of 4 weeks post-injury
- Symptoms include
  - Pain on the ulnar side of the wrist or hypothenar eminence
  - Discomfort with tight grip activities
  - Decreased grip strength and limited ulnar deviation
- Neurovascular findings
  - Paresthesia along the ulnar nerve distribution
  - Positive Tinel's sign over Guyon's canal
  - Weakness in intrinsic hand muscles

22.2.6 Provocative Test

- Hook of Hamate Pull Test
  - Wrist held in ulnar deviation as patient flexes DIP joints of the ring and little fingers against resistance
  - Pain indicates possible fracture due to tension from the flexor tendons at the fracture site
- Pain may also worsen with dorsoulnar deviation of the wrist

22.2.7 Imaging

- Standard views PA, lateral, and carpal tunnel view
- CT scan Preferred if X-rays are inconclusive or when better detail is needed for chronic or nondisplaced fractures
- MRI Most sensitive imaging modality, especially useful when clinical suspicion is high despite normal radiographs

22.2.8 Management

22.2.8.1 Nonoperative

- Immobilization in a cast for 6 weeks
- Suitable for acute, nondisplaced fractures
- Though nonunion occurs in 40–50%, many patients remain asymptomatic with full range of motion

22.2.8.2 Operative

- Excision of the hook is indicated for
  - Symptomatic chronic nonunions
  - Presence of ulnar neuritis
  - High-demand patients, especially athletes
- ORIF (Open Reduction and Internal Fixation)
  - Considered for displaced fractures or when grip strength is significantly impaired and reduction is necessary

22.2.9 Complications

- Nonunion
- Ulnar nerve entrapment or neuritis
- Flexor tendon rupture, particularly to the small finger
- Chronic pain and grip weakness

22.2.9.1 Hamate Body Fracture

Fractures of the hamate body are extremely rare, often resulting from direct trauma and may be associated with injuries to the bases of the 4th and 5th metacarpals.

22.2.10 Epidemiology

- Account for less than 2% of carpal bone injuries

22.2.11 Mechanism of Injury

- Caused by a direct blow with a clenched fist, often against a hard object

22.2.12 Associated Injuries

- Base fractures or dislocations of the 4th and 5th metacarpals
- Concurrent hook of hamate fracture

22.2.13 Clinical Features

- Pain and swelling on the ulnar side of the wrist
- Tenderness localized over the hamate body

22.2.14 Imaging

- Radiographs PA, lateral, external rotation oblique (best view), and carpal tunnel views
- CT scan Helps to define fracture geometry, guide surgical decision-making, and assess intra-articular extension
- Differential diagnoses include
  - Hook of hamate fracture
  - Pisiform fracture
  - Metacarpal shaft fractures

22.2.15 Management

22.2.15.1 Non-operative

- Immobilization is appropriate for extra-articular, non-displaced fractures

22.2.15.2 Operative (ORIF)

- Most intra-articular fractures require open reduction and fixation for anatomical alignment and joint preservation

22.2.16 Complications

- Stiffness
- Malunion
- Infection
- Persistent pain or instability if inadequately treated

22.3 Pisiform Fracture

Fractures of the pisiform, a small sesamoid bone within the flexor carpi ulnaris (FCU) tendon, are rare and often missed on initial evaluation, especially when associated with falls on an outstretched hand.

22.3.1 Epidemiology

- Represent less than 1% of all carpal fractures
- Frequently underdiagnosed due to overlapping symptoms and subtle radiographic findings

22.3.2 Mechanism of Injury

- Typically caused by a direct blow to the volar-ulnar wrist, such as a fall on an outstretched hand or impact against a hard surface

22.3.3 Associated Injuries

- Occur in isolation in 50% of cases
- In the remaining 50%, found alongside other carpal fractures or distal radius fractures

22.3.4 Clinical Presentation

- Ulnar-sided wrist pain following trauma

- Swelling and tenderness over the hypothenar eminence
- Weak grip strength may be present
- Important to assess for concurrent injuries to carpal bones and distal radius

22.3.5 Imaging Evaluation

22.3.5.1 Radiographs

- Standard views PA and lateral
- External oblique and carpal tunnel view are most effective for visualizing the pisiform

22.3.5.2 CT Scan

- Helps delineate the fracture pattern, especially in complex or subtle injuries
- Aids in treatment planning

22.3.5.3 MRI

- Useful when X-rays are negative but suspicion remains high
- May reveal bone marrow edema within the pisiform suggestive of an occult fracture

22.3.6 Differential Diagnosis

- Hook of hamate fracture
- Hamate body fracture
- Flexor carpi ulnaris (FCU) tendinitis

22.3.7 Management

22.3.7.1 Nonoperative

- Immobilization in a short-arm cast for 6–8 weeks
- Cast is typically applied with the wrist in 30° flexion and ulnar deviation
- Appropriate for nondisplaced and minimally symptomatic fractures

22.3.7.2 Operative

- Pisiformectomy is indicated in cases of
  - Displaced fractures with persistent symptoms
  - Painful nonunion not resolving with conservative measures

22.3.8 Potential Complications

- Malunion or nonunion
- Chronic pain on the ulnar side of the wrist
- Reduced grip strength
- Persistent discomfort during resisted wrist flexion or ulnar deviation

22.4 Scapholunate Ligament Injury & DISI)

Injury to the scapholunate interosseous ligament (SLIL) is a common cause of dorsoradial wrist pain, especially after trauma. If left untreated, chronic scapholunate injuries can result in carpal instability, most notably the DISI deformity.

22.4.1 Epidemiology

- Acute SLIL injuries are seen in up to 10–30% of intra-articular distal radius or carpal fractures
- Degenerative SLIL injuries are present in over 50% of individuals above the age of 80
- Incomplete tears are more frequent than full-thickness ruptures

22.4.2 Mechanism of Injury

- Most commonly due to a high-energy force applied to the wrist in extension, ulnar deviation, and carpal supination
- Often occurs during a fall on an outstretched hand (FOOSH)

22.4.3 Associated Pathology

- May lead to dissociation between the scaphoid and lunate, producing DISI

- In DISI, the scaphoid flexes volarly while the lunate tilts dorsally
- Chronic instability can progress to SLAC (Scapholunate Advanced Collapse) wrist
- DISI can also result after distal pole scaphoid excision performed for STT arthritis

22.4.4 Clinical Presentation

- History of trauma or degenerative wrist pain, depending on age and activity level
- Symptoms include
  - Pain over the dorsal, radial wrist
  - Worsening pain during weight-bearing activities (e.g., push-ups)
  - Clicking or catching sensations
  - Swelling over the dorsal wrist
  - Tenderness near the scapholunate interval (just distal to Lister's tubercle)

22.4.5 Provocative Test – Watson Test

- Wrist is moved from ulnar to radial deviation while pressure is applied to the volar scaphoid
- A painful clunk may be felt as the scaphoid subluxes dorsally and reduces—suggestive of ligament insufficiency

22.4.6 Imaging Studies

22.4.6.1 Radiographs

- Standard views PA and lateral, along with radial/ulnar deviation, flexion-extension, and clenched fist views

22.4.7 Key findings

- SL gap >3 mm on AP (Terry Thomas sign)
- Cortical ring sign (rotated scaphoid)
- DISI pattern SL angle >70°, capitolunate angle >20°
- Humpback deformity may indicate a concurrent scaphoid fracture

22.4.7.1 Arthrography

- May help identify communication between joints but lacks specificity

22.4.7.2 MRI

- Often overused, and interpretation requires a skilled radiologist
- Has low sensitivity for SLIL tears

22.4.7.3 Arthroscopy

- Gold standard for both diagnosis and staging of scapholunate ligament injuries

22.4.8 Differential Diagnosis

- Lunotriquetral ligament (LT) injury with VISI deformity
- Carpal instability nondissociative (CIND)

22.4.9 Treatment Approach

22.4.9.1 Non-operative

- Indicated for acute partial tears without malalignment or for chronic asymptomatic findings
- Includes rest, NSAIDs, and possible immobilization

22.4.9.2 Operative Options

1. Primary Repair
   - Best suited for acute injuries (<18 months) without carpal misalignment and when ligament structure is amenable to repair
2. Reconstruction
   - Indicated when ligament is non-repairable or injury is older than 18 months
   - Can also be used in reducible chronic instability
3. Scaphoid ORIF/CRPP
   - Used when scaphoid fracture is the underlying cause of the ligament disruption
4. Partial Wrist Fusions (e.g., Scaphoid Trapezoid Trapezium, Scaphoid Lunate Capitate)
   - Reserved for non-reducible deformities or those with degenerative changes

22.4.10 Complications

- Progression to SLAC wrist
- Postoperative stiffness and pain
- Weakened grip strength
- Development of carpal arthritis

22.5 Lunotriquetral Ligament Injury & VISI

Injuries to the lunotriquetral (LT) ligament are rare but clinically significant causes of ulnar-sided wrist pain. When combined with damage to the dorsal radiocarpal and volar radiolunate ligaments, these injuries can lead to volar intercalated segment instability (VISI)—a type of carpal instability dissociative (CID).

22.5.1 Epidemiology

- Less common than scapholunate ligament injuries
- VISI may also occur in the absence of trauma in individuals with generalized ligamentous laxity, unlike DISI, which is always considered pathologic

22.5.2 Mechanism of Injury

- Typically results from hyperextension of the wrist or extension with radial deviation
- The scaphoid flexes, causing the lunate to follow into volar flexion, while the triquetrum extends, disrupting the LT ligament

22.5.3 Pathophysiology of VISI

- VISI involves volar tilting of the lunate due to
  - Injury to the lunotriquetral ligament
  - Disruption of dorsal radiotriquetral and volar radiolunate ligaments
- Radiologically, VISI presents with volar rotation of the lunate and a reduced scapholunate angle

22.5.4 Clinical Presentation

- Ulnar wrist pain, particularly aggravated by pronation and ulnar deviation during power grip activities
- May be accompanied by weakness and instability symptoms

22.5.5 Physical Examination

22.5.5.1 LT Shuck Test (Ballottement Test)

- Lunate is stabilized while alternating palmar and dorsal pressure is applied to the triquetrum
- A positive test produces pain, clicking, or excessive laxity

22.5.5.2 Kleinman's Shear Test

- The radiolunate joint is stabilized, and the triquetrum is sheared in an anteroposterior direction
- Pain or a palpable clunk suggests an LT tear

22.5.5.3 Lunotriquetral Compression Test

- During radioulnar deviation, displacement of the triquetrum induces pain over the LT joint

22.5.6 Imaging

22.5.6.1 Radiographs

- Lateral view shows
  - Volar flexion of the lunate
  - Scapholunate angle <30° (normal ~47°)
  - Capitolunate angle >15°, indicative of the zig-zag deformity of VISI
- AP view may reveal
  - Disruption of Gilula's arc
  - Possible LT overlap or proximal translation of the triquetrum
  - No significant LT interval widening, unlike scapholunate dissociation

22.5.6.2 Arthroscopy

- Most accurate diagnostic tool, especially when radiographs appear normal

22.5.7 Differential Diagnosis

- Scapholunate ligament injury with DISI
- TFCC tear
- Carpal instability nondissociative (CIND)

22.5.8 Treatment Options

22.5.8.1 Nonoperative

- Initial conservative management with observation in mild or asymptomatic cases

22.5.8.2 Operative Interventions

1. Acute Tears
   - Closed reduction and percutaneous pinning (CRPP) using K-wires
   - Primary repair of LT ligament ± dorsal capsulodesis
2. Chronic Instability
   - LT Fusion for persistent instability
   - Arthroscopic debridement combined with ulnar shortening osteotomy in cases of ulnar positive variance causing chronic overload
   - Often associated with TFCC degeneration

22.5.9 Complications

- Progression to chronic instability
- Degenerative arthritis
- Persistent pain and limited wrist function

22.6 Distal Radioulnar Joint (DRUJ) Injuries

Injuries to the distal radioulnar joint (DRUJ) often accompany distal radius fractures, although isolated DRUJ injuries can also occur. These injuries are frequently overlooked, yet they are a significant source of wrist pain and restricted forearm rotation, especially following trauma.

22.6.1 Anatomy

The DRUJ comprises the articulation between the ulnar head and the sigmoid notch of the distal radius. Its stability is maintained by

- Dorsal and volar radioulnar ligaments
- The Triangular Fibrocartilage Complex (TFCC)

22.6.1.1 TFCC Components

- Volar and dorsal radioulnar ligaments
- Central articular disc
- Meniscal homologue
- Ulnolunate and ulnotriquetral ligament origins
- Sheath floor of the extensor carpi ulnaris (ECU) tendon

22.6.2 Clinical Features

22.6.2.1 Acute Injury

- Pain and instability of the ulnar wrist
- May be associated with a visible dislocation or subluxation

22.6.2.2 Chronic Cases

- Dorsal-sided wrist pain
- Snapping, crepitus, or feeling of looseness during motion
- Limited pronation and supination
- Decreased grip strength

22.6.3 Imaging Studies

22.6.3.1 Plain Radiographs

- AP view may show DRUJ widening
- Lateral view can reveal dorsal displacement of the ulna relative to the radius

22.6.3.2 Dynamic CT Scan

- Best for identifying subtle or chronic instability
- Allows evaluation of joint congruency in various wrist positions

22.6.3.3 MRI

- Highly effective for detecting TFCC tears or ligamentous disruptions

22.6.4 Management Approach

22.6.4.1 Nonoperative Treatment

- Suitable for purely ligamentous injuries without significant instability
- Includes closed reduction followed by immobilization (e.g., in a long arm cast)

22.6.4.2 Operative Intervention

1. Indicated for unstable DRUJ dislocations or ligamentous disruption
2. May involve
   - Percutaneous DRUJ pinning (e.g., K-wire stabilization)
   - Surgical repair of radioulnar ligaments or TFCC reconstruction

Multiple Choice Questions

1. Most common carpal bone to fracture is
   (a) Lunate
   (b) Scaphoid
   (c) Hamate
   (d) Trapizium
2. Which is true for scaphoid?
   (a) distal pole is most common fractured location
   (b) least common carpal bone fracture
   (c) proximal pole is most common fractured location
   (d) more common in male
3. Which is false for DISI?
   (a) associated with scapholunate Ligament Injury
   (b) painful pushup position
   (c) complete tears are more common than incomplete tears
   (d) watson provocative test is used
4. The following are the radiologica signs of DISI except
   (a) capitolunate angle $\leq 20°$
   (b) Terry Thomas sign
   (c) Cortical ring sign
   (d) SL angle >70° on lateral view
5. Not a component of TFCC
   (a) floor of the FCU tendon sheath
   (b) volar and dorsal radioulnar ligaments
   (c) meniscal homologue
   (d) central articular disc

Answers: 1. (b), 2. (d), 3. (c), 4. (a), 5. (a)

Hand Injuries

23

Sanny Kumar Singh and Mahesh Prasad

23.1 Flexor Tendon Injuries

Flexor tendon injuries involve damage to the flexor digitorum superficialis (FDS) and flexor digitorum profundus (FDP) tendons, most often caused by trauma or sharp laceration to the volar aspect of the hand. These injuries are relatively rare, with an incidence of approximately 4.83 per 100,000 people. Neurovascular injury may be present due to the anatomical proximity of structures.

23.1.1 Mechanism of Injury

- Most commonly due to penetrating trauma or lacerations on the volar hand or fingers
- May also occur from crush injuries or closed avulsions
- Often accompanied by nerve or vessel injury

S. K. Singh (✉)
Department of Orthopaedics, Postgraduate Institute of Medical Education & Research, Chandigarh, India

M. Prasad
Department of Orthopaedics, Patna Medical College & Hospital, Patna, India

23.1.2 Tendon Healing Pathways

Healing occurs through two biological mechanisms

- Intrinsic healing
  - Mediated by tenocytes within the tendon substance
- Extrinsic healing
  - Involves surrounding synovial fluid and inflammatory cells
  - More likely to produce adhesions and scar tissue

23.1.3 Phases of Tendon Healing

1. Inflammatory phase (0–5 days)
   - Cellular proliferation
   - No mechanical strength
2. Fibroblastic phase (5–28 days)
   - Fibroblast activity and collagen deposition
   - Collagen is disorganized, but mechanical strength improves
3. Remodeling phase (after 28 days)
   - Linear collagen alignment
   - Tendon can begin to tolerate controlled active motion

V. Kumar et al. (eds.), *A Quick Guide to Essential Orthopedics*,
https://doi.org/10.1007/978-981-95-2676-5_23

23.1.4 Relevant Anatomy

- *Camper's chiasm*
  - Location where FDP passes through the FDS at the level of the proximal phalanx
- *Pulley system in digits 2–5*
  - Five annular pulleys (A1 to A5)
  - Three cruciate pulleys (C1 to C3)
  - Cruciate pulleys are flexible and allow approximation of annular pulleys during flexion
- *Pulley system in the thumb*
  - A1 pulley
  - Av pulley (prevents bowstringing, functionally most important)
  - A2 pulley
  - A1 and Av pulleys are supported by the oblique pulley

23.1.5 Blood Supply

Flexor tendons receive nutrients from two main sources

- Diffusion through synovial fluid in tendon sheaths
- Direct vascular supply for portions outside of tendon sheaths

23.1.6 Clinical Presentation

- *Symptoms*
  - Inability or weakness of active digital flexion
  - Loss of grip strength
- *Inspection and Examination*
  - Assess hand posture and digital cascade
  - Observe skin integrity for laceration or arthrotomy
  - Test passive wrist movements to evaluate tenodesis effect
    - Wrist extension should cause passive flexion at MCP, PIP, and DIP
    - Failure to observe this suggests tendon discontinuity
  - Check active flexion at each joint in isolation
  - Evaluate neurovascular status of each digit

23.1.7 Imaging

- Radiographs
  - May reveal fractures or foreign bodies
- Ultrasound
  - Helpful in detecting suspected tendon lacerations
- MRI is not routinely required but may aid in chronic or complex injuries

23.1.8 Treatment Options

- *Nonoperative Management*
  - Indicated for partial tendon lacerations involving less than 60% of the tendon width
  - Includes local wound care and early range of motion
  - Risks include tendon gapping and potential for triggering
- *Operative Management*
  - Indicated for tendon injuries greater than 60% or full-thickness lacerations
  - Includes tendon repair with early controlled mobilization
  - Reconstruction is considered in chronic cases or failed primary repair
  - In chronic flexor pollicis longus ruptures, FDS transfer from the ring finger may be done as a single-stage procedure

23.1.9 Common Complications

- Adhesions and scarring
- Tendon rupture
- Decreased finger range of motion
- Triggering or gap formation after partial lacerations
- Stiffness or loss of digital glide despite rehabilitation

23.2 Jersey Finger

Jersey finger is a flexor tendon injury resulting from avulsion of the flexor digitorum profundus (FDP) tendon from its insertion at the base of the distal phalanx. It typically occurs when a player grabs another's jersey, and the finger is forcibly extended while actively flexed.

23.2.1 Commonly Affected Finger

- The ring finger is involved in approximately 75% of cases
- During gripping, the ring fingertip tends to protrude about 5 mm more than the others in most individuals
- This anatomical position subjects the ring finger to higher forces during sudden extension

23.2.2 Mechanism of Injury

- The injury occurs when the FDP muscle is strongly contracted while the distal interphalangeal (DIP) joint is suddenly extended
- This causes the tendon to pull away from its insertion

23.2.3 Clinical Features

- Pain and swelling over the volar aspect of the distal phalanx
- Inability to actively flex the DIP joint
- Affected finger may appear slightly extended compared to other fingers at rest
- In some cases, the retracted tendon can be felt along the flexor sheath

23.2.4 Imaging

- Plain radiographs may reveal a small avulsion fragment from the distal phalanx
- In cases without a visible fragment, clinical examination remains the mainstay for diagnosis

23.2.5 Treatment Options

- *Acute injuries (within 3 weeks)*
  - Direct repair of the tendon or reinsertion using a dorsal button technique
  - Open reduction and internal fixation for avulsion fractures involving large fragments (type III and IV)
  - Type IV cases may need combined fracture fixation and tendon repair
- *Chronic injuries (more than 3 months)*
  - Two-stage flexor tendon grafting for patients who retain passive range of motion at the DIP
  - Arthrodesis of the DIP joint is a salvage procedure in cases with chronic stiffness and poor motion

23.2.6 Possible Complications

- Quadrigia effect may occur if the repaired tendon is advanced more than 1 cm
  - This results in limited flexion of adjacent digits due to tension imbalance

23.2.7 Extensor Tendon Injuries

Extensor tendon injuries affect the tendons on the dorsal aspect of the hand and fingers. These injuries may result from lacerations, blunt trauma, or repetitive overuse. Due to the superficial location of these tendons, they are more prone to injury than flexor tendons.

23.2.8 Most Common Site

- The long finger is the most frequently affected
- Zone VI, located over the dorsum of the hand, is the zone most commonly injured

23.2.9 Nonoperative Treatment Options

- *Early protected mobilization*
  - Appropriate when less than half of the tendon width is lacerated
  - Applicable to all zones if the patient can actively extend the digit against resistance
- *Splinting methods based on injury zone*
  - DIP joint extension splint
    - Used for acute mallet finger (Zone I), including cases with nondisplaced avulsion fractures
    - Also useful in chronic mallet finger if the joint remains flexible and aligned
  - PIP joint extension splint
    - Used for closed injuries to the central slip (Zone III)
  - MCP joint extension splint
    - Applied for sagittal band injuries in Zone V presenting with subluxation or tendon instability

23.2.10 Surgical Treatment Options

- *Primary tendon repair*
  - Indicated when more than half of the tendon width is damaged
  - Used in all anatomical zones when conservative management is inadequate
- *Fixation of avulsion fractures*
  - Required when bony mallet finger is accompanied by volar subluxation of the distal phalanx
- *Tendon reconstruction procedures*
  - Considered for chronic tendon ruptures or when direct repair is not feasible
  - Central slip reconstruction is performed when the injury involves the central band and has resulted in a boutonnière deformity
  - Extensor indicis proprius (EIP) to extensor pollicis longus (EPL) tendon transfer
    - Done for chronic EPL tendon rupture

23.3 Mallet Finger

Mallet finger refers to a deformity caused by disruption of the terminal portion of the extensor tendon, typically where it inserts on the distal phalanx. This results in the inability to actively extend the distal interphalangeal (DIP) joint.

23.3.1 Common Risk Groups

- Most often occurs in individuals involved in manual labor or contact sports
- Frequently seen in young to middle-aged men and older women
- The long, ring, and small fingers of the dominant hand are most commonly affected

23.3.2 Mechanism of Injury

- *Traumatic impaction*
  - Caused by sudden forced flexion of the extended fingertip, such as being struck by a ball
- *Dorsal laceration*
  - Less commonly, a sharp or crushing injury over the dorsal DIP joint may disrupt the extensor mechanism

23.3.3 Typical Presentation

- *Symptoms*
  - Pain and swelling at the DIP joint following direct trauma
- *On examination*
  - Finger tip rests in a flexed posture, typically around 45°
  - Patient is unable to actively extend the DIP joint

23.3.4 Imaging Findings

- Radiographs may reveal a small avulsion fragment from the dorsal base of the distal phalanx
- In some cases, no bony injury is seen and the injury is purely ligamentous
- Normal alignment of the joint rules out subluxation

23.3.5 Treatment Options

- *Nonoperative management*
  - Continuous splinting of the DIP joint in extension for 6–8 weeks
  - Suitable for acute soft tissue injuries (less than 12 weeks old)
  - Also indicated for small or minimally displaced bony avulsions when joint alignment is preserved
- *Surgical management*
  - Required in cases with joint subluxation, large fracture fragments, or chronic deformity
  - Techniques include closed reduction with percutaneous pinning (CRPP), open fixation, tendon reconstruction, or DIP joint fusion
  - Swan neck deformities resulting from chronic mallet finger may require surgical correction

23.3.6 Potential Complications

- Persistent extensor lag of the DIP joint
- Development of swan neck deformity due to imbalance between flexor and extensor forces across the PIP and DIP joints

23.4 Phalanx Fractures

Phalanx fractures are among the most frequent injuries of the hand, involving the distal, middle, or proximal phalanges. These fractures can result from various mechanisms depending on age and are often seen in trauma clinics and emergency settings.

23.4.1 Epidemiology

- Represent around 10% of all skeletal fractures
- More frequent in males with a ratio of approximately two to one
- Distribution by location
  - Distal phalanx is most commonly fractured
  - Followed by middle and then proximal phalanx
- The small finger is most often affected, accounting for nearly 40% of all hand fractures

23.4.2 Mechanism of Injury

- Varies by age group
  - Sports injuries are the leading cause in individuals aged 10–29
  - Machinery-related trauma is more common in those aged 40–69
  - Falls are the primary cause in patients over 70

23.4.3 Associated Injuries

- Nail bed injuries are frequently seen with distal phalanx fractures
- Soft tissue and tendon damage may coexist
- Open wounds can occur in high-energy injuries

23.4.4 Clinical Presentation

- Pain and tenderness localized to the injured finger
- Swelling and visible deformity
- Crepitus may be present
- Rotational deformity observed through scissoring on finger flexion

- Neurovascular assessment is essential
  - Sensory changes suggest digital nerve involvement
  - Doppler exam may be used to evaluate digital artery perfusion

23.4.5 Radiographic Evaluation

- Standard imaging includes posteroanterior, lateral, and oblique views
- In proximal phalanx fractures
  - The apex tends to angle volarly
  - This occurs due to flexion of the proximal fragment (by interossei) and extension of the distal fragment (by the central slip)
- In middle phalanx fractures
  - Fractures distal to the flexor digitorum superficialis (FDS) insertion tend to angulate volarly
  - Fractures proximal to the FDS insertion show dorsal angulation
- Orthogonal views are essential for accurate diagnosis and surgical planning

23.4.6 Treatment Options

- Management depends on the type, location, displacement, and stability of the fracture
- Nondisplaced and stable fractures are treated with splinting or buddy taping
- Unstable, displaced, or intra-articular fractures may require surgical fixation
- Early motion is emphasized post-treatment to minimize stiffness

23.4.7 Complications

- Loss of range of motion is the most frequent long-term issue
- Malunion may develop due to angulation, shortening, or rotational misalignment
- Nonunion is rare but may occur in cases of poor vascularity or inadequate stabilization

23.5 Phalanx Dislocations

Phalanx dislocations are frequent hand injuries, often affecting the proximal interphalangeal joint (PIP) or distal interphalangeal joint (DIP). These injuries are especially common in athletes and result from direct trauma or combined avulsion and shear forces.

23.5.1 Causes and Associated Injuries

- Commonly caused by direct impact or axial loading
- Often linked to fracture-dislocations from impaction or ligament avulsion
- Can occur with swan neck deformities or nail bed injuries, especially when the distal phalanx is involved

23.5.2 Clinical Features

- Pain and noticeable finger deformity
- Skin puckering may suggest soft tissue interposition
- Joint stability is assessed through passive and active range of motion tests
- Neurovascular evaluation is essential to detect any digital nerve traction injuries

23.5.3 Stability Tests

- Lateral stress in extension and 30-degree flexion helps assess collateral ligaments and secondary stabilizers
- Hyperextension test evaluates the volar plate
- Elson's test checks for central slip integrity
- Flexion and extension help gauge active joint stability

23.5.4 Imaging

- X-rays in standard views (AP, lateral, oblique)
- A widened joint space or subtle misalignment (V sign) may suggest subluxation

- Diagnosis is confirmed through history, clinical examination, and imaging

23.5.5 PIP Joint Dislocations

These are the most frequently dislocated joints in the hand. Dislocations can be dorsal, volar, or lateral.

23.5.6 Dorsal PIP Dislocations

- Caused by hyperextension and axial load
- Collateral ligaments and volar plate are disrupted
- May present with avulsion fractures at the base of the middle phalanx
- Categorized into
  - Simple dislocations with partial contact between phalanges
  - Complex dislocations with complete displacement and soft tissue entrapment

23.5.7 Volar PIP Dislocations

- May result from central slip rupture
- Rotational injuries may occur when only one collateral ligament is torn, causing one phalangeal condyle to rotate or buttonhole

23.5.8 Management of PIP Dislocations

23.5.8.1 Nonoperative

- Closed reduction followed by buddy taping or splinting
- Indicated for stable dorsal, volar, or lateral dislocations

23.5.8.2 Operative

- Open reduction may be needed when soft tissue blocks reduction
- In dorsal dislocations, the volar plate is the usual obstruction
- In volar dislocations, the flexor digitorum profundus may prevent reduction
- Lateral dislocations may involve interposed lateral bands

23.5.8.3 Possible Complications

- Flexion contracture at the PIP joint (pseudo-boutonnière), often temporary
- Swan neck deformity after dorsal dislocation due to volar plate injury
- Extensor lag more common after volar dislocation

23.5.8.4 PIP Fracture Dislocations

Fractures can occur along with PIP dislocations, usually from avulsion or shear forces. Volar lip fractures are frequently associated with dorsal dislocations. Highly comminuted injuries are known as pilon-type fractures.

23.5.8.5 Mechanism

- Hyperextension causes failure of the volar plate and avulsion of the volar lip
- Hyperflexion causes central slip failure and dorsal lip avulsion
- Axial loading with the PIP flexed or extended leads to dorsal or volar fracture-dislocations

23.5.9 Management

23.5.9.1 Nonoperative

- Closed reduction and splinting if less than 40% of the joint surface is involved and the joint is stable

23.5.9.2 Operative

- Fixation with pins or screws if more than 40% is involved and the joint is unstable
- External fixator for severely comminuted fractures
- Arthroplasty or fusion for chronic cases

23.5.9.3 DIP Dislocations and Fracture -Dislocations

These are less common than PIP dislocations and are usually dorsal or lateral. Volar dislocations are rare and often involve soft tissue injury due to tight skin coverage.

23.5.10 Management

23.5.10.1 Nonoperative

- Closed reduction and splinting are usually attempted first

23.5.10.2 Operative

- Required when reduction is not successful after two attempts
- In dorsal dislocations, the volar plate or FDP tendon may block reduction
- In volar dislocations, the terminal extensor tendon may obstruct realignment
- Arthroplasty if a large part of the joint is damaged
- Fusion in comminuted injuries with joint preservation
- Amputation may be considered if there is severe bone and soft tissue destruction

23.5.10.3 Complications

- Joint stiffness
- Mallet finger deformity, more likely after volar dislocations

23.6 Base of Thumb Fractures

Fractures at the base of the first metacarpal are classified into extra-articular fractures, partial intra-articular fractures like Bennett fractures, and complete intra-articular fractures such as Rolando fractures.

23.6.1 Epidemiology and Mechanism

- Approximately 80% of thumb fractures involve the base of the first metacarpal
- The most frequent type is an extra-articular epibasal fracture
- Bennett and Rolando fractures usually result from an axial load to the thumb while it is in a flexed position
- Poor alignment or reduction can increase joint contact forces and lead to early arthritis
- Excessive angulation may result in metacarpophalangeal joint hyperextension deformity

23.6.2 Classification

Fractures of the first metacarpal are categorized into

- Extra-articular transverse or oblique fractures
- Bennett fractures involve a single volar-ulnar fragment at the base of the metacarpal that articulates with the trapezium
- Rolando fractures are comminuted, typically Y-shaped or T-shaped, representing complete intra-articular involvement
- Severely comminuted intra-articular fractures may also be seen

23.6.3 Clinical Features

- Sudden pain, swelling, and bruising at the thumb base
- Pain worsens with thumb movement
- Loss of normal thumb motion and grip strength may occur

23.6.4 Imaging and Diagnosis

- Standard radiographic evaluation includes Robert's view (true AP with full forearm pronation), lateral view with slight hand pronation and angled beam, and a 30-degree pronated oblique view
- Bennett fractures may show a small metacarpal base fragment in contact with the trapezium
- Rolando fractures often present with a classic Y-shaped splitting of the base
- Diagnosis is made through clinical examination and imaging

23.6.5 Treatment Approach

23.6.5.1 Nonoperative Management

- Thumb spica casting may be used when extra-articular fractures show less than 30° of angulation after reduction
- Minimally displaced Bennett fractures (less than 1 mm of step-off) can also be managed conservatively

23.6.5.2 Operative management

- Closed reduction with K-wire fixation is suitable when extra-articular fractures exceed 30° of angulation, if reduction cannot be maintained, or for Rolando fractures with small fragments
- Open reduction and internal fixation are advised when Bennett or Rolando fractures have more than 1 mm of displacement and fragments are large enough for fixation
- External fixation with or without traction is reserved for cases with major soft tissue damage, highly comminuted injuries, or small fracture fragments unsuitable for screws

23.6.5.3 Complications

- Potential long-term issues include joint stiffness, instability, posttraumatic arthritis, and malunion

23.6.5.4 Prognosis

- Better outcomes are associated with early treatment and less complex fracture patterns
- Factors such as delayed intervention, intra-articular extension, and comminution typically result in less favorable recovery

23.7 Thumb CMC Dislocation

Dislocations at the base of the thumb CMC joint are rare and usually result from trauma involving axial force on a flexed thumb.

23.7.1 Epidemiology and Mechanism

- These injuries represent less than 1% of all hand injuries
- Most dislocations are dorsal, while volar dislocations are uncommon
- Commonly caused by an axial load applied to a flexed thumb
- Less frequently, a direct dorsal force to the first web space may cause the injury, such as when a handlebar impacts the thumb during a motorcycle accident
- The dorsoradial ligament is usually ruptured, and the anterior oblique ligament may peel off from the base of the first metacarpal but remains connected

23.7.2 Anatomy and Ligament Support

Four key stabilizing ligaments of the thumb CMC joint include

- Anterior oblique ligament, often involved in Bennett or Rolando fractures
- Dorsoradial ligament, frequently disrupted in dislocations
- Posterior oblique ligament
- Intermetacarpal ligament

23.7.3 Clinical Presentation

- Patients typically report trauma involving impact on a fixed object or direct force on the flexed thumb
- Common symptoms include pain, swelling, and bruising near the thenar region
- Difficulty or inability to form a fist may also be noted

23.7.4 Imaging

- Radiographs should include PA, lateral, and Robert's view for evaluating displacement or associated base fractures
- Findings may reveal widening of the joint space and dorsoradial displacement of the first metacarpal
- MRI is useful when instability persists after reduction and helps in planning ligament reconstruction

23.7.5 Diagnosis

- Established through clinical history, physical examination, and imaging findings

23.7.6 Treatment Options

23.7.6.1 Nonoperative

- Closed reduction followed by immobilization with the thumb in extension and pronation
- Appropriate for stable joints post-reduction, suggesting the anterior oblique ligament remains intact

23.7.6.2 Operative

- Closed reduction with temporary percutaneous pinning for unstable joints
- In more severe cases, reconstruction of the dorsal ligament complex using a tendon graft along with pinning may be required
- This is particularly recommended when both the dorsoradial and anterior oblique ligaments are compromised

23.7.6.3 Complications

- Anterior osteophyte formation may be seen in follow-up imaging
- Recurrence of dislocation is rare
- Persistent instability or early degenerative changes may occur in some cases

23.8 Thumb Collateral Ligament Injury

These are injuries to the ligaments that stabilize the metacarpophalangeal (MCP) joint of the thumb, most often involving the ulnar collateral ligament (UCL). They reduce grip and pinch strength and are commonly seen in athletes.

23.8.1 Epidemiology and Terminology

- Injuries to the UCL occur ten times more often than those affecting the radial collateral ligament (RCL)
- UCL injuries represent over 80% of thumb injuries in sports
- Acute UCL injuries are often called Skier's thumb, while chronic degenerative injuries are referred to as Gamekeeper's thumb
- RCL injuries are less frequent and tend to result in joint subluxation rather than instability

23.8.2 Mechanism of Injury

- Most commonly caused by a force that drives the thumb into radial deviation and hyperabduction
- This typically happens during falls or sports-related trauma, such as hitting a fixed object with the thumb while skiing
- UCL tears may lead to a Stener lesion, where the torn ligament gets trapped above the adductor aponeurosis, preventing natural healing
- RCL injuries rarely result in Stener-like lesions due to protective overlying structures

23.8.3 Clinical Presentation

- History of trauma involving the thumb, such as falls or impact from sports equipment
- Ulnar-sided thumb MCP pain that worsens with pinch or grip suggests a UCL injury
- Radial-sided pain is more suggestive of RCL involvement
- Joint deformity is not usually visible
- A tender mass near the UCL may indicate a Stener lesion
- Stress testing in extension and at 30° of flexion helps evaluate for collateral ligament instability
- A difference greater than 15° in side-to-side comparison may indicate a complete tear
- Additional tests like anterior and posterior drawer maneuvers may help assess joint stability

23.8.4 Imaging

- Standard radiographic views include posteroanterior, lateral, oblique, and stress views
- UCL injuries may show small avulsion fractures or dorsal subluxation on lateral views
- RCL injuries may show pronation of the proximal phalanx relative to the metacarpal
- MRI is highly sensitive and specific and is used when the diagnosis is unclear
- Ultrasound may be used if available, although accuracy depends on the operator

23.8.5 Diagnosis

- Based on history and clinical examination, particularly stress testing of the MCP joint
- Confirmed with imaging, typically MRI

23.8.6 Treatment

23.8.6.1 Nonoperative Management

- Immobilization in a thumb spica splint for 4–6 weeks
- Suitable for partial tears or complete tears with less than 15° of instability

23.8.6.2 Surgical Management

- Repair is recommended for complete ligament ruptures with significant instability or for confirmed Stener lesions
- Delayed injuries or failed repairs may require reconstruction using tendon grafts
- In cases with chronic instability or failed prior surgery, MCP joint fusion or adductor advancement may be considered as salvage options

23.8.6.3 Complications

- Joint stiffness at the MCP and interphalangeal joints is the most frequent problem after treatment
- Persistent instability may occur in higher-grade tears treated without surgery
- Superficial radial nerve symptoms such as numbness may be noted near the incision site

23.8.6.4 Metacarpal fractures

Fractures of the metacarpal bones are among the most frequent injuries of the hand, often resulting from trauma, falls, or sports injuries. They can affect any of the five metacarpals and may involve the head, neck, shaft, or base.

23.8.6.5 Epidemiology and Common Sites

- Metacarpal fractures account for approximately 30–40% of all hand fractures
- The most commonly fractured metacarpal is the fifth (little finger), especially at the neck
- Males are more commonly affected than females, particularly in the younger age groups

23.8.6.6 Mechanism of Injury

- Direct blow to the hand, such as punching a wall or another person (typical for fifth metacarpal neck fractures)
- Falls on an outstretched hand
- Crush injuries from machinery or accidents
- Axial loading of the metacarpal shaft during forceful grip or trauma

23.8.6.7 Anatomic Classification

- Head fractures
- Neck fractures (common site for boxer's fracture)
- Shaft fractures
- Base fractures (intra-articular and extra-articular)

23.8.6.8 Clinical Presentation

- Pain, swelling, and bruising over the injured area
- Deformity such as angulation, shortening, or rotational malalignment
- Tenderness over the fracture site
- Limited range of motion and pain with gripping
- Rotational deformities may cause finger overlap during flexion (scissoring)

23.8.6.9 Physical Examination

- Observe for swelling, visible angulation, or rotational alignment
- Test digital cascade by asking the patient to flex all fingers
- Check neurovascular status, especially for sensation and capillary refill
- Evaluate extensor and flexor tendon function

23.8.6.10 Imaging

- Standard radiographs include anteroposterior, oblique, and lateral views of the hand
- Rotational deformities are best assessed clinically
- CT may be considered for intra-articular base fractures or comminuted injuries

23.8.7 Treatment

23.8.7.1 Nonoperative Management

- Most metacarpal fractures can be managed with closed reduction and splinting
- Indications include fractures with minimal angulation, shortening, or rotational deformity
- Common immobilization methods include ulnar gutter splints or functional bracing
- Acceptable angulation varies by digit (up to 40° for the fifth metacarpal neck, 10° for the index)

23.8.7.2 Operative Management

- Indicated for fractures with significant angulation, rotation, or shortening
- Open fractures or intra-articular involvement often require surgical fixation
- Techniques include percutaneous pinning, plate and screw fixation, or intramedullary devices
- Early motion is encouraged postoperatively to minimize stiffness

23.8.7.3 Complications

- Malunion with rotational deformity or angulation
- Stiffness of metacarpophalangeal joints
- Extensor lag or loss of grip strength
- Nonunion or delayed union (less common)
- Post-traumatic arthritis, especially in intra-articular fractures

Multiple Choice Questions

1. Camper chiasm is located at the level of:
   (a) Distalal phalanx
   (b) Proximal phalanx
   (c) Middle phalanx
   (d) Meta-tarso phalyngeal joint
2. Which is true for Mallet Finger?
   (a) caused by disruption of the terminal flexor tendon
   (b) occurs at PIP joint
   (c) ring finger is most commonly involved
   (d) caused by disruption of the terminal extensor tendon
3. Which is true for Jersey Finger?
   (a) traumatic extensor tendon injury
   (b) avulsion injury of the FDS from the insertion

(c) avulsion injury of the FDP from the insertion
(d) middle finger is most commonly involved

4. True for Seymour Fractures are
(a) displaced distal phalangeal physeal fractures
(b) more common in old age
(c) most common finger involved is index finger
(d) more common in female than male

5. True for Sagittal Band Ruptures are:
(a) lead to dislocation of the extensor tendons
(b) ring finger is most commonly involved
(c) not caused by chronic inflammatory process
(d) lead to dislocation of the flexor tendons

Answers: 1. (b), 2. (d), 3. (c), 4. (a), 5. (a)

Fractures and Dislocations Around the Hip

24

Tushar Gupta

24.1 Hip Dislocation

Hip dislocation is a commonly seen entity in trauma and emergency settings. Owing to the bony socket and the surrounding soft tissue anatomy, the hip joint is well contained. A force of at least 400N is required to displace the femoral head out of its socket.

24.1.1 Mechanism of Injury

High-velocity injuries and motor vehicle accidents, especially in a setting of polytrauma. It has been known to be present with associated fractures of femur.

The position of the limb at the time of the impact dictates the direction of hip dislocation and hence is classified accordingly as:

- Posterior: *Most common*
- Anterior
- Central

T. Gupta (✉)
Department of Orthopedics, All India Institute of Medical Sciences, Rishikesh, Uttarakhand, India

24.2 Posterior Dislocation

24.2.1 Mechanism of Injury

High-impact injury to the knee head on, with the limb in slight flexion, adduction, and internal rotation (For instance: dashboard injury—Fig 24.1) can lead to a posterior dislocation of the hip. It may be associated with a common posterior wall acetabular fracture.

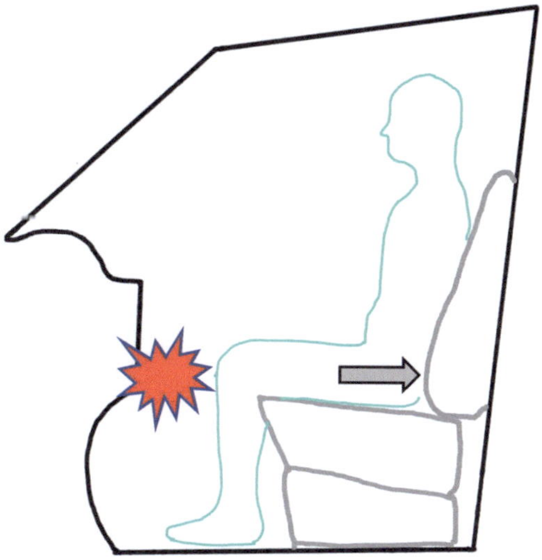

Fig. 24.1 Dashboard injury—arrow shows the line of impact and hence the femoral head dislocates posteriorly out of the acetabular socket

V. Kumar et al. (eds.), *A Quick Guide to Essential Orthopedics*,
https://doi.org/10.1007/978-981-95-2676-5_24

24.2.2 Clinical Features

The limb would be found in a FAdIR attitude (Flexion, Adduction, and Internal rotation) along with an abnormal solid globular mass palpable in the gluteal region (femoral head) with possible limb shortening. However, this position may be affected by presence of shaft femur fracture.

Neurovascular examination is pertinent in such settings, with special focus on the sciatic nerve. Proceeding with imaging is the next logical step in case of clinical suspicion.

24.2.3 Radiology

A pelvis with bilateral hip joint radiograph in the anteroposterior projection (Fig. 24.2) will show us a high riding and smaller head as compared to the other side. Other noteworthy findings may be of associated fractures such as those of the pelvis, posterior wall acetabulum and femoral head or shaft.

A CT scan of the pelvis is routinely performed in all such cases, particularly to rule out all the associated fractures and to look at the integrity of the socket. It also helps us rule out any intra articular loose bodies or incarcerated fragments.

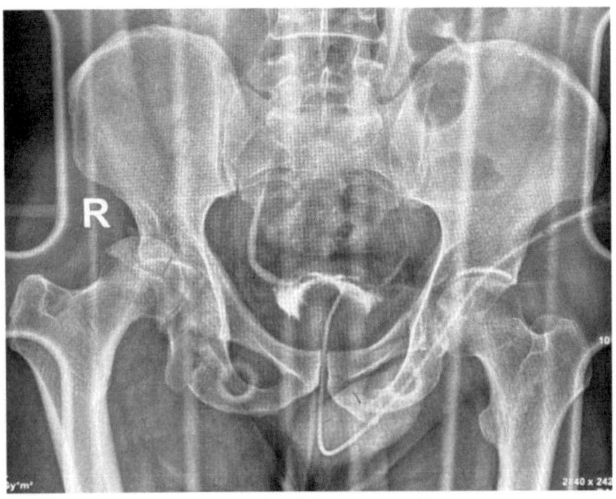

Fig. 24.2 Posterior hip dislocation with associated fractures

24.2.4 Classification

Thompson and Epstein classification

- Type I—dislocation with no more than minor chip fractures
- Type II—dislocation with single large fragment of posterior acetabular wall
- Type III—dislocation with comminuted fragments of posterior acetabular wall
- Type IV—dislocation with fracture through acetabular floor
- Type V—dislocation with fracture through acetabular floor and femoral head.

24.2.5 Treatment

The dislocated hip must be reduced as soon as possible (ideally within 6 h) as the chances of the femoral head going into avascular necrosis increase with the hip staying outside the joint for prolonged periods. This can be done under sedation or general anesthesia. This should be avoided in cases of concomitant femoral fractures in the neck area or distal to it.

Most commonly used manoeuvre is the Allis manoeuvre wherein the pelvis is stabilized and an inline traction is given with the hip in flexion. The hip is reduced with gentle rotations.

A clunk and disappearance of the globular swelling (of head) would indicate the reduction of the hip joint. A pre-reduction assessment and documentation of the sciatic nerve status is imperative in these cases.

Other Reduction Manoeuvres:

1. Bigelow
2. Captain Morgan
3. East Baltimore lift
4. Stimson
5. Lefkowitz
6. Rocket launcher/Piggyback
7. Rochester

The stability of this reduced hip joint is assessed by checking the rotations gently and giving provocative forces to the hip joint. The

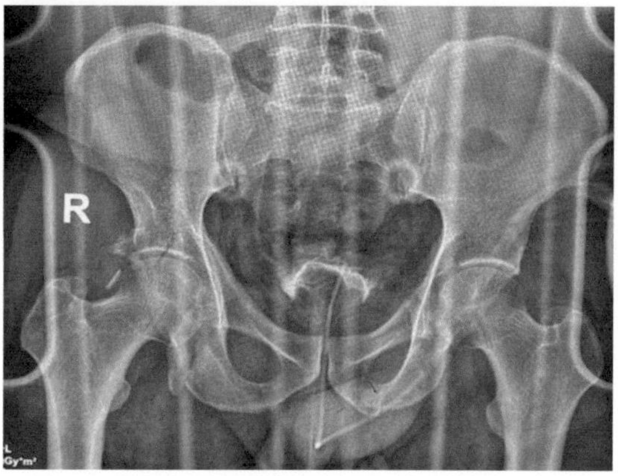

Fig. 24.3 Reduced posterior hip dislocation with associated fractures

limb is to be kept in skeletal traction after reduction and further plan be decided after check x-ray (Fig. 24.3) and getting the post reduction CT.

Indications of Surgery:
1. Persistent dislocation
2. Unstable reduction
3. Non concentric reduction
4. Associated fractures warranting surgical fixation
5. Intra articular loose bodies

Early Complications:
1. Sciatic nerve injury
2. Vascular injury—superior gluteal artery
3. Associated fractured femoral shaft

Late Complications:
1. Osteonecrosis of the femoral head
2. Myositis ossificans
3. Unreduced dislocation
4. Secondary osteoarthritis
5. Recurrent instability

24.3 Anterior Dislocation X-Ray Showing Pubic and Obturator Dislocation

Rare injuries accounting for up to 20% of all hip dislocations.

24.3.1 Mechanism of Injury

High energy trauma with the limb in abduction and external rotation

24.3.2 Clinical Features

It is worth noting that anterior dislocations are more commonly associated with femoral head impaction and chondral injury. The limb is found in the FAbER attitude (Flexion, abduction and external rotation).

24.3.3 Radiology

Pelvis with bilateral hip joint radiograph in the anteroposterior projection—the affected head appears to be larger than the other femoral head and is found medial or inferior to the acetabulum.

CT scan of the pelvis is routinely performed in all such cases particularly to rule out all the associated fractures.

24.3.4 Classification

Anatomical classification:

- type I—pubic (superior)
- type II obturator (inferior) injuries

24.3.5 Treatment

Closed/Open reduction

24.4 Central Dislocation

24.4.1 Mechanism of Injury

Femoral head maybe displaced medially by a blow on the greater trochanter or a fall on the side. This 'dislocation' occurs through the 'fractured' acetabulum (Fig. 24.4).

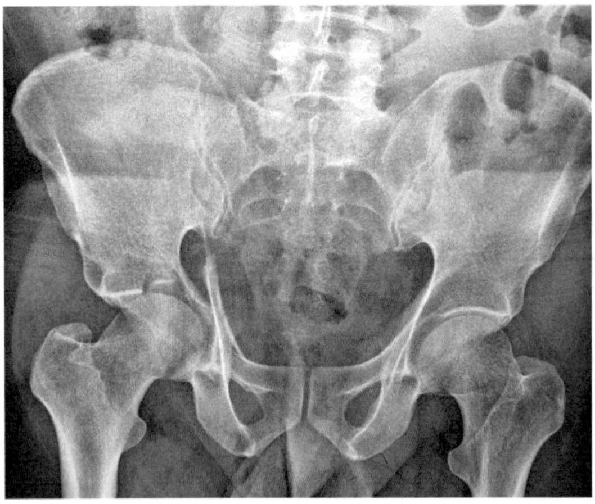

Fig. 24.4 Central hip dislocation with associated fractures

24.4.2 Treatment

Reduction is achieved by means of a distal femoral pin with or without a lateral trochanteric pin.

24.5 Femoral Head Fracture

These are commonly seen in association with femoral head dislocation. It is worth noting that it is more commonly associated with posterior hip dislocation; however, the chances of femoral head getting fractured are more when the hip dislocates anteriorly.

24.5.1 Associated Injuries:

- Acetabular fractures
- Femoral shaft fractures
- Femoral neck fractures
- Knee ligament injuries
- Sciatic nerve injuries

24.5.2 Pipkin Classification

Type I—The fracture line is inferior to the fovea
Type II—The fracture fragment includes the fovea
Type III—As with types I and II but with an associated femoral neck fracture
Type IV—Any pattern of femoral head fracture and an acetabular fracture

Femoral head fractures must be fixed operatively if the fragment is large enough. Headless/Herbert screws are commonly used for fixation. Herbert and headless screws xray

24.5.3 Complications:

- Osteoarthritis
- Osteonecrosis
- Sciatic nerve palsy
- Fracture malreduction
- Non-union
- Heterotopic ossification

24.6 Proximal Femoral Fractures

Classified as Intracapsular (Femur neck fracture) and Extracapsular (Intertrochanteric and Subtrochanteric fractures). Mostly occur secondary to low velocity injury such as fall from standing height in elderly population and high-energy trauma in young healthy adult. Other causes affecting the balance of the patient maybe contributory such as alcoholism, parkinsonism, etc.

They are important to be dealt with care as they determine the morbidity and mortality in the elderly patient.

24.7 Femur Neck Fracture

24.7.1 Anatomical Classification: Figures 24.5, 24.6, 24.7 and 24.8

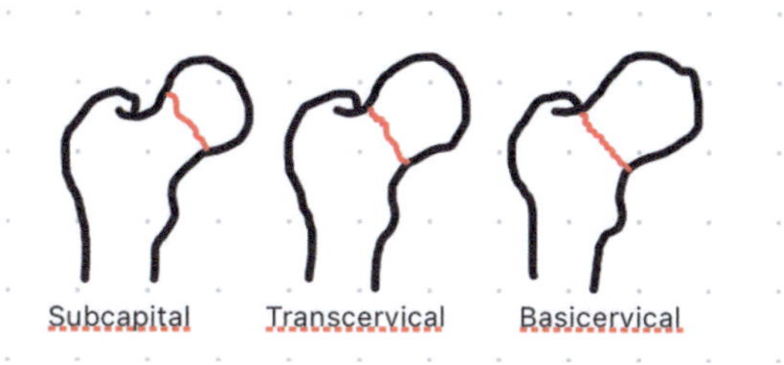

Fig. 24.5 Anatomical classification of fracture neck femur

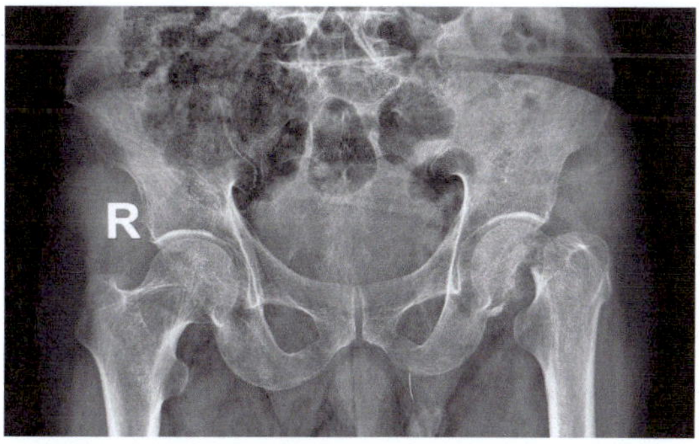

Fig. 24.6 Subcapital neck femur fracture

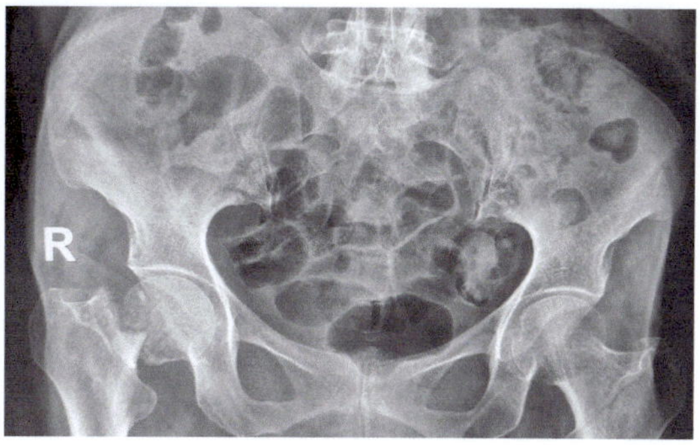

Fig. 24.7 Transcervical neck femur fracture

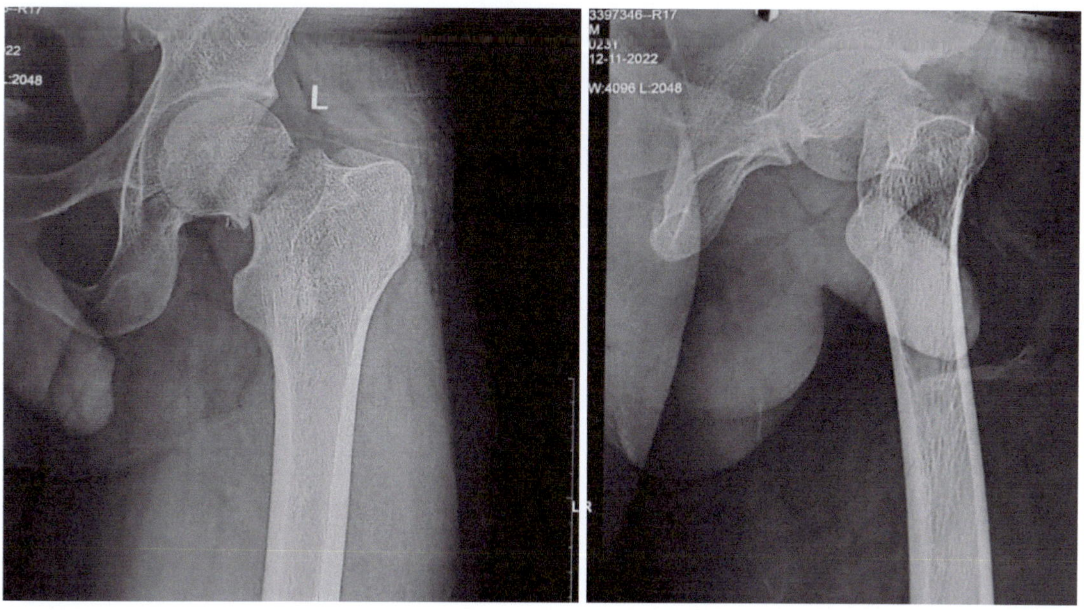

Fig. 24.8 Basicervical neck femur fracture

24.7.2 Pauwell Classification: Fig. 24.9

24.7.3 Garden Classification: Figure 24.10

- Stage I—an incomplete impacted fracture, including the so-called ‘abduction fracture’ in which the femoral head is tilted into valgus in relation to the neck
- Stage II—a complete but undisplaced fracture
- Stage III—a complete fracture with moderate displacement
- Stage IV—a severely displaced fracture

24.8 Intertrochanteric Fractures

Fracture present in the intertrochanteric region (Fig. 24.11). Commonly divided as:

Stable
Unstable

- severe comminution: fractured fragments are very small
- posteromedial cortex fractured: fracture line extending into the posteromedial part of proximal femur
- reverse oblique type: fracture line extends from proximal-medial to distal-lateral through intertrochanteric region
- subtrochanteric extension: fracture line extending below the intertrochanteric region

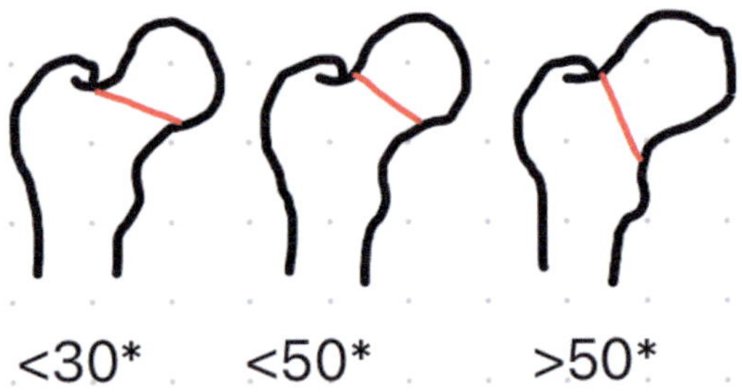

Fig. 24.9 Pauwell classification of neck femur fracture (Red line indicates site and orientation of fracture line and the angle it forms with the horizontal plane)

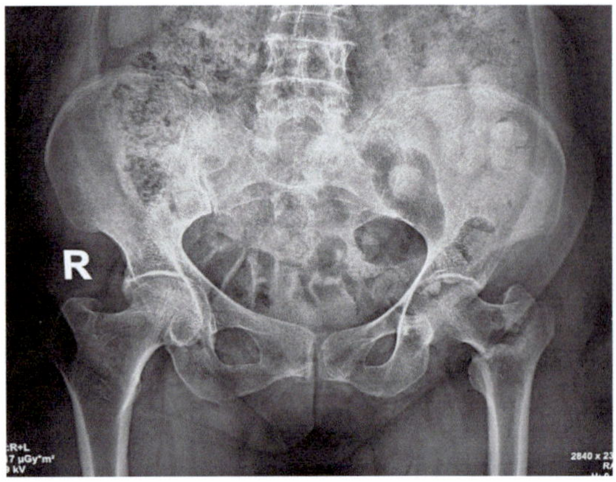

Fig. 24.11 Intertrochanteric femur fracture

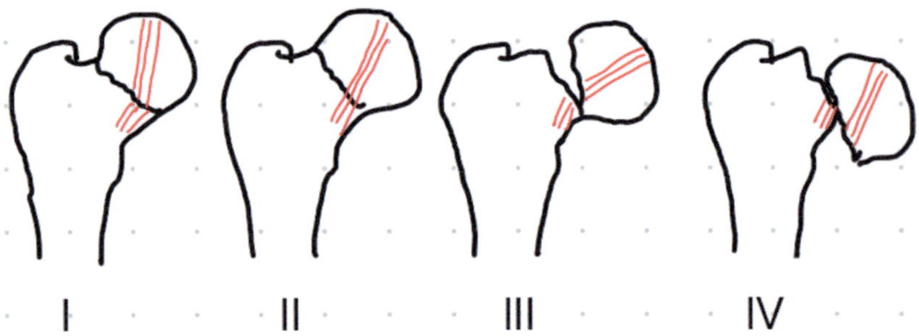

Fig. 24.10 Garden classification of neck femur fracture

24.9 Subtrochanteric Hip Fractures

Fractures found within 5 cm from the lesser trochanter. They occur secondary to high-energy trauma in young or in the setting of 'atypical' fractures secondary to osteoporosis, osteomalacia, Paget's disease, metastatic deposits or the atypical changes seen in association with bisphosphonate use.

24.9.1 Clinical Features of Proximal Femur Fractures

1. Pain in the hip/proximal thigh
2. Swelling in hip/proximal thigh
3. Limb deformity—FAbER (Flexion, Abduction and External Rotation deformity)
4. Limb length discrepancy
5. Associated fractures of acetabulum/lower limb

It is noteworthy that the degree external rotation deformity can act as a guide to differentiate fracture neck femur (lesser deformity or the lateral border of foot does not touch the bed) from Intertrochanteric fracture (more deformity or the lateral border of foot touches the bed). This is because the hip joint capsule is attached to the intertrochanteric line of femur and acts as a restraint to the external rotation in case of fracture neck femur.

24.9.2 Investigations

1. Pelvis with bilateral hip X-ray—will show obvious fractures (Fig. 24.12)
2. NCCT—to rule out associated pelvis fractures
3. MRI—to rule out occult fractures

24.9.3 Treatment

1. Patient stabilization as per ATLS protocol
2. Adequate analgesia
3. Splintage/traction
4. Non-surgical: Traction/Boot and bar application (Fig. 24.13)
   (a) Extremely comorbid patients who are not fit for surgery
   (b) Patient refusal
5. Surgical: Kindly refer to next section

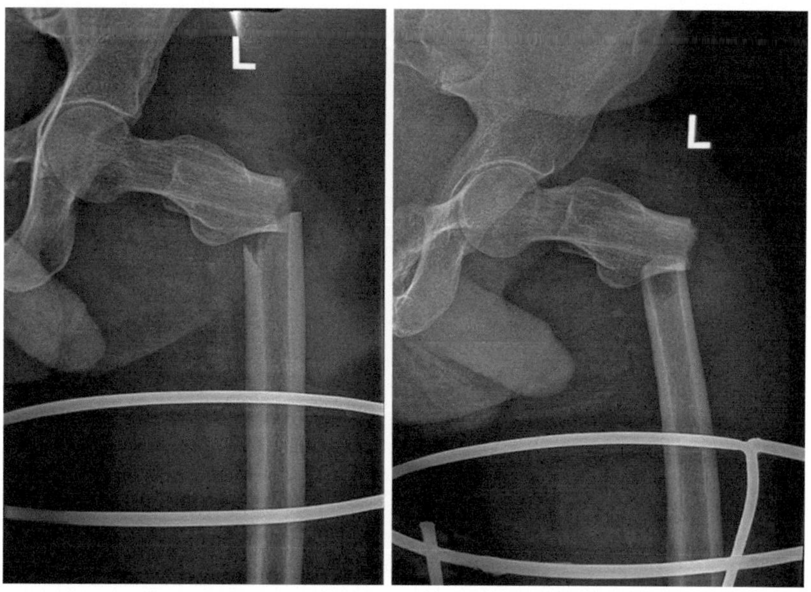

Fig. 24.12 Subtrochanteric femur fracture

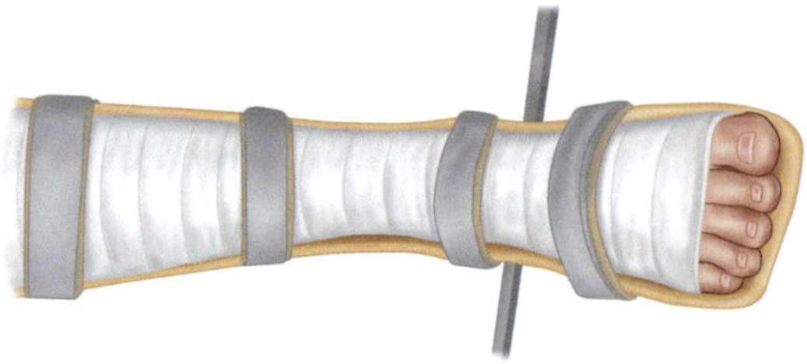

Fig. 24.13 Boot and bar splint—to avoid rotation of proximal fragment

24.10 Surgery

24.10.1 Fracture Neck Femur

1. Cannulated cancellous (CC) screw fixation:

Fixation of choice in young patients with good bone quality in whom osteosynthesis is anticipated to give positive outcomes.

Three screws are used to fix the fracture in an inverted triangle pattern (Fig. 24.14).

2. Prosthetic Replacement

Patients who are >60 years old or have a poor bone stock/are anticipated to have poor bone healing are advised to undergo prosthetic replacement.

Patients who were active pre-injury and have a significant life expectancy remaining or are desirous of activities beyond community ambulation are advised a total hip replacement (THR) (Fig. 24.15).

Patients who are frail or are homebound/community ambulator pre-injury or have a limited life expectancy are advised a modular bipolar hemi replacement (Fig. 24.16).

24.10.2 Intertrochanteric Fracture

Must undergo internal fixation by means of

1. Dynamic hip screw

X-ray image

Used in stable patterns

2. Intramedullary nailing—proximal femoral nailing system Fixation of choice in all fractures of this type (Fig. 24.17).

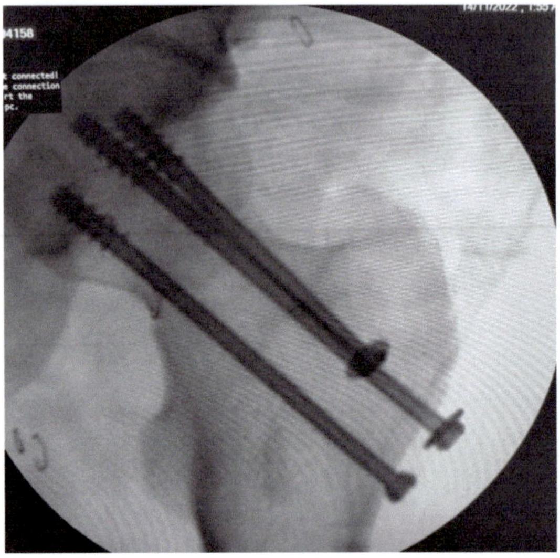

Fig. 24.14 Neck femur fracture fixed with CC screws in an inverted triangle pattern

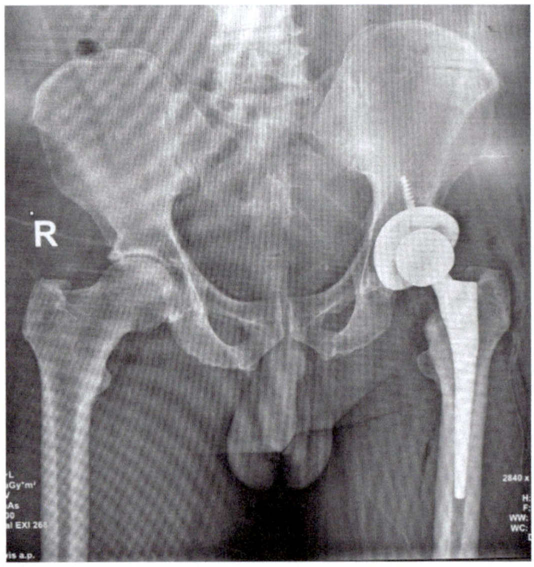

Fig. 24.15 THR done in case of fracture neck femur

24.10.3 Subtrochanteric Fracture

Must undergo internal fixation by means of

1. Dynamic condylar screw

Used in cases where intramedullary fixation cannot be done

X-ray image

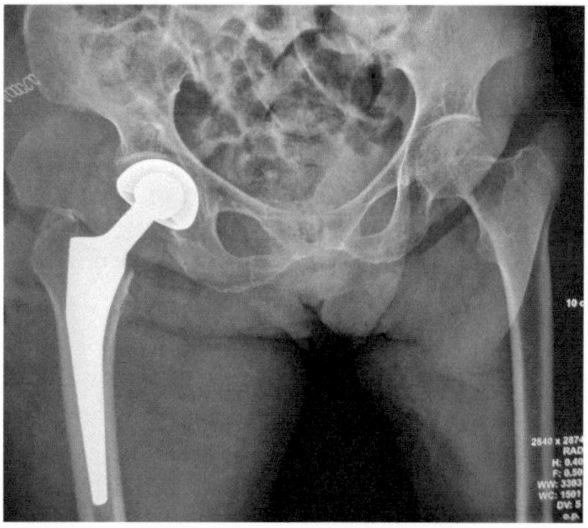

Fig. 24.16 Bipolar hemi replacement done in case of fracture neck femur

2. Intramedullary nailing—long proximal femoral nailing system

Fixation of choice in all fractures of this type (Fig. 24.18)

3. Proximal femoral plating with locking screws

24.10.4 Complications

1. Osteonecrosis
2. Non-union
3. Osteoarthritis
4. Failed fixation
5. Malunion
6. Non-union

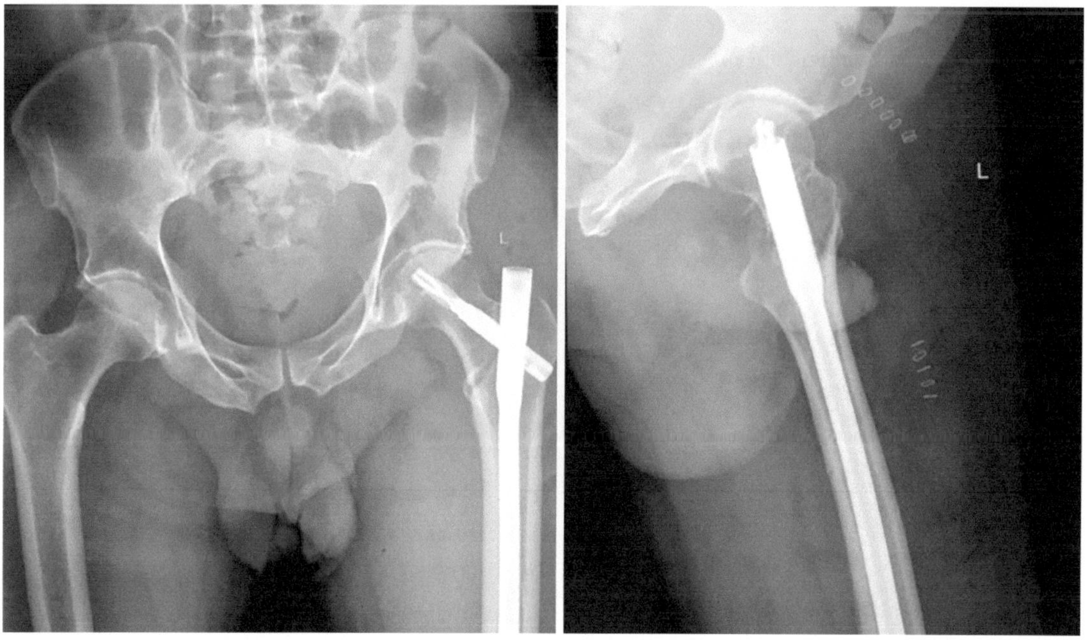

Fig. 24.17 Intramedullary nailing done in case of Intertrochanteric fracture femur

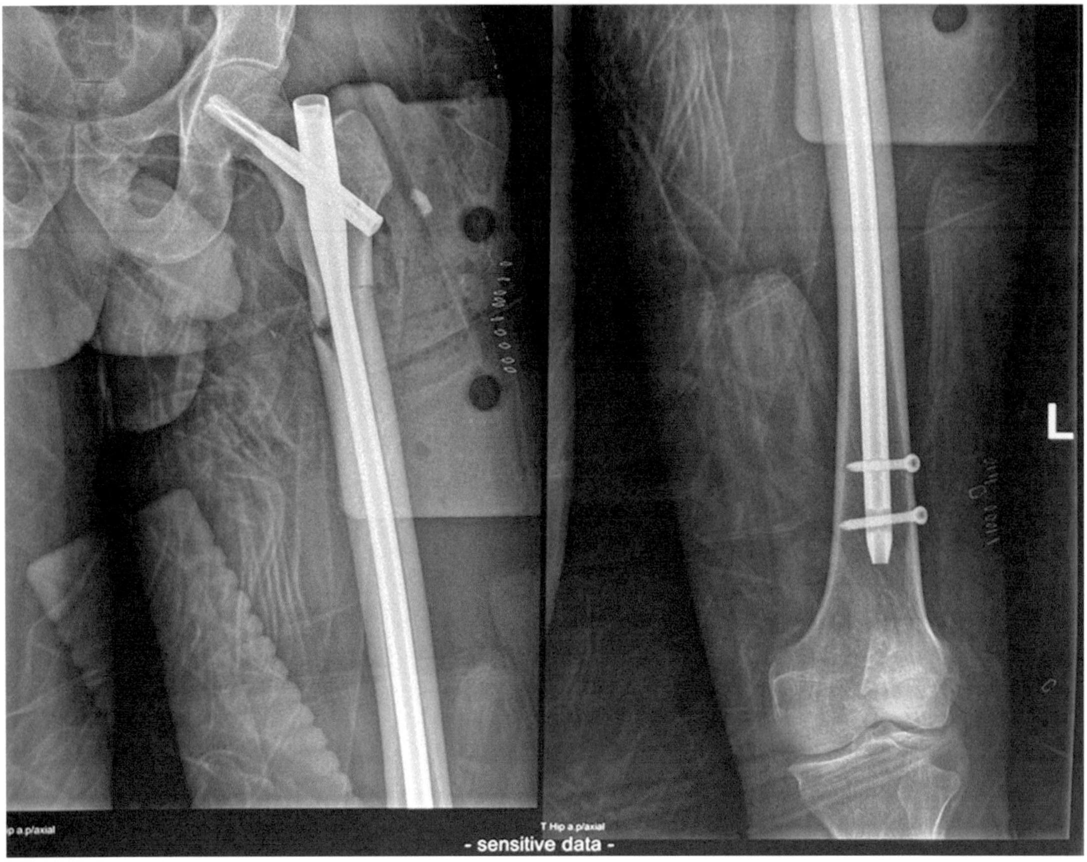

Fig. 24.18 Subtrochanteric fracture fixed with Intramedullary nailing

Multiple Choice Questions

1. Which of the following is not a complication of hip dislocation?
   (a) Osteonecrosis of the femoral head
   (b) Myositis ossificans
   (c) Unreduced dislocation
   (d) Primary osteoarthritis
2. Which of the following is correct order of reduction of dislocated hip?
   (i) Neurological examination
   (ii) CT
   (iii) X-ray
   (iv) Stability check
   (v) Skeletal traction
   (a) i,ii,iii,iv,v,ii
   (b) i,iii,iv,i,iii,v,ii
   (c) v,iv,iii,ii,i
   (d) none of these
3. A 68-year-old extremely active male undergoes stroke and residual hemiparesis with fracture left neck femur. The patient is fit for surgery although his weakness is not expected to recover and he is expected to stay dependent. What is the most suitable method of management for him?
   (a) Boot and bar
   (b) Bipolar hemiarthroplasty
   (c) Total hip replacement
   (d) Patient/family should decide
4. Which of the following areas is predilected to have atypical fractures caused due to an anti-osteoporotic drug taken once weekly?
   (a) Head femur
   (b) Intertrochanteric femur
   (c) Subtrochanteric femur
   (d) Shaft femur

5. Dynamic condylar screw is used to fix:
   (a) Fracture lateral condyle femur
   (b) Facture lateral condyle tibia
   (c) Fracture subtrochanteric femur
   (d) Any condylar fracture can be fixed with DCS

Answers: 1. (d), 2. (b), 3. (b), 4. (c), 5. (c)

References for Further Reading

Masiewicz S, Mabrouk A, Johnson DE. Posterior hip dislocation. [Updated 2023 Jul 31]. In: StatPearls [Internet]. Treasure Island (FL): StatPearls Publishing; 2023. Available from: https://www.ncbi.nlm.nih.gov/books/NBK459319/.

Kazley J, Bagchi K. Femoral neck fractures. [Updated 2023 May 8]. In: StatPearls [Internet]. Treasure Island (FL): StatPearls Publishing; 2023. Available from: https://www.ncbi.nlm.nih.gov/books/NBK537347/.

Attum B, Pilson H. Intertrochanteric femur fracture. [Updated 2023 Aug 8]. In: StatPearls [Internet]. Treasure Island (FL): StatPearls Publishing; 2023. Available from: https://www.ncbi.nlm.nih.gov/books/NBK493161/.

Giannoudis PV, Kontakis G, Christoforakis Z, Akula M, Tosounidis T, Koutras C. Management, complications and clinical results of femoral head fractures. Injury. 2009;40(12):1245–51. https://doi.org/10.1016/j.injury.2009.10.024. Epub 2009 Nov 7. PMID: 19897188.

Kellam P, Ostrum RF. Systematic review and meta-analysis of avascular necrosis and posttraumatic arthritis after traumatic hip dislocation. J Orthop Trauma. 2016;30(1):10–6. https://doi.org/10.1097/BOT.0000000000000419. PMID: 26849386.

25 Femur Fracture

Tushar Gupta and Vishal Kumar

25.1 Introduction & Epidemiology

Femur shaft fractures are common fractures encountered by trauma surgeons and orthopedic surgeons. Its annual incidence is 10 per 1,00,000 person-years. The incidence of shaft femur fracture is common among the young, decreases after age 20, and significantly increases in the elderly. The force causing the femoral shaft fracture may be:

- direct trauma: forceful blow to the thigh
- indirect trauma: twisting or bending forces acting on the femur

It is associated with high-velocity trauma in the young, such as motor vehicle accidents. In contrast, in the elderly, the fracture is associated with low-energy trauma, such as falls, and with conditions like smoking, long-term steroid use or any other condition leading to osteopenia.

T. Gupta (✉)
Department of Orthopedics, All India Institute of Medical Sciences, Rishikesh, Uttarakhand, India

V. Kumar
Department of Orthopaedics, PGIMER, Chandigarh, Chandigarh, India

25.2 Clinical Anatomy

Clinically the femur is divided into three parts: the proximal femur (including head, neck, intertrochanteric area, and subtrochanteric area), the shaft of the femur, and distal femur (includes metaphyseal-diaphyseal junction to the articular surface of the knee, involving the distal 15 cm of the femur). Among the proximal femur, subtrochanteric femur fracture occurs within 5 cm of the lesser trochanter (Fig. 25.1).

The femoral shaft is a cylindrical structure. It is expanded inferiorly and narrowest in the middle. It has a convexity directed anteriorly and is oriented obliquely downwards and medially. The femur shaft has three borders (lateral, medial, and posterior) and three surfaces (anterior, medial, and lateral). The two medial and lateral borders are smooth, and the posterior border has a broad, roughed ridge known as linea aspera with a distinct medial and lateral ridge. The Linea Aspera in the upper 1/3rd diverges to form an additional posterior surface. And in the lower 1/3rd, the Linea Aspera diverges to form a posterior popliteal surface.

The blood supply of the shaft and distal part of the femur is by perforating branches of the deep femoral artery.

V. Kumar et al. (eds.), *A Quick Guide to Essential Orthopedics*,
https://doi.org/10.1007/978-981-95-2676-5_25

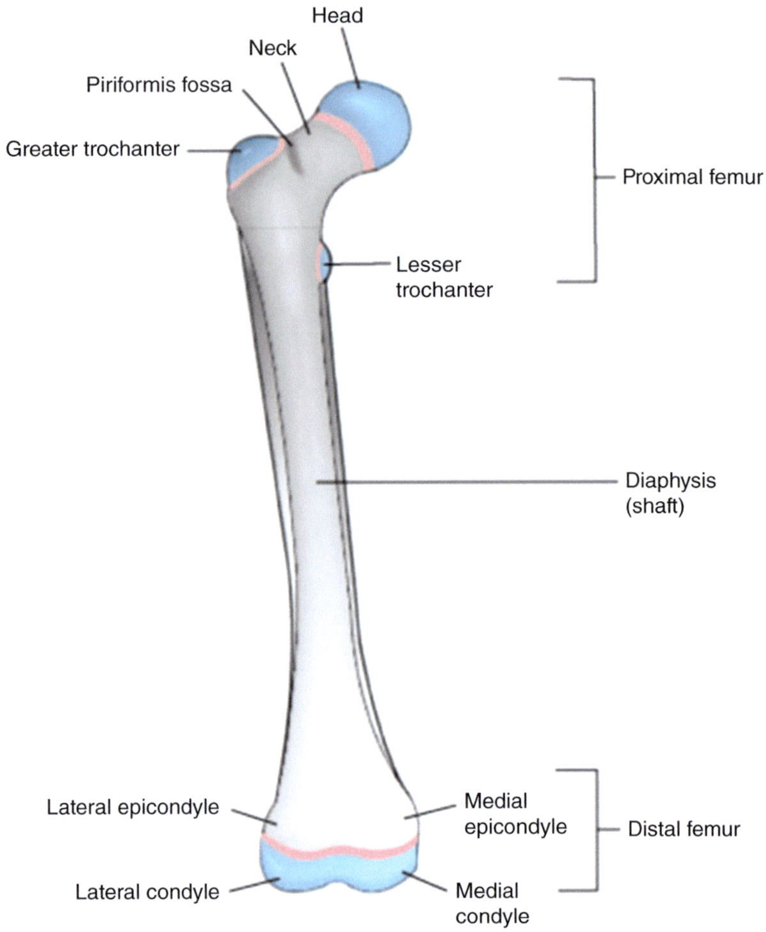

Fig. 25.1 Anatomy of the femur

25.3 Clinical Features

(A) History: H/o high velocity trauma (motor vehicle accident >100 kmph) in young adults and trivial trauma/fall (not otherwise known to cause fracture) in elderly.

(B) Symptoms:
   (a) Pain and swelling in the affected thigh
   (b) Unable to bear weight on the affected limb
   (c) Visible deformity, either shortening or externally rotated
   (d) Could be associated with an open wound
   (e) Associated fractures (pelvis, sacrum, bones of upper extremity)

(C) Signs:
   (a) Tenderness at the fracture site
   (b) Palpable deformity at the fracture site with abnormal mobility and crepitus
   (c) Restricted ROM at affected hip and knee

It is essential to check for distal pulses at ATA (anterior tibial artery), PTA (posterior tibial artery), and DPA (Dorsalis Pedis artery).

25.3.1 Deformity at Thigh Following Shaft of Femur Fracture

The proximal fragment has a specific deformity at the hip. Due to the pull of stronger muscles like hip flexors, abductors, and external rotators, the proximal fragment is flexed, abducted, and externally rotated. The distal fragment is adducted due to the pull of adductors (Fig. 25.2).

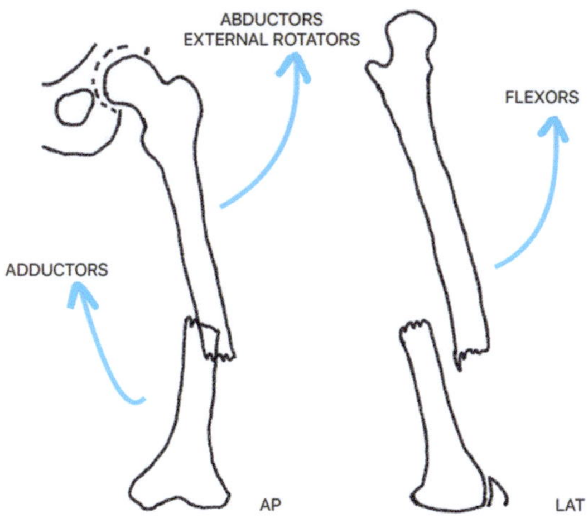

Fig. 25.2 Depiction of the muscular forces in fracture shaft of femur

25.4 Investigations

(A) X-ray:
 (a) X-ray is the first line of investigation. X-ray of the thigh, including hip and knee, in both the anteroposterior and lateral view is advised (Fig. 25.3).
 (b) Also, chest and pelvis X-rays should be advised to the patient as a part of ATLS protocol to rule out other injuries associated with trauma. In high-velocity trauma, there is an incidence of 2.5–9% of ipsilateral shaft and neck femur fractures, especially in young adults and associated with multiple injuries.

(B) E-fast: To assess additional injuries

Fig. 25.3 Xray showing fracture of right femur in AP and lateral projection

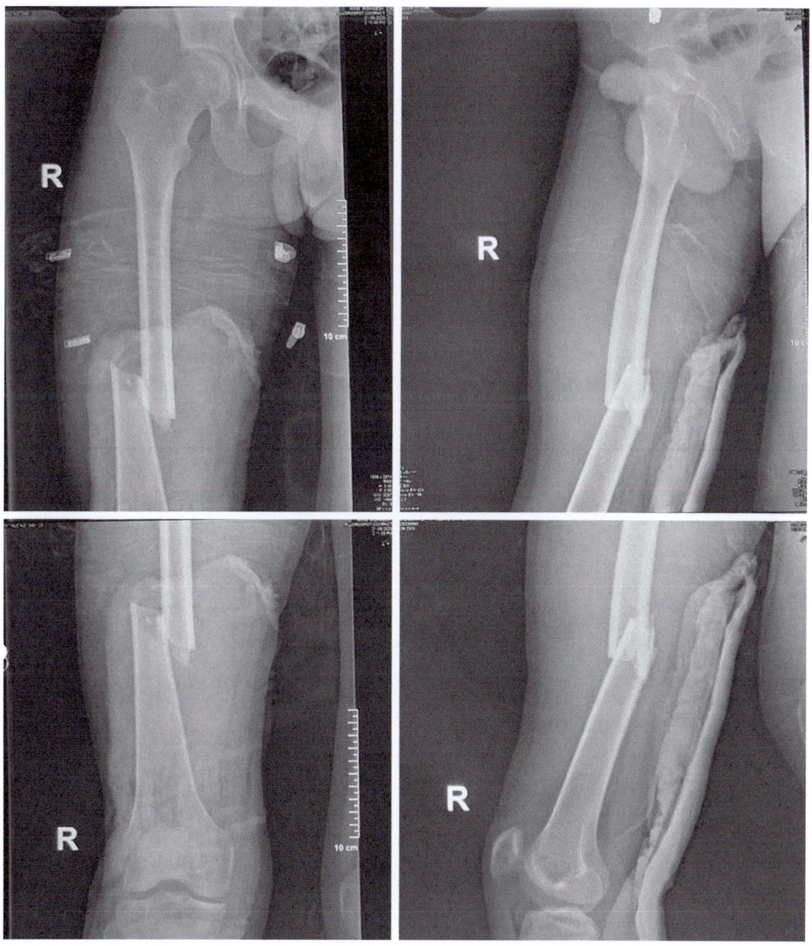

(C) Additional investigations:
 (a) Complete blood count: As the femur fracture is associated with up to 1 L of blood loss in the thigh, a complete blood count assessment is necessary. If associated with pelvic injury or polytrauma, the patient may present with anemia and shock.
 (b) Other tests: Kidney function test, Liver function test, Prothrombin time, Viral Markers, ECG, may be done for initial assessment and preoperative anesthetic checkup.
 (c) CT scan: to assess other associated injuries such as head injury, injury of chest, abdomen, and pelvis

25.5 Treatment

(A) Conservative Management:
 (a) Pavlik Harness: for immobilization of fractures in children <6 months.
 (b) Bryant's traction: Historically used for children <3 years or weight <10 kg (Fig. 25.4). The child is placed on a splint bedframe with the hip flexed at 90° and traction applied at the leg. The vascularity of the limbs should be monitored.
 (c) Hip spica casting: It is applied for the pediatric population, positioned at 30° abduction, 30° to 40° flexion, and external rotation. Opted for children between 3 and 5 years.

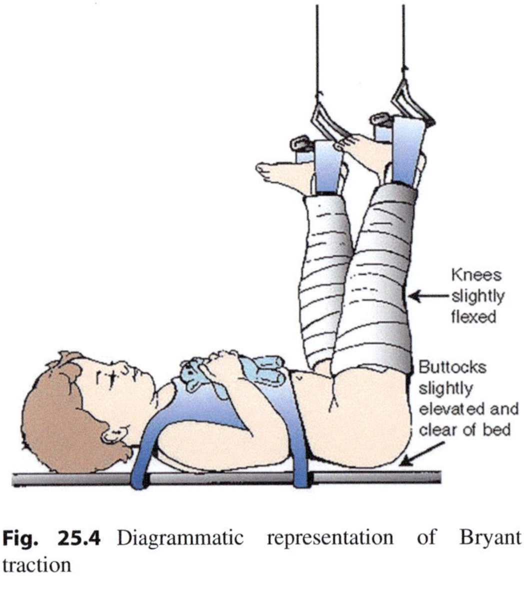

Fig. 25.4 Diagrammatic representation of Bryant traction

(B) Surgical Management:
 (a) Flexible Intramedullary nailing is usually the most preferred procedure and is opted for the shaft of femur fracture, which is of closed type in patients (Fig. 25.5).
 (b) Submuscular plating: Preferred in unstable fractures, very proximal or distal and severely comminuted fractures in children of age >5 years and weight >49 kg (Fig. 25.6).
 (c) External fixation: It can act as definitive fixation as well as temporary fixation and is preferred for open and contaminated wounds, neurovascular injury associated with shaft of femur fracture as part of damage control orthopedics.
 (d) Rigid intramedullary nailing: A titanium or stainless-steel rod designed with prebend according to the axis of the femur is placed antegrade into the medullary canal of the femur, usually through the greater trochanter or piriformis, and locked with screws both proximally and distally (Fig. 25.7). In another type of intramedullary fixation of fracture of the shaft of the femur, a nail can be introduced distally through the distal femur also in a retrograde fashion.
 (e) Plate fixation: It is the preferred method of fixation for the comminuted shaft of femur fracture or femur fractures with the extension of fracture line into distal femur or intraarticular extension.

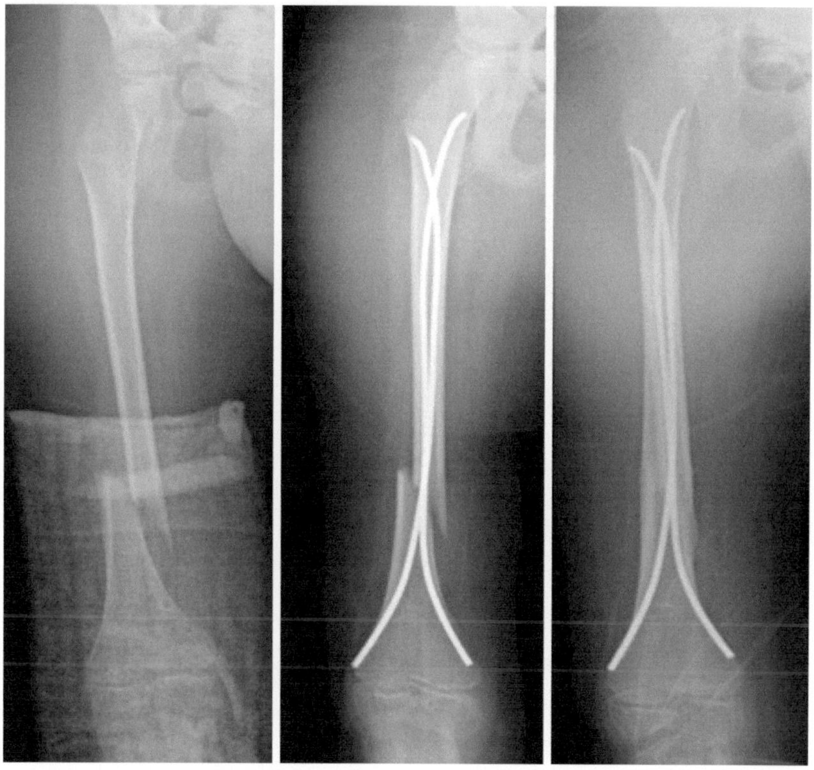

Fig. 25.5 Flexible intramedullary nail in a case of fracture shaft of femur

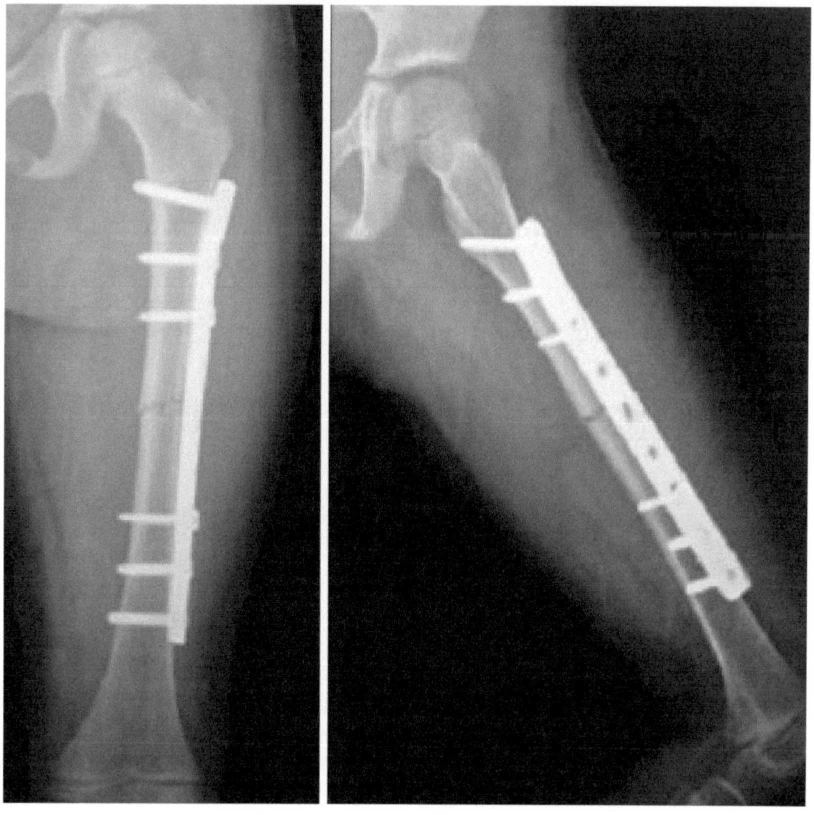

Fig. 25.6 Submuscular plating

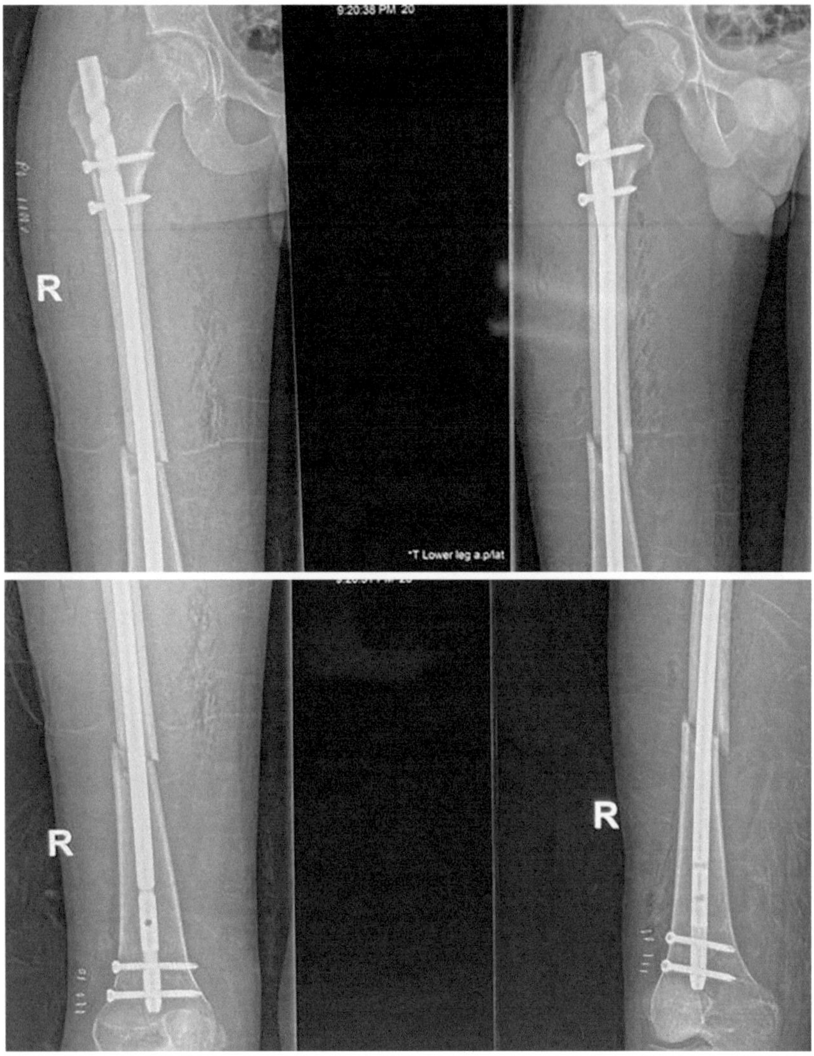

Fig. 25.7 Xray showing post operative antegrade rigid intramedullary nailing

25.6 Complications

1. Early:
   (A) Neurovascular injury: Femur shaft fracture is associated with bleeding and neurovascular injury. Blood loss up to 1L can be expected in an isolated femur fracture. If other damages, such as internal organ injury or pelvic girdle fracture, are associated with the shaft of femur fracture, the patient may present with shock. External fixation and vascular repair may become necessary in these circumstances.
   (B) Wound infection (if associated with wound) – Intravenous antibiotics
   (C) Fat Embolism and ARDS—Patients may have hypoxemia, petechiae, and non-specific neurological symptoms. Early immobilization and external fixation can help reduce the incidence. In the setting of established FES, supplemental treatment with oxygen inhalation and intravenous fluids is known to help.
   (D) Sciatic Neuropraxia—resolves with time
2. Late:
   (A) Delayed union and Nonunion
   (B) Malunion

(C) Joint stiffness
(D) Shortening of limb
(E) Osteomyelitis
(F) Quadriceps Contracture

Multiple Choice Questions

(1) Injury to the popliteal artery in fracture of lower end femur is due to?
 (a) Distal fragment pressing the artery
 (b) Proximal fragment pressing the artery
 (c) Tight plaster
 (d) Hematoma

(2) Which of the following is not a complication of fracture shaft femur?
 (a) Sciatic Neuropraxia
 (b) Lengthening of limb
 (c) Osteomyelitis
 (d) Quadriceps Contracture

(3) Which is not a major criterion of Gurd's fat embolism syndrome?
 (a) Petechial rash
 (b) Respiratory insufficiency
 (c) Cerebral involvement in non-head injury patients
 (d) Fat macroglobulinemia

(4) Which of the following is not a criterion to diagnose the most dreaded complication of long bone fracture?
 (a) Gurd
 (b) Wilson
 (c) Schoenfeld
 (d) Ghent

(5) Which of the following has no role in the management of FES?
 (a) Pharmacotherapy
 (b) Superior Vena Cava Filter
 (c) Operative Measures
 (d) Supportive Care

Answers: 1. (a), 2. (b), 3. (d), 4. (d), 5. (b)

Further Reading

Denisiuk M, Afsari A. Femoral shaft fractures. [Updated 2023 Jan 2]. In: StatPearls [Internet]. Treasure Island (FL): StatPearls Publishing; 2023. Available from: https://www.ncbi.nlm.nih.gov/books/NBK556057/.

Medda S, Unger T, Halvorson J. Diaphyseal femur fracture. [Updated 2023 Feb 20]. In: StatPearls [Internet]. Treasure Island (FL): StatPearls Publishing; 2023. Available from: https://www.ncbi.nlm.nih.gov/books/NBK493169/.

Duan X, Li T, Mohammed AQ, Xiang Z. Reamed intramedullary nailing versus unreamed intramedullary nailing for shaft fracture of femur: a systematic literature review. Arch Orthop Trauma Surg. 2011;131(10):1445–52. https://doi.org/10.1007/s00402-011-1311-8. Epub 2011 May 19. PMID: 21594571.

Poolman RW, Kocher MS, Bhandari M. Pediatric femoral fractures: a systematic review of 2422 cases. J Orthop Trauma. 2006;20(9):648–54. https://doi.org/10.1097/01.bot.0000247073.79430.87. PMID: 17088672.

Nahm NJ, Vallier HA. Timing of definitive treatment of femoral shaft fractures in patients with multiple injuries: a systematic review of randomized and nonrandomized trials. J Trauma Acute Care Surg. 2012;73(5):1046–63. https://doi.org/10.1097/TA.0b013e3182701ded. PMID: 23117368.

26 Injuries Around Knee

Arkesh Madegowda and Mosharaf Hossain Sarkar

26.1 Distal Femur Fracture

Distal femur fractures are traumatic injuries involving the region extending from the distal metaphyseal–diaphyseal junction to the articular surface of the femoral condyles. It has a bimodal age distribution, with a high incidence in young males due to road traffic accidents and a second peak in elderly women resulting from minor falls [1].

Anatomical Considerations The distal femur widens from a cylindrical shaft to form medial and lateral condyles separated by an intercondylar groove. The medial condyle extends more distally and is more convex than the lateral condyle, resulting in physiologic valgus of 9°. In the lateral view, the posterior halves of both condyles are posterior to the posterior cortex of the femoral shaft. The muscular attachments to the distal femur result in characteristic displacement patterns. Gastrocnemius flexes the distal fragment, causing posterior displacement and angulation. Quadriceps and hamstrings exert proximal traction, resulting in the shortening of the lower extremity (Fig. 26.1).

Mechanism of Injury Distal femur fractures typically result from severe axial load with a varus, valgus, or rotational force. In young adults, this force is usually the result of high-energy trauma like a fall from height or a road traffic accident, whereas in the elderly with weak bone, it may result from a minor slip and fall [2].

A. Madegowda (✉) · M. H. Sarkar
All India Institute of Medical Sciences,
Raipur, Chhattisgarh, India

26.1.1 Clinical Evaluation

Patients may present with pain, swelling and variable deformity in the lower thigh and knee. Due to the proximity of neurovascular structures to the distal femur area, it is mandatory to thoroughly assess neurovascular status in these fractures. Rupture of a major vessel is indicated by tense swelling in the popliteal area and lack of distal pulse. Examination of the ipsilateral hip, knee, leg and ankle is essential, especially in obtunded or polytrauma patients.

26.1.2 Radiographic Evaluation

Anteroposterior, lateral and two 45-degree oblique radiographs of the distal femur are recommended to evaluate the fracture pattern. Radiographic evaluation should include the entire femur. Computed Tomography scan with 3D reconstruction may be necessary to better understand the fracture morphology, fragment displacement, articular evaluation and for preoperative planning (Fig. 26.2).

V. Kumar et al. (eds.), *A Quick Guide to Essential Orthopedics*,
https://doi.org/10.1007/978-981-95-2676-5_26

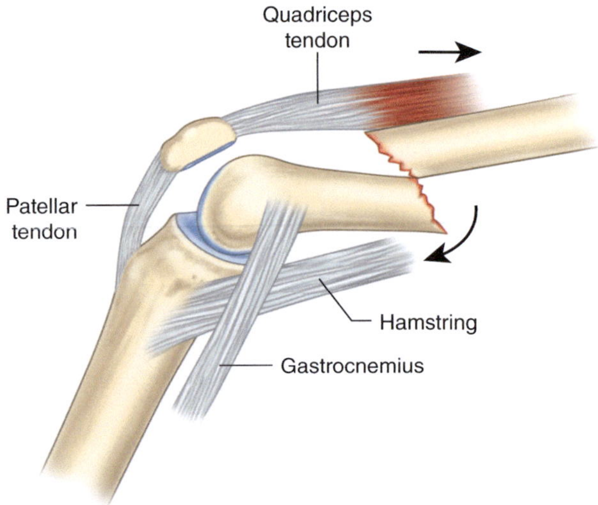

Fig. 26.1 Side view of distal femur with knee showing muscular attachments and its deforming forces. Gastrocnemius pulls the distal fragment into flexion, and hamstrings and quadriceps cause overlap of the fragments

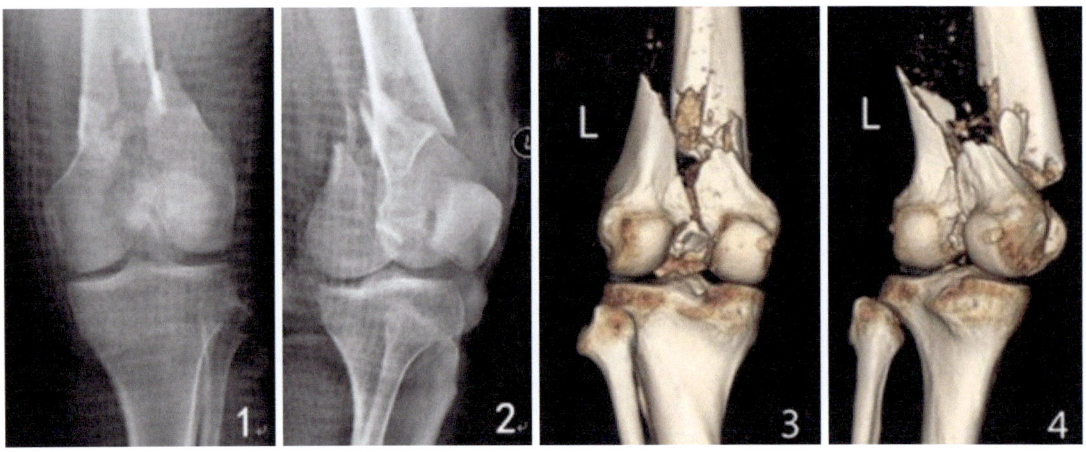

Fig. 26.2 X-ray and computed tomography with 3D reconstruction of distal femur fracture showing fracture pattern, displacement of fragments and articular extension

Magnetic resonance imaging may be helpful in evaluating associated ligament or meniscal injuries. Arteriography may be indicated in fractures associated with suspected vascular injury.

26.1.3 Treatment

26.1.3.1 Non-operative

Indications for non-operative management include stable, non-displaced fractures, a non-ambulatory patient and a patient with significant comorbidities presenting a high degree of surgical/anesthetic risk.

The treatment includes immobilisation of the extremity with above-knee cast for a period of 8–12 weeks, followed by gradual knee mobilisation. Disadvantages of this treatment include malunion, knee stiffness and the necessity of prolonged bed rest.

26.1.3.2 Operative

External Fixation As a temporary measure to restore alignment and stability in unstable, polytrauma patients, open fractures with severe soft tissue injury [3].

Open Reduction and Internal Fixation Indications include displaced fractures, intra-articular fractures and fractures with severe metaphyseal comminution. Anatomically countered locking plates are preferred to achieve fracture reduction and stability.

Retrograde Intramedullary Nail These nails which are inserted through the knee into the shaft are preferred in extra-articular fractures, simple intra-articular fractures.

Distal Femoral Replacement Indicated in low-demand patients with unreconstructable fractures, osteoarthritis, fractures around prior total knee arthroplasty. It allows immediate mobilisation of the patient.

26.1.3.3 Post-operative Management

The injured extremity may be placed on a continuous passive motion device in the immediate post-operative period to start knee joint mobilisation.

Physical therapy consists of active range-of-motion exercises and non-weight-bearing mobilisation with crutches in the immediate postoperative period. Weight-bearing may be advanced with radiographic evidence of healing (6–12 weeks).

26.1.3.4 Complications

- Loss of knee motion: Most common complication which may result from articular disruption, quadriceps damage, or scarring
- Malunion: This usually results from malalignment of fragments during cast immobilisation or at the time of surgery.
- Fixation failure: This may result from non-union, poor bone stock, improper surgical planning and execution.
- Post-traumatic osteoarthritis
- Infection: open fractures are more susceptible to infection, require thorough debridement, intravenous antibiotics and fracture stabilisation with an external fixator.

26.2 Patella Fracture

Patella fractures represent 1% of all skeletal injuries with a male-to-female ratio of 2:1. They most commonly occur in 20–50 years of age.

Anatomy The patella is the largest sesamoid bone in the body. The quadriceps tendon inserts on the superior pole, and the patellar ligament originates from the inferior pole of the patella. The superior 3/4 of posterior surface of patella is covered by articular cartilage and is divided into two large facets (medial and lateral). The retinacula are strong longitudinal expansions of the quadriceps and insert directly onto the tibia contributing to the strength of extensor mechanism.

The function of the patella is to increase the mechanical advantage and leverage of the quadriceps tendon, aid in the nourishment of the femoral articular surface, and protect the femoral condyles from direct trauma.

26.2.1 Mechanism of Injury

Indirect Eccentric Contraction Most common injury pattern, occurs from rapid knee flexion against contracted quadriceps muscle. The pull of musculotendinous structure exceeds the intrinsic strength of patella resulting in transverse fracture.

Direct Trauma to the patella may produce incomplete, simple, stellate, or comminuted fracture patterns. The medial and lateral retinacula expansions remain intact, so displacement is less. Active knee extension may be preserved.

26.2.2 Clinical Evaluation

Patients may present with pain, swelling and tenderness of the involved knee with difficulty in standing or walking. A palpable defect may be felt at the patella. Hemarthrosis (collection of blood) may be noted in the knee joint. Active knee extension should be evaluated to determine injury to the extensor and retinacular mechanism [4].

26.2.3 Radiographic Evaluation

Anteroposterior (AP) and lateral views of the knee should be obtained.

The lateral view helps to evaluate transverse fractures and should be obtained in 30^0 knee flexion to see articular step-off.

Computed tomography may be used to understand fracture patterns, identify marginal fractures, or free osteochondral fragments.

26.2.4 Classification

Pattern Based on the fracture morphology, patella fractures can be divided into transverse, vertical (marginal), stellate, comminuted, polar osteochondral types (Fig. 26.3).

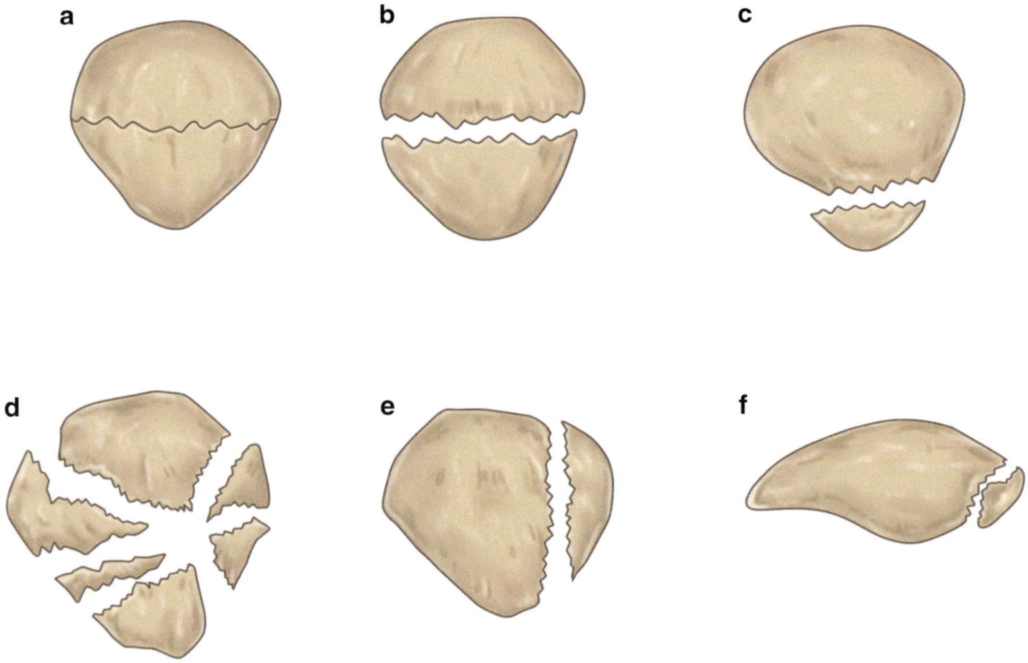

Fig. 26.3 Types of patella fracture: (**a**) undisplaced, (**b**) transverse, (**c**) lower pole, (**d**) comminuted, (**e**) vertical and (**f**) osteochondral

26.2.5 Treatment

Indication	Management
Non-displaced or minimally displaced Articular incongruity (<2 mm) Intact extensor mechanism	Non-operative: cylinder cast or knee immobiliser for 4–6 weeks followed by early weight-bearing in extension Rehabilitation plan: Early straight leg raising and isometric quadriceps strengthening exercises should be started within few days With radiographic evidence of healing, active flexion and extension strengthening exercises are continued with a hinged knee brace
Loss of active extension with extensor lag Articular incongruity >2mm Displacement of fragments >3mm Open fractures	Open reduction and internal fixation Tension band wiring (TBW). The principle behind TBW is to convert distraction force into compressive force at the fracture site
Non-salvageable smaller, comminuted polar fragments	Partial patellectomy
Non-salvageable extensive, and severely comminuted patella fractures	Total patellectomy (rare)

26.2.6 Complications

- Loss of knee movements: due to prolonged immobilisation [5]
- Non-union: Most patients retain good knee function. Painful non-union may need revision surgery.
- Post-operative infection.
- Prominent hardware: Due to subcutaneous nature of the fixation, it may need implant removal if painful.
- Post-traumatic osteoarthritis: may result in anterior patellofemoral pain.

26.2.7 Ligamentous Injuries Around Knee

Ligament injuries of the knee are common and are often associated with a twisting injury or a direct blow to the medial or lateral aspect of the knee [6].

26.2.8 Anatomic Considerations

The knee is a complex hinge joint and is made up of a synovial capsule, bony articular surfaces, menisci, ligaments and tendons. Medial and lateral menisci are the semilunar fibrocartilaginous structures located between the femoral and tibial condyles. These act as a filler between incongruous articulating surfaces, providing shock absorption, lubrication and nutrition.

The cruciate and collateral ligaments are the primary stabilisers of the knee. The anterior cruciate and posterior cruciate ligaments are intra-articular and provide stability by preventing anterior and posterior displacement of the tibia over the femur, respectively. Medial and lateral collateral ligaments are extrinsic to the joint and prevent valgus or varus deviation of the knee.

26.2.9 Medial Collateral Ligament (MCL)

Injury to the medial collateral ligament occurs due to valgus force applied to the knee with external tibial rotation. They can occur in isolation or in association with an ACL or meniscal injury [7].

Clinical Symptoms Pain on the medial side of the knee. Knee giving way into valgus may be seen with complete tears.

Examination Positive valgus stress test; on giving valgus stress, the injured knee will yield more gap on the medial side compared to the opposite side.

Investigation Magnetic resonance imaging (MRI) is the investigation of choice.

26.2.10 Treatment

Grade I and II Sprains These patients are treated with rest, ice pack application, compression bandage and limb elevation (RICE protocol) and functional rehabilitation.

Grade III Sprain (Complete Ligament Tear) Surgery may be indicated for complete MCL tears in association with other ligament injuries. Isolated Grade III sprains are also managed with RICE and rehabilitation.

26.2.11 Lateral Collateral Ligament (LCL)

Injury to lateral collateral ligament is caused by a varus or twisting force applied to the knee. LCL injuries may be associated with injury to posterolateral structures like popliteus tendon, iliotibial band, popliteofemoral ligament and peroneal nerve when there is a blow to anteromedial tibia with knee in hyperextension.

Clinical Symptoms Patients experience pain over the lateral aspect of knee. Patients with chronic posterolateral injury may also complain of giving way of knee into hyperextension while standing and walking.

Examination Positive varus stress test; at 30° of knee flexion, applying varus stress results in increased lateral joint opening.

Investigation Anteroposterior radiograph of the knee may show a Segond fracture, which is the avulsion fracture of the insertion of the iliotibial band onto the proximal lateral tibia. This sign likely indicates presence of an associated ACL injury. MRI of the knee is the standard investigation of choice for LCL injuries.

26.2.12 Treatment

Grade I and II Sprains Patients with mild grade sprains are treated with RICE, crutch mobilisation and rehabilitation.

Grade III Sprain (Complete Ligament Tear) Surgical repair is usually preferable if injury involves posterolateral structures along with LCL.

26.2.13 Anterior Cruciate Ligament

ACL injury is the second most common ligament injury in the knee. The injury is often the result of twisting of a hyperextended knee. ACL may be torn from femur or tibia, or torn in its midportion. In young patients, it may avulse from tibial spine [8].

Clinical Symptoms A patient with an ACL injury often feels a ‘pop’ in the knee and presents with an immediate hemarthrosis. In chronic injuries, patients experience giving way on twisting, pivoting and cutting.

26.2.14 Examination

Lachmann Test It is the most sensitive examination for acute ACL injuries. With patient being supine and knee flexed to 30°, stabilise femur with 1 hand and gently apply anterior force on tibia with opposite hand. Excessive anterior translation of tibia compared to opposite knee.

Anterior Drawer Test With patient supine, hip flexed to 45° and knee to 90°, foot is kept flat on bed. Stabilise femur with 1 hand and apply anterior force on tibia with opposite hand. Excessive anterior translation of tibia compared to normal knee indicates positive test.

Investigation On plain radiographs of knee, associated tibial spine avulsion fracture may be seen in young patients. MRI has high accuracy rates to confirm diagnosis and evaluate injuries to other structures.

26.2.15 Treatment

Treatment decisions are individualised based on age, activity level, instability and associated injuries. Initial management consists of protection, rest, ice, compression and rest. This is followed by physiotherapy to regain range of movement.

Surgical treatment involves arthroscopic-assisted reconstruction of the ligament using either autologous hamstring tendons (semitendinosus and gracilis) or patella tendon or donor tissue (allograft).

26.2.16 Posterior Cruciate Ligament

Injury to the posterior cruciate ligament occurs due to valgus/varus force applied to a fully extended knee or due to a direct blow to the proximal tibia.

Clinical Symptoms Swelling of the knee in acute injuries. Patients also experience the feeling of the femur sliding anteriorly off the tibia when descending slopes or stairs.

26.2.17 Examination

- Posterior drawer test: With the patient supine, hip flexed to 45° and knee to 90° and foot kept flat on the table, a rapid posterior force is applied to the tibia. Excessive posterior translation of the tibia indicates a positive test.
- Posterior sag sign test: with patient in supine position, flex hip to 45° and knee to 90°. Posterior sagging of the tibia indicates a positive sign.

Investigation MRI helps to confirm the diagnosis of PCL injuries and also to evaluate other associated injuries.

Treatment Patients with mild laxity may be treated with protection, rest and functional rehabilitation. For moderate or severe laxity, surgical repair/reconstruction is usually required.

26.2.18 Meniscus Tears

Medial meniscus and lateral meniscus consist mainly of fibrocartilage, attached to the joint capsule at the periphery. The main functions of menisci are shock absorption, load sharing and stability.

They have limited vascular supply and healing potential. The outer third (red-red zone) of meniscus is vascular, while the inner third (white-white zone) is avascular and the middle third (red-white zone) has an intermediate blood supply. The common mechanism of acute meniscus injury is twisting or hyperflexion force to the knee. Chronic injuries are associated with degenerative osteoarthritis.

26.2.19 Clinical Symptoms

Patients may present with acute pain with or without swelling. There might be associated mechanical symptoms like locking episodes. Audible pop may be heard at the time of injury.

26.2.20 Examination

- *McMurray test*: With the patient supine, flex the thigh and hyperflex the knee. Grip the knee with one hand and hold the foot with the other hand. Flex and extend the knee while simultaneously internally and externally rotating the lower leg (varus and valgus stress). Pain in the joint line or audible clicking or locking of the knee indicates a positive test.

- *Apley grinding test*: With the patient prone, flex the knee to 90°. Apply axial pressure to the knee, holding the heel (compression) while rotating the leg internally (for the lateral meniscus) and externally (for the medial meniscus). Pain or clicking indicates a positive test.

Investigations Meniscal tear pattern and displacement can often be determined by magnetic resonance imaging (MRI). Multiple types of meniscal tears may be appreciated on MRI, like vertical tears, horizontal tears, radial tears and root tears.

Treatment Initial treatment with rest, ice, compression and elevation helps to decrease swelling and pain. Young patients with acute meniscal tears may require arthroscopic repair. Patients with degenerative meniscal tears may benefit from partial meniscectomy if symptoms are not responsive to conservative treatment.

26.3 Multiple Choice Questions

1. Patella provides attachment to all the following structures except
   (a) quadriceps tendon
   (b) patellar tendon
   (c) retinaculum
   (d) iliotibial band
2. The commonest mechanism of injury of distal femur fractures in young adults
   (a) fall from height
   (b) twisting injury while playing
   (c) motor vehicle accident
   (d) slip and fall at home
3. All the following clinical tests may be positive in ACL tear patient except
   (a) Lachmann test
   (b) pivot shift test
   (c) anterior drawer test
   (d) valgus stress test
4. The most common mechanism of medial collateral ligament injury is
   (a) varus stress
   (b) valgus stress
   (c) hyperextension
   (d) twisting force
5. Healing of meniscal tears is better if it involves
   (a) outer 1/3rd
   (b) middle 1/3rd
   (c) inner 1/3rd
   (d) root tears

Answers: 1. (d), 2. (c), 3. (d), 4. (b), 5. (a)

References

1. Gwathmey FW Jr, Jones-Quaidoo SM, Kahler D, Hurwitz S, Cui Q. Distal femoral fractures: current concepts. J Am Acad Orthop Surg. 2010;18(10):597–607.
2. Higgins TF. Distal femoral fractures. J Knee Surg. 2007;20(1):56–66.
3. Dugan TR, Hubert MG, Siska PA, Pape HC, Tarkin IS. Open supracondylar femur fractures with bone loss in the polytraumatized patient – timing is everything! Injury. 2013;44(12):1826–31.
4. Melvin JS, Mehta S. Patellar fractures in adults. J Am Acad Orthop Surg. 2011;19(4):198–207.
5. LeBrun CT, Langford JR, Sagi HC. Functional outcomes after operatively treated patella fractures. J Orthop Trauma. 2012;26(7):422–6.
6. Gupte C, St Mart JP. The acute swollen knee: diagnosis and management. J R Soc Med. 2013;106(7):259–68.
7. Knutson T, Bothwell J, Durbin R. Evaluation and management of traumatic knee injuries in the emergency department. Emerg Med Clin North Am. 2015;33(2):345–62.
8. Micheo W, Hernández L, Seda C. Evaluation, management, rehabilitation, and prevention of anterior cruciate ligament injury: current concepts. PM R. 2010;2(10):935–44.

27 Fractures of the Tibia and Fibula

Arkesh Madegowda and Mosharaf Hossain Sarkar

27.1 Proximal Tibia Fracture

27.1.1 Introduction

Proximal tibia fractures are also known as tibial plateau fractures. These constitute 1% of all fractures and involve a wide spectrum of fracture patterns which may involve the lateral tibial plateau, medial tibial plateau, or both [1].

27.1.2 Anatomical Considerations

The tibial plateau comprises the articular surfaces of the medial and lateral tibial plateaus, on which the menisci are located. The two plateaus are separated from each other by the intercondylar eminence, which serves as an attachment to the cruciate ligaments.

The lateral condyle of the proximal tibia and its articular surface are weaker than the medial counterpart. This, along with the common direction of the injuring force from the lateral side, explains more incidence of lateral tibial plateau fractures.

A. Madegowda (✉) · M. H. Sarkar
All India Institute of Medical Sciences, Raipur, Chhattisgarh, India

27.1.3 Mechanism of Injury

Tibial plateau fractures are commonly caused by motor vehicle accidents in young individuals. Elderly patients with osteopenic bone may sustain these injuries following a simple fall. The mechanism of injury is by valgus or varus force coupled with axial loading. The magnitude and direction of the injuring force, bone quality, and position of the knee determine the pattern of fracture, amount of comminution.

27.1.4 Clinical Features

Patients with tibial plateau fractures present with pain, swelling, deformities around the knee, restricted joint movements, and inability to bear weight. On clinical examination, special attention should be given to assess the soft tissue status, open communicating wounds, neurovascular status of the limb, and compartment syndrome. A significant proportion of tibial plateau fractures are associated with injuries to menisci, collateral ligaments, and cruciate ligaments. These should be evaluated thoroughly [2].

27.1.5 Investigations

Anteroposterior and lateral views of the knee joint help to identify the fracture pattern.

V. Kumar et al. (eds.), *A Quick Guide to Essential Orthopedics*,
https://doi.org/10.1007/978-981-95-2676-5_27

Computed tomography with three-dimensional reconstruction aids in delineating the amount of comminution and depression of the articular surface. It also helps in preoperative planning of fracture fixation. Arteriography may be indicated when there is suspicion of vascular compromise.

27.2 Classification of Proximal Tibia Fracture:

Schatzker Classification (1979) A morphological system based on AP radiographs, distinguishing six types of fractures ranging from simple split fractures to complex fractures (Fig. 27.1) [3].

27.2.1 Treatment

Non-operative treatment with a hinged knee brace is indicated for non-displaced or minimally displaced fractures. Isometric quadriceps exercises, early range of knee motion exercises are recommended in minimally displaced fractures.

Operative treatment is indicated in open fractures, fractures associated with compartment syndrome or vascular injury, articular gap or depression more than 10 mm, and malalignment more than 10°.

A knee-spanning external fixator may be applied temporarily in patients with significant soft tissue injury. The external fixator helps in initial soft tissue management and maintains fracture reduction until definitive surgery is done.

Operative treatment aims at the reconstruction of the articular surface along with the reconstruction of tibial alignment. The depressed articular segments can be elevated and buttressed with bone graft or bone graft substitutes. The fixation of a fracture can be achieved with screws, plates, or an external fixator.

Following surgery, the patients are encouraged to do an active range of motion exercises and non-weight-bearing mobilization. Weight-bearing is allowed after 8–12 weeks, depending on radiological union.

27.3 Complications

- Infection: This may be due to surgical interventions through compromised soft tissues or extensive dissection.
- Compartment syndrome
- Neurovascular injury to the peroneal nerve and/or popliteal artery
- Malunion or non-union: this is commonly associated with severe grade fractures due to comminution, unstable fixation, or infection.
- Arthrofibrosis: Joint stiffness is due to prolonged immobilization, scarring, and improper exercise protocol.
- Posttraumatic arthritis.

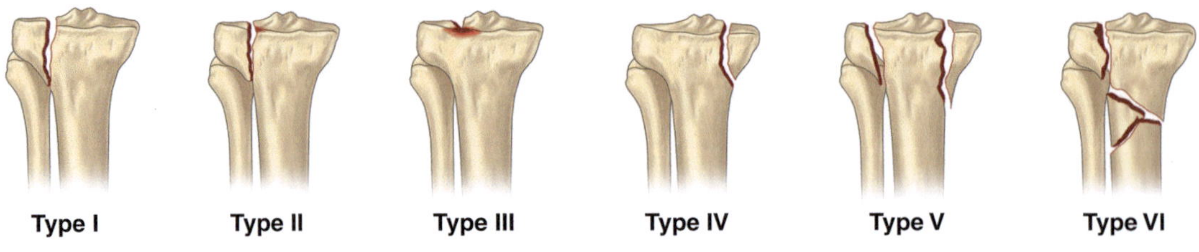

Fig. 27.1 Schatzkar's classification of proximal tibia fractures. Type I: split fracture lateral plateau, Type II: split & depression lateral plateau, Type III: lateral depression, Type IV: medial plateau fracture, Type V: Bicondylar tibial plateau fracture, and Type VI: metaphysis-diaphysis dissociation

27.3.1 Tibia and Fibula Shaft Fractures

Fractures of the tibial and fibular shafts are the most common long-bone fractures. These fractures are commonly seen in the second or third decade of life following motor vehicle accidents. Severe open fractures are often associated with high complication rates and poor long-term outcomes [4].

27.3.2 Anatomical Considerations

The tibia is a long tubular bone with triangular cross-section and is surrounded by tight fascial compartments. Minimal soft tissue coverage over the anteromedial shaft predisposes tibial shaft fractures to be open injuries. Also, the entire diaphysis of the tibia is supplied by a single nutrient artery arising from the posterior tibial artery, with limited contribution from periosteal branches. These factors risk impaired healing of diaphyseal fractures of the tibia.

The fibula is a smaller and thinner bone located posterolaterally parallel to the tibia and is responsible for 6–17% of weight-bearing load. Its major function is to provide support and attachment to leg muscles.

27.3.3 Mechanism of Injury

Fractures of the tibia and fibula shaft occur by direct and indirect mechanisms. Common mechanisms are bumper injuries, gunshot wounds, and bending or torsional injuries with a firmly planted foot. High-energy injuries are often associated with extensive soft tissue damage leading to compartment syndrome.

27.3.4 Clinical Features

Patients with tibial shaft fractures often present with pain, swelling, deformity of the leg, and inability to bear weight. The surrounding soft tissues should be carefully examined for signs of open injuries, blisters, and contusions. These patients should be monitored for compartment syndrome. Pain out of proportion to the injury might be the early, reliable sign of compartment syndrome. In the presence of compartment syndrome, an urgent fasciotomy must be done.

27.3.5 Investigations

X-rays of the leg in Anteroposterior and lateral views should reveal the diagnosis in the majority of cases. The X-rays should include the entire length of the tibia with visualization of the knee and ankle joints to evaluate comminution, displacement of fragments, extension of fracture into joints, and presence of knee osteoarthritis.

27.3.6 Treatment

Non-operative Low-energy fractures with minimal displacement and comminution can be treated with application of an above-knee cast. The acceptable fracture reduction for cast immobilization is varus/valgus angulation of less than 5°, anteroposterior angulation of less than 10°, rotational malalignment of less than 10°, and shortening of less than 1 centimeter with more than 50% cortical contact. After 4–6 weeks of above-knee cast, it may be converted to patella-bearing cast till radiological union is seen.

27.3.7 Operative Treatment

An external fixator can be temporarily applied to severe open fractures, fractures associated with compartment syndrome, undergoing fasciotomy. This is commonly converted to definitive fixation once the soft tissue condition improves.

Intramedullary interlocking (IMIL) nailing is the preferred choice for tibial shaft fractures as it provides biomechanical control of alignment, translation, and rotation. It also helps in preserving the periosteal blood supply and limits soft tissue damage. Flexible nails are recommended for fractures in children or adolescents with open physes [5].

27.3.8 Complications

Immediate

- Infection: These are commonly associated with open fractures.
- Compartment syndrome: The anterior compartment of the leg is most involved following high velocity injuries.
- Neurovascular injury: Less commonly seen with tibial shaft fractures. The anterior tibial artery and common peroneal nerve are at risk in grossly displaced fractures.

Delayed

- Malunion: commonly seen with non-operative treatment of fractures with deformities outside the acceptable range.
- Non-union: associated with high-energy injuries, open fractures, infection, and fractures treated with inadequate fixation.
- Knee and ankle stiffness: Following prolonged cast immobilization.

Multiple Choice Questions

1. The most common variety of tibial plateau fractures is?
   (a) medial plateau
   (b) lateral plateau
   (c) bicondylar
   (d) bicondylar with metaphyseal comminution
2. The following injuries are commonly associated with tibial plateau fractures except
   (a) tibial nerve injury
   (b) meniscal tears
   (c) common peroneal nerve injury
   (d) cruciate ligament injury
3. All of the following are indications for non-operative treatment in tibial plateau fractures except
   (a) minimally displaced split or depressed fractures
   (b) open fractures
   (c) non-ambulatory patients
   (d) patient with significant co-morbidities
4. All these signs suggest compartment syndrome in a patient with tibial shaft fracture except
   (a) pain out of proportion
   (b) blisters
   (c) pallor
   (d) paraesthesia
5. All the following are recommended in severe grade open tibia shaft fractures except
   (a) antibiotics
   (b) wound debridement
   (c) fixation with nail
   (d) external fixator application

Answers: 1. (b), 2. (a), 3. (b), 4. (b), 5. (c)

References

1. Rudran B, Little C, Wiik A, Logishetty K. Tibial plateau fracture: anatomy, diagnosis and management. Br J Hosp Med (Lond). 2020;81(10):1–9.
2. Thomas C, Athanasiov A, Wullschleger M, Schuetz M. Current concepts in tibial plateau fractures. Acta Chir Orthop Traumatol Cech. 2009;76(5):363–73.
3. Prat-Fabregat S, Camacho-Carrasco P. Treatment strategy for tibial plateau fractures: an update. EFORT Open Rev. 2017;1(5):225–32.
4. Mundi R, Chaudhry H, Niroopan G, Petrisor B, Bhandari M. Open tibial fractures: updated guidelines for management. JBJS Rev. 2015;3(2):e1.
5. Keller CS. The principles of the treatment of tibial shaft fractures: a review of 10,146 cases from the literature. Orthopedics. 1983;6(8):993–9.

Ankle Injuries

28

Balgovind S. Raja and Anusree Akshay

28.1 Introduction

Injuries in and around ankle are the most common lower limb traumatic injuries one sees in the outpatient and emergency. Owing to a large variety of forces (twisting, bending, and compression) and position of the foot following trauma, the presentation of these injuries varies. An immediate identification and prompt treatment of these injuries often result in good clinical outcomes. A basic understanding of the core anatomy, classification of injuries, radiology, and treatment would be ideal.

28.2 Basic Anatomy

The foot and ankle always work in unison. The complex consists of 26 bones and 9 joints, out of which the tibiotalar joint forms the ankle joint (Fig. 28.1). The ankle joint is formed by tibial plafond (articular surface of distal tibia), medial malleolus, lateral malleolus and talus. Its a modified hinge joint with the superior articular dome of the talus articulating with the tibial plafond and the two malleoli. The principal motion in the joint is plantar flexion and dorsiflexion (Fig. 28.2). Inversion and eversion also occur in ankle joint, but it also involves the subtalar joint. The ankle motion and the muscles responsible are listed in Table 28.1.

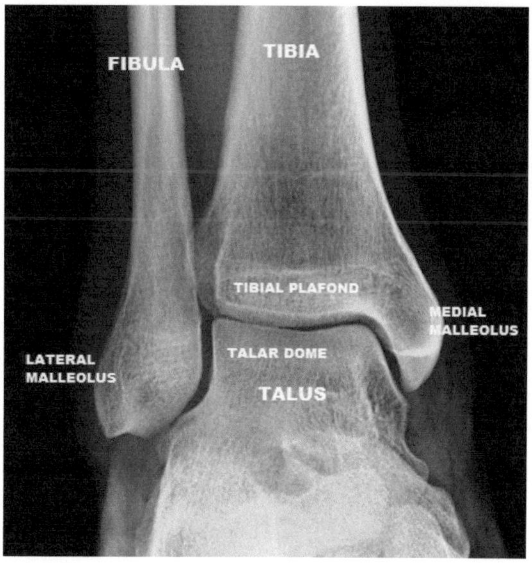

Fig. 28.1 Normal ankle anatomy

B. S. Raja (✉)
Department of Orthopedics, AIIMS,
Patna, Bihar, India

A. Akshay
All India Institute of Medical Sciences, Raipur, India

V. Kumar et al. (eds.), *A Quick Guide to Essential Orthopedics*,
https://doi.org/10.1007/978-981-95-2676-5_28

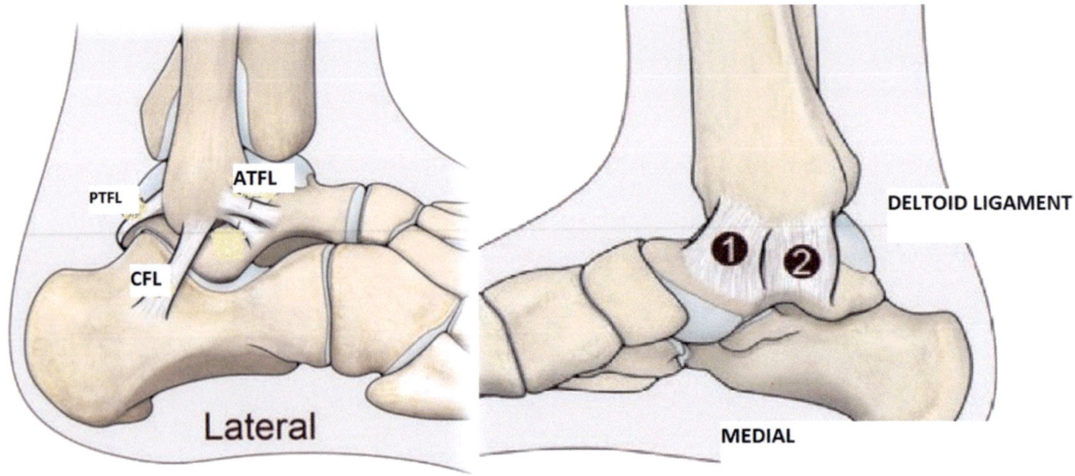

Fig. 28.2 Ankle ligaments (ATFL anterior talofibular ligament, CFL calcaneofibular ligament, PTFL posterior talofibular ligament)

Table 28.1 Ankle movements and muscles responsible

Ankle motion	Muscles responsible
Plantar flexion	*Soleus* *Gastrocnemius* Tibialis posterior Peroneus longus Peroneus brevis Flexor digitorum longus Flexor hallucis longus
Dorsiflexion	*Tibialis anterior* Extensor digitorum longus Peroneus tertius Extensor hallucis longus
Inversion	*Tibialis anterior* *Tibialis posterior* Soleus Gastrocnemius
Eversion	*Peroneus longus* *Peroneus brevis* *Peroneus tertius*

Prime movers are highlighted in italics

28.3 Ankle Ligaments

The collateral ligaments of the ankle include medial and lateral complexes (Fig. 28.2). These ligaments are aligned coronally and prevent the medial and lateral translation of the ankle. The medially located ligament is the deltoid ligament, which consists of superficial and deep parts. The lateral ankle ligamentous complex includes ATFL (anterior talofibular ligament), PTFL (posterior talofibular ligament), and CFL (calcaneofibular ligament). The syndesmosis or the ligaments connecting the distal tibia and fibula keep the ankle mortise intact throughout the range of motion and during gait (Fig. 28.2). High ankle sprains refer to injury to syndesmosis. The ligaments are briefly described in Table 28.2.

Table 28.2 Ankle ligaments, attachments, and function

Lateral ligaments	Function	Attachments
Anterior talofibular (Weakest of the lateral ligaments)	1. Primary restraint to inversion in plantar flexion 2. Resists anterolateral translation of talus in the mortise	Extends from the anteroinferior border of the fibula to the neck of the talus
Posterior talofibular (Strongest of the lateral ligaments)	Restrains posterior displacement of talus Resists talar external rotation	Posterior border of fibula to posterolateral tubercle of the talus
Calcaneofibular	Restrains inversion of calcaneus	Anterior border of fibula 9 mm proximal to distal tip to calcaneus 13 mm distal to subtalar joint
Medial ligament (Deltoid)	Primary restraint to valgus tilting of the talus	
Superficial	Resists valgus tilting and eversion	Crosses both ankle and subtalar joints
Deep (Functions as the primary stabilizer of the medial ankle)	Prevents lateral displacement and external rotation of the talus	Crosses only ankle joint Origin from inferior & posterior aspects of medial malleolus and inserts to medial and posteromedial aspects of the talus

28.4 Injuries Around Ankle

The injuries around the ankle can be broadly classified into

(A) Ligament injuries (ankle sprains)
(B) Fractures around the ankle
(C) Chronic injuries

28.4.1 Ankle Sprain

The ligament injuries of ankle are the most common ligament injury in athletic population. The ATFL is the most commonly injured. The force acting on the ankle and the direction of the foot dictate the injury pattern. Ankle sprain refers to disruption of the ankle ligaments. A low ankle sprain involves the medial or the lateral ligament complexes and high ankle sprains involve the syndesmosis. The injuries involving ligaments are classified on the basis of the degree of disruption of the fibers (Table 28.3).

- *Grade 1 (Mild)*: The ligament fibers are stretched slightly, or there is a very small tear. The ankle will have minor swelling and tenderness to the touch.
- *Grade 2 (Moderate)*: The ligament is torn, but it isn't a complete tear. The ankle has swelling over the injury and will hurt to move.
- *Grade 3 (Severe)*: The ligament is torn completely. The ankle has significant swelling and is painful, and walking would be difficult.

28.4.1.1 Mechanism of Injury

- The lateral ankle ligament injuries:
  - A combination of plantarflexion and inversion.
  - ATFL is most commonly injured. Instability often ensues once the calcaneofibular ligament is disrupted with ATFL.
  - Posterior talofibular ligament is considered the strongest of the three in the lateral ligamentous complex and rarely gets injured in an inversion sprain.

Table 28.3 Summary of ankle sprain (features, treatment, and complications)

Sprain Low ankle sprain	Features	Treatment	Complications
Grade I	No ligament disruption Minimal pain on weight bearing Minimal ecchymosis or bruising (bluish discoloration)	PRICE[a] Exercise (ankle specific) +/− Physio	Pain and recurrent instability Stretch neuropraxia
Grade II	Partial ligament tear Restricted ROM, localized tenderness (medial or lateral) Bruising & swelling present Abnormal laxity +/−	PRICE[a] Bracing, Tapping, or casting (below knee) Exercise (ankle specific) and Physio If unstable even after conservative management: Surgery	
Grade III	Complete ligament tear Restricted ROM, localized tenderness (medial or lateral) Diffuse swelling and ecchymosis Abnormal laxity ++	PRICE[a] Bracing, Tapping, or casting (below knee) Exercise (ankle specific) and Physio If unstable even after conservative management: Surgery	
High ankle sprain (affects distal Tibio-fibular ligaments & Syndesmosis) Often associated with fractures around the ankle	External rotation Injury Tenderness over the syndesmosis Difficulty in weight bearing Hopkin's test +ve External rotation stress test +ve	PRICE[a] Non-weight-bearing cast or brace for 2–3 weeks Surgery if ankle instability or diastasis is present	Chronic ankle pain Post-traumatic tibiofibular synostosis ankle arthritis (if missed)

[a]PRICE - Protect, Rest, Ice, Compression, and Elevation

- Injuries to the deltoid ligament or the medial ligament:
  - Excessive eversion and ankle dorsiflexion.
  - The deltoid ligament is strong, and its deep division is the primary restraint for valgus stability of the ankle.
  - They may often coexist with medial malleolus fractures.
- Syndesmotic injuries (less common):
  - External rotation and dorsiflexion of the ankle.

28.4.1.2 Clinical Presentation

- Patient would be able to walk, albeit carefully, with pain.
- All patients will give a history of twisting of the ankle. An inversion injury for lateral ligament injury and an eversion injury for medial or syndesmotic injury
- A history suggesting a sudden increase in pain associated with the rapid onset of swelling and bruising indicates a ruptured ligament
- Neurovascular compromise may be suspected only in cases of cold sensation and or history of paraesthesia.

28.4.1.3 Physical Examination (Fig. 28.3)

- Localized tenderness over the ligaments
- No bony tenderness (if present, suspect fracture)
- Ecchymosis or bruising (not specific)
- Swelling or edema over the ankle (if significant, suspect fracture)
- Complete tears or Grade III tears may have a restricted range of motion
- Active ROM needs to be assessed at all times, as Tendoachilles rupture can mimic ankle ligament injury

28.4.1.4 Imaging

- *Radiographs*:
  - Simple Anteroposterior (AP) and lateral X-rays help to rule out fractures or bony abnormalities (Fig. 28.4)
  - Weight-bearing AP and lateral radiographs of the ankle for syndesmotic injuries, valgus or varus stress radiographs for deltoid or lateral ligament stability, respectively (Fig. 28.4)
  - Every ankle injury patient must get radiographs to rule out foot injuries and disruption of the proximal tibiofibular joint, also
- *Magnetic resonance imaging*: Ideal investigation for finding out ligamentous injuries. Associated conditions such as osteochondral fragments, hairline fractures, or tendon injuries can be identified (Fig. 28.5).
- *Computed tomography*: No role in ankle sprains except in conditions associated with fractures.

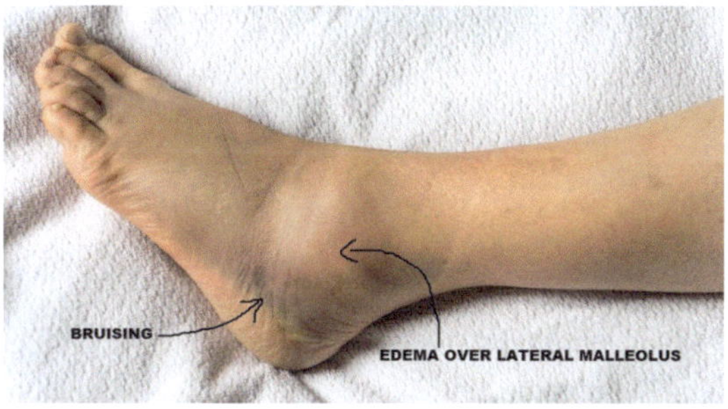

Fig. 28.3 Clinical picture of patient ankle injury

28.4.1.5 Treatment

Chronic ankle injuries are persistent instability beyond 3 months following the initial episode of trauma. These conditions necessitate surgical treatment. However, even in these conditions, a 3-month conservative trial is preferred.

For the sake of completion, the major surgical options available for lateral ankle instability are Brostrom repair, tendon transfers, or reconstruction with autografts. Deltoid ligaments are often repaired and, if needed, are reconstructed with autografts. Syndesmosis injuries are often fixed with the help of screws or using anchors.

28.4.2 Fractures Around Ankle

Ankle fractures are caused by twisting mechanism and or compression/impaction injury. The fractures can be of

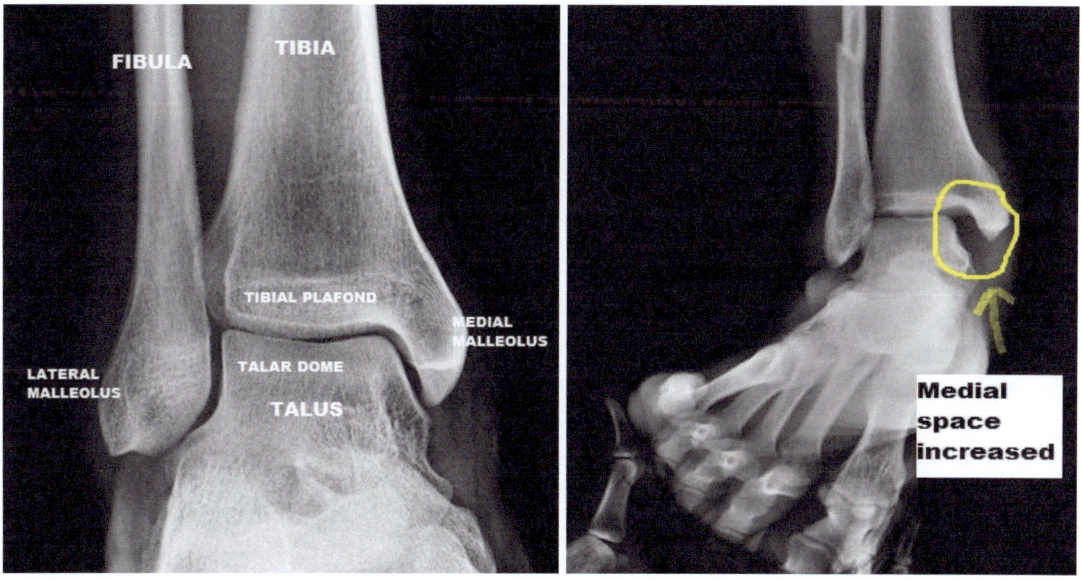

Fig. 28.4 Radiograph of normal ankle mortise view and stress radiograph showing medial space opening up and distal fibula fracture

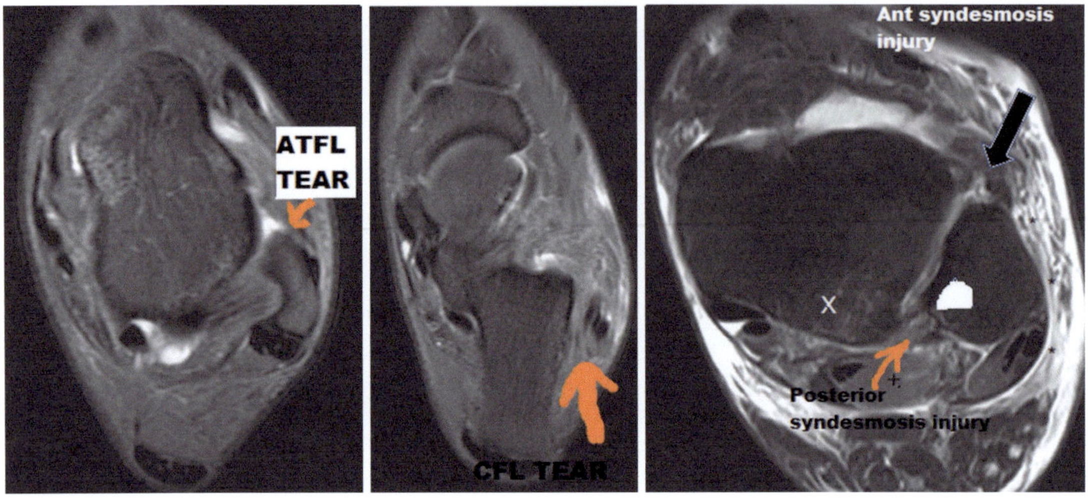

Fig. 28.5 MRI sections showing ankle ligament injuries

- Malleolus
- Pilon fractures
- Talus

28.4.3 Malleolar Fractures

28.4.3.1 Epidemiology

Malleolar fractures involve the medial and or lateral malleolus. Potts' fracture refers to a bimalleolar fracture. These fractures have a bimodal distribution pattern with high incidence in the age groups 15–24 and 75–84 years. Isolated fractures are the most common with an incidence of 70%, followed by bimalleolar fractures 20%, and trimalleolar fractures 7%. Coexisting conditions include open fractures 2%, syndesmotic injury 10%, osteochondral injury, and peroneal tendon injury.

28.4.3.2 Mechanism of Injury

The position of the foot and direction of the force at the time of injury determine the type of ankle fracture. Lauge-Hansen classification describes the clinical varieties with their associated mechanisms (Table 28.4). Weber classification is detailed in Table 28.5 and Fig. 28.6.

Table 28.4 Lauge-Hansen classification of ankle fractures

Lauge-Hansen Stages	Findings
Supination Adduction (SAD)	Transverse fracture of lateral malleolus Vertical fracture of medial malleolus
Supination External Rotation (SER)	Injury to anterior inferior talofibular ligament (AITFL) Low oblique/short spiral fracture of lateral malleolus Injury of posterior inferior talofibular ligament (PITFL) Deltoid ligament injury or medial malleolus fracture
Pronation External Rotation (PER)	Deltoid ligament injury or medial malleolus fracture Injury to anterior inferior talofibular ligament (AITFL) High oblique/short spiral fracture of distal fibula Injury of posterior inferior talofibular ligament (PITFL) or posterior malleolus
Pronation Abduction (PAB)	Deltoid ligament injury or medial malleolus fracture Injury to anterior inferior talofibular ligament (AITFL) Transverse or comminuted fracture of distal fibula

Table 28.5 Weber's classification

Dennis–Weber types	Fracture of distal fibula
Type A	Infra-syndesmotic (SAD)
Type B	Trans-syndesmotic (SER)
Type C	Supra-syndesmotic (PER, PAB)

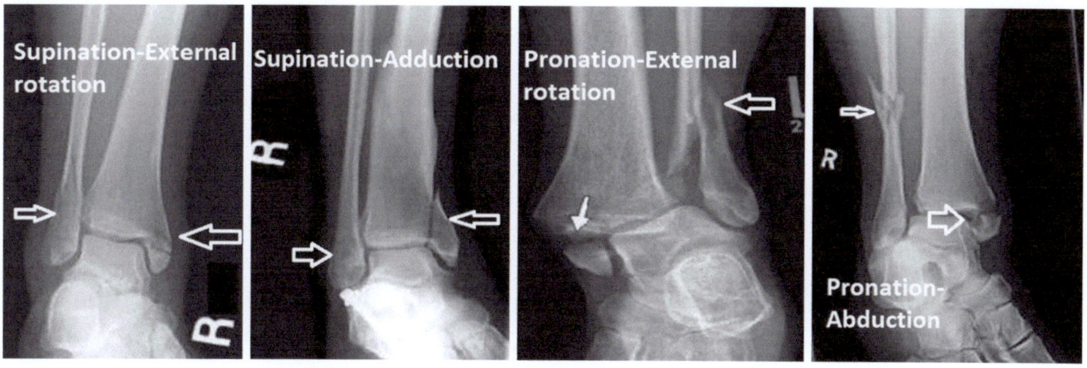

Fig. 28.6 Radiographs showing various varieties of ankle

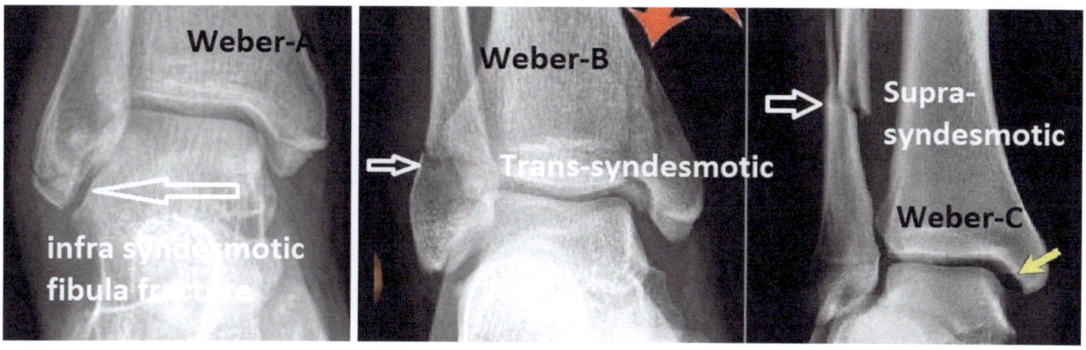

Fig. 28.7 Weber classification

Dennis Weber Classification (Fig. 28.7)

28.4.3.3 Clinical Presentation

Patients with ankle fracture presents with

- Severe ankle pain
- Inability to weight bear or ambulate
- Bony tenderness
- Deformity
- Edema +/– ecchymosis

Physical examination often reveals

- Ecchymosis and swelling around the ankle
- Deformity in case of displaced fractures
- Bony tenderness
- Soft tissue assessment may show blisters in case of displaced fractures, tenting of skin, or open wounds
- Range of motion restricted
- Neurovascular compromise in rare cases of displaced fractures or fractures with compartment syndrome

28.4.3.4 Imaging

- Routine ankle AP and lateral views along with mortise view (AP view in 10° internal rotation)

- Full-length tibia radiographs to rule out Maisonneuve-type fracture (proximal fibula fracture)
- Weight-bearing X-rays and stress views not possible in majority of cases
- CT scans are indicated in suspected cases of trimalleolar fractures, supination adduction injury (to assess plafond injury), and look for comminution.
- MRI is indicated to assess soft tissue or cartilage injuries.

28.4.3.5 Treatment

Initial management of all ankle fractures includes RICE protocol with analgesics. Elevation of lower limb is essential in decreasing edema around ankle. Bohler Braun's splint may be used (Fig. 28.8).

Non-operative or conservative management is indicated in these conditions

1. Stable ankle fracture
   - Stable medial or lateral malleolus fracture
   - Small avulsion tip fractures of medial or lateral malleolus
   - Posterior malleolar fracture with <25% joint involvement or <2 mm step-off
2. Unfit for surgery

The options available include (Fig. 28.9)

- Cam boot
- Below-knee slab or cast
- Short leg splint

Operative management includes open reduction and internal fixation (ORIF) and external fixation. Anatomic reduction with restoration of ankle mortise is aimed for during the surgery. Direct lateral approach is used for fibular fractures. Direct medial approach is used for an isolated medial fracture. The posterolateral approach is used for fibula and posterior malleolus fractures. The posteromedial approach is used for medial malleolus and posterior malleolus fractures.

ORIF is indicated in fractures with

- Talar displacement
- Bimalleolar fracture or its equivalent
- Posterior malleolar fracture with >25% joint involvement or >2 mm step-off
- Maisonneuve fracture
- Open fracture
- Symptomatic malleolar nonunions

The implant options include (Fig. 28.10)

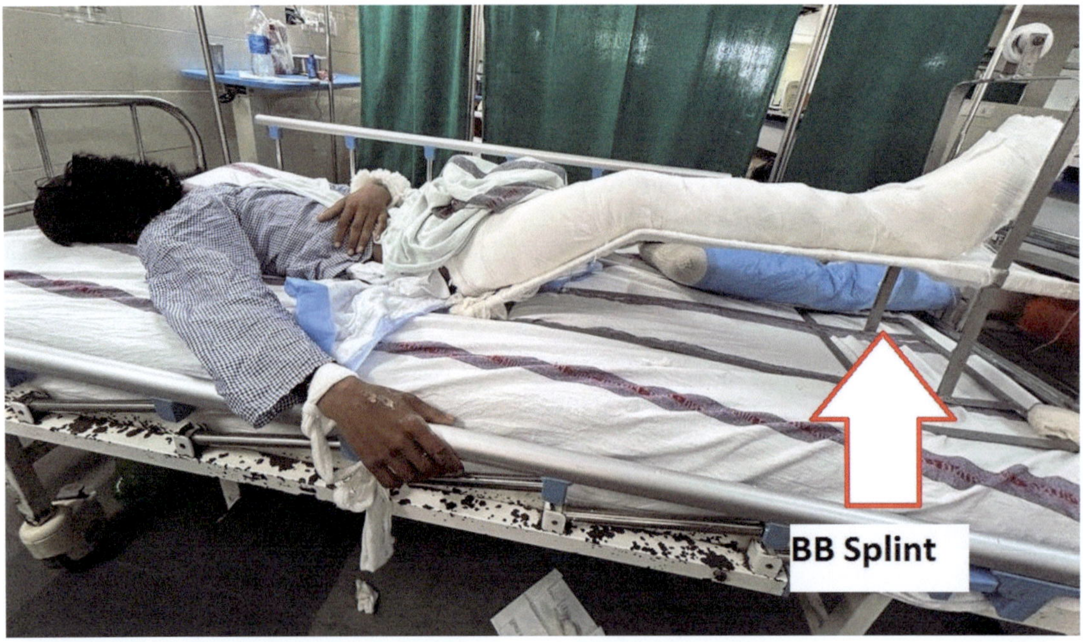

Fig. 28.8 Bohler–Braun splint

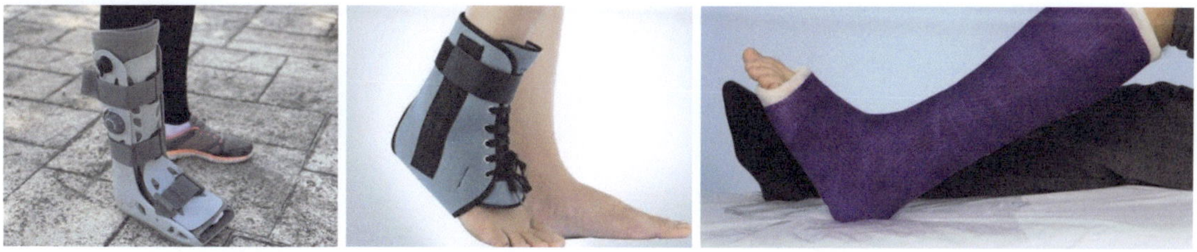

Fig. 28.9 Options available for conservative management

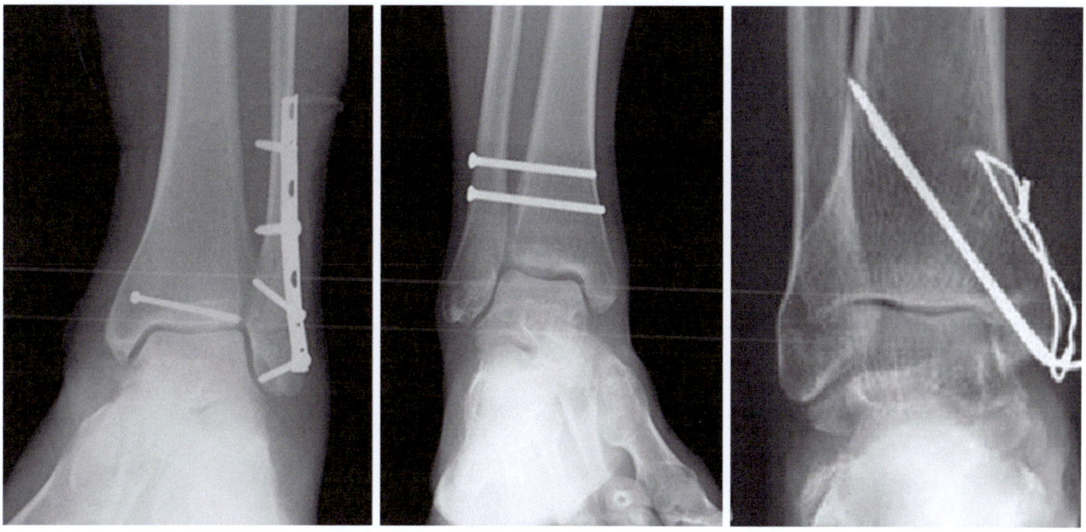

Fig. 28.10 Implant options for ORIF in ankle fractures (screws, plates, and tension bank wiring)

- Lag screws (medial and lateral malleolus fractures)
- Antiglide plate (for medial malleolus fractures—Supination adduction type)
- Tension band fixation (medial malleoulus feacrutes)
- Associated syndesmosis, if found unstable, is fixed with the help of screws or using suture anchors.

The overall success rate is 90%.

External Fixation

It is indicated

- In ankle fractures in scenarios wherein there are open fractures with severe contamination, poor soft tissue envelope (skin impending necrosis, severe blisters, neurovascular injury)
- In cases of unstable reduction

Ankle spanning fixator's or Ilizarov (ring fixators), or hybrid fixators are the most common varieties. Pin tract infection is the most common complication. Moreover, the majority of these fractures are operated in a staged manner with the first stage being External fixation, followed by definitive ORIF later when the soft tissue covet and other factors are favourable (Fig. 28.11).

Complications

- Nonunion
- Malunion

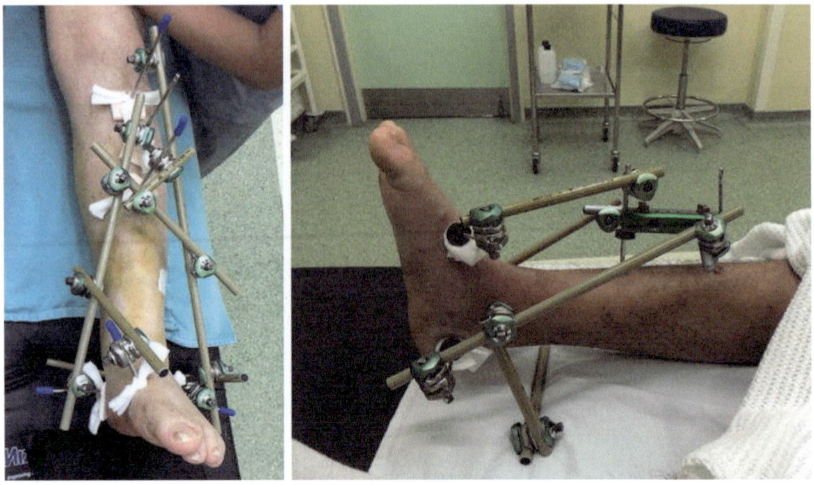

Fig. 28.11 External fixator

- Compartment syndrome
- Implant failure or breakout
- Infection
- Skin necrosis and CRPS

28.4.4 Pilon Fractures

28.4.4.1 Epidemiology

Pilon fractures are fractures of the distal tibia characterized by high-energy injury leading to dissociation of the articular surface from the tibia shaft. Plafond refers to the distal tibial articular surface, which forms the roof of ankle joint. It accounts for 5–10% of all tibial fractures, usually seen in age group 35–45 with male preponderance over females.

28.4.4.2 Mechanism of Injury

The most common mechanism is abnormally high axial load, leading the talus to drive into the plafond (motor vehicle accidents or fall from heights). The fracture often contains three fragments, mainly medial malleolar, posterolateral, and anterolateral fragments. Associated injuries include fibula fractures, open injury, and compromised soft tissues.

28.4.4.3 Classification

The classification most commonly used is AO/OTA classification, which broadly divides the fracture into extra-articular, partial-articular, and complete-articular (Fig. 28.12).

28.4.4.4 Clinical Presentation

- Severe ankle pain
- Inability to weight bear or ambulate
- Bony tenderness, deformity, and edema with ecchymosis.
- Swelling around the ankle, deformity in case of displaced fractures
- Soft tissue assessment may show blisters, tenting of skin or open wounds, and severe range of motion restriction. (Fig. 28.13)
- Neurovascular compromise in cases of displaced fractures or fractures with compartment syndrome may be seen.

28.4.4.5 Imaging

- Routine ankle AP and lateral views, along with mortise view (AP view in 10° internal rotation), along with full-length tibia radiographs with knee joint is performed

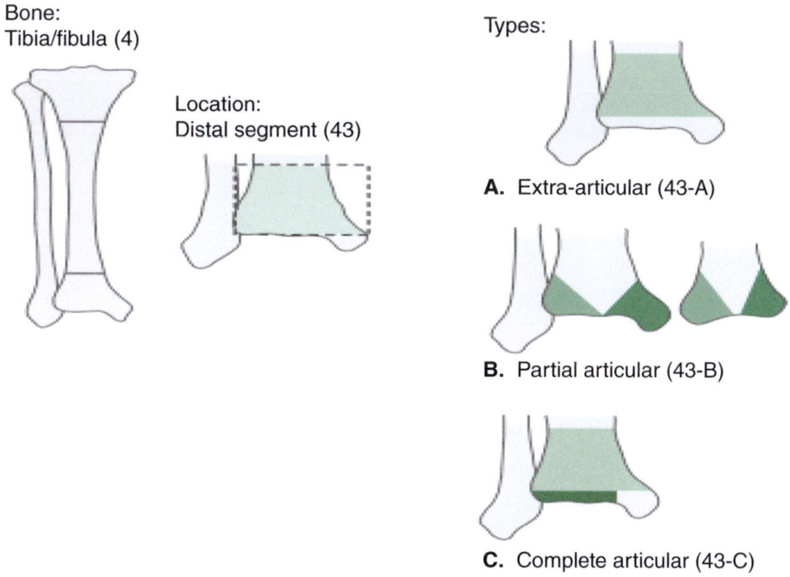

Fig. 28.12 AO/OTA classification of tibial pilon fracture (AO surgery)

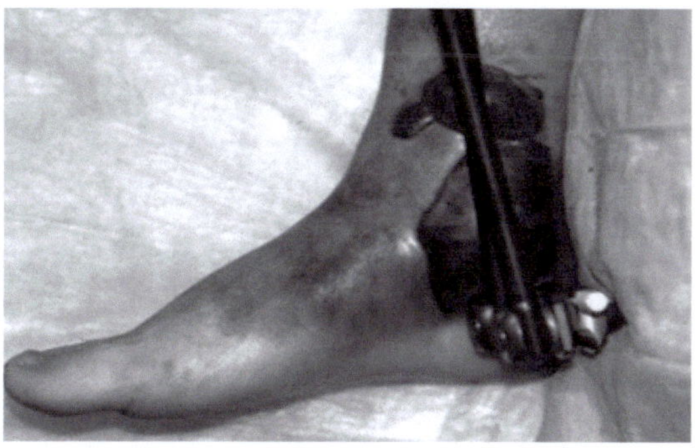

Fig. 28.13 Clinical picture of a patient with a pilon fracture and compromised soft tissues. Note the fixator applied to stabilize the patient

- CT scans are important in preoperative planning to assess articular involvement, fracture displacement and fracture comminution. 'Mercedes-Benz sign' seen in axial view (3 parts visible)

28.4.4.6 Treatment

Management includes

- RICE protocol with analgesics
- Elevation of lower limb is essential in decreasing edema around ankle.
- Bohler Braun's splint may be used.
- If significant soft tissue compromise is expected or when open fractures are encountered, external fixation followed by staged open reduction and internal fixation can be attempted
- ORIF with locking plates are the treatment of choice in displaced fractures. Extra-articular variety can be treated with intramedullary nails, and severe fracture fragment comminution may require arthrodesis.

28.4.5 Talus Fracture

28.4.5.1 Clinical Anatomy

Talus is the osseous link between leg and foot. It consists of a head, neck, and body and articulates with the tibia to form the ankle joint, with calcaneum to form subtalar joint, and with the naviculum to form a talonavicular joint.

28.4.5.2 Epidemiology and Mechanism of Injury

Fractures of talus accounts for 3–6% of fractures of foot and are associated with high-velocity injuries (motor vehicle accidents or falls from height). They have a high propensity for avascular necrosis owing to their precarious blood sup-

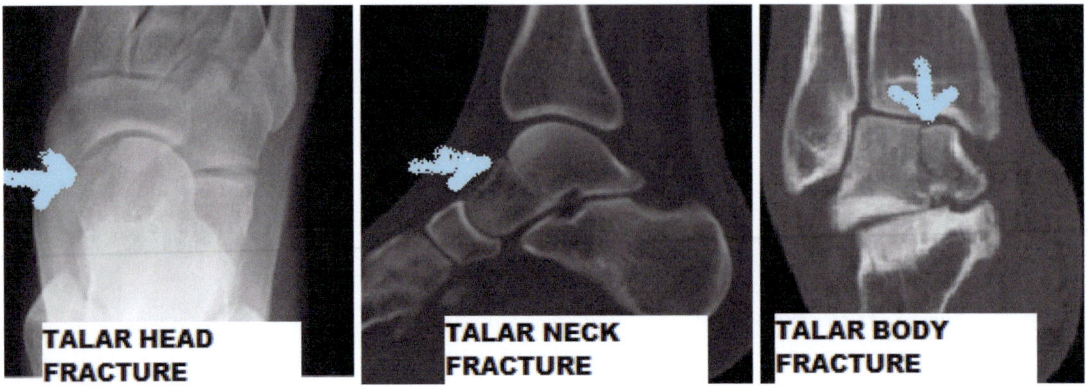

Fig. 28.14 Morphology of talus fractures

ply. Fractures of talus can be of the body or neck or head (Fig. 28.14). Talar head fractures occur at the articular surface of the talonavicular joint. No classification exists for this type of fracture; however, they may be associated with subluxation or dislocation of talus.

28.4.5.3 Clinical Presentation

- Pain, inability to weight bear or ambulate
- Swelling and hematoma involving ankle.
- Physical examination may reveal significant ecchymosis and swelling around the ankle
- Deformity in case of displaced fractures
- Bony tenderness,
- Soft tissue assessment may show blisters in case of displaced fractures, tenting of skin or open wounds, and severe range of motion restriction.
- Neurovascular compromise in cases of displaced fractures or fractures with compartment syndrome may be seen.

28.4.5.4 Imaging

- Anteroposterior (AP), mortise, and lateral views of the ankle
- AP, oblique, and lateral views of the foot.
- Special views—Canale radiographic view for talar neck fractures

Hawkins sign refers to a thin linear subcortical radiolucency on post-treatment images, indicating preserved blood flow to the talar body in the setting of talar neck fractures.

Computed tomography aids in surgical planning, evaluating clinically suspected radiographically occult talar fracture, assessing displacement, and detecting additional fractures.

28.4.5.5 Treatment

Talus receives its blood supply from the posterior tibial artery, dorsalis pedis artery, and perforating peroneal artery. Non-displaced talar fractures receive conservative treatment, and displaced fractures are an indication for surgical intervention.

Talus body or neck or head fractures: treated conservatively if its undisplaced and displaced fractures require ORIF. Higher grades of neck fractures are prone to avascular necrosis (Fig. 28.15). Type 1 neck fractures are treated conservatively if its undisplaced, and ORIF is preferred when fracture is displaced. Type 2–4 fractures are treated with ORIF. Body fractures have good outcomes except for comminuted or crushed type.

The implant options include cannulated screws, headless (Herbert) screws, and mini-fragment plates. Arthrodesis as a primary option may be viable in severe communition. Patients with soft tissue compromise are treated with a two-stage protocol wherein the first stage is damage control with the help of external fixators and the second stage is definitive fixation once the soft tissue is viable.

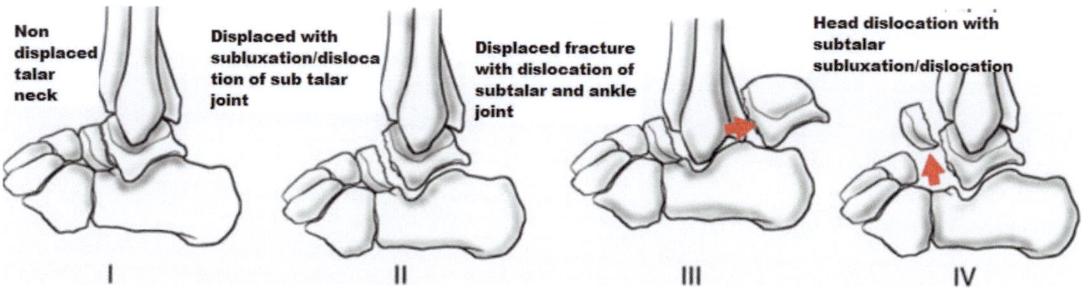

Fig. 28.15 Hawkins classification of Talar neck fractures

28.4.5.6 Complications

Secondary osteoarthritis of subtalar or tibiotalar joints in unreduced fractures, malunion, and avascular necrosis.

28.4.6 Chronic Injuries

28.4.6.1 Tendoachilles Rupture

The Achilles tendon is formed by the confluence of soleus tendon and medial and lateral gastrocnemius tendons.

28.4.6.2 Mechanism of Injury

Injury occurs due to sudden dorsiflexion of a plantarflexed foot. It occurs often as an athletic injury. It can be seen also with road traffic injuries.

28.4.6.3 Clinical Presentation

It may present as an acute or chronic presentation. Rupture usually occurs 4–6 cm above the calcaneal insertion in the hypovascular region. The presentation includes

- A history of a popping sensation associated with weakness and difficulty in walking and pain in heel.

28.4.6.4 Physical Examination

- Increased resting ankle dorsiflexion in prone position with knees bent
- A papable gap (Fig. 28.16)

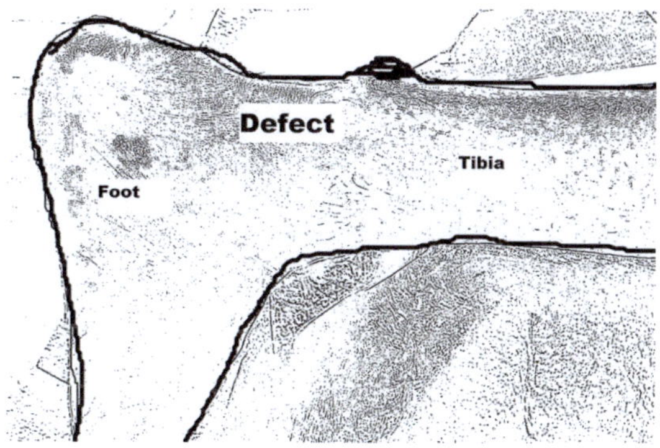

Fig. 28.16 Representation of Tendoachilles tear

- Calf atrophy may be evident in chronic conditions.
- Weakness in ankle plantar flexion and increased passive dorsiflexion.
- Thompson test (lack of plantarflexion when calf is squeezed)
- Inability to stand on toes on the affected side and inability to perform single limb hops

28.4.6.5 Imaging

Radiographs can be used to rule out other pathologies like trauma or fractures.

USG or ultra sonography may be useful in determining complete vs partial tears.

MRI is the investigation of choice and is used to measure the size of the defect, the quality of the tissue, retraction of the tendon, and coexisting conditions.

28.4.6.6 Treatment

- Non operative management is indicated in conditions
  (a) medically frail patients
  (b) sedentary patients
  (c) acute injury with minimal tear.

- Operative techniques include
  (a) End-to-end repair (acute injuries < 6 weeks)
  (b) reconstruction with VY advancement (defect <3 cm) and
  (c) FHL transfer (>3 cm defect).

28.4.6.7 Complications

(a) re-rupture
(b) wound complications
(c) infection
(d) sural nerve injury.

Multiple Choice Questions

1. Hawkins sign is seen with which of the following fractures
   (a) Talus fracture
   (b) Calcaneum fracture
   (c) Pilon fracture
   (d) All of the above
2. Mercedes-Benz sign is seen with following fractures
   (a) Talus fracture
   (b) Calcaneum fracture
   (c) Pilon fracture
   (d) Medial malleolus fracture
3. The most commonly injured ankle ligament is
   (a) ATFL
   (b) PTFL
   (c) CFL
   (d) Deltoid ligament
4. Launge–Hausen classification SER is a type of which Weber?
   (a) Weber-A
   (b) Weber-B
   (c) Weber-C
   (d) All of the above
5. Which bone fracture near the ankle and foot often proceeds to AVN?
   (a) Talus
   (b) Calcaneum
   (c) Naviculum
   (d) Cuboid

Answers: 1. (a), 2. (c), 3. (a), 4. (b), 5. (a)

Foot Injuries

29

Balgovind S. Raja and Anusree Akshay

Each human foot is made up of 26 bones, 30 joints and a large number of muscles, ligaments and tendons, which all work in unison to bear weight and aid in body propulsion during gait. The human foot can be functionally divided into three parts (Fig. 29.1): Forefoot, Midfoot and Hindfoot. The hindfoot consists of talus and calcaneum. The midfoot consists of the tarsal bones. The forefoot consists of metatarsals and phalanges.

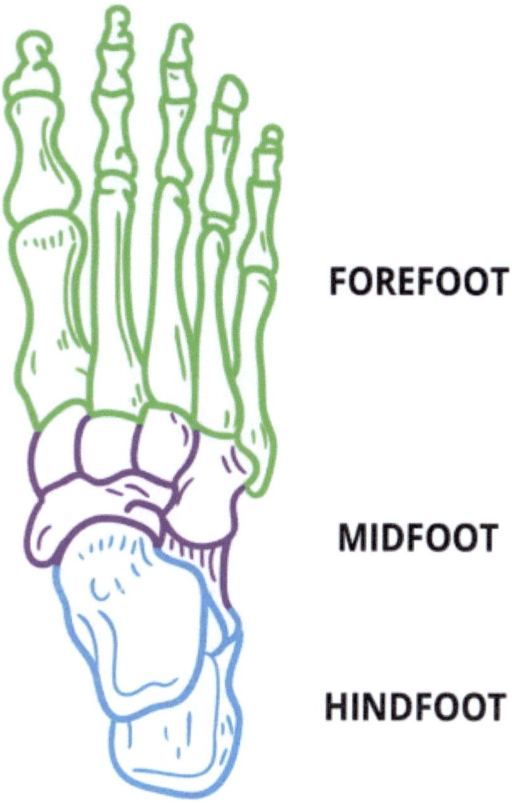

Fig. 29.1 Functional division of foot

B. S. Raja (✉)
Department of Orthopedics, AIIMS,
Patna, Bihar, India

A. Akshay
All India Institute of Medical Sciences, Raipur, India

V. Kumar et al. (eds.), *A Quick Guide to Essential Orthopedics*,
https://doi.org/10.1007/978-981-95-2676-5_29

29.1 Foot Arches

The foot comprises three arches: one transverse arch (anterior) and two longitudinal arches (medial and lateral). The tarsal and metatarsal bones form them, and the foot's ligaments and tendons support them. By virtue of their design, they can support the body's weight and absorb the shock caused by movement in a manner similar to that of a spring. These arches give the foot flexibility, which makes activities like walking and running easier (Table 29.1).

Two abnormalities can be seen with foot arch. First is pes planus or flat-foot (Fig. 29.2), the other pes cavus or an increase in arch (Fig. 29.3).

Table 29.1 Arches of foot

Arch	Bony support
Medial longitudinal	Calcaneum, talus, navicular, three cuneiforms and the first three metatarsal bones
Lateral longitudinal	Calcaneum, cuboid, 4th and 5th metatarsal
Transverse	Metatarsal bases, cuboid and three cuneiform bones

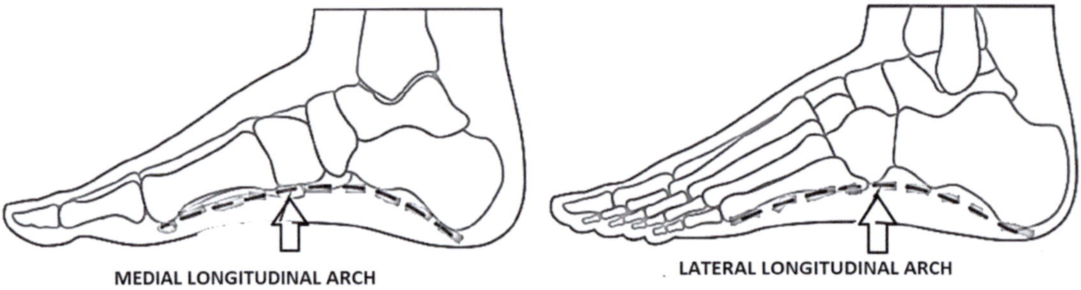

Fig. 29.2 Two longitudinal arches of foot

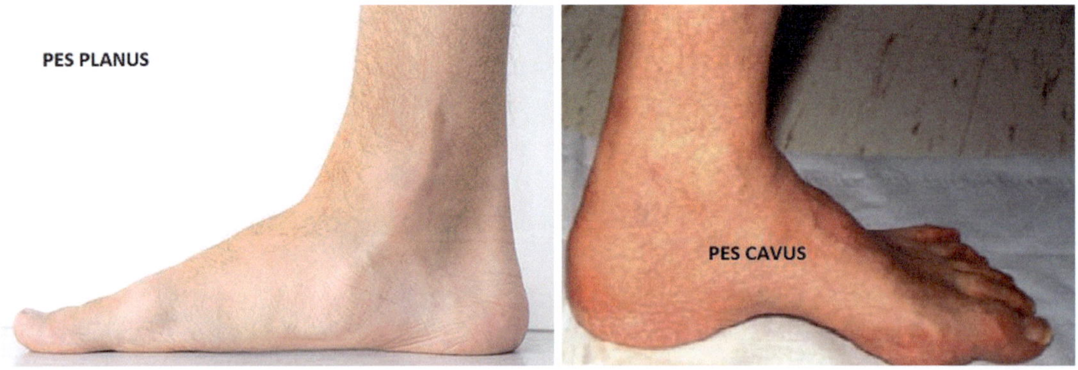

Fig. 29.3 Pathological varieties of arches

29.2 Fractures of Foot

(A) Hind foot
- Fractures of Calcaneum
- Fractures of Talus (described in detail in Chap. 28)

(B) Midfoot
- Cuneiforms, Cuboid
- Navicular

(C) Forefoot
- Fractures of metatarsals and phalanges

29.2.1 Fractures of Hind Foot

29.2.1.1 Fractures of Calcaneum

Epidemiology

Calcaneum is the most commonly fractured bone among tarsal in the foot. It provides support for weight-bearing, transmits weight to the sole and acts as a lever to improve the efficiency of the calf muscles. The longitudinal arch of the foot at the posterior aspect is formed by this bone. Calcaneum articulates with the talus via three facets out of which the main joint is subtalar joint. It also articulates with the cuboid forming the calcaneo-cuboid joint (Fig. 29.4).

Mechanism of Injury

The most common mechanism of injury is high velocity trauma with axial loading (fall from height, road traffic accidents). About 17% of these fractures are open injuries. Calcaneal tuberosity fractures are seen in osteoporotic bones with a history of violent contractions of the triceps surae or tendoachilles against forced dorsiflexion. Anterior process fractures occur due to twisting injury mechanism. Often, these fractures are seen with poly trauma including fractures of pelvis, chest and spine.

Classification

The fractures can be broadly classified as extra-articular and intra-articular fractures.

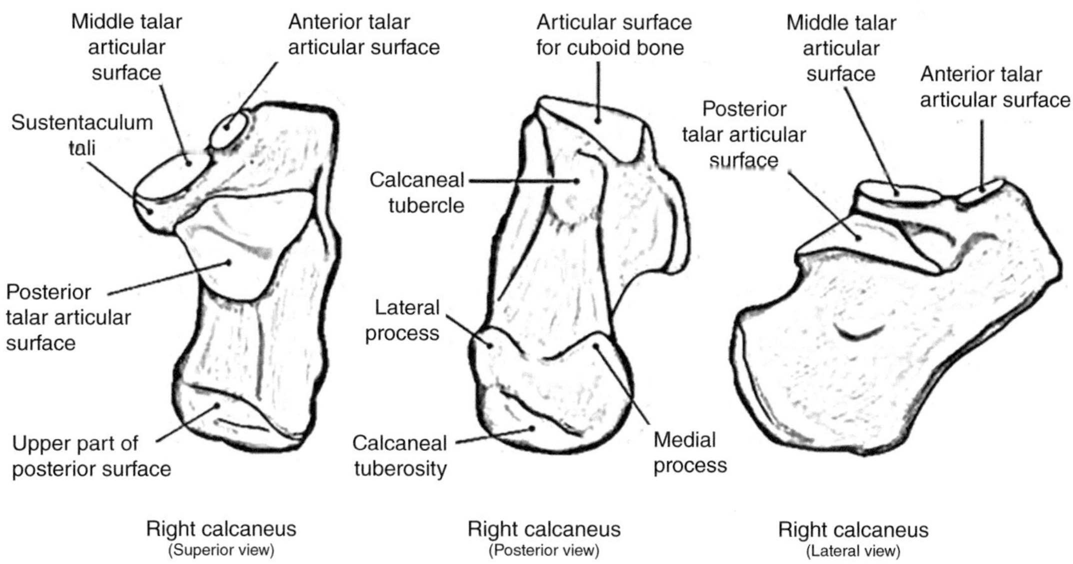

Fig. 29.4 Calcaneum morphology

- Extraarticular fractures accounts for 25% of calcaneal fractures
  - Calcaneal tuberosity fractures
  - Sustentaculum tali fractures
  - Body fractures
  - Anterior process fractures
- The intra-articular fracture classification (Table 29.2).
  - Sanders classification (CT scan coronal slice)
  - Essex–Lopresti classification based on fracture lines seen on lateral radiographs

Clinical Presentation

- Diffuse pain, oedema and ecchymosis at the heel and ankle
- Inability to weight-bear
- Any disability of the Achilles tendon should raise the suspicion of a calcaneum injury
- Skin or soft tissue may be compromised

Table 29.2 Calcaneum fracture classification

Fracture	Classification
Extra-articular	Calcaneal tuberosity fracture Sustentaculum tali fracture Body fracture Anterior process fracture
Intra-articular	
(a) Essex-Lopresti classification a diagram 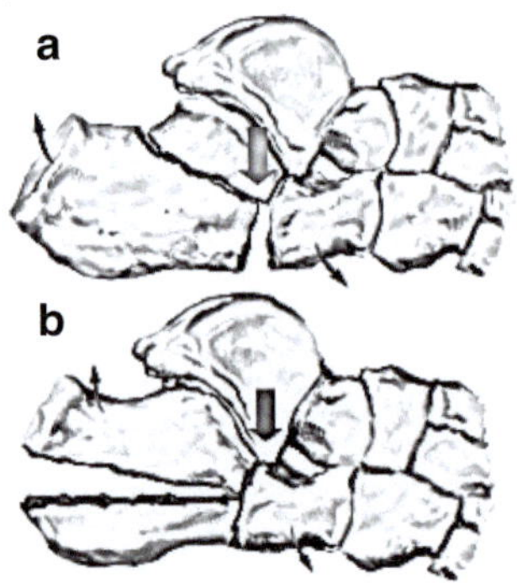	(a) Joint depression type: A single vertical fracture line through the angle of Gissane, separating the anterior and posterior portions of the calcaneus (b) Tongue type: A vertical fracture line as a depression type with another horizontal fracture line running posteriorly, creating a postero-superior fragment
(b) Sanders classification 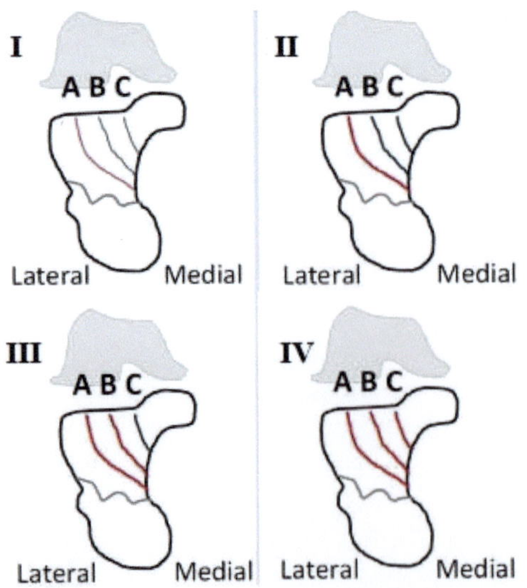	(a) Type I fractures: 1 Undisplaced or minimally displaced bony fragment (b) Type II fractures: 2 bony fragments involving the posterior facet (c) Type III fractures: 3 bony fragments, including an additional depressed middle fragment (d) Type IV fractures: 4 comminuted bony fragments

Physical examination

- Oedema at the ankle or foot associated with ecchymosis
- Restriction of ankle or foot movements
- Should be evaluated for compartment syndrome
- Tenderness at the heel

Imaging

Radiographic investigation includes

- Anteroposterior view of ankle, anteroposterior view of foot
- Lateral view of ankle
- Oblique views of foot
- Harris view or Canale view for axial calcaneal orientation
  - Bohler's angle: the angle between two lines, the first line is between the highest point on the tuberosity and the highest point of posterior facet, and the second is the highest point on the anterior process and the highest point on the posterior facet. Normal is 20–40° (Fig. 29.5)
  - Critical angle of Gissane: the angle between two lines, the first along the anterior downward slope of the calcaneus and the second along the superior upward slope. A normal critical angle of Gissane is 130–145° (Fig. 29.5)
- *Mondor's Sign* is a haematoma identified along the sole and is considered pathogenomic for calcaneal fracture.
- In calcaneal fractures, usually, the Bohler's angle is decreased and the angle of Gissane is increased. However, normal Bohler's and Gissane's angles do not rule out a fracture

Computed tomography: 'Gold standard'

- Preoperative planning
- Classification of fractures

Treatment

Open fractures may require debridement and external fixators as first stage, followed by second stage, definite ORIF or flap coverage with K-wire fixation and continuation of fixator.

Extra-articular fractures

- Conservative in majority—Casts with non-weight-bearing
- Tuberosity avulsion, displaced sustentaculum tali and large substantial calcaneal body fractures may require operative management.

Intra-articular fractures

- With significant loss of joint surfaces, altered angles: Surgical intervention.

The implant options: ORIF with locking calcaneum plates or screws for tongue-type fragment or avulsion fractures (Fig. 29.6).

Complications Compartment syndrome, Osteomyelitis, postoperative wound infection, mal-

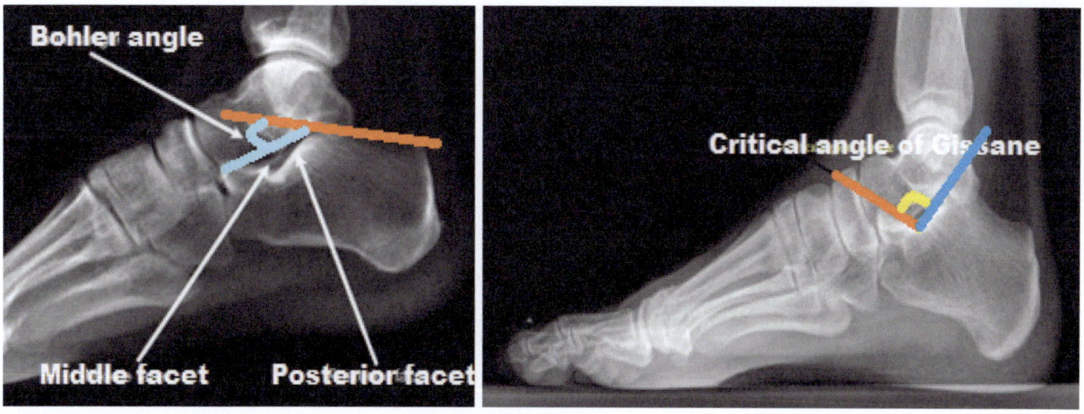

Fig. 29.5 Radiographic angles in lateral radiograph of ankle

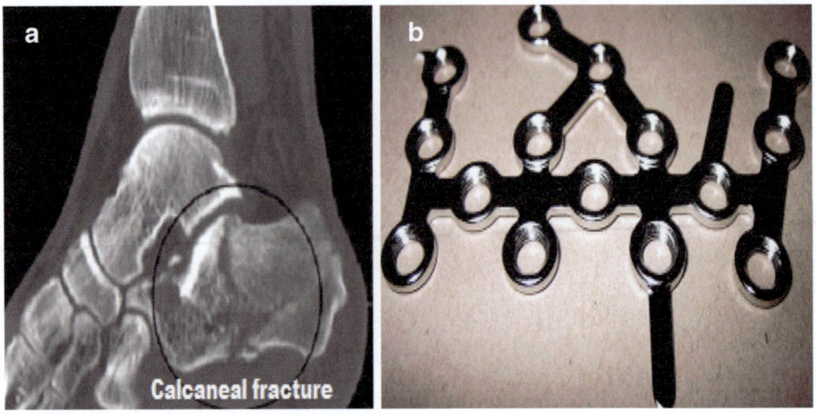

Fig. 29.6 Calcaneal fracture extending into the subtalar joint (**a**) along with the plate (**b**) used for osteosynthesis

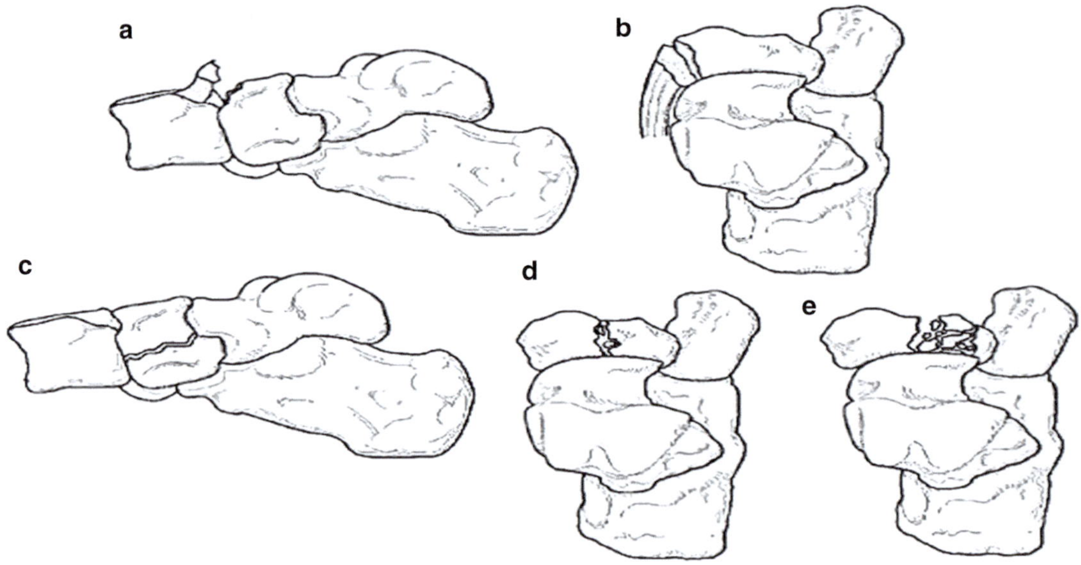

Fig. 29.7 Fracture of the navicular—avulsion (**a**, **b**), body (**c**, **d**, **e**)

union and subtalar arthritis. Sural nerve injury and peroneal tendon dysfunction can also be seen. Unreduced calcaneum fractures can lead to flat-foot.

29.2.2 Fractures of Midfoot

29.2.2.1 Fractures of Naviculum

Provide headings of mechanism of injury, classification, clinical features, imaging and treatment

29.2.2.2 Mechanism of Injury

Navicular fractures are rare fractures that occur mostly due to direct trauma or due to repetitive microstress.

Classification

- Avulsion fractures with a mechanism of plantarflexion with eversion/inversion
- Tuberosity fractures caused by eversion with simultaneous contraction of PTT
- Body fractures by axial loading (Fig. 29.7).

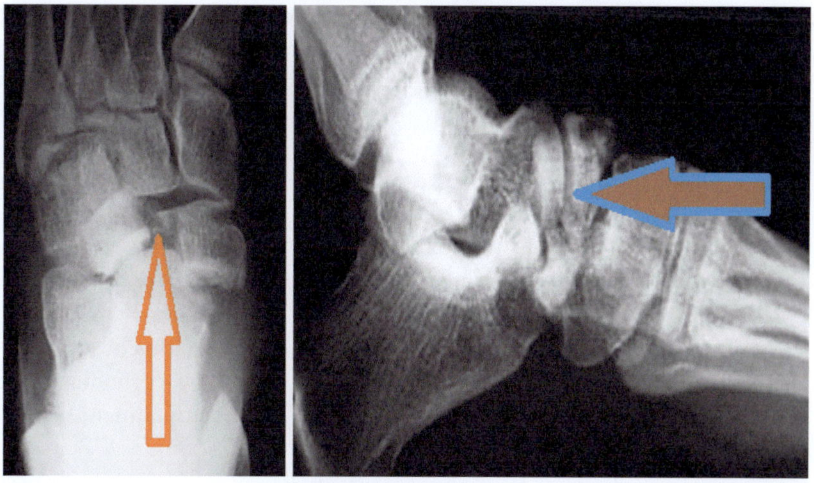

Fig. 29.8 Navicular fracture radiograph

Clinical Presentation

- Pain on the medial aspect of dorsum of foot associated with swelling and difficulty in walking
- Point tenderness over navicular bone along with midfoot swelling and full ROM of ankle and subtalar joints can be observed.

Radiographic initial evaluation: AP, lateral and oblique plain films of the foot and ankle (Fig. 29.8).

Kohler's disease is a self-limiting rare condition characterised by avascular necrosis of navicular bone.

Treatment

- Nondisplaced fractures—immobilisation in short leg cast with non-weight-bearing for 6–8 weeks.
- Unstable fractures usually need surgery and screw fixation is preferred.

29.2.2.3 Injuries to the Cuneiforms

The three cuneiforms are present on the medial side of the midfoot. Fractures are rare and are often associated with metatarsal injuries. Direct crushing forces or axial load through the foot leads to this fracture. Clinical presentation is that of a patient with midfoot pain on weight-bearing and possible ecchymosis over the dorsum of the midfoot. Palpation often reveals tenderness over

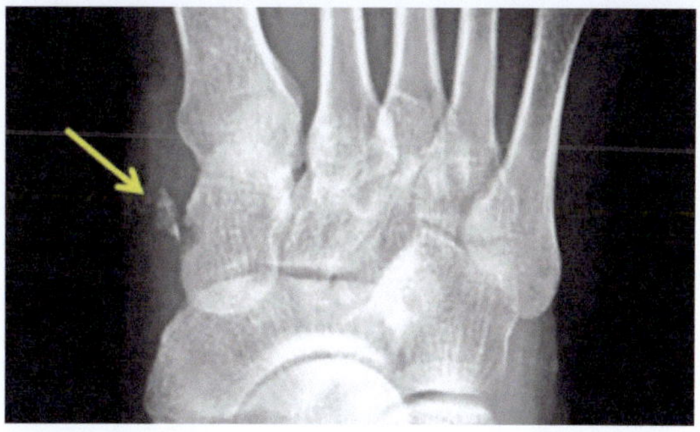

Fig. 29.9 Cuneiform fracture

the medial dorsal aspect. Radiographs (AP and oblique foot) show the fracture lines (Fig. 29.9). Treatment for stable, non-displaced cuneiform fractures is below knee cast. Fractures with structural displacement or instability need open reduction through a dorsal approach combined with rigid internal fixation.

29.2.2.4 Lisfranc Injury or Dislocation

Provide headings of mechanism of injury, classification, clinical features, imaging and treatment

29.2.2.5 Anatomy

This injury describes a spectrum of injuries involving the tarsometatarsal (TM) joints of the foot. The articulations between the first, second and third metatarsal bones and the cuneiform bones form the Lisfranc joint. The 'Lisfranc ligament' is an isolated ligament that connects the medial cuneiform to the second metatarsal (Fig. 29.10).

29.2.2.6 Mechanism of Injury

- Direct mechanism: Crush injuries to the joint region during a motor vehicle collision.
- Indirect mechanism: Sports participation involves a longitudinal force while the foot is plantar flexed with a medial or lateral rotational force.

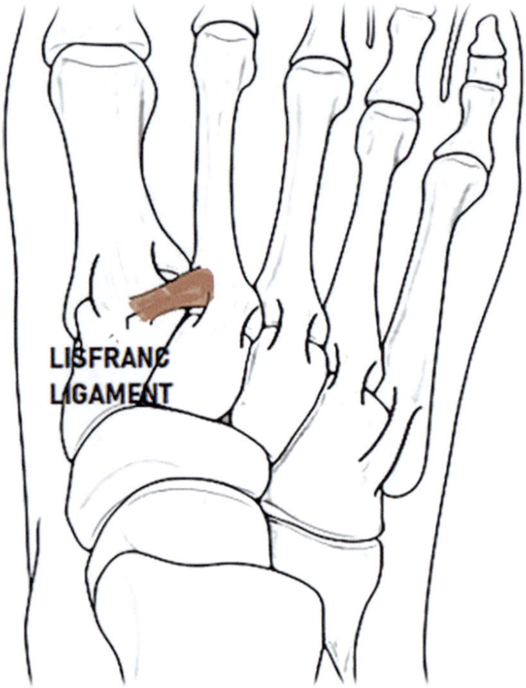

Fig. 29.10 Lisfranc ligament

29.2.2.7 Clinical Presentation

- Midfoot pain associated with difficulty in weight-bearing
- Pain is classically increased on weight-bearing, especially in push-off phase of gait
- Oedema of foot
- Late or undiagnosed cases can present with compartment syndrome

29.2.2.8 Classification

'Myerson classification': Based on the displacement of rays or metatarsals (Fig. 29.11).

- Type A: total incongruity (all the rays are displaced in one direction)
- Type B: partial incongruity (lateral four rays can be displaced laterally or medial 1st ray displaced medially)
- Type C: divergent (1st ray displaced medially and lateral 4 rays displaced laterally)

29.2.2.9 Imaging

- Anteroposterior
- 30-degree oblique and lateral weight-bearing radiographs of foot

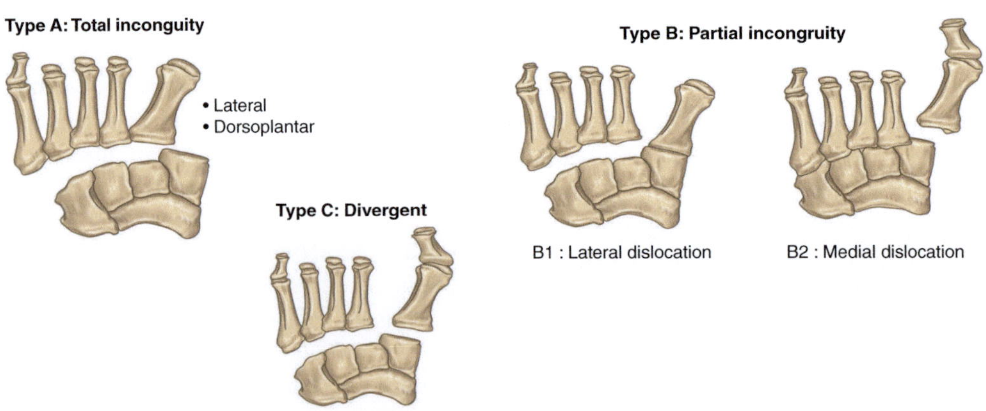

Fig. 29.11 Classification of Lisfranc injury

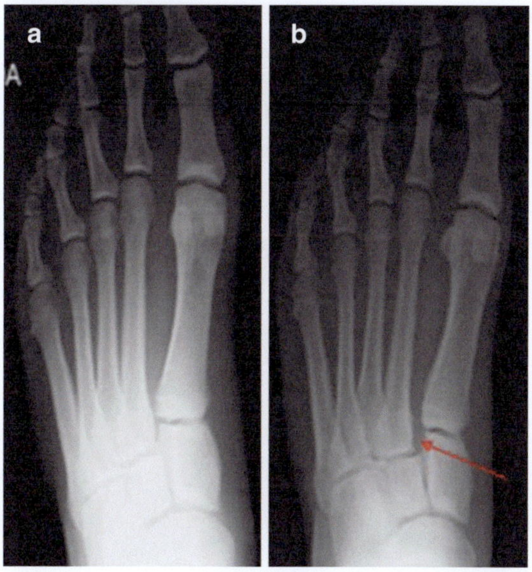

Fig. 29.12 Importance of weight-bearing. (**a**) shows non-weight-bearing radiographs, (**b**) weight-bearing shows diastasis between the 1st and 2nd metatarsal

Weight-bearing rays are essential in diagnosing the condition (Fig. 29.12).

The findings in X-rays:

- Malalignment of the lateral margin of the first metatarsal base with the lateral edge of the medial cuneiform
- Malalignment of the medial aspect of the second metatarsal base with the medial edge of the middle cuneiform, and/or small avulsion fragments of one of the metatarsal or cuneiform bones (Fleck sign)
- A displacement of more than 2 mm between the first and second metatarsal bases is strongly suggestive of a Lisfranc injury
- On oblique views, the medial aspect of the cuboid should line up with the medial aspect of the 4th metatarsal base.
- On the lateral weight-bearing radiographs, the dorsal cortex of the 1st metatarsal and medial cuneiform should be aligned.

Computed tomography is diagnostic and can be helpful in surgical planning and assessing minor fractures. MRI is useful in investigating ligamentous injury.

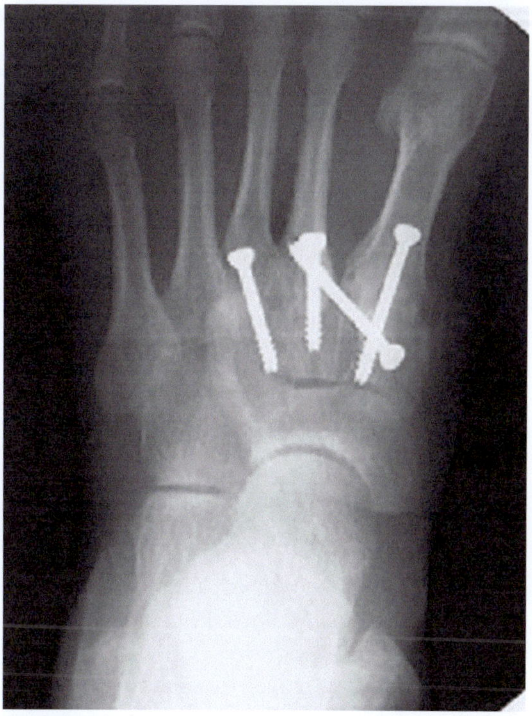

Fig. 29.13 Screw fixation in a Lisfranc injury

29.2.2.10 Treatment

- Initial treatment: RICE regimen with emphasis on reduction of injury, below-knee slab and aggressive limb elevation
- Conservative treatment: Only reserved for anatomically stable and non-displaced injuries, wherein the patient is immediately made non-weight-bearing and put in a cast or boot. After at least six weeks, if clinically on tender and radiographs are negative weight-bearing can be started along with physiotherapy.
- Any displacement requires surgical fixation.

Implant options include screws, K-wires and small mini plates (Fig. 29.13).

Complications include compartment syndrome, post-traumatic arthrosis, skin necrosis, infection and loss of normal foot contour if untreated.

29.2.3 Injuries to the Forefoot

29.2.3.1 Metatarsal Fractures

Mechanism of Injury Usually results from the direct blow of a heavy object dropped onto the forefoot. They can also be seen with motor vehicle accidents. A direct force can result in the fracture of any metatarsal at any point, and indirect forces, such as twisting the body with the toes fixed, produce fractures of the metatarsal shafts (spiral fractures).

Clinical Presentation Presence of pinpoint tenderness, palpable non-pitting oedema and crepitus. Deformity is readily apparent when there is displacement.

Investigations Radiographs (AP and oblique foot) show the fracture lines (Fig. 29.14).

Treatment Conservative (extended below-knee cast or slab with non-weight-bearing for 3–4 weeks) in all situations other than grossly displaced fractures, unstable fractures, multiple metatarsal injuries and open fractures (Fig. 29.15). In these instances, K-wire fixation is the preferred method.

29.2.3.2 Phalangeal Injuries

Traumatic phalangeal injuries are often isolated injuries. These fractures are also associated with

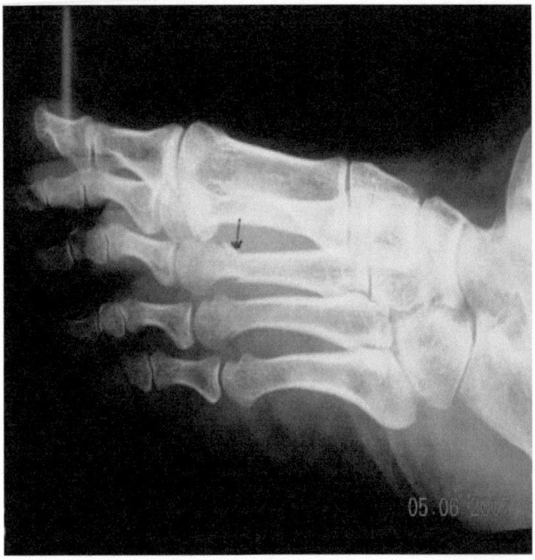

Fig. 29.14 Metatarsal fracture

Fig. 29.15 Unstable injuries require K-wire fixation

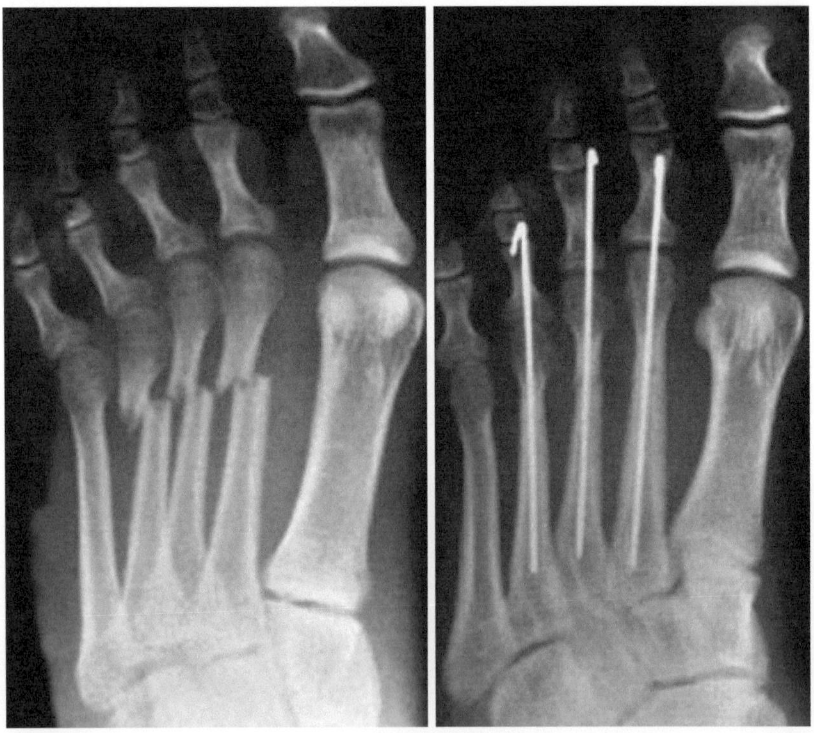

motor vehicle accidents with multiple injuries. They are easy to diagnose with complaints of local pain in the affected toe and are visible in plain radiographs (AP or oblique foot). If displaced, they can be associated with deformity. Most can be treated by buddy taping, with K-wire or needle fixation needed in open fractures or gross deformity.

29.3 Midfoot Injuries

29.3.1 Navicular Stress Fracture

Stress fractures of navicular bone are associated with significant morbidity as there is a high chance of non-union (Fig. 29.16). Patients complain of dorsal foot pain and have tenderness over the navicular bone. Most of these patients require MRI or CT scans or radioisotope scanning to confirm the diagnosis. A well-moulded cast with non-weight-bearing for 6–8 weeks is treatment of choice. Non-unions may require fixation.

29.3.2 Extensor Tendonitis

Tendonitis of the extensor tendons will present as an ache over the dorsal aspect of the midfoot and insertion of tibialis anterior. Weakening is noted among extensor tendons, and the extensor and strengthening is essential (Fig. 29.17).

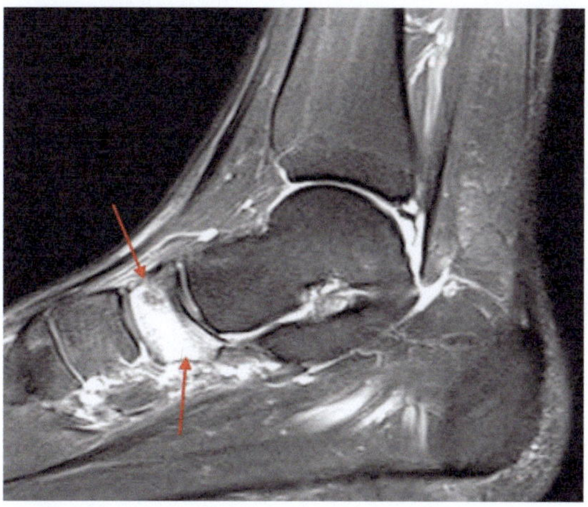

Fig. 29.16 Navicular stress fracture (MRI)

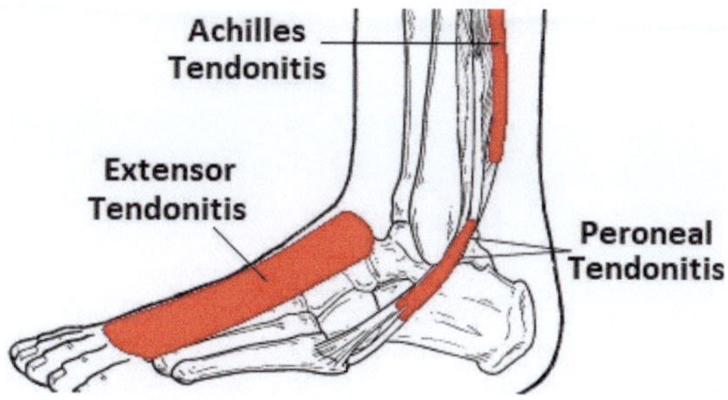

Fig. 29.17 Tendonitis around ankle and foot

29.3.3 Midtarsal Joint Sprains

The sprains of the midtarsal joints are rarely injured except in cases of high velocity or motor vehicle accidents. These injuries are also predisposed in individuals with a history of foot instability. The most commonly involved ligament is the calcaneo-navicular ligament. Treatment is conservative with non-weight-bearing casting for a period of 3–4 weeks.

29.4 Forefoot Injuries

29.4.1 Metatarsal Stress Fractures

Stress fractures of the metatarsals are frequent complaints of athletes, who complain of forefoot pain, aggravated by running or weight-bearing activities. The most common site of injury is the second metatarsal. Often, one requires a bone scan to identify these conditions. The stress fracture of the base of 5th metatarsal is known as a Jones fracture (Fig. 29.18).

The most difficult to treat stress fractures are the second metatarsal fracture, proximal shaft fracture of 5th metatarsal and those affecting the sesamoid bones (Fig. 29.19). Treatment involves non-weight-bearing cast for 4–6 weeks in cases of metatarsal stress fractures. However, in cases of non-union internal fixation may be needed.

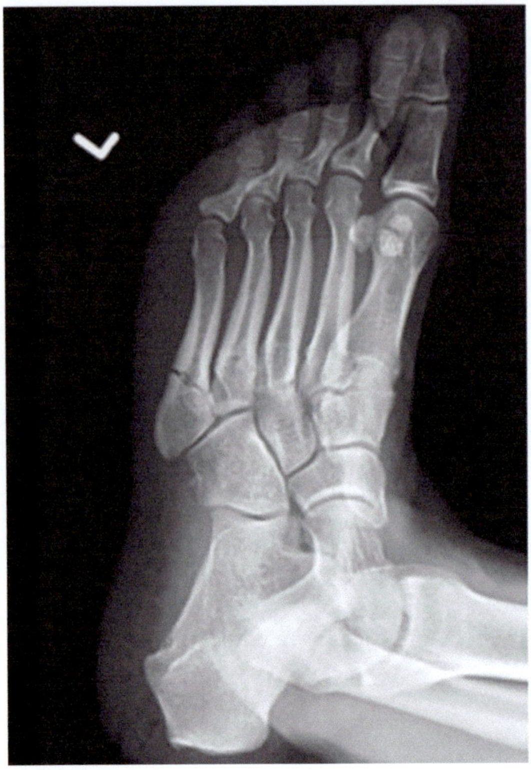

Fig. 29.18 Jones fracture

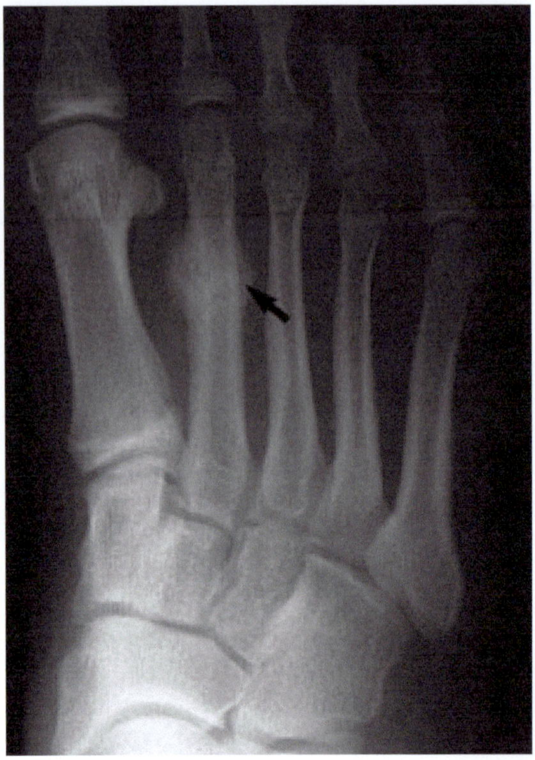

Fig. 29.19 Stress fracture metatarsal

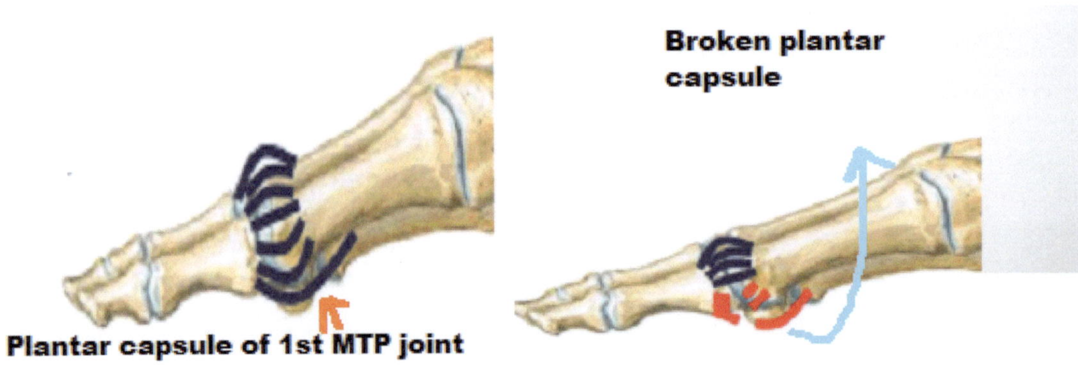

Fig. 29.20 Turf toe mechanism. (Courtesy: Netters anatomy)

29.4.2 First Metatarsophalangeal Joint Sprain

Turf toe or first MTP sprain occurs as a result of excessive forced dorsiflexion of the first MTP joint (Fig. 29.20). Patients often have a history of vigorous 'bending' at the first MTP joint and presents with pain on movement. Plantar capsule and ligament are sprained. Conservative management with focus on weight-bearing restriction along with physiotherapy and orthotic correction may be required.

29.4.3 Sesamoid Injuries

Traumatic fracture, stress fracture and sprain of a bipartite sesamoid are considered as sesamoid

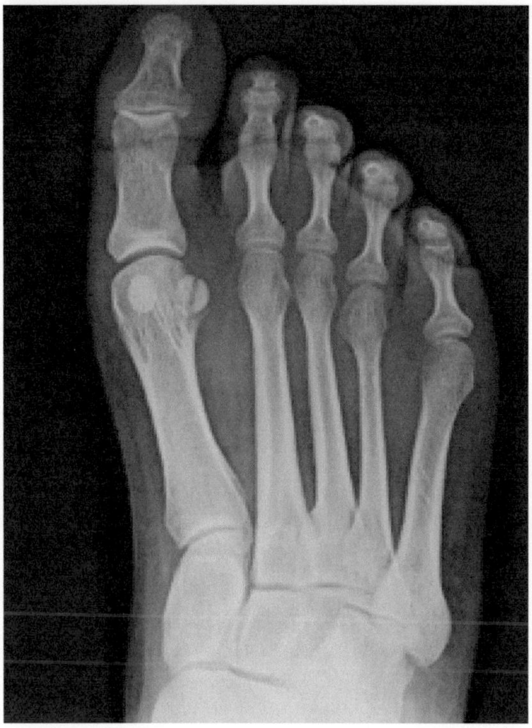

Fig. 29.21 Sesamoid fracture

injuries (Fig. 29.21). Patients present with marked tenderness and swelling in the sesamoid region affected and often walk with their weight borne laterally to compensate. Treatment is conservative and aims to decrease pain and oedema. Rehabilitation includes physiotherapy, padding to distribute the weight and corticosteroid injections. Stress fractures have a propensity for chronicity.

Multiple Choice Questions

1. Sanders classification is utilised in fractures of
   (a) Talus
   (b) Calcaneum
   (c) Navicular
   (d) Tibia
2. Turf toe refers to joint sprain of
   (a) Ist MTP
   (b) 2nd MTP
   (c) 3rd MTP
   (d) 5th MTP
3. Lisfranc ligament connects
   (a) 1st to 2nd MT
   (b) 2nd to 3rd MT
   (c) 3rd to 4th MT
   (d) 4th to 5th MT
4. Jones fracture refers to fracture of
   (a) 1st MT base
   (b) 2nd MT base
   (c) 3rd MT base
   (d) 5th MT base
5. Kohler's disease affects
   (a) Talus
   (b) Cuneiform
   (c) Navicular
   (d) Calcaneum

Answers: 1. (b), 2. (d), 3. (a), 4. (d), 5. (c)

Pelvis Injuries

30

Balgovind S. Raja and Anusree Akshay

30.1 Anatomy

Pelvis is a ring structure formed by sacrum, coccyx, and the innominate bones (ilium, ischium and pubis). The innominate bones articulate posteriorly with the sacrum and anteriorly through pubic symphysis (Fig. 30.1). Acetabulum is formed by fusion of these three innominate bones, and in paediatric age group, they are connected by the triradiate cartilage. The pelvis contains blood vessels, nerves, urogenital organs, and the rectum. True pelvis is the space below the pelvic brim, and false pelvis is the space above pelvic brim (Fig. 30.2).

Fractures of any of these bones leading to pelvic ring disruption are known as pelvic ring fractures. Stability depends upon the integrity of the surrounding ligament complex. Displacement occurs when there is a ring disruption in two places. It can be either through the joints or bone fractures. Neurovascular structures are in proximity to posterior pelvic ligaments, and high index of suspicion should be kept in cases of disruption.

Epidemiology: Injuries to pelvis are not common. The pelvic ring and the bones are solid structures which are held together by strong ligament complexes. These ligament complexes are so strong that a great deal of forces is required. Hence, the injuries to pelvic bones occur as a result of motor vehicle accidents, falls from height, or a skiing accident. Pelvic fractures account for about 10% of fractures in blunt trauma patients. The importance of these fractures is the occurrence of a high rate of associated injuries in about 12–62% of patients. About 40% of associated injuries are related to urogenital system. Urethral injuries are the most common, followed by bladder injuries. Rectal and vaginal injuries are relatively rare, with about 2% incidence each.

B. S. Raja (✉)
Department of Orthopedics, AIIMS,
Patna, Bihar, India

A. Akshay
All India Institute of Medical Sciences, Raipur, India

V. Kumar et al. (eds.), *A Quick Guide to Essential Orthopedics*,
https://doi.org/10.1007/978-981-95-2676-5_30

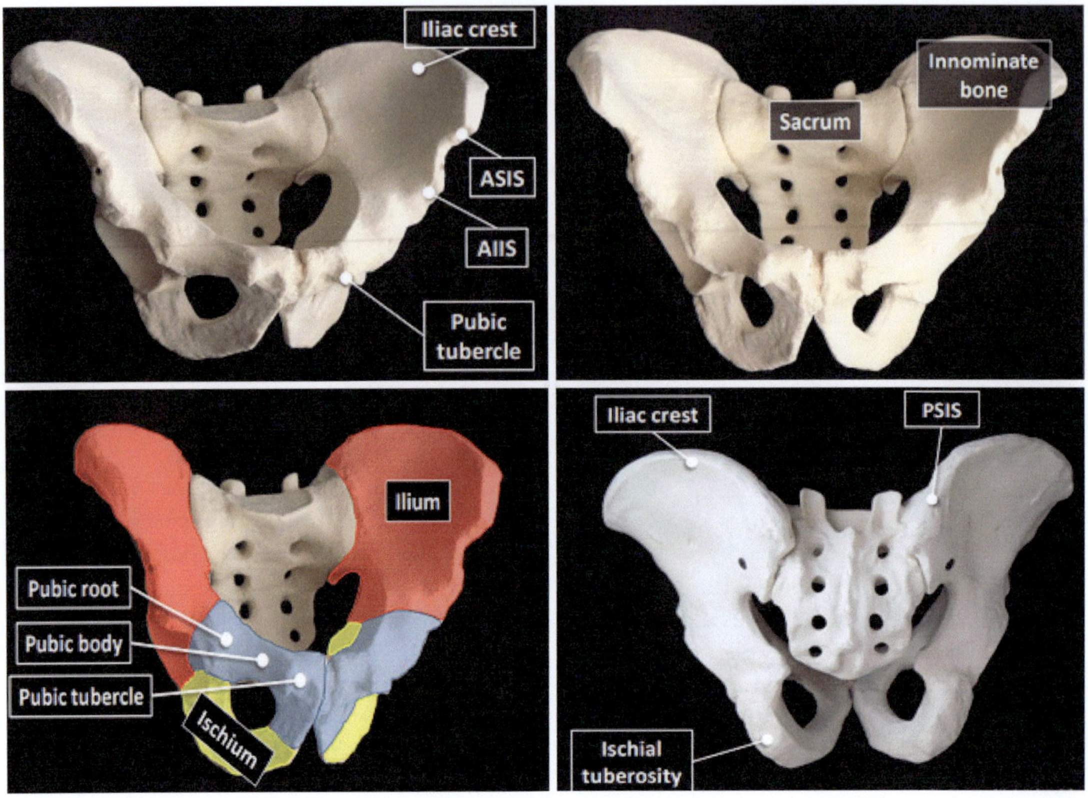

Fig. 30.1 Pelvis anatomy. (Pic courtesy: Rohen et al. [1])

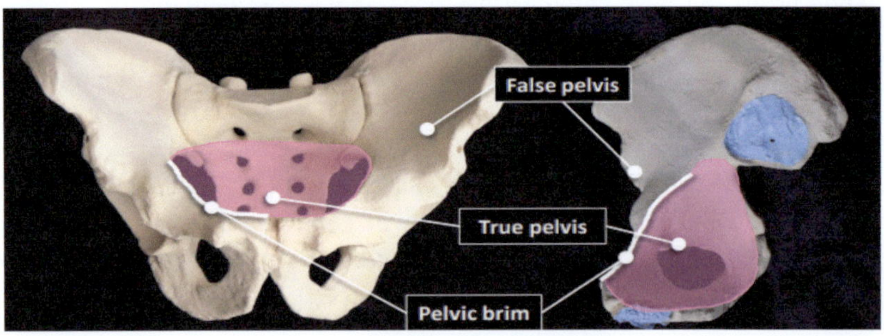

Fig. 30.2 True and false pelvis. (Pic courtesy: Rohen et al. [1])

30.2 Clinical Anatomy

A number of vascular structures exist within the pelvic cavity. The major blood vessel aorta divides into common iliac arteries at the level of L4, and these common iliac arteries further divide into internal and external iliac branches at the level of sacroiliac joints (Fig. 30.3). Branches from these internal and external iliac arteries bleed during pelvic injuries. The superior gluteal artery is the most commonly injured arterial vessel in pelvic trauma. The arteries are in proximity to the veins. The presacral and prevesical veins are the most commonly injured. Hence, combined injury to arteries and veins is of common occurrence. The importance of understanding the above vasculature helps one to understand the seriousness of pelvic trauma, wherein high chance exists for haematoma, especially in retroperitoneal region and haemorrhagic shock. Haemorrhage or blood loss from pelvic fractures is a major cause of morbidity and mortality for

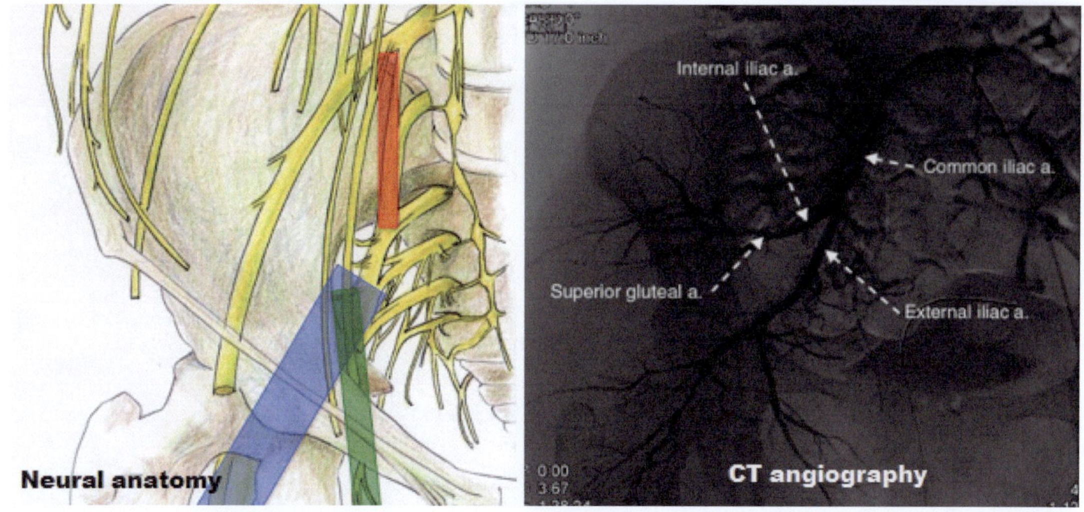

Fig. 30.3 Neurovascular structures in pelvis

the patient. The lumbosacral plexus lies in proximity to the sacrum and sacroiliac joints. Disruptions of the sacrum and sacroiliac (SI) joints often lead to neurologic injuries. L5 nerve root is commonly affected as it's close to the SI joint. Injury often occurs due to a traction or compression injury, leading to displacement of sacral fracture fragments or SI joint disruption.

In this chapter, we will discuss the pelvic injuries in two segments. First, fractures of the pelvic ring and second, acetabular fractures in a brief.

30.3 Pelvic Ring Fractures

The anatomy described here can be moved to the previous section. Finish all details about anatomy in one section itself. We start directly with the mechanism of injury, associated injuries, classification, imaging and treatment and complications.

30.3.1 Mechanism of Injury

The fractures of pelvic ring are 'high energy fractures'. These occur as a result of blunt trauma to the pelvic region. Road traffic accidents and falls from height are the two common mechanisms of injury.

30.3.2 Associated Injuries

The associated injuries include

- Chest injury (63%), long bone fractures (50%), fractures of spine (25%), head and abdominal injury (40%) and sexual dysfunction (50%).

In children, the triradiate cartilage is open. Here, the ligaments are stronger than bones, and hence, bone disruption is seen more than pelvic ring disruptions.

30.3.3 Classification

Being a ring structure, any fracture can disrupt the ring. So, classifications look at the integrity of the pelvic ring rather than the morphology of individual fractures. Tile classification (Fig. 30.4) and Young–Burgess classification (Fig. 30.5) are the two named classification systems. They are explained in Tables 30.1 and 30.2.

Young–Burgess Classification is based on the force mechanisms and the injury pattern. It can be antero-posterior compression (APC) force, lateral compression (LC) force and vertical shear (VS) force. The classification, hence, has APC injury, LC injury and VS injury. Subdivisions are too complex for undergraduate level and hence not added.

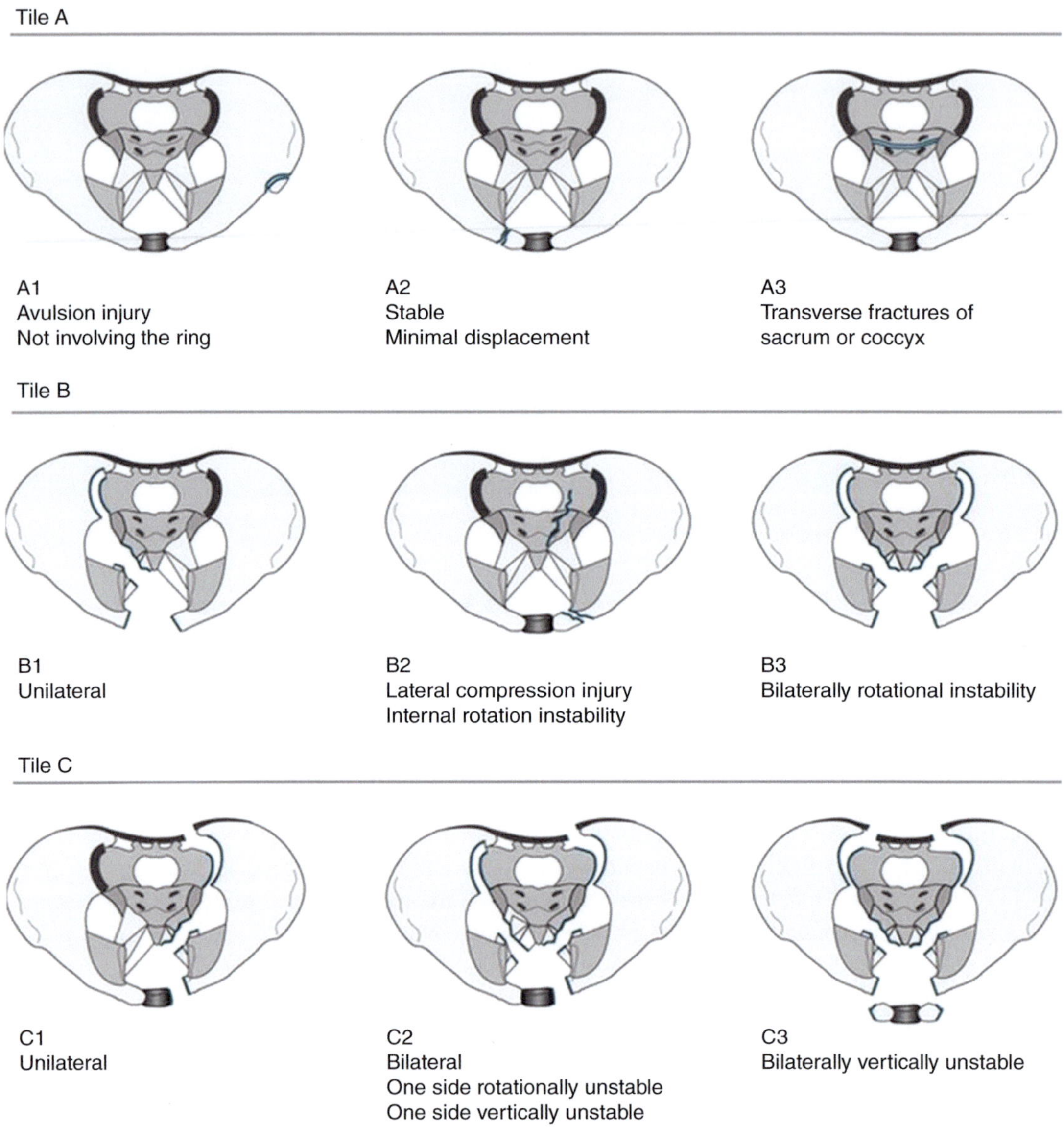

Fig. 30.4 Tile classification

30.3.4 History and Clinical Examination

Patients present with

- History of pain and inability to bear weight following a history of trauma.
- He or she may have significant blood loss and may have haemorrhagic shock.
- The initial approach to a patient with pelvic injury is as per advanced trauma life support (ATLS) protocol. It's designed to recognize and stabilize life-threatening injuries first (Airway, Breathing, Circulation, Disability and Exposure).
- Detailed history is obtained after stabilization of the patient.

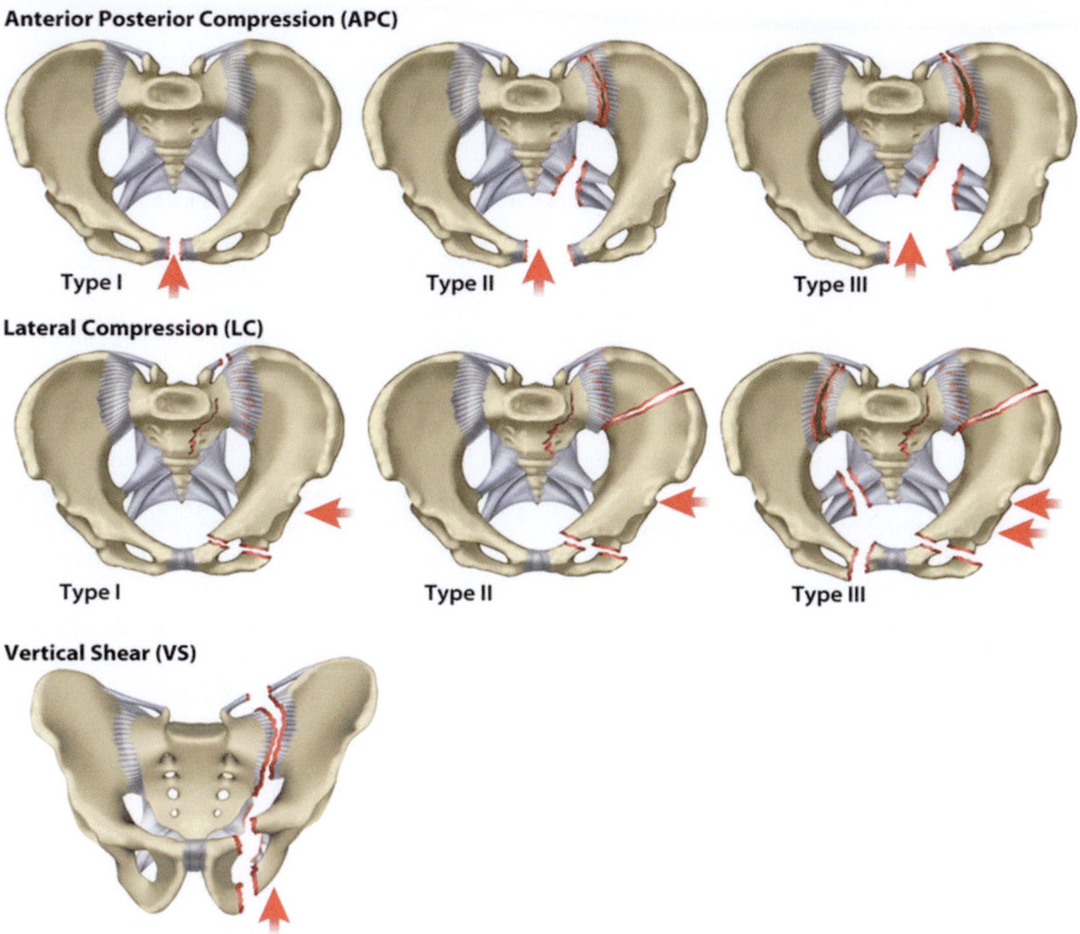

Fig. 30.5 Young–Burgess classification

Table 30.1 Tile classification

Tile classification	
Type A	'Stable' Fracture not involving the ring (ASIS/AIIS avulsion or iliac wing fracture), Stable or minimally displaced fracture of the ring or Transverse sacral fracture (Denis zone III sacral fracture)
Type B	Rotationally unstable and vertically stable Open book injury (anterior opening up of the ring), lateral compression injury, bilateral
Type C	Rotationally and vertically unstable Both anterior and posterior disruption present Often associated with sacral fracture, SI joint disruption Can be unilateral or bilateral

Patient is inspected for

- Any visible scrotal, labial or perineal haematoma, swelling or ecchymosis, flank haematoma, lacerations of perineum and degloving injuries (Morel–Lavallee lesion).
- A thorough neurological examination is done to rule out lumbosacral plexus injuries (L5 and S1 are the most commonly involved nerve roots).
- Rectal examination is also performed to evaluate sphincter tone and perirectal sensation, as

Table 30.2 Young–Burgess classification

Young–Burgess classification	
Anteroposterior compression (APC)	Antero-posterior compression leads to disruption of pubic symphysis, first leading to pubic diastasis. Further force then injures Anterior SI ligaments, followed by posterior SI joints
Lateral compression (LC)	Lateral compression force or force from sides leads to fracture of ipsilateral pubic rami, followed by ipsilateral sacrum fracture. If force still persists, opposite side is also involved
Vertical shear (VS)	Posterior and superior directed force ↓ Vertical translation of the hemipelvis 'Associated with the highest risk of hypovolemic shock (63%); mortality rate up to 25%'

up to 10–15% of patients will sustain neurologic injury.

- Blood in urethral meatus is suggestive of urethral injury.
- Any abnormal positioning of the lower limb (external rotation of limb or limb length discrepancy) is looked for, and if present, may suggest associated long bone injury or acetabular fractures.
- The pelvis stability is assessed with a single attempt of anteroposterior compression. Any instability indicates a pelvic fracture.

Investigations include

- CBC, Hb, PT and aPTT, RFT, LFT (If Hb is low, transfusions may be needed).
- Ultrasound of abdomen can be done to perform a Focused Assessment with Sonography in Trauma (FAST) in pelvic injuries for any intra-abdominal injury.
- Serum lactate and base deficit can be used to monitor resuscitation.

Imaging (Includes radiographs and CT scan)

- *Anteroposterior (AP)* pelvis with both hips: To look for asymmetry, rotation or displacement of each hemipelvis and any fracture lines (Fig. 30.6).
- *Lateral view of each hip*: To see the hip joint and the pelvis for any fractures or displacements.
- *Inlet view*: X-ray beam angled 40° caudad or to foot side. The inlet view shows the pelvic inlet. It's ideal for visualising anterior or posterior translation of the hemipelvis, internal or external rotation of the hemipelvis, widening of the SI joint and sacral ala impaction (Fig. 30.7).
- *Outlet view*: X-ray beam angled 40° cephalad or to head side. The outlet view shows the pelvic outlet. It is useful for finding out vertical translation of the hemipelvis, flexion/extension of the hemipelvis and disruption of sacral foramina and location of sacral fractures (Fig. 30.7).

All these views are needed in a pelvic injury. If an associated acetabular injury is present, additional oblique views (iliac oblique and obturator oblique) are required.

Computed tomography is a routine part of investigation in any patient with pelvic injury. It is useful in

- Better understanding of posterior ring injuries (sacrum and SI joint)
- Fracture comminution
- Fragment rotation
- Classification of injuries
- Preoperative planning for surgical management

Additional investigations include

- Urethrogram: in case of suspected urethral injury
- CT angiography: in case of occult haemorrhage or vascular complications

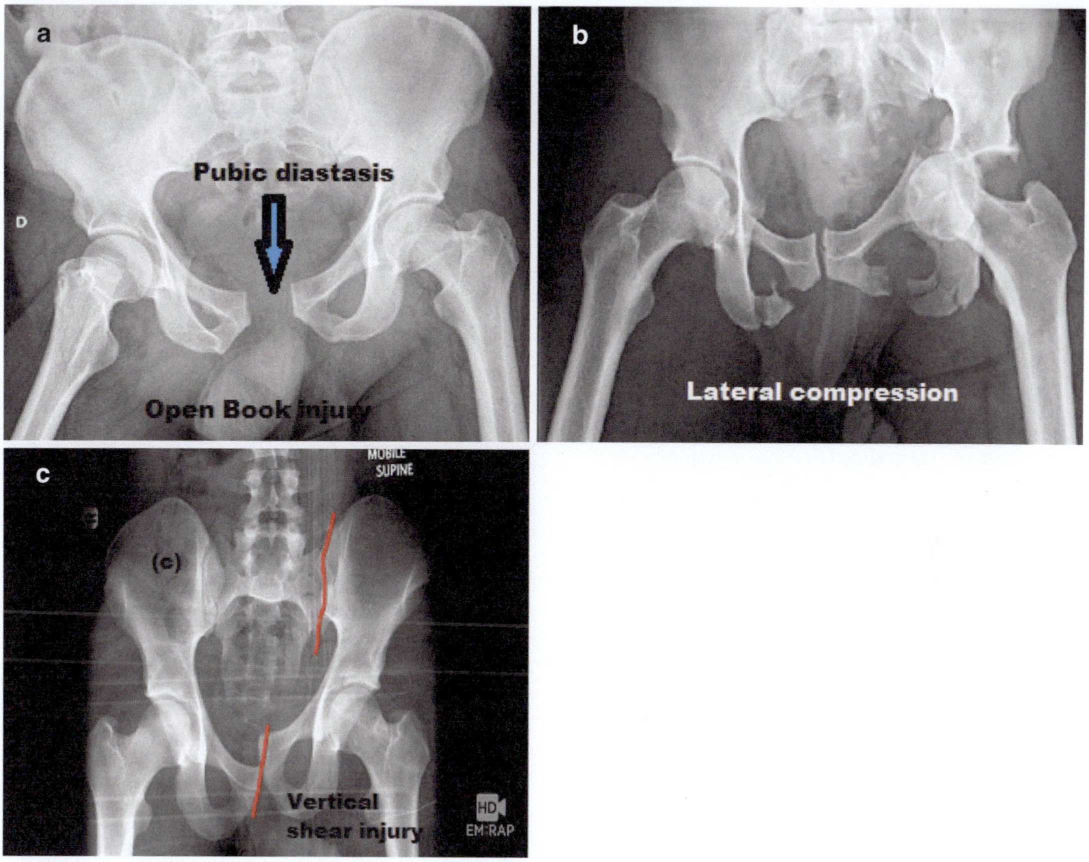

Fig. 30.6 Pelvic fractures—Pubic diastasis (**a**), Lateral compression (**b**), and vertical translation (**c**)

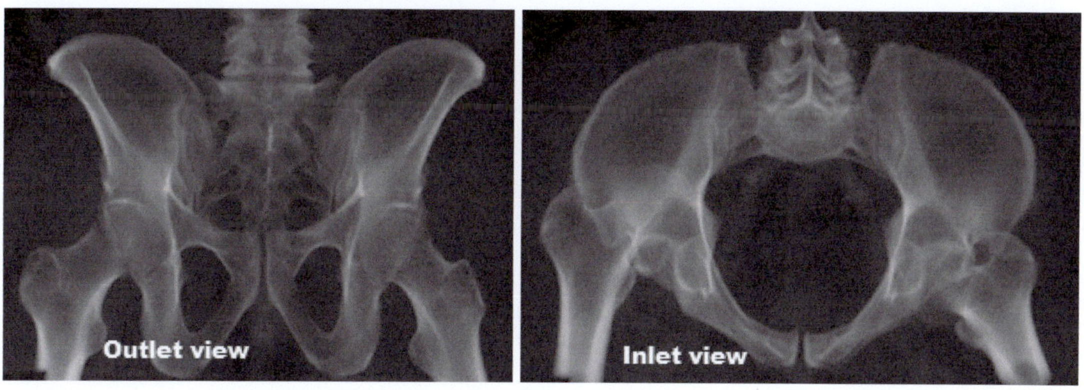

Fig. 30.7 Inlet and outlet views

30.3.5 Treatment/Management

Pelvic fractures have a propensity to be life-threatening. Treatment for any fracture starts with

- ABCs (airway, breathing and circulation) during the primary survey
- Adequate resuscitation (Two large-bore IV cannula, hypotension addressed with fluids, blood transfusion if needed)

- Pelvic binders: In patients where there is a sign of pelvic ring disruption (stable or unstable patients). It compresses bleeding bones, decreases the volume in pelvis (creates a tamponade effect) and is a temporary measure. Adequate application is necessary for it to act. It is kept around greater trochanter and pubic symphysis. Contraindicated in lateral compression injury (it can increase bleeding).
- If haemodynamically unstable, CT angiography to look for the cause of bleeding and angioembolisation or emergency laparotomy should be carried out.

30.3.6 Definitive Treatment

Please make the bullets uniform.

Definitive treatment of pelvic injury starts, once patient is haemodynamically and clinically stable.

Options include

- Conservative management: indicated in mechanically stable pelvic ring injuries
  - Traumatic widening of pubic symphysis <1 cm
  - Isolated pubic rami fractures
  - Isolated sacral fractures

  Patient is advised bed rest with or without traction. If a stable pattern, protected weight-bearing can be advised. In all others, bed rest may be advised.
- External fixation (Fig. 30.8): indicated in conditions
  - Unstable ring injury with ongoing blood loss (applied before laparotomy)
  - Pelvic ring injuries with an external rotation component
  - Open fractures

  Contraindicated (relative) in acetabular fractures and ilium fractures
- Open reduction internal fixation (Fig. 30.9): when the ring is disrupted and is unstable
  - Anterior ring stabilisation: Plate across the symphysis pubis (superior surface)

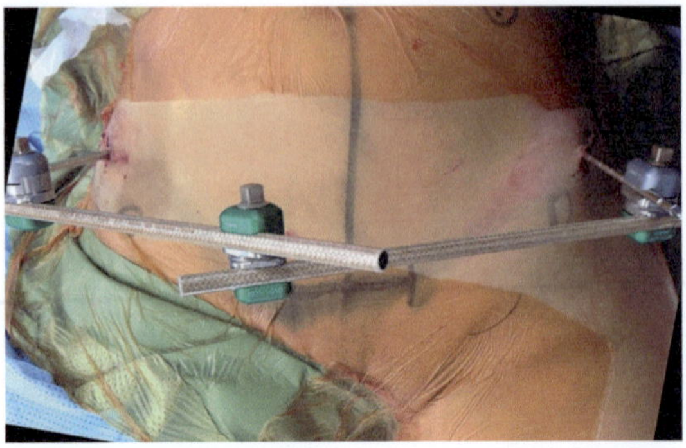

Fig. 30.8 External fixator

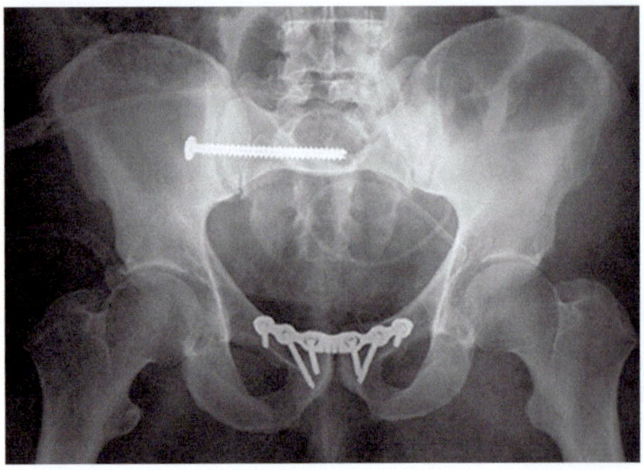

Fig. 30.9 ORIF of anterior ring disruption and Iliosacral screw

  - Posterior ring stabilisation:
    - Anterior SI joint plating (rarely done)
    - Iliosacral screws: for SI joint disruptions and sacral fractures. The L5 nerve root is commonly injured
    - Posterior SI plating: can have hardware complications
  - Anterior and posterior plating or stabilisation: In vertical shear fractures
  - Concomitant acetabulum and pelvic ring fracture: treat pelvic ring first, then acetabulum

Rehabilitation consists of slow mobilisation and physiotherapy once the ring has been stabilised. Post pelvic injury, there is a high incidence of chronic pain. Poor outcomes are usually associated with SI joint incongruity of >1 cm, high degree initial displacement, malunion or residual displacement, leg length discrepancy >2 cm, non-union, neurologic injury and urethral injury

30.3.7 Complications

The complications following pelvic fractures include

- Urogenital injury: The most common is a posterior urethral tear. Bladder rupture is associated with disruption of pubic symphysis. May require suprapubic catheterisation or repair
- Neurologic injury: L5 is the most commonly involved nerve root. It can also be involved with Iliosacral screw. Fixator pins can injure lateral femoral cutaneous nerve.
- Deep vein thrombosis (60%), pulmonary embolism (27%). Prophylaxis is essential for every pelvic injury patient.
- Chronic instability: rare
- Infection: prolonged ICU stay, open wounds and bladder injury are risk factors
- Vascular injury: may require CT angiography and embolisation

30.4 Acetabular Fractures

30.4.1 Epidemiology

Pelvic fractures that involve the articular surface of the hip joint and may involve one or two columns, one or two walls, or the roof within the pelvis are known as acetabular fractures. They can be better understood as a deep, cup-shaped structure that encloses the head of the femur at the hip joint. The incidence is around 4 per 100,000. It can be associated with high-energy trauma in younger individuals and low-energy injury in older individuals. Fracture patterns are influenced by bone quality, position of the femoral head and force vector at the time of injury. Clinical anatomy. Acetabulum is the socket of the hip joint and has six components. (1) anterior, or iliopubic, column, (2) posterior, or ilioischial, column, (3) anterior wall, (4) posterior wall, (5) acetabular dome/roof and (6) medial wall or quadrilateral plate. The anterior and posterior column forms an inverted Y and are connected to sacrum through sciatic buttress (Fig. 30.10).

The anterior column is comprised of anterior ilium (gluteus medius tubercle), anterior wall and dome, iliopectineal eminence and lateral superior pubic ramus. The posterior column is comprised of quadrilateral surface, posterior wall and dome, ischial tuberosity, and greater/lesser sciatic notches (Fig. 30.11). The mean acetabular inclination in coronal plane is 40–50°, and anteversion in axial plane is 18–21°. Corona mortis refers to the anastomosis of external iliac (epigastric) and internal iliac (obturator) vessels, which is at risk with lateral dissection over superior pubic ramus.

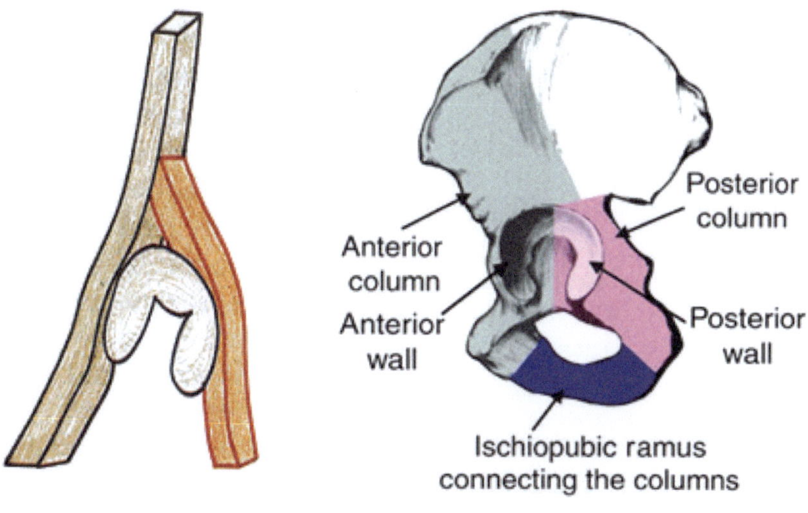

Fig. 30.10 Acetabular columns representation

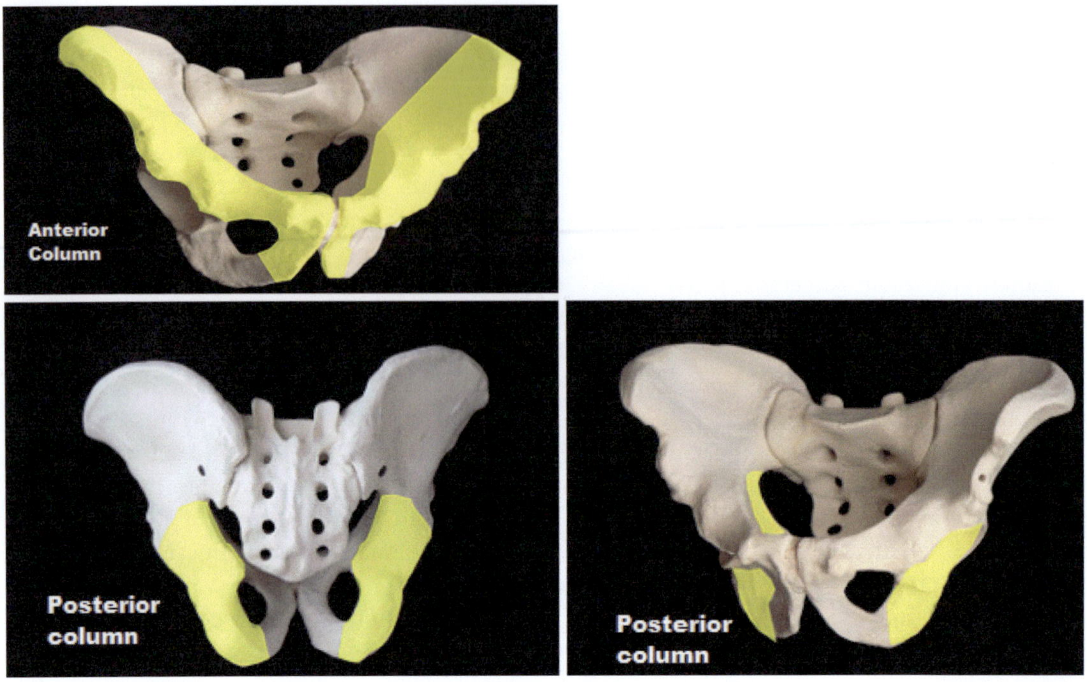

Fig. 30.11 Anterior and posterior columns

Table 30.3 Judet and Letournel classification

Judet and Letournel classification	
Elementary classification	Posterior wall (most common) (Gull sign in X-ray) Anterior wall Anterior column Posterior column Transverse
Associated patterns	Associated with both column fractures (spur sign in X-ray) Transverse with posterior wall (most common associated fracture) (highest risk of nerve injury) T-type Anterior column or wall + posterior hemitransverse (most common in elderly) Posterior column + posterior wall

30.4.2 Classification

Acetabular fractures are classified as per Judet and Letournel classification (Table 30.3). It includes '5' elementary and '5' associated fractures (Figs. 30.12 and 30.13). The most common fractures in younger individuals are posterior wall followed by transverse fractures. In elderly, anterior column fractures are common.

30.4.3 History and Clinical Examination

Clinical history and presentation are similar to pelvic injuries detailed before. All basic investigations and resuscitation need to be followed till patient is clinically and haemodynamically stable (Fig. 30.14).

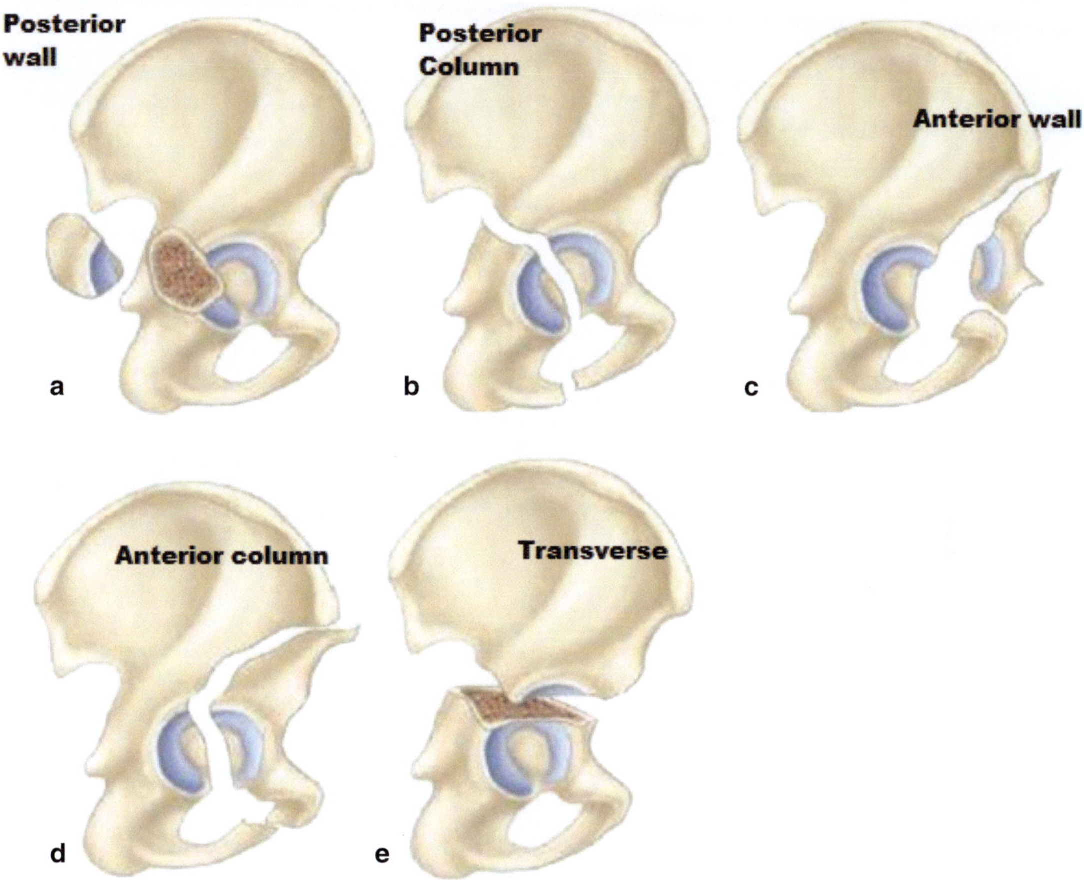

Fig. 30.12 Elementary fractures—Posterior wall (**a**), Posterior column (**b**), Anterior wall (**c**), Anterior column (**d**) and Transverse (**e**)

30.4.4 Imaging

Only additional investigation that one would order for acetabular fractures is special radiographic views: Iliac oblique and Obturator oblique views, aka Judet views (Fig. 30.15). Inlet and outlet views are optional if pelvis is not disrupted.

- Obturator oblique: shows profile of obturator foramen and anterior column and posterior wall are visible
- Iliac oblique: shows profile of involved iliac wing and posterior column and anterior wall are visible

Radiographic findings of interest include

- Spur sign: both column fractures
- Gull sign: posterior wall fracture (impaction injury)
- Iliopectineal line broken in anterior column fracture
- Ilioischial line broken in posterior column fracture
- Shenton's line broken in hip dislocation
- Roof: superior articular surface
- Tear drop: relationship of columns

Computed tomography is the gold standard investigation of choice. It's useful in

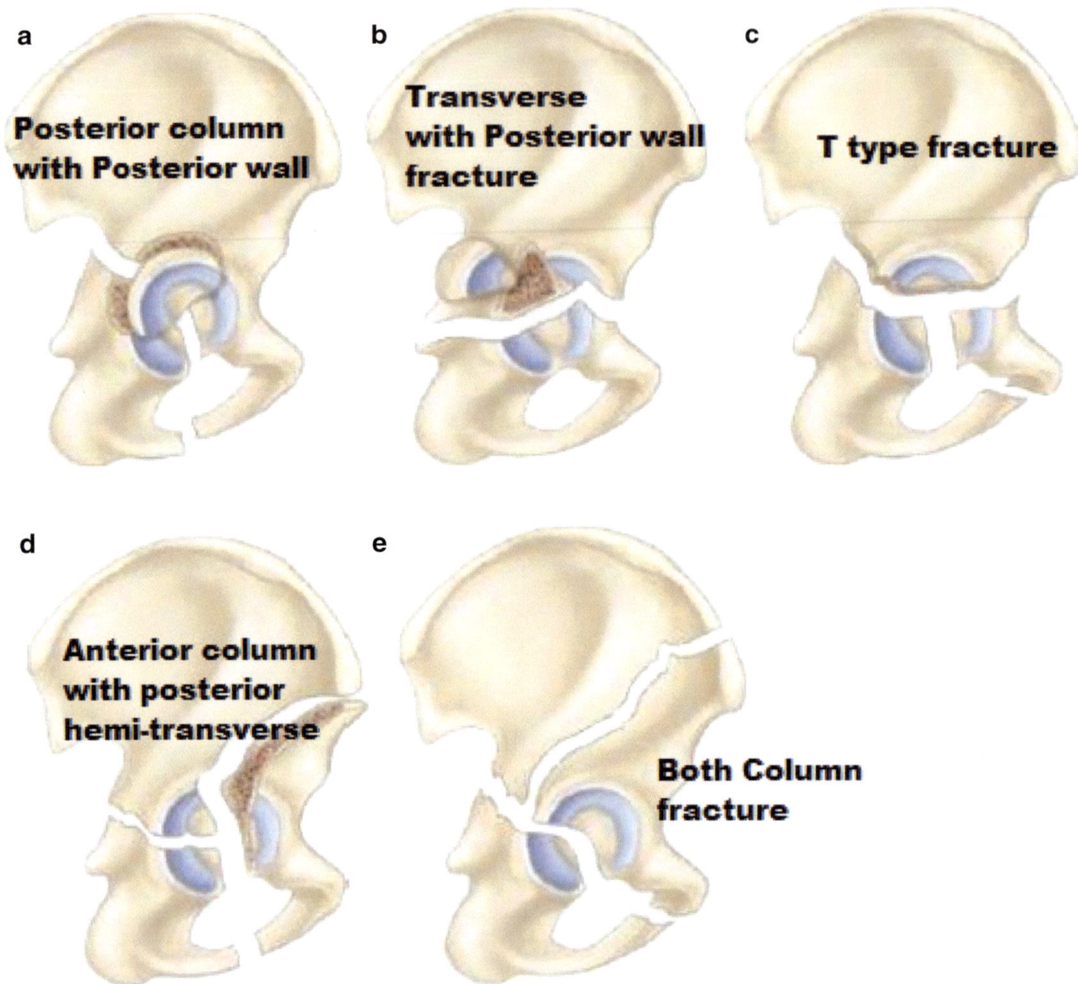

Fig. 30.13 Associated fracture—Posterior colomn with posterior wall (**a**), Transverse with posterior wall (**b**), T type (**c**), Anterior column with posterior hemi-transverse (**d**) and both column (**e**) fracture

Fig. 30.14 Normal radiographic findings

1. ILIOPECTINEAL LINE
2. ILIOISCHIAL LINE
3. TEAR DROP
4. ROOF OF ACETABULUM
5. EDGE OF ANTERIOR WALL OF ACETABULUM
6. EDGE OF POSTERIOR WALL OF ACETABULUM

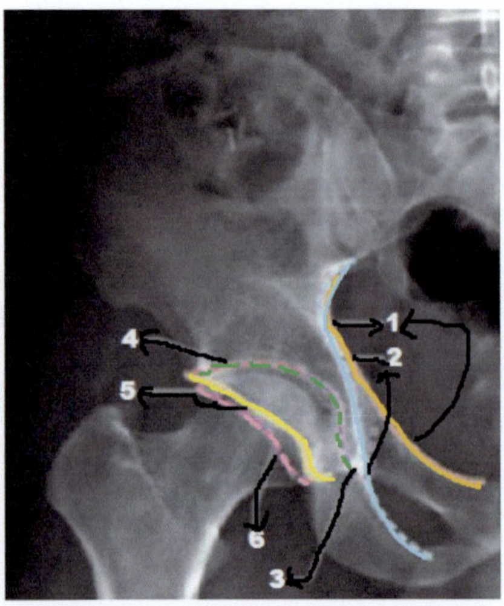

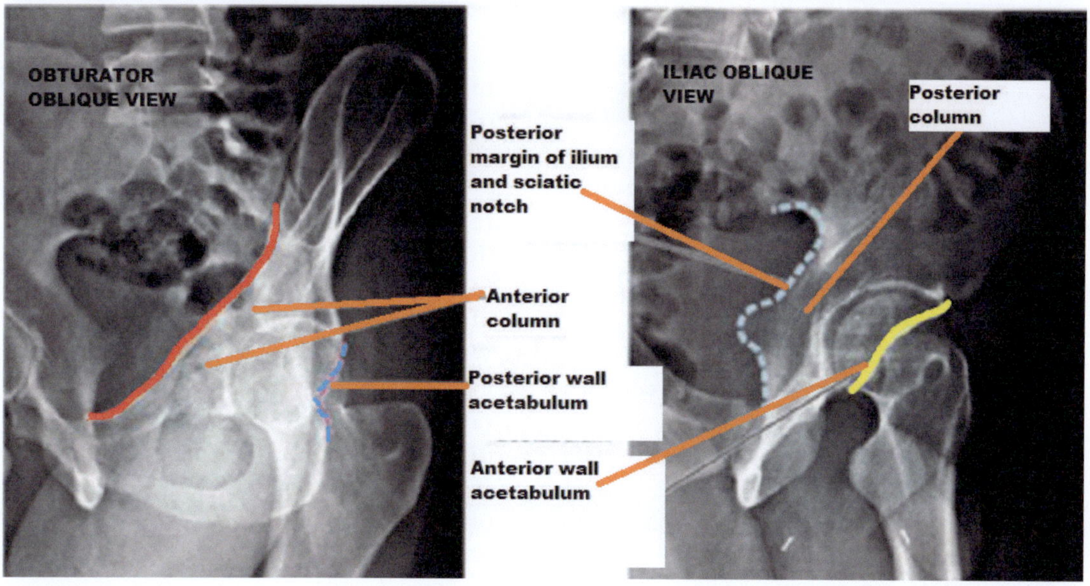

Fig. 30.15 Judet views

- Fracture pattern orientation
- Define fragment size and orientation
- Identify marginal impaction
- Identify loose bodies (e.g. post-reduction)
- Look for an articular gap or step-off

30.4.5 Treatment

Evaluation and initial management are similar to that of pelvic injury management. An emphasis is kept on DVT prophylaxis or PE prevention.

Treatment options for acetabular fractures include

- Conservative
- Protected weight-bearing is advised for 6–8 weeks. Skeletal traction is utilised for unstable or displaced fractures and may be continued in frail patients. Indications for conservative management include
  - High operative risk or frail patients (e.g. elderly patients, presence of DVT)
  - Morbid obesity
  - Late presentation (>3 weeks)
  - Minimally displaced fracture of roof <2 mm displacement
  - Posterior wall fractures with no head dislocation and size <20%
- Operative (Fig. 30.16)
- ORIF
  - displacement of roof >2 mm
  - Unstable fracture pattern (e.g. posterior wall fracture involving >40–50%)
  - Presence of marginal impaction
  - Presence of intra-articular loose bodies
  - Irreducible fracture-dislocation

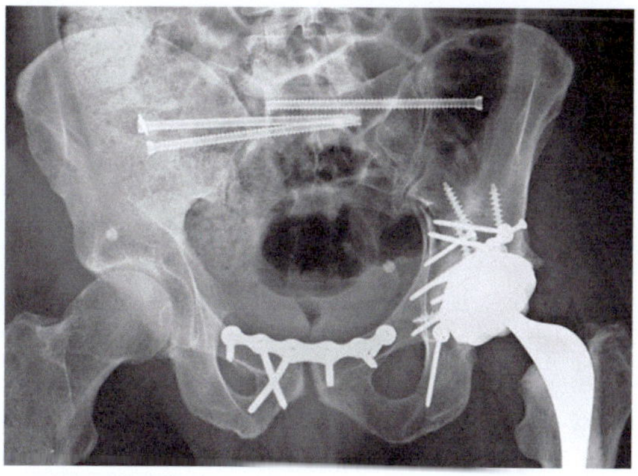

Fig. 30.16 Implant options

Implant options include screws, plates and cables. Common approaches are anterior (ilioinguinal, Stoppa), posterior (Kocher–Langenbeck)

- Total hip arthroplasty
  Indicated in elderly patients with fracture comminution or pre-existing arthritis
- External fixator
  Indicated in unstable patients, or patients with associated pelvic ring disruption, as first-stage stabilization

30.4.6 Complications

- Post-traumatic arthritis (most common complication)
- Heterotrophic ossification (associated with surgery)
- Osteonecrosis of femoral head (more with column and wall fractures)
- Deep vein thrombosis and pulmonary embolism
- Infection
- Neurovascular injury
- Abductor muscle weakness

Prognosis of acetabular fractures depends upon the initial fracture morphology, comminution and the reduction achieved. 70-80% of patients have good outcomes. A large number of patients develop post-traumatic arthritis. Overall, poor outcomes are associated with multi-system trauma, increasing age, poor articular congruency, associated femoral head articular injury and post-traumatic arthritis.

Multiple Choice Questions

1. Young–Burgess Classification is used for classifying which injury?
   (a) Acetabular fracture
   (b) Pelvic injury
   (c) Proximal humerus fracture
   (d) Proximal tibial fracture
2. Tile classification consists of all the following except?
   (a) Vertical shear
   (b) Lateral compression
   (c) Antero-posterior compression
   (d) Posterior acetabular wall fracture
3. What are the treatment options for pelvic injuries?
   (a) Conservative
   (b) External fixation
   (c) Internal fixation
   (d) All of the above
4. Radiographic investigations in acetabular fractures include
   (a) Antero-posterior pelvis X-ray
   (b) Iliac oblique view
   (c) Obturator oblique view
   (d) All of the above
5. Gull sign is seen in?
   (a) Posterior wall fracture
   (b) Anterior wall fracture
   (c) Anterior column fracture
   (d) Posterior column fracture

Answers: 1. (b), 2. (d), 3. (d), 4. (d), 5. (a)

References

1. Rohen JW, Yokochi C, Lutjen-Drecoll E. Color atlas of anatomy: a photographic study of the human body (Color Atlas of Anatomy (Rohen)). 6th ed. Lippincott Williams & Wilkins; 2006.

Spine Injuries and Traumatic Paraplegia

31

Aman Verma and Narayan Prasad Mishra

31.1 Introduction

Trauma is the most common cause of spinal injuries. This can be devastating, often resulting in severe morbidity and can lead to permanent disability. Injuries of the spine can be divided into five distinct anatomic regions, like cervical, cervicothoracic, thoracic, thoracolumbar, and low lumbar segments. Most of the injuries occur in the thoracolumbar area, followed by the lower cervical region. The clinical outcomes of spinal cord injuries (SCIs) depend on the severity and location of the injury. They may include partial or complete loss of sensory and/or motor function below the level of injury. The neurological deficit can be paraplegia in thoracolumbar injuries or quadriplegia in cervical spine injuries. It has devastating consequences for patients' physical, emotional, social, and vocational well-being.

31.2 Anatomy

The vertebral column is structured in a top-to-bottom sequence, starting with seven cervical vertebrae, followed by twelve thoracic vertebrae, five lumbar vertebrae, the fused sacrum (resulting from five vertebrae), and the fused coccyx (formed from four vertebrae). These vertebrae are held together by ligaments and strong muscles at the back, which play a crucial role in maintaining an individual's posture.

The movable vertebrae share a relatively consistent anatomical design. Each vertebra consists of an anterior vertebral body and a posterior bony arch, known as the neural arch. Between these structures lies the vertebral foramen. When the vertebrae are aligned in the spine, their vertebral foramina create the spinal canal. Within the upper two-thirds of the spinal canal resides the spinal cord, which reaches its end point at the level of the first lumbar vertebra in adults.

Extending out laterally from the neural arch are the transverse processes, while projecting backward from the arch's posterior midline is the spinous process. The segment of the neural arch positioned between the bases of the transverse and spinous processes is called the lamina, due to its thick, plate-like appearance. The right and left laminae meet at the posterior midline where the spinous process originates (Figs. 31.1 and 31.2).

On each side, the foremost section of the neural arch, where it connects with the back of the vertebral body, is referred to as the pedicle. The height of each pedicle is approximately half that of the vertebral body. Consequently, there is a substantial gap between consecutive pedicles,

A. Verma (✉)
Department of Orthopaedics, All India Institute of Medical Sciences, Rishikesh, India

N. P. Mishra
Department of Orthopaedics, All India Institute of Medical Sciences, Jodhpur, India

V. Kumar et al. (eds.), *A Quick Guide to Essential Orthopedics*,
https://doi.org/10.1007/978-981-95-2676-5_31

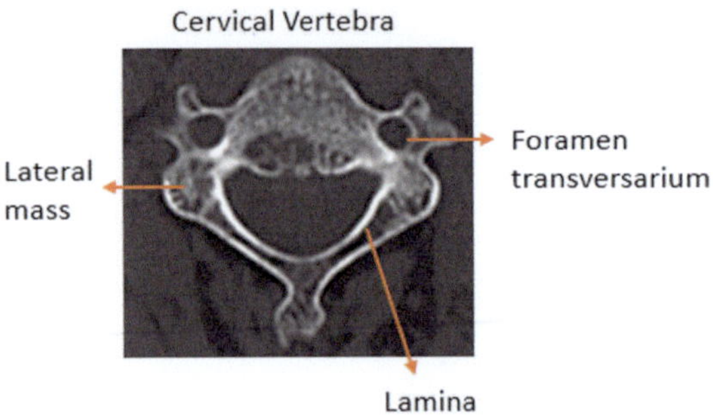

Fig. 31.1 Anatomy of the cervical vertebra

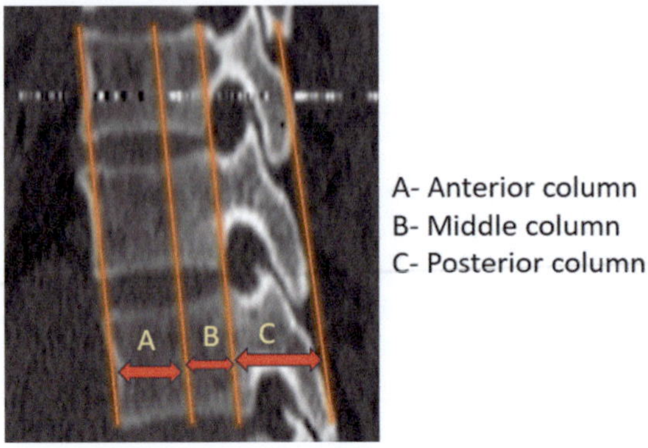

Fig. 31.3 Three-column concept of the spine

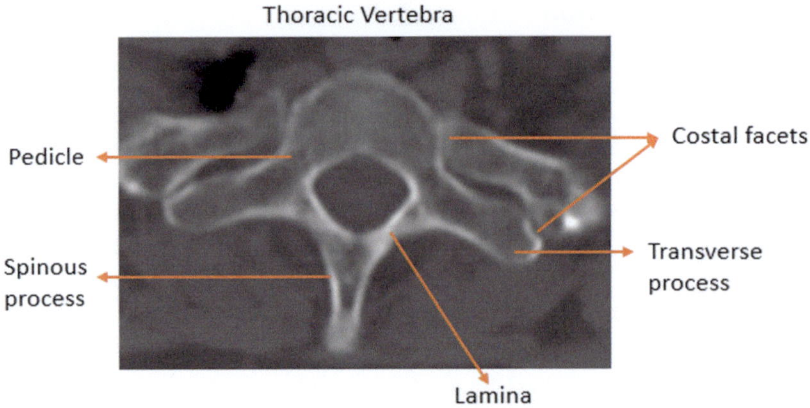

Fig. 31.2 Anatomy of the thoracic vertebra

known as the intervertebral foramen. This opening contains the spinal nerve on either side.

The spinal motion segment is the functional (biomechanical) unit of the spine and can be defined as any two successive, moveable vertebrae, including the structures and articulations that unite them. The following structures confer the stability, integrity, and flexibility of a spinal motion segment and hence of the entire vertebral column:

1. The intervertebral disc (reinforced by the anterior and posterior longitudinal ligaments)
2. Facet joints
3. Ligaments between adjacent vertebral arches

The three-column concept given by Denis and Ferguson is widely accepted and it helps to formulate treatment algorithms of thoracolumbar injuries based on the inherent stability of the spinal column (Fig. 31.3).

31.2.1 Anterior Column

- Anterior longitudinal ligament (ALL)
- Anterior two-thirds of the vertebral body and annulus fibrosus

31.2.2 Middle Column

- Posterior one-third of the vertebral body and annulus
- Posterior vertebral wall
- Posterior longitudinal ligament (PLL)

31.2.3 Posterior Column

- All structures posterior to the PLL, including the posterior bony arch and the posterior ligamentous complex (supraspinous ligament, interspinous ligament, capsule, and ligamentum flavum)

31.3 Types of Spine Injuries

Based on the mechanism of injury and the structures involved the injuries are further classified as:

31.3.1 Compression

Structures involved:

- Fracture of the anterior column of the vertebral body with an intact middle column
- Failure of the anterior column in compression
- May involve the superior or inferior endplate, or both

31.3.1.1 Mechanism of Injury
Anterior flexion and axial loading (Fig. 31.4)

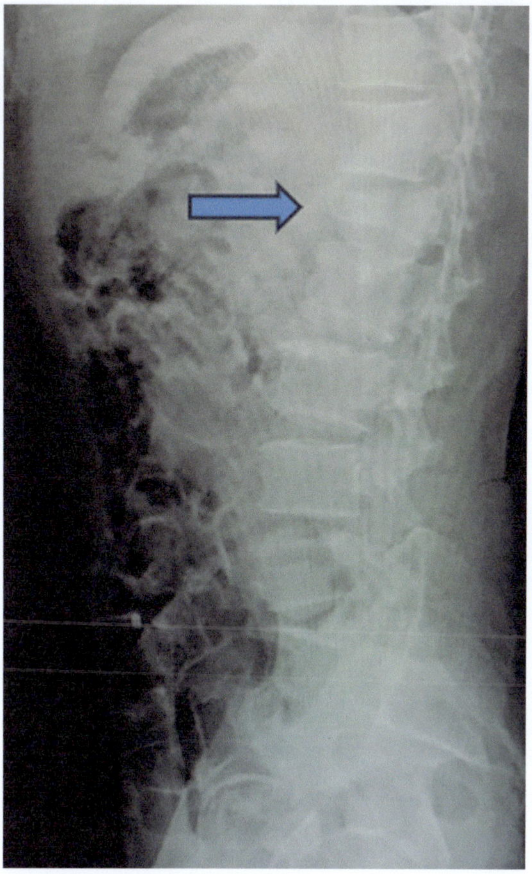

Fig. 31.4 Compression fracture

31.3.2 Burst

Structures involved:

- Compression fractures of the anterior and middle columns. The posterior column may or may not be involved if lamina fractures are present or if dural tears or nerve entrapments occur
- May involve the superior or inferior endplate, or both

31.3.2.1 Mechanism of Injury
Axial compression (Fig. 31.5)

31.3.3 Flexion-Distraction (Seatbelt-Type)

Structures involved:

- Usually involves all three columns
- No associated translation

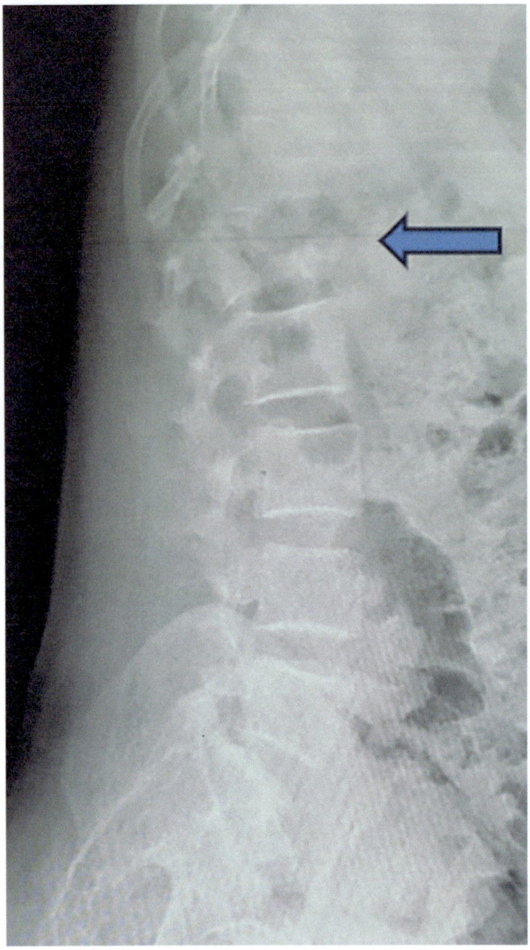

Fig. 31.5 Burst fracture

31.3.3.1 Mechanism of Injury

Flexion injuries to the middle and posterior columns with distraction posteriorly from tensile forces. The ALL serves as the axis of rotation, and the anterior column may fail secondary to compression (Fig. 31.6).

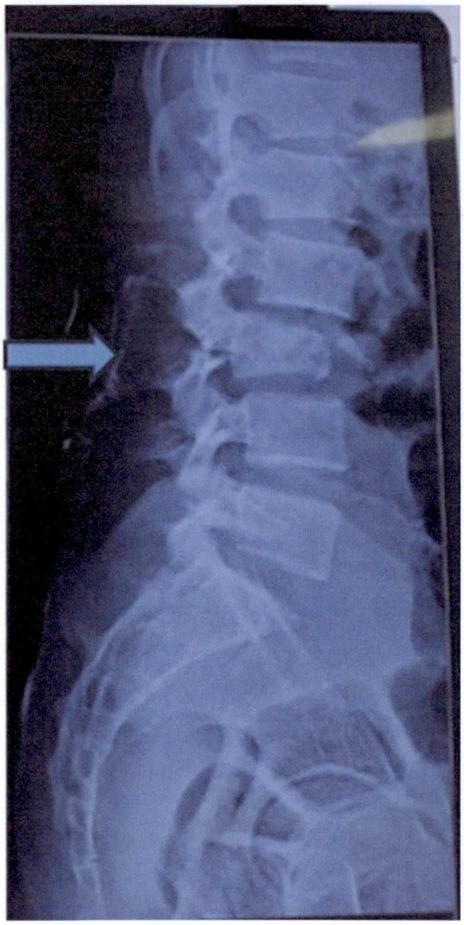

Fig. 31.6 Flexion-distraction injury

31.3.4 Fracture-Dislocation

Structures involved:

- Involvement of all three columns

31.3.4.1 Mechanism of Injury

Variable mechanisms: shear, rotation, compression, and tension (Fig. 31.7).

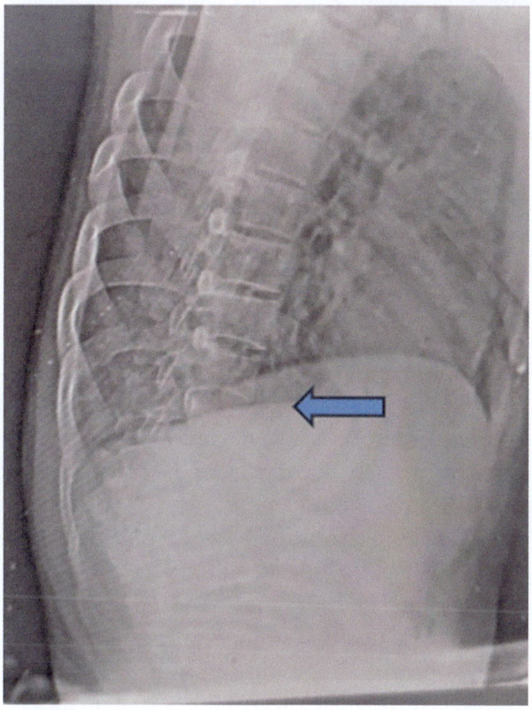

Fig. 31.7 Fracture-dislocation

31.4 Spine Examination

31.4.1 Sensory Examination

It includes testing of anterior, anterolateral, and posterior column sensations.

Ventral column sensation: Light touch
Lateral column sensation: Pain and temperature
Dorsal column sensation: Vibration, Joint position sense and two-point discrimination

The ASIA impairment scale is a standardized assessment that includes a myotomal-based motor examination, a dermatomal-based sensory examination, and an anorectal examination. The results of these evaluations are used to determine the severity (grade) and neurological level of the spinal cord injury (Refer ASIA chart).

31.4.2 Motor Examination

The muscle groups, their functions, and motions associated with different myotomes are as follows:

Root	Action	Reflex
C5	Elbow flexors, shoulder abductors, and external rotators	Biceps
C6	Elbow flexors, wrist extensors and pronators, and shoulder external rotators	Brachioradialis
C7	Elbow extensors and wrist pronators	Triceps
C8	Extension of index finger, finger abduction and flexion, and abduction of thumb	–
T1	Finger abduction	–
L2	Hip flexion	–
L3	Hip flexion, hip adduction, and knee extension	–
L4	Knee extension and ankle dorsiflexion	Knee
L5	Ankle dorsiflexion, great toe extension, ankle eversion, hip abduction, and internal rotation	Medial hamstring
S1	Ankle plantarflexion and toe flexion	Ankle

The muscle strength is graded as per medical research council (MRC) scale of 1–5 as follows:

Grade	Ability to move
0	No muscle contraction seen or identified with palpation; paralysis.
1	Muscle contraction is seen or identified with palpation, but it is insufficient to produce joint motion even with elimination of gravity.
2	The muscle can move the joint it crosses through a full range of motion only if the part is properly positioned so that the force of gravity is eliminated.
3	The muscle can move the joint it crosses through a full range of motion against gravity, but without any resistance.
4	The muscle can move the joint it crosses through a full range of motion with moderate resistance.
5	The muscle can move the joint it crosses through a full range of motion against gravity and against full resistance applied by the examiner.

Generally, SCI can be classified as either complete or incomplete. The first classification system, "Frankel Grade," was developed by Frankel and colleagues in 1969. They assessed the severity and prognosis of SCI using numerical sensory and motor scales. This was a five-grade system.

Frankel grade	Motor	Sensory
A	Complete loss	Complete loss
B	Complete loss	Preserved
C	Incomplete motor function (nonambulatory)	Preserved
D	Fair to good motor function (ambulatory)	Preserved
E	Normal	Normal

31.4.3 American Spinal Injury Association (ASIA) Scoring System

This system scores sensory function from 0 to 2 and motor function from 0 to 5. The ASIA impairment score (AIS) ranges from complete loss of sensation and movement (AIS = A) to normal neurological function (AIS = E).

ASIA Impairment Scale		
Grade	Type of injury	Definition of a type of injury
A	Complete	No motor or sensory function below the level of injury
B	Incomplete	Sensory but not motor function is preserved below the level of injury
C	Incomplete	Motor function is preserved, but more than 50% of key muscles below the neurological level have a muscle grade < 3
D	Incomplete	Motor function is preserved, but at least 50% of key muscles below the neurological level have a muscle grade ≥ 3
E	Normal	Motor and sensory functions are normal

It's crucial to distinguish between a complete spinal cord injury and a state known as spinal shock. Spinal shock can occur immediately after the injury and may last anywhere from 2 days to a few weeks. Spinal shock shares many characteristics with a complete cord injury, but has an additional feature, the absence of the bulbocavernosus reflex, which is not present in a complete cord injury. In contrast, an incomplete injury involves the partial preservation of sensory or motor functions below the level of the injury. Incomplete spinal cord injuries include

- Anterior cord syndrome
- Brown-Sequard syndrome
- Central cord syndrome
- Posterior cord syndrome
- Conus medullaris syndromes
- Cauda equina syndrome

31.5 Cervical Spine Injuries

Injuries to the cervical spine are highly perilous, especially when accompanied by neurological harm, as the consequences can be profoundly catastrophic. Despite notable advancements in diagnostic and therapeutic approaches over time, cervical spine injuries remain a formidable test of the expertise and discernment of orthopedic and neurosurgeons. Approximately 40% of cases exhibit neurological impairment, while in 10% of cases, X-ray images appear normal.

31.5.1 Applied Anatomy

The cervical spine, comprising the first seven vertebrae of the vertebral column, plays a vital role in supporting the head's weight, facilitating movement, and protecting the spinal cord. Each cervical vertebra possesses unique features that contribute to its function. Starting at the top, the first cervical vertebra, called the atlas (C1), lacks a traditional vertebral body. It consists of an anterior and posterior arch, and it articulates with the skull, allowing for nodding movements. The second cervical vertebra, the axis (C2), features a peg-like projection called the odontoid process (dens), which articulates with the atlas, enabling rotational movement.

31.5.2 Nerve Root Anatomy

The cervical nerve roots exit above the corresponding pedicle. For example, C5 nerve root exits above C5 pedicle. The nerve roots travel horizontally to exit the spinal canal. The cervical spine has an extra C8 nerve root that does not have a corresponding vertebral body, and as a result, it exits above T1 pedicle.

The phrenic nerve is the most important nerve, which originates from C3–C5 nerve roots and provides the primary motor supply to the diaphragm. Any injury involving C3–C5 can result in an abnormal breathing pattern or respiratory arrest.

31.5.3 Clinical Features

The patient usually presents with a history of trauma, resulting in pain and restricted neck movements, which may or may not be associated with a neurological deficit. In the presence of neurological deficit, a detailed physical examination is a must, which helps determine the level of the injury. However, the mere absence of neurological deficit doesn't rule out cervical spine fracture. As per the recent ATLS guidelines, all trauma patients are considered to have cervical spine injury, unless proven otherwise.

31.5.4 Physical Examination

A complete motor and sensory examination is performed with the cooperative patient. Once this information has been obtained, the American Spinal Injury Association (ASIA) score can be assigned to the patient's neurological physical exam. It is critical to evaluate the bulbocavernosus reflex to determine if the patient is in spinal shock. If hyperactive, it represents a complete spinal cord injury. A rectal exam is done to assess tone. If the patient is critically ill and on mechanical ventilation, with associated head injuries such as traumatic brain injury (TBI), the rectal tone may be the only objective finding of the neurological physical exam in patients with SCI.

31.5.5 Radiological Investigations

Plain radiographs are the initial investigation of choice. Both anteroposterior and lateral views are crucial to assess for any fracture or dislocation. Additionally, an Open-mouth view and swimmer's view are crucial in cases where upper or lower cervical spine injury is suspected.

A CT scan helps in accurately diagnosing fractures in the upper and lower cervical spine as these regions are often not clearly visible on plain radiographs. It helps to accurately assess the bony morphology and helps in classifying the type of fracture; however, it offers little or no information regarding cord injury or soft tissue injury.

Magnetic resonance imaging (MRI) is the investigation of choice to assess the status of the cord, soft tissue structure, and posterior ligamentous structures, which is essential for deciding the management of the fracture.

31.5.6 Management

The initial management of all trauma patients is done as per the ATLS guidelines. All patients with suspected cervical spine injury should have cervical immobilization by a hard collar (Philadelphia collar). After stabilizing the cervical spine, assessment for airway and breathing of the patient is done. Utmost care should be taken while transporting the patient from the site of trauma to the hospital. In the absence of a hard collar, care must be taken to restrict any kind of unnecessary neck movements.

The primary treatment goals in cervical spine injury are to realign the spine and prevent any further neurological damage by maintaining the stability. Based on the stability of the fracture, the management can be conservative or operative.

31.5.7 Indications of Nonoperative Treatment

1. Stable compression fractures of vertebral body without neurological deficit
2. Isolated fractures of lamina, lateral masses, and spinous process
3. Undisplaced fractures involving the facet joint
4. Unilateral facet dislocations that can be reduced with traction

31.5.8 Indications of Operative Treatment

1. Unstable compression fractures with or without neurological deficit
2. Flexion distraction and translation injuries
3. Fractures associated with an injured disc or posterior ligaments
4. Irreducible unilateral facet dislocation

31.5.9 Methods of Fixation

Preoperatively, patients with unstable fracture dislocations and neurological deficits, skeletal traction can be applied to achieve a closed reduction, which will prevent any further neurological damage (Fig. 31.8).

Commonly used devices for skeletal traction:

1. Crutchfield tongs
2. Mayfield
3. Garden-well tongs

An anterior-based surgery is indicated in cases where there is significant cord compression anteriorly, either from the fractured vertebral body or prolapsed intervertebral disc. Anterior corpectomy (removal of the vertebral body) or discectomy (removal of intervertebral disc) followed by fusion using anterior cervical plates and filling the bony defect using a cortical bone graft or Cage (PEEK or titanium) is the most commonly done procedure in recent times.

Posterior-based surgeries are done in cases with injured posterior ligamentous structures. The cervical spine is fixed via pedicle or lateral mass screws which are interconnected using rods which provide stability to the spine. The posterior base surgeries are biomechanically weaker as compared to anterior-based surgeries, often requiring more instrumented vertebrae and potentially increasing patient morbidity.

A combined anterior and posterior surgery is indicated in cases where there is anterior compression along with injured posterior ligaments.

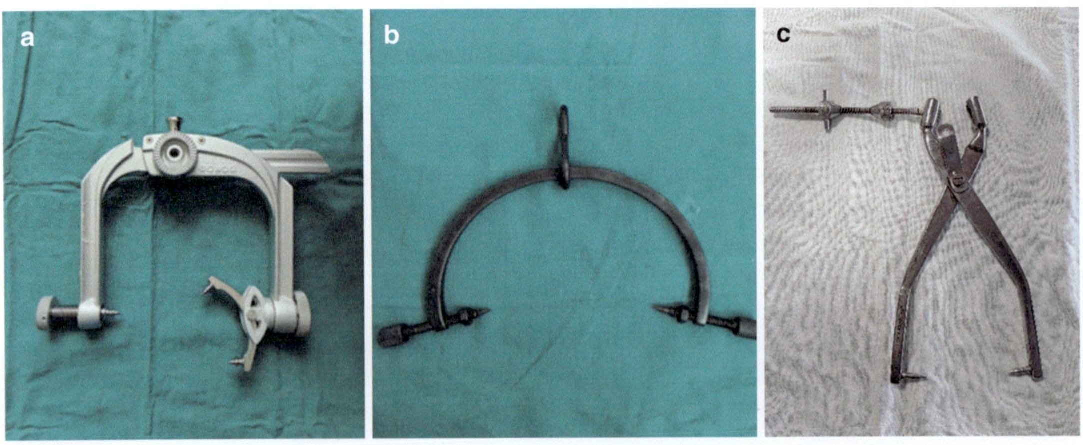

Fig. 31.8 Skeletal traction: (**a**) Mayfield fraction, (**b**) Garden-well tongs, and (**c**) Crutchfield tongs

31.6 Named Cervical Spine Fractures

31.6.1 Jefferson Fracture (C1 Fracture)

A vertebral compression fracture of C1 occurs, when the force is transmitted through the occipital condyles to the superior articular surfaces of the lateral masses of C1. It results from axial loading (Fig. 31.9).

31.6.1.1 Treatment

Stable fracture: Four-post collar for 8–12 weeks
Unstable fracture: Posterior C1–C2 instrumented fusion or occipitocervical fusion

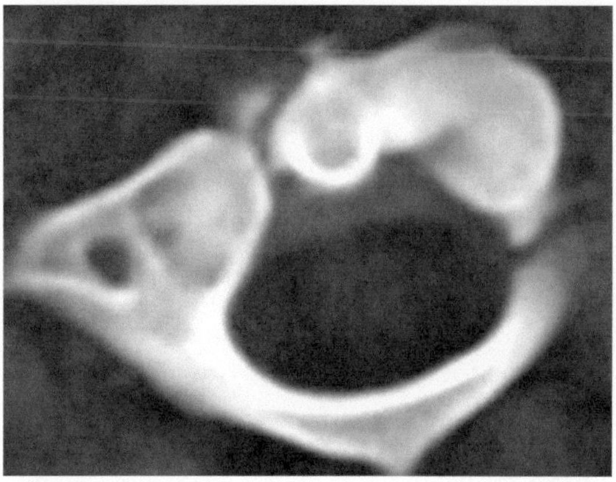

Fig. 31.9 Jefferson fracture

31.6.2 Hangman's Fracture (C2 Fracture)

The "Hangman's fracture" is a bilateral fracture of the pars interarticularis of C2 caused by hyperextension of the spine. In this fracture, the skull, atlas, and axis function as a unit during hyperextension. Since the AP diameter of the neural canal is greatest at C2, cord damage is uncommon or minimal (Fig. 31.10).

31.6.2.1 Treatment

Stable fracture: Hard collar or halo immobilizer
Unstable fracture: Anterior or posterior stabilization

31.6.3 Odontoid Fracture

The typical mechanism is flexion movement. Anderson and D'Alonzo classified odontoid fractures into the following types:

Type I: Fracture of the tip of the odontoid process; usually stable.
Type II: Fracture through the waist of the odontoid process; more commonly seen and unstable, and often complicated by non-union.
Type III: Fracture of the base extending laterally into the body of the axis; stable (Fig. 31.11).

Fig. 31.10 Hangman's fracture

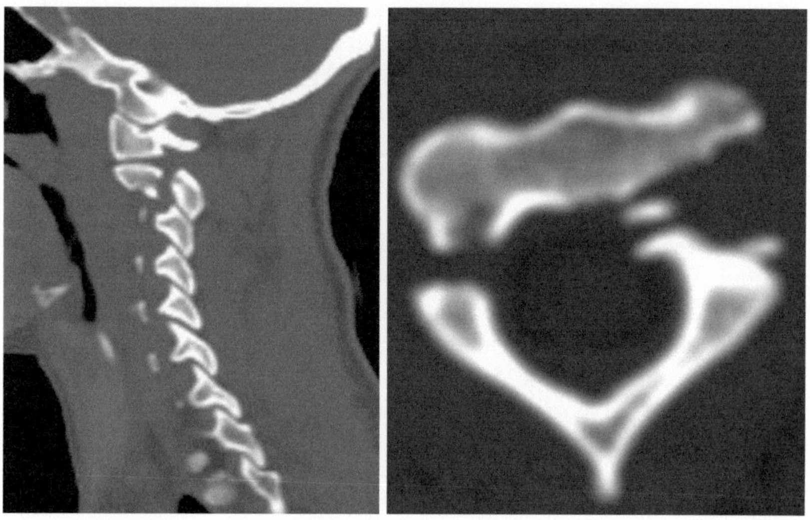

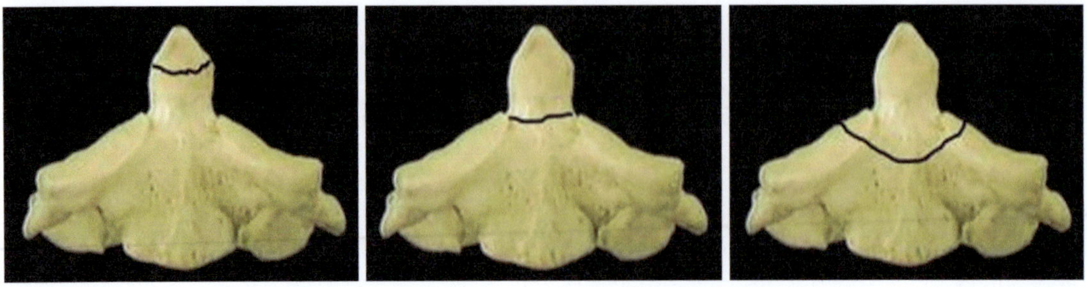

Fig. 31.11 Anderson and D'Alonzo classification of odontoid fracture

31.7 Thoracic and Lumbosacral Spine Injuries

The thoracic spine consists of 12 vertebrae (T1–T12) which is followed by 5 lumbar vertebrae (L1–L5). The thoracolumbar spine (T10–L2) is the most common region of the spine affected by trauma due to the specific biomechanics of this segment. It is highly susceptible to injury because it is a transition area from the rigid and less mobile thoracic spine, due to the attached ribs bilaterally, to a more flexible caudal lumbar spine.

Injury to the thoracolumbar spine can occur from motor vehicle accidents, falls from height, recreational accidents, and occupational injuries. In the event of high-velocity spine injuries, there is an associated 25% risk for accompanying spinal cord injury (SCI), which can have devastating effects on the patient, with loss of individual productive years and an associated high cost to society. As many as 25% of thoracolumbar fractures have another spine fracture elsewhere, most commonly the cervical spine.

31.7.1 Applied Anatomy

Typically, the spinal cord ends at the level of L1 vertebra. An injury above L1 has the potential to injure the spinal cord; however, injury below L1 can result in a permanent neurological deficit due to compression of the conus medullaris or the descending nerve roots and warrants immediate attention and assessment. The visceral organs of thorax and abdomen receive the sympathetic supply, which originates from the T3–T11 segments; hence, an injury in this region can lead to visceral organ paralysis in these regions. The segment from T12–L2 segments innervate the lower extremities and pelvic viscera, which can lead to sexual dysfunction and variable lower limb weakness if the injury involves this region.

31.7.2 Nerve Root Anatomy

It is important to decipher the level of cord injury based on the level of vertebral injury. The following method is most commonly used to correlate the bone segment to the cord segment

T1–T5: Add 2 to the vertebral level
T6–T11: Add 3 to the vertebral level
T11: Corresponds to epiconus region
T12–L1: Conus medularis region
Below L1: Cauda equina region

31.7.3 Physical Examination

As discussed earlier.

31.7.4 Clinical Features

The patient who suffered a thoracolumbar junction fracture may present on a physical exam with intact function, incomplete deficits, or complete neurological deficits. The level of injury in the conus region can determine the deficit that the patient presents with. If the affected area is in the transition area, it can cause symptoms of both upper and lower motor neuron dysfunction.

If the lesion is above the conus, only upper motor signs and symptoms will be elicited; if the lesion is below, then lower motor signs and symptoms will be found. Patients usually have a mix of upper and lower motor neuron symptoms due to many exiting nerve roots from the conus medullaris in this region. Injuries above T10 are more likely to result in complete neurological deficits, while injuries below L1 are more likely to result in radicular symptoms. This is due to the anatomic position of the spinal cord, where the conus medullaris usually does not extend below the level of L1.

There may be overt signs on the physical exam, such as widened spaces between spinous processes or displacement of spinous processes from the midline, which can be seen in the patient's physical exam on palpation and inspection when the patient is rolled over in the primary trauma survey.

31.7.5 Radiological Investigations

Plain radiographs usually do not provide the detail to characterize the fracture type and are not routinely used. In some situations, plain radiographs can detect fractures or evaluate bone instability if they are the only modality available.

Computed tomography (CT) scan adequately assess bony structures, including the vertebral bodies, pedicles, laminae, facets, and transverse and spinous processes.

MRI provides a higher resolution of structures. It allows an understanding of the type of fracture, which will subsequently influence the proposed treatment options. It provides a better evaluation of the ligamentous and neural structures, including the spinal cord, cauda equina, conus medullaris, and spinal nerve roots. If there is a documented neurological deficit on the patient's physical exam and initial CT scan images are negative for fractures or dislocations, it is essential to perform an MRI. The MRI can identify bone marrow oedema associated with an occult fracture, soft tissue changes, annular disruption, disruption of the posterior ligamentous complex, hemorrhage, herniated disc material, and the status of the spinal cord.

31.7.6 Management

Spinal precautions should be implemented in all trauma patients until a spine fracture is ruled out. Limiting flexion, extension, rotation, and twisting of the spine can help avoid exacerbating an injury to the spinal cord. Maintaining perfusion to the spinal cord with supportive care, including airway, breathing, and circulation management with a mean arterial pressure above 85 mmHg, is essential to enhance spinal cord perfusion. The patient may require emergency surgery based on the amount of instability or neurological involvement.

Although very common, injuries at the thoracolumbar junction comprise a heterogeneous group of injuries that has led to an increased discrepancy over the ideal surgical or nonsurgical management. The concept of spine stability is one of the most critical factors in deciding if the thoracolumbar junction fracture requires surgical treatment or can be managed conservatively. Disruption of the posterior ligamentous complex integrity raises the likelihood of instability when identified by MRI. Even without neurologic injury, many of these fractures will require operative intervention for stabilization due to the degree of bony or ligamentous injury that may be present.

Conservative management techniques include thoracolumbar orthosis, plaster cast, Jewett brace, and a plastic body cast for approximately 12 weeks. The majority of the compression fractures are stable and are treated with simple observation or an orthosis.

31.8 Management of Different Types of Fractures

31.8.1 Compression Fractures

Nonoperative:
 Bracing, kyphoplasty/vertebroplasty
Operative:
 Posterior instrumentation and fusion
- Indications:
  - 30 degrees of traumatic kyphosis
  - 50% vertebral body height loss

31.8.2 Burst Fractures

Nonoperative:
 Bracing
Operative:
 Anterior/posterior decompression and instrumented fusion
- Indications:
  - Neurologic deficit
  - Spinal canal compromise
  - Degree of deformity
  - Disruption of the posterior ligamentous complex

31.8.3 Flexion-Distraction Injuries

Nonoperative:
 Bracing
- Indications: minimally displaced bony or ligamentous injuries

Operative:
 Posterior instrumentation, with or without fusion
- Indications: kyphotic deformity greater than 20 degrees

31.8.4 Fracture Dislocation Injuries

Operative:
 All require open reduction with instrumented fusion

31.8.5 Surgical Interventions

For surgical intervention, approach alternatives include anterior, posterior, lateral, or combined approaches. The operative planning and stabilization of these fractures usually include a multifactorial decision-making process. The key factor for deciding an anterior versus a posterior approach is the location of the pathology to be addressed. Different techniques include posterior segmental instrumentation and fusion with or without posterior decompression, percutaneous pedicle screw instrumentation, lateral interbody fusion, and anterior column fusion. Spinal neuromonitoring is routinely used during surgery in patients with intact neurology. Postoperative bracing can be used for 8–12 weeks following surgery.

31.8.6 Complications

1. Pulmonary complications: Pneumonia, Atelectasis, URTI
2. Bedsores
   - Primary goal is prevention
   - Do not leave the patient on the spine board
   - Start log rolling early
   - Proper bedding
   - Remove garments that can cause circumferential compressions
3. Venous Thromboembolism.
   - Can be prevented with immediate DVT prophylaxis
4. Urinary tract infections
   - Common cause of death
   - Strict aseptic technique when placing a catheter
   - Don't let the bladder become overly distended
5. Sinus bradycardia
   - Most common cardiac arrhythmia in the acute stage following SCI
6. Orthostatic hypotension
   - Occurs as a result of a lack of sympathetic tone
7. Autonomic dysreflexia

- Potentially fatal
- Presents with headache, agitation, and hypertension
- Caused by unchecked visceral stimulation
- Check Foley
- Radiographs of the lower extremity if there is concern for an undiagnosed fracture

8. Major depressive disorder (MDD)
   - ~11% of patients with spinal cord injuries suffer from MDD
   - MDD in spinal cord injury patients is highly associated with suicidal ideation in both the acute and chronic phases

31.9 Rehabilitation in Spinal Cord Injury

The rehabilitation of the paraplegics and quadriplegics is a multimodal approach that plays a pivotal role in restoring independence and providing an improved quality of life for individuals with spinal cord injury. It involved physical therapy, occupational therapy, and psychological support. Physical therapy plays a crucial role in the rehabilitation of spinal cord injury (SCI) patients by improving strength, mobility, and overall function. The various methods used are passive or active range of motion exercises, strength training, functional electrical stimulation, and body weight support treadmill training. Respiratory muscle training to improve breathing and lung function is done particularly in patients with high cervical spine injuries.

Multiple Choice Questions

1. Which of the following sentences correctly defines anterior, middle, and posterior columns of the three-column concept in spine.
   (a) Anterior column—anterior one-third of vertebral body, middle column—posterior two-third of vertebral body, and posterior column—structures posterior to PLL.
   (b) Anterior column—anterior half of vertebral body, middle column—middle half of vertebral body, and posterior column—structures posterior to PLL.
   (c) Anterior column—anterior two-thirds of vertebral body, middle column—posterior one-third of vertebral body, and posterior column—structures posterior to PLL.
   (d) Anterior column—vertebral body, middle column—spinal canal and posterior column—structures posterior to spinal canal.
2. Denis and Ferguson classified the spinal into how many columns
   (a) 2 column
   (b) 3 column
   (c) 4 column
   (d) 5 column.
3. Compression fracture of C1 vertebra is also known as
   (a) Jefferson fracture
   (b) Hangman Fracture
   (c) Clay shoveler fracture
   (d) Jones fracture
4. What is the mechanism of injury in Hangman's fracture
   (a) Compression
   (b) Distraction
   (c) Hyperflexion
   (d) Hyperextension
5. In an adult spine, at what level does the spinal cord end
   (a) D12
   (b) L1
   (c) L2
   (d) L3

Answers: 1. (c), 2. (b), 3. (a), 4. (d), 5. (b)

References for Further Reading

1. Mahadevan V. Anatomy of the vertebral column. Surgery (Oxford). 2018;36(7):327–32.
2. Zhang A, Chauvin BJ. Denis classification. In: StatPearls [Internet]. Treasure Island (FL): StatPearls Publishing; 2023. Available from: http://www.ncbi.nlm.nih.gov/books/NBK544310/.
3. Essential orthopaedics, J Maheswari, 5th edition.
4. The spine, Rothman-simeone, 6th edition.
5. American Spinal Injury Association. International Standards for Neurological Classification of Spinal Cord Injury. Atlanta, GA, Revised 2011, Updated 2015.

32 Brachial Plexus Injuries

Suresh Chand

Applied Anatomy The brachial plexus is a pair of complex networks of nerves supplying both the upper limbs. It is formed by the contribution of the **anterior rami** of cervical spinal nerves C5, C6, C7 and C8, and the first thoracic spinal nerve, T1.

For description, brachial plexus may be divided into the following parts: roots, trunks, divisions, cords, and branches *(mnemonic **R**ead **T**hat **D**isney **C**omic **B**ook)*. The diagrammatic representation of brachial plexus and its branches is shown in Fig. 32.1.

Branches of Posterior Cord (Mnemonic 'ULTRA')

Upper subscapular nerve
Lower subscapular nerve
Thoracodorsal nerve
Radial nerve
Axillary nerve

Branches of Lateral Cord: (Mnemonic 'LML')

Lateral pectoral nerve
Musculocutaneous nerve
Lateral root of median nerve

Branches of Medial Cord: (Mnemonic 'M4U')

Medial Pectoral nerve
Median root of median nerve
Medial cutaneous nerve of arm
Medial cutaneous nerve of forearm
Ulnar nerve

Causes of brachial plexus injury include:

1. Obstetrical brachial plexus palsy (OBPP): traction injury during birth
2. Traumatic: accidents and fractures around the shoulder, stab or bullet injuries
3. Idiopathic/inflammatory: Idiopathic brachial neuritis (IBN), also known as 'Parsonage Turner syndrome'

Brachial plexus injury may be classified as follows:

1. *Pre–/post-ganglionic:* Lesion proximal to dorsal root ganglion, that is, avulsion of nerve root from its origin at the spinal cord, is termed as a preganglionic lesion (Fig. 32.2). However, injury to nerve roots distal to dorsal root ganglion is a post-ganglionic lesion.

   Diagnostic features of pre-ganglionic lesions include:

   (i) Horner's syndrome (ptosis, miosis, enophthalmos, anhidrosis)
   (ii) Flare response on the histamine test is intact
   (iii) Pseudo meningomyelocele on MRI

   Pre-ganglionic lesions have a poor prognosis and are practically irreparable.
2. *Upper/lower/pan—plexus:*
   (i) Upper plexus injury or *Erb's palsy* is caused by injury C5 & C6 nerve roots

S. Chand (✉)
Department of Paediatric Orthopaedics, King George's Medical University, Lucknow, India

V. Kumar et al. (eds.), *A Quick Guide to Essential Orthopedics*,
https://doi.org/10.1007/978-981-95-2676-5_32

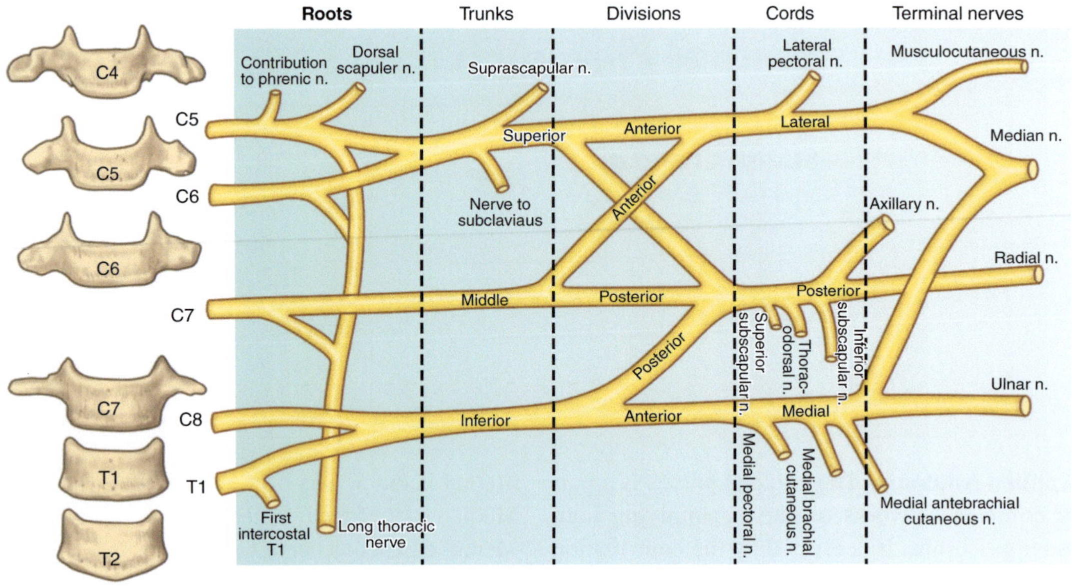

Fig. 32.1 Brachial plexus

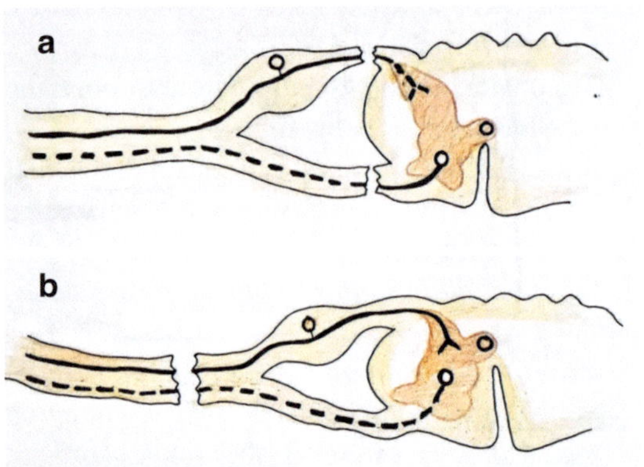

Fig. 32.2 (**a**) Pre- and (**b**) post-ganglionic lesion

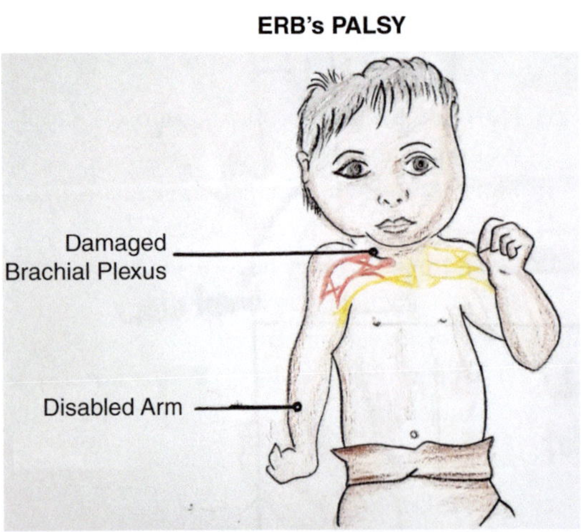

Fig. 32.3 Erb's palsy

and is the commonest. Clinically, it may present with the classical 'Policeman tip' posture of the affected side (Fig. 32.3). The arm is held to the side, internally rotated and pronated.

(ii) *Lower plexus injury or Klumpke's palsy* is caused by injury to C8 and T1 nerve roots. There may be associated Horner's syndrome and claw hand deformity due to paralysis of hand intrinsic muscles (Fig. 32.4).

(iii) *Pan plexus injury* presents with paralysed arm, forearm and hand. It may be associated with Horner's syndrome. Lower and pan plexus injuries have a poorer prognosis compared to upper plexus injury.

3. *Narakas classification*

Group	Type	Roots affected	Region affected
1	Upper	C5,C6	Shoulder abduction/ external rotation, elbow flexion
2	Extended upper	C5,C6,C7	As above + wrist drop

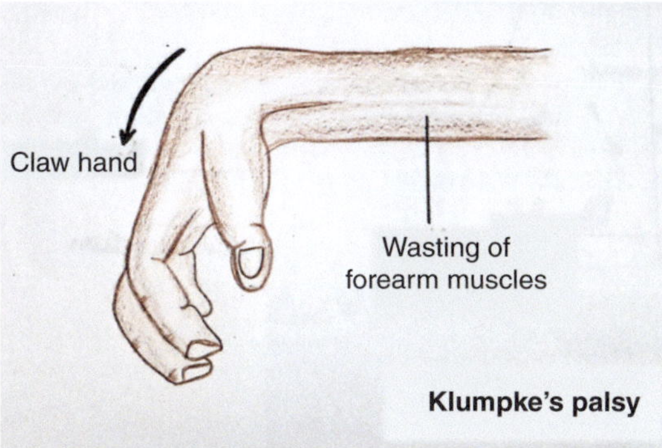

Fig. 32.4 Klumpke's palsy

Group	Type	Roots affected	Region affected
3	Pan-plexus palsy without Horner's syndrome	C5 to T1	Complete upper limb paralysis
4	Pan-plexus palsy with Horner's syndrome	C5 to T1	As above + Horner's syndrome

32.1 Management of Brachial Plexus Injuries

Most of the treatment strategies are directed towards maintaining shoulder abduction, external rotation, elbow flexion, wrist extension and finger flexion. While waiting for spontaneous recovery (which is seen in most of the upper plexus injuries), physiotherapy and splints are utilized as a conservative method.

If there is no recovery (no activity noted in Biceps muscle) after at least 3–6 months, a surgical exploration with nerve repair or transfer may be advised by a microsurgical or peripheral nerve surgeon. Results of primary nerve repair or nerve transfer may not be fruitful after 12 months of injury due to loss of neuromuscular junctions at the muscle level. Late presenters or sequelae may need contracture release, free functional muscle transfer, rotational osteotomy of Humerus or arthrodesis at the elbow/shoulder.

Multiple Choice Questions

1. The Brachial plexus is formed by contribution of
   (a) anterior rami of spinal nerves C5, C6, C7, C8 and T1
   (b) posterior rami of spinal nerves C5, C6, C7, C8 and T1
   (c) anterior horn cells of cervical spinal nerves
   (d) anterior branch of the first seven cranial nerves
2. Pseudo meningomyelocele with brachial plexus palsy is a hallmark feature of
   (a) associated congenital malformation
   (b) high-energy trauma
   (c) pre-ganglionic lesion
   (d) chronic injury to brachial plexus
3. Horner's syndrome refers to a combination of
   (a) ptosis, miosis, enophthalmos, hyperhidrosis
   (b) ptosis, miosis, enophthalmos, anhidrosis
   (c) ptosis, miosis, exophthalmos and clavicle fracture
   (d) bilateral brachial plexus injury
4. Erb's Palsy is characterised by:
   (a) 'Policeman's tip' deformity
   (b) Injury to C5 and C6 Cervical nerve roots
   (c) Both of the above
   (d) Flail upper limb
5. Which of the following is true regarding management of brachial plexus palsy:
   (a) 3–6 months of observation is an acceptable approach
   (b) Nerve repair beyond 12 months is generally not recommended
   (c) Nerve repair should be done by a microsurgical or peripheral nerve surgeon
   (d) All of the above

Answers: 1. (a), 2. (c), 3. (b), 4. (c), 5. (d)

References for Further Reading

1. Limthongthang R, Bachoura A, Songcharoen P, Osterman AL. Adult brachial plexus injury: evaluation and management. Orthop Clin North Am. 2013;44(4):591–603. https://doi.org/10.1016/j.ocl.2013.06.011. Epub 2013 Sep 6. PMID: 24095074

2. Yang LJ. Neonatal brachial plexus palsy—management and prognostic factors. Semin Perinatol. 2014;38(4):222–34. https://doi.org/10.1053/j.semperi.2014.04.009. PMID: 24863029
3. Moran SL, Steinmann SP, Shin AY. Adult brachial plexus injuries: mechanism, patterns of injury, and physical diagnosis. Hand Clin. 2005;21(1):13–24. https://doi.org/10.1016/j.hcl.2004.09.004. PMID: 15668062
4. Pulos N, Shaughnessy WJ, Spinner RJ, Shin AY. Brachial plexus birth injuries: a critical analysis review. JBJS Rev. 2021;9(6) https://doi.org/10.2106/JBJS.RVW.20.00004. PMID: 34102666

33 Peripheral Nerve Injuries

Suresh Chand

33.1 Anatomy

Peripheral nerves are a group of *axons* bundled together in the form of an electric cable. It conducts efferent (motor) signals from cells in the anterior horn of the spinal cord to a particular muscle or group of muscles, and afferent (sensory) signals from peripheral receptors via cells in the posterior root ganglia to the spinal cord. Humans have a total of 31 pairs of spinal nerves, which connect with all the skin and muscles of the limbs and trunk. Before supplying to the limbs, these nerves may form a particular arrangement called *plexus* (brachial plexus for the upper limb and lumbar plexus for the lower limb).

All peripheral nerves are mixed, and each nerve fibre or axon is either myelinated or unmyelinated. In the myelinated type, axons are coated with *myelin* sheath, a lipoprotein membrane formed by *Schwann* cells. Every few millimetres where Schwann cell ends, the myelin sheath is interrupted, leaving short segments of uncovered axon called the *nodes of Ranvier*. The nerve signals leap from node to node at the speed of electricity.

Outside the Schwann cell membrane, the axon is covered by a connective tissue, the *endoneurium*. A group of axons covered with endoneurium are bundled together to form fascicle which in turn is covered with dense layer of *perineurium*. The groups of fascicles together make up a peripheral nerve are enclosed in an even thicker connective tissue coating, the *epineurium* (Fig. 33.1).

The peripheral nerves are supplied by blood vessels that run longitudinally in the epineurium before penetrating the various layers.

S. Chand (✉)
Department of Paediatric Orthopaedics,
King George's Medical University, Lucknow, India

V. Kumar et al. (eds.), *A Quick Guide to Essential Orthopedics*,
https://doi.org/10.1007/978-981-95-2676-5_33

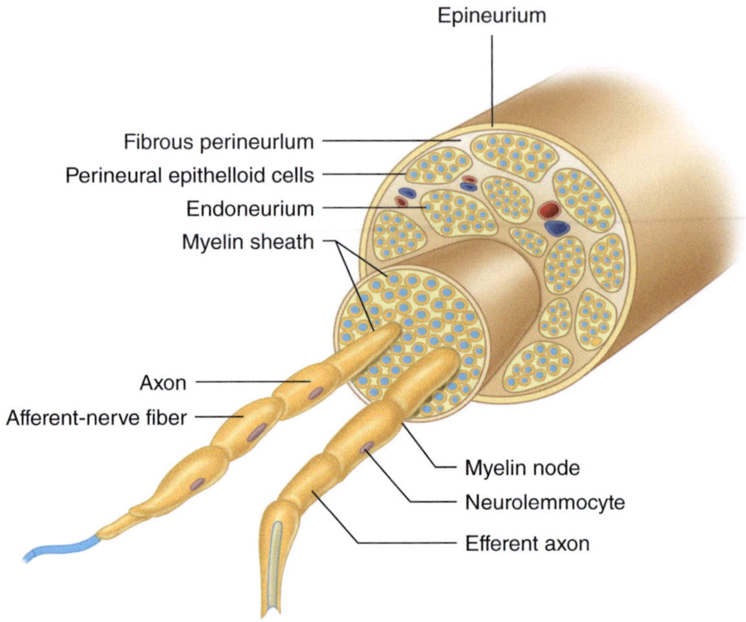

Fig. 33.1 Structure of Nerve

33.2 Pathology: Neuronal Degeneration and Regeneration

If any part of an axon is damaged due to injury and there is loss of conduction, the axons get disintegrated by phagocytes. This process of nerve degeneration proximal to the site of injury is called primary or retrograde degeneration. The disintegration distal to the point of injury is called secondary or *Wallerian* degeneration (named after August Waller, who described it in 1851). The disintegration starts 24–36 h after injury and is completed by 3–4 weeks. It is associated with the proliferation of Schwann cells and fibroblasts lining the endoneurial tubes and forming a hollow tube covering the debris.

Axonal regeneration starts within hours of injury, encouraged by growth factors from Schwann cells that form the hollow tube. There are numerous unmyelinated axonal sprouts from the proximal stump, many of which reach the distal end and grow into it at about 1 mm per day. The newly formed axons slowly acquire the myelin coat and eventually innervate the target tissue. A gentle tap along the course of a nerve (distal to proximal) may elicit a tingling sensation in the patient due to hyperexcitability of newly formed unmyelinated axons. This is called *Tinel's sign*, and a progressive positive Tinel's sign is clinical evidence of regeneration. During this regeneration process, the muscle nearest to the point of injury gets reinnervated first, followed by the next, and so on. This sequential process of reinnervation of muscles from proximal to distal is called *motor march* and is another sign of recovery.

Sometimes, in cases with more severe injury, the sprouting nerves fail to enter the distal tube. These nerve ends grow aimlessly and form a *neuroma*.

33.3 Classification of Nerve Injuries

33.3.1 Seddon's Classification

33.3.1.1 Neuropraxia

Seddon coined the term 'Neuropraxia' to describe a reversible and physiological blockage of transmission of nerve impulses in an anatomically intact nerve. It is due to mechanical pressure leading to loss of sensation & muscle power, which gets recovered completely in few days to weeks. There is no Wallerian degeneration, so no advancing Tinel's sign or motor march is seen in neuropraxia.

33.3.1.2 Axonotmesis

There is a more serious injury to axons; however, endoneurial tubes and Schwann cells are preserved. Wallerian degeneration followed by spontaneous regeneration with advancing Tinel's sign and motor march are noted in axonotmesis.

33.3.1.3 Neurotmesis

It refers to total anatomical cut injury to a nerve. There is rapid Wallerian degeneration, and spontaneous recovery is unlikely unless the nerve is surgically repaired.

33.3.2 Sunderland's Classification

Many times, nerve injuries fall in between axonotmesis and neurotmesis. Therefore, Sunderland described a more comprehensive classification to include the whole spectrum of injury:

(i) *First degree:* This includes transient ischaemia and neurapraxia, which is a completely reversible injury.
(ii) *Second degree:* This injury is akin to Seddon's axonotmesis. As the endoneurium is intact, complete regeneration is possible without surgical intervention.
(iii) *Third degree:* Here, the endoneurium is disrupted, but the perineurial sheaths are intact. During regeneration, the growing axons might reach the distal target. However, recovery may remain suboptimal due to fibrosis and cross-connections.
(iv) *Fourth degree:* Only the epineurium is intact. Although the nerve is in continuity, the internal damage is severe, and spontaneous recovery is unlikely.
(v) *Fifth degree:* The nerve is divided completely and will need surgical repair.

33.4 Assessment for Suspected Nerve Injury

Nerve injuries are easily overlooked, especially in an acute trauma setting associated with a fracture or dislocation. A detailed history and thorough examination are a must to identify a nerve injury.

Ask: Ask the patient about the mechanism of injury, duration and symptoms suggesting numbness, paraesthesia or muscle weakness.

Look: Observe the attitude of the injured limb that may be of diagnostic significance, for example, wrist drop in case of radial nerve palsy. Disuse atrophy or wasting may be noted in specific muscle groups in chronic cases.

Feel: This includes sensory examination to map the areas of altered sensation. Each spinal nerve supplies a specific dermatome, as shown in Fig. 33.2. Area supplied by a peripheral nerve exclusively is called as the *autonomous zone*, while the large area supplied along with the overlap of adjacent nerves is called the *maximal zone* (Fig. 33.3). In case of nerve injury, there will be a complete loss of sensation in the autonomous zone.

Move: This includes motor examination to test the strength of a muscle supplied by the nerve of interest. Also, check for the reflexes in the area of nerve distribution.

Neurological examination is a continued evaluation and must be repeated to identify changes following fracture reduction or surgery, or delayed changes after injury.

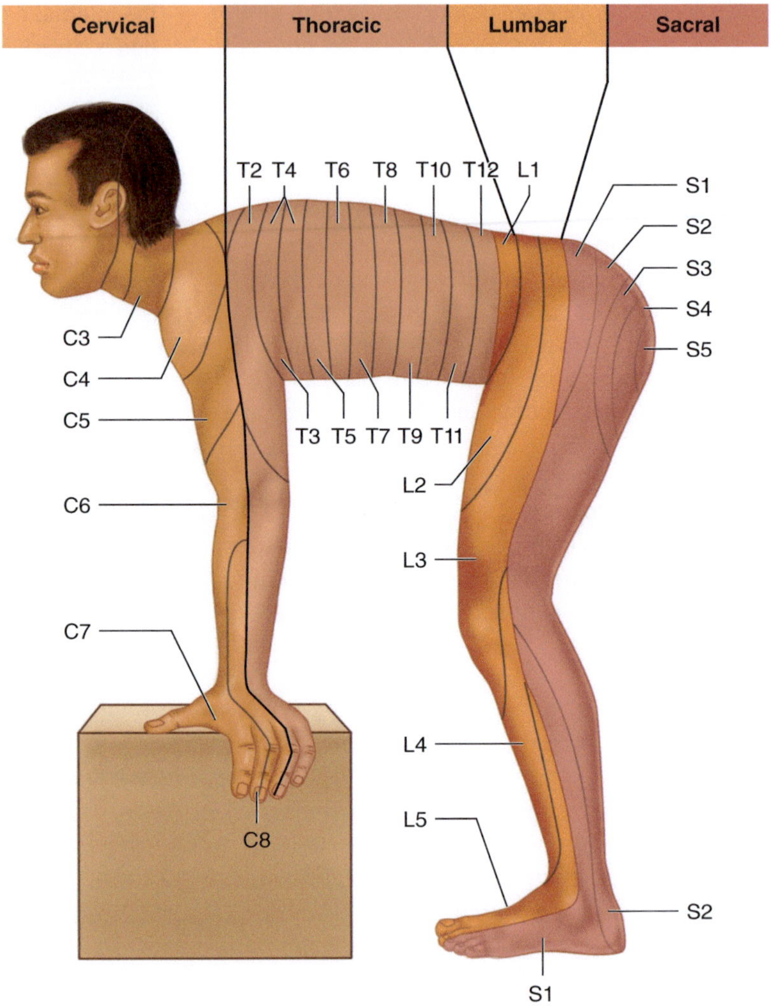

Fig. 33.2 Spinal nerve dermatomes

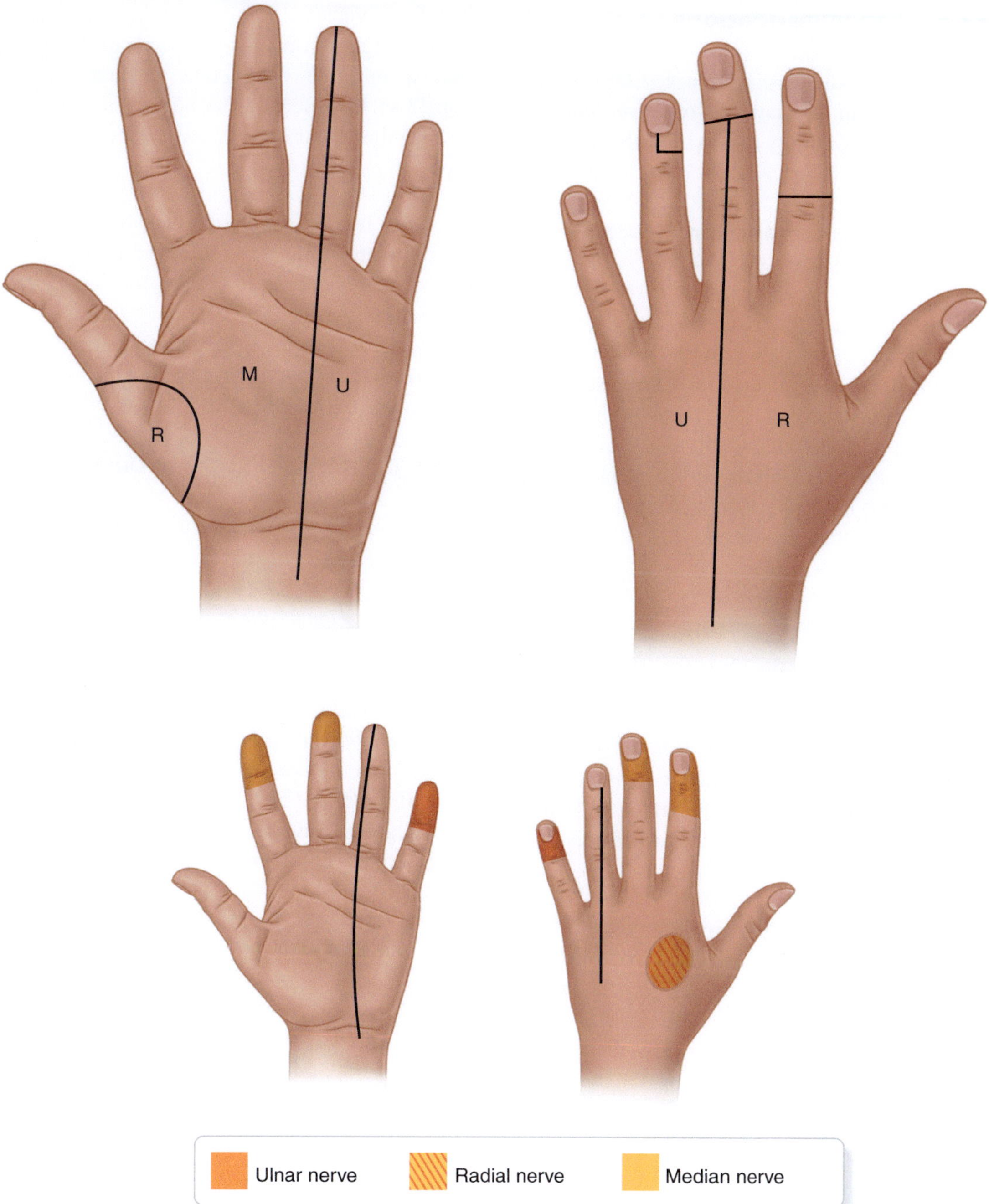

Fig. 33.3 Autonomous and maximal zones

33.5 Lab Investigations

Various electrodiagnostic studies (EDS) are utilised to confirm the diagnosis of nerve injury, the site and extent of injury and to track the recovery.

33.5.1 Nerve Conduction Velocity (NCV) Test

A nerve conduction velocity (NCV) test, also called a nerve conduction study (NCS), simply measures how fast an electrical impulse travels through a nerve being tested. During this test, the nerve is stimulated with an electrode patch on the skin over the nerve under test. The other electrode records it distally. The velocity, latency and amplitude are then measured.

33.5.2 Electromyography

During Electromyography (EMG) a needle electrode is placed through the skin into the muscle to be tested. EMG measures the electrical activity of muscle during rest, slight contraction and forceful contraction. The recording is presented in the form of a graph and analysed to reach a diagnosis.

33.5.3 Strength Duration Curve

The strength–duration curve is a graphical representation of the relationship between the intensity of an electrical stimulus (Y-axis of graph) and the length of time taken (X-axis of graph) to elicit a minimal contraction in that muscle (Fig. 33.4). It is used to determine the nerve damage and the amount of recovery that has taken place.

Rheobase: It is the minimum intensity of current required to stimulate a muscle at infinite duration. The rheobase is greater for denervated muscles.

Chronaxie: It is the minimum time required for a current of double the intensity of rheobase to stimulate a muscle.

33.5.3.1 Analysis of Strength Duration Curve

Normal Innervation: This is also called a 'nerve curve'. The shape of the curve is a continuous rectangular hyperbola.

Complete Denervation: This is also called a 'muscle curve'. As all the nerve fibres supplying the muscle have degenerated, the curve is shifted to the right and is steep.

Partial Denervation/ Recovering Pattern: It lies between the nerve and muscle curve. Since a few of the nerve fibres supplying the muscles have degenerated while others are intact, a characteristic kink is present in the curve (Fig. 33.5).

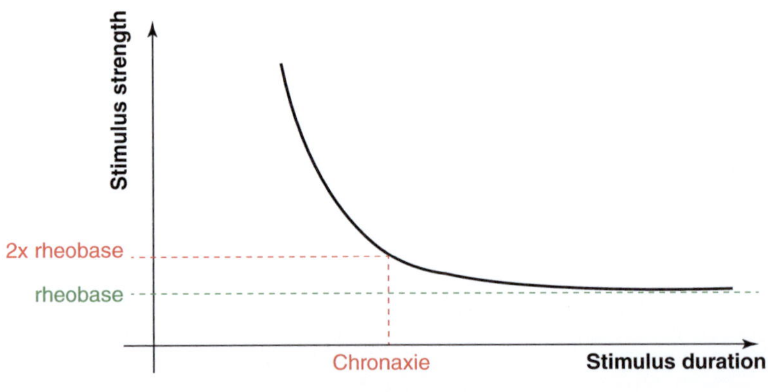

Fig. 33.4 Strength–Duration curve

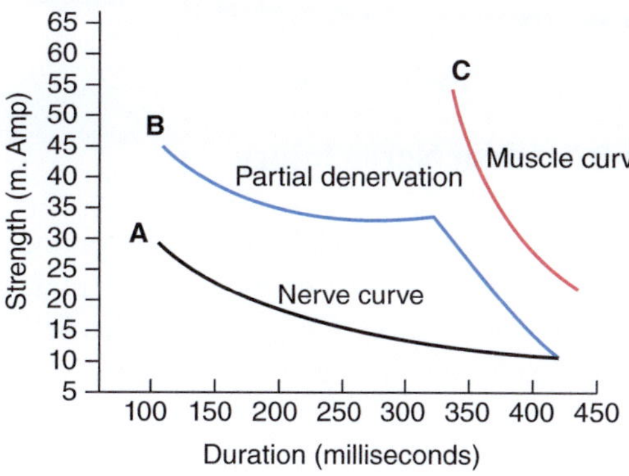

Fig. 33.5 Pattern of curve in injuries

33.6 Management of Nerve Injuries

As described in the previous section, a detailed history and clinical examination are the first step in the management of nerve injuries. Associated injuries may play a vital role in deciding the further course of management. Low-energy, closed injuries (without open wounds) have high chances of spontaneous recovery and may be observed for signs of recovery. However, if there are no signs of recovery by 6–12 weeks, nerve exploration may be warranted. Other indications for nerve exploration may include: open injuries, associated fracture/dislocation requiring open surgery.

Primary Repair: If the nerve is found clean cut, it can be repaired end-to-end with fine (10/0) sutures under magnifying loops or an operating microscope. The repair should be tension-free, and the limb is splinted to avoid undue traction on the repaired section.

Delayed Repair: Repair of the nerve weeks to months after primary injury is called delayed or secondary repair. The indications may include: failed primary repair, missed or neglected nerve injury and failure to recover after primary conservative management.

Nerve Grafting: While doing nerve repair, especially during delayed repair, if the nerve ends cannot be brought together without tension even after sufficient mobilisation, a nerve graft is used. The sural nerve is most commonly utilised as a free autogenous graft for nerve grafting, and up to 40 cm can be harvested from each leg in an adult.

Tendon Transfers: At times, motor recovery may not be possible due to neglect or even despite the best efforts of repair. The neuromuscular junctions generally degenerate after 18–24 months. In these situations, tendon transfers may be considered to achieve the best possible function. Some principles of tendon transfer are as follows:

The recipient site must be stable and have mobile joints.

The donor muscle must be powerful (power grade 4 or above), expandable and agonist/synergist.

The transferred tendon must be placed in a straight line of pull through the subcutaneous plane.

The patient must understand the procedure and the important role of rehabilitation after surgery.

Role of Supportive Management While recovery is awaited, the affected part/limb must be taken care of. Gentle therapy to prevent deformity or contractures, care of skin from sores or callosities is advised. Dynamic splints may be helpful during this recovery phase.

33.7 Peripheral Nerve Injuries Of Lower Limb

33.7.1 Lumbosacral Plexus Injury

It must always be suspected in a patient with pelvic injury. The patient may present with bladder/bowel involvement, loss of sensation in the perineal area and some part of the lower limb. Management is mostly directed to pelvic injury, and conservative management is done for plexus injury.

33.7.2 Sciatic Nerve Injury

Complete transaction of the sciatic nerve is rare except in gunshot injuries. Injury may occur in fracture-dislocation of the hip, iatrogenic injuries during surgical procedures around the hip, for example, total hip replacement or intramuscular injections in buttocks. The common peroneal nerve part is affected most commonly due to the outermost arrangement of its fibres in the sciatic nerve. The common peroneal nerve may be injured directly at the knee level, where it is superficial and more prone to injury.

In complete injury of the sciatic nerve, all the muscles of the leg will be paralysed, and sensation is lost except the medial aspect, which is supplied by femoral nerve. The ankle jerk is absent. The patient walks with a 'foot drop' or 'high stepping gait' in an attempt to clear the paralysed foot off the ground.

Treatment may include surgical repair of the nerve with or without grafting. Tendon transfer may be required for late-presenting or not-recovered cases. A foot drop splint is utilised while waiting for recovery to avoid fixed equinus contracture formation.

33.7.3 Femoral Nerve Injury

Due to its anatomical location, the femoral nerve is rarely injured and may be associated with arterial injuries. The causes of injury may be gunshot or blast injury, fracture-dislocations around the hip joint and iatrogenic injury during surgeries around the hip joint and thigh region. The patient may present with weakness of knee extension, numbness in the medial and anterior aspect of the thigh, and loss of knee reflex. However, identifying these clinical features may be difficult in an acute trauma setting, and a high index of suspicion is necessary. Clean-cut injuries may be repaired with a guarded prognosis. Tendon transfers or callipers may be utilised to stabilise the knee.

33.8 Peripheral Nerve Injuries of Upper Limb

33.8.1 Ulnar Nerve Injury

The ulnar nerve (Musician's nerve) is a continuation of the medial cord of the brachial plexus. Being a mixed nerve, it supplies muscles in the forearm and hand and provides sensory supply over the medial half of the fourth digit and the entire fifth digit and the ulnar portion of the posterior aspect of the hand (as shown in Fig. 33.3).

Ulnar nerve may be injured or compressed at the arcade of Struthers in the arm, behind the medial epicondyle at the elbow and Guyon's canal (under the piso-hamate ligament) at the hand. Although open injuries may damage nerves at any level.

The patient may present with wasting of the hypothenar and interosseous muscles. Due to weakness of intrinsic muscles, there is 'ulnar claw hand deformity'—hyperextension of the MCP joint of the ring and little fingers. The book test or Froment's sign is positive, and the Egawa test or card test may demonstrate the weakness of interossei (Fig. 33.6a, b). The loss of sensation may be tested over the autonomous zone of the ulnar nerve, which includes the tip of the little finger.

33.8.1.1 High Lesion, Low Lesion and the Ulnar Paradox

In *high lesions*, the nerve injury is above the level of elbow, for example, elbow fracture dislocations. Thus, all the muscles supplied by the ulnar nerve are paralysed. In *low lesions*, the injury is distal to elbow, and the ulnar half of flexor digitorum profundus and flexor carpi ulnaris muscle are spared.

The hand is markedly deformed and clawed in low lesions when compared to high lesions, which is labelled as *'ulnar paradox'*. This is because of sparing of FDP and FCU in low lesions, causing more pronounced flexion of DIP joints and resultant more severe clawing in low lesions.

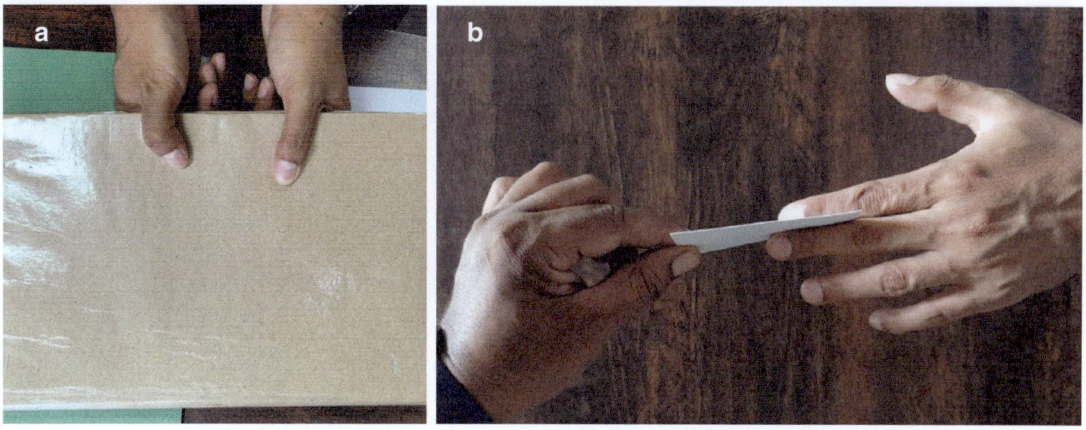

Fig. 33.6 (**a**) Book test. (**b**) Card test

33.8.2 Median Nerve Injury

The Median nerve (Labourer's nerve) is formed by the medial and lateral cords of brachial plexus. It supplies the muscles of forearm, hand and thumb and provides sensory supply to the skin of palmar and distal dorsal aspects of lateral three and a half digits.

Median nerve may be injured or compressed at the distal arm (paediatric supracondylar humerus fractures), at the level of proximal forearm (pronator syndrome, lacertus syndrome), and most commonly at the level of the wrist (carpal tunnel syndrome).

The patient may present with inability to abduct the thumb (positive pen test), inability to flex the index finger (pointing index or Osner's clasping sign) and inability to make 'OK sign' (Fig. 33.7).

In chronic cases, there may be wasting of the thenar muscles. The loss of sensation may be tested over the autonomous zone of the median nerve, which includes the tips of the index and middle fingers.

33.8.2.1 High and Low Lesions with Median Nerve Injury

High lesion may be due to proximal forearm fractures or elbow dislocation and is basically a lesion proximal to the origin of the anterior interosseous nerve. Low lesion is at the level of the wrist due to direct cut, wrist and carpal injuries.

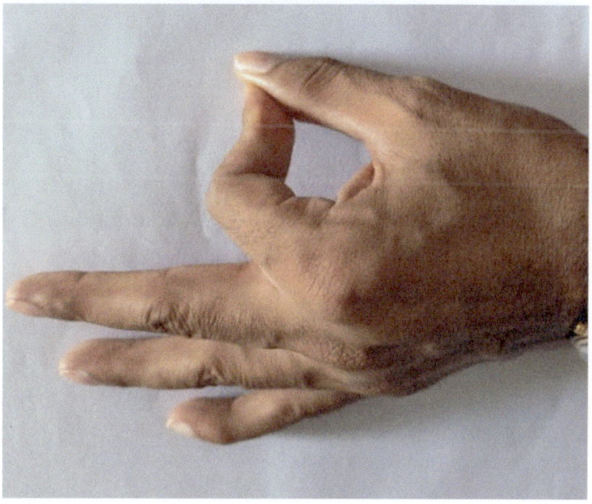

Fig. 33.7 Classical 'OK sign'

In low lesions, only the hand function is affected, while in high lesions, all muscles innervated by the median nerve would be affected.

33.8.3 Radial Nerve Injury

The radial nerve is one of the terminal branches of the posterior cord of the brachial plexus. It supplies the muscles of the dorsal aspect of the arm and forearm and provides sensory supply to the dorsal aspect of the arm, forearm and hand, with the autonomous zone being the dorsal aspect of the 1st web space.

The patient typically presents with the 'wrist drop' sign (high radial nerve palsy) or 'finger

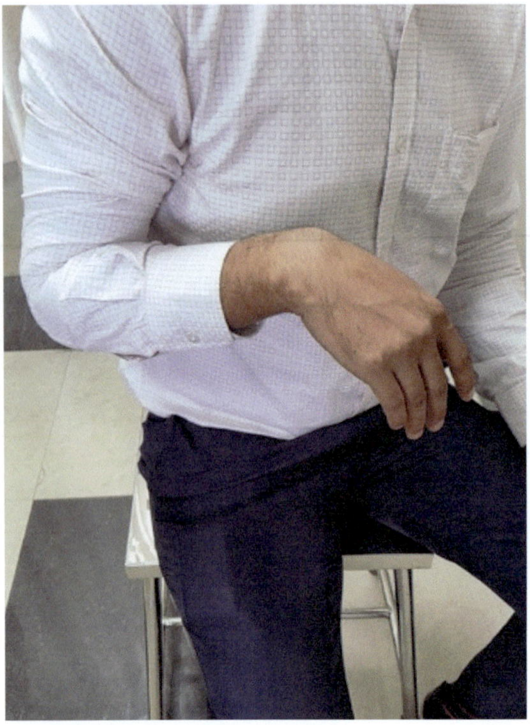

Fig. 33.8 Typical 'Wrist drop' sign

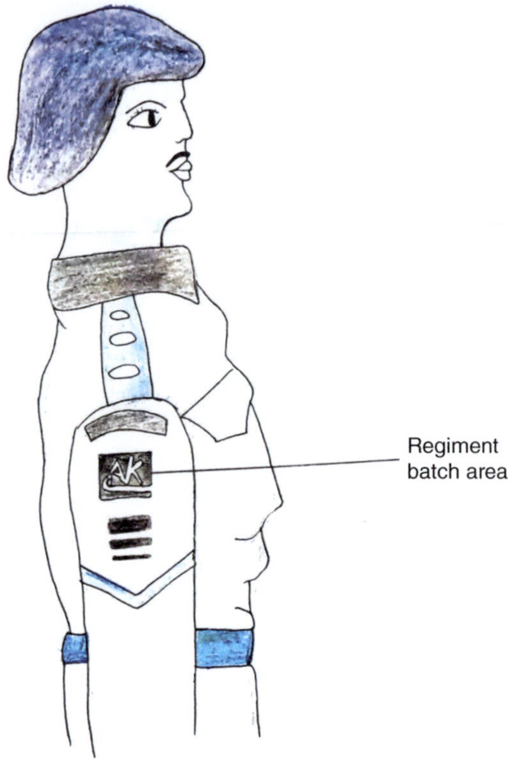

Fig. 33.9 Regiment batch area

drop' sign or inability to extend metacarpophalangeal joints (posterior interosseous nerve palsy) (Fig. 33.8).

33.8.3.1 Very High, High or Low Radial Nerve Palsy

In '*Very high radial nerve palsy*', the injury is above the spiral groove, affecting all the muscles. It may be seen in open injuries or surgeries around the shoulder, alcoholics or drug addicts due to compression over the chair (Saturday night palsy) or chronic compression in axilla (crutch palsy). In addition to wrist drop, elbow extension is also affected due to triceps paralysis.

'*High radial nerve palsy*' is at or below the spiral groove, and the triceps muscle is spared.

'*Low radial nerve palsy*' involves injury at or below the elbow affecting the posterior interosseous nerve part. The presence of intact wrist extension with loss of MCP joint extension is the hallmark of this injury.

33.8.4 Axillary Nerve Injury

It is a small branch of posterior cord of brachial plexus and supplies deltoid and teres minor muscle. The nerve may be injured in shoulder dislocations, proximal humerus fractures or surgeries.

The patient may present with shoulder weakness and loss of active abduction at the shoulder beyond 20° (action of supraspinatus intact). There may be a loss of contour of the shoulder due to deltoid wasting. Sensory examination will reveal numbness over the lateral aspect of the shoulder and upper arm (regimental badge sign) (Fig. 33.9).

33.8.5 Long Thoracic Nerve Palsy

The long thoracic nerve of 'Bell' is derived from ventral rami of C5, 6,7 roots of brachial plexus and supplies the serratus anterior muscle.

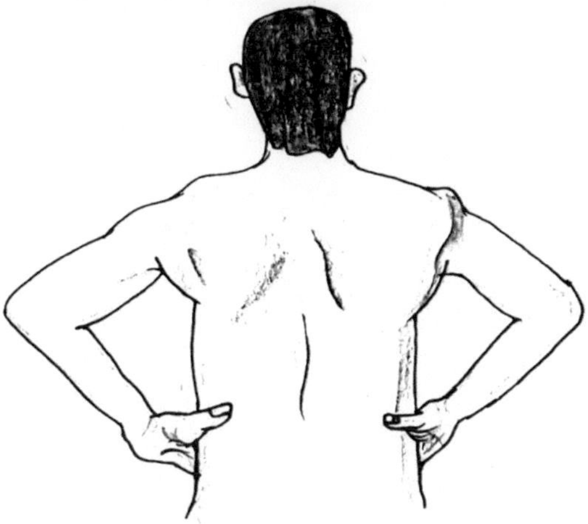

Fig. 33.10 Winging of right scapula

The patient complains of difficulty in lifting the arm above the shoulder and presents with '*winging of scapula*'. Clinically, this sign is demonstrated by asking the patient to push forwards against a wall (Fig. 33.10).

Multiple Choice Questions

1. Wallerian degeneration refers to:
   (a) Degeneration of neuromuscular junction after nerve injury
   (b) Degeneration of nerve distal to site of injury
   (c) Idiopathic disintegration of nerves
   (d) Post-surgery remodelling of grafted nerve
2. Reversible blockage of nerve function after injury is classified as:
   (a) Axonotmesis
   (b) Neurotmesis
   (c) Neuropraxia
   (d) Tinel's sign
3. An area supplied exclusively by a peripheral nerve is called:
   (a) Autonomous zone
   (b) Maximal zone
   (c) Node of Ranvier
   (d) Seddon's area
4. Ulnar Paradox refers to:
   (a) Ulnar nerve injury recovers earlier than radial nerve injury
   (b) The hand appears more deformed in low ulnar nerve injury
   (c) There is a mismatch in muscles paralysed after ulnar nerve injury
   (d) None of the above
5. Inability to make 'OK' gesture with hands may be a sign of:
   (a) Ulnar nerve injury
   (b) Median nerve injury
   (c) Brachial plexus palsy
   (d) Parsonage–Turner syndrome

Answers: 1. (b), 2. (c), 3. (a), 4. (b), 5. (b)

Further Reading

1. Flores AJ, Lavernia CJ, Owens PW. Anatomy and physiology of peripheral nerve injury and repair. Am J Orthop (Belle Mead NJ). 2000;29(3):167–73. PMID: 10746467.
2. Campbell WW. Evaluation and management of peripheral nerve injury. Clin Neurophysiol. 2008;119(9):1951–65. https://doi.org/10.1016/j.clinph.2008.03.018. Epub 2008 May 14. PMID: 18482862.
3. Janjic JM, Gorantla VS. Peripheral nerve nanoimaging: monitoring treatment and regeneration. AAPS J. 2017;19(5):1304–16. https://doi.org/10.1208/s12248-017-0129-x. Epub 2017 Aug 4. PMID: 28779380.
4. Loewenstein SN, Adkinson JM. Tendon transfers for peripheral nerve palsies. Clin Plast Surg. 2019;46(3):307–15. https://doi.org/10.1016/j.cps.2019.02.004. Epub 2019 Apr 12. PMID: 31103075.
5. Li R, Liu Z, Pan Y, Chen L, Zhang Z, Lu L. Peripheral nerve injuries treatment: a systematic review. Cell Biochem Biophys. 2014;68(3):449–54. https://doi.org/10.1007/s12013-013-9742-1. PMID: 24037713.

Part IV

Infections in Orthopedics

Acute Osteomyelitis

34

Sourabh Kumar Sinha

34.1 Introduction

Infections of the musculoskeletal system can present as osteomyelitis (infection of bone), septic arthritis (infection of joints), pyomyositis (infection of muscle) or a combination of these.

Acute osteomyelitis is an infection of the bone presenting within 2 weeks of symptom onset [1, 2].

34.2 Etiopathogenesis

The most common route of inoculation of infection is by the hematogenous route with a focus of infection elsewhere in the body (sinusitis, pharyngitis, otitis media, etc.). Direct inoculation by injection or penetrating wound and contiguous spread from adjacent joints are the other modes of infection [3, 4]. The sluggish blood flow in the hairpin loops and deficient tissue macrophages in the metaphyseal region of bone make it the commonest site for osteomyelitis [5]. Staphylococcus aureus is the most common causative organism [6]. The common causative organism in various age groups and underlying conditions is listed in Table 34.1.

Table 34.1 Common causative organism in various age groups

Patient characteristics	Causative organisms
Neonates	S. aureus, Streptococcus species, Enterobacteriaceae, Candida species
Infant	S. aureus, K. kingae, S. pneumoniae, N. meningitidis, H. influenzae type b
1–3 years	S. aureus, K. kingae, S. pneumoniae, N. meningitidis, H. influenzae type b
3–12 years	S. aureus, Group A Beta Hemolytic Streptococcus (GABHS)
12–18 years	S. aureus, GABHS, Neisseria gonorrhoeae

Once infection is established, local immune response leads to inflammation and exudation. The exudate in the form of pus collects in the medullary cavity. It may breach the bony cortex and form a subperiosteal abscess. This may further spread into the muscle plane as pyomyositis. As the pus lifts the endosteum and periosteum off the bone, the bone becomes devascularised, leading to "sequestrum" formation. New bone formation occurs around the sequestrum, called "involucrum" as a result of subperiosteal deposition of new bone. The intramedullary pus drains across the bone through channels in the involucrum called "cloaca." If left untreated, the abscess may burst through the skin, leading to sinus formation (Fig. 34.1).

S. K. Sinha (✉)
Department of Orthopaedics, All India Institute of Medical Sciences, Bhopal, India

V. Kumar et al. (eds.), *A Quick Guide to Essential Orthopedics*,
https://doi.org/10.1007/978-981-95-2676-5_34

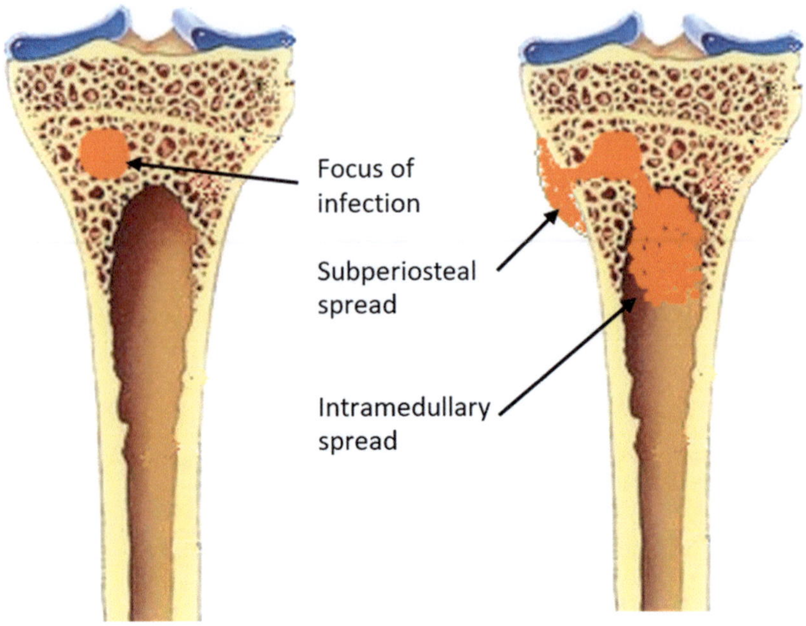

Fig. 34.1 A schematic representation of the metaphyseal focus of acute osteomyelitis and its subperiosteal spread

34.3 Clinical Features

A child with acute osteomyelitis presents with an acute onset of pain, redness and swelling over the affected limb associated with systemic features of high-grade fever and malaise. Local rise of temperature and tenderness is present over the affected bone. The child may refuse to move the affected limb due to pain, and this phenomenon is termed "pseudoparalysis" [7, 8].

34.4 Investigations

Routine blood workup shows elevated total leukocyte counts, C-reactive protein levels and ESR. High-resolution ultrasound is used to detect the presence of a subperiosteal abscess [9]. Radiographs may reveal loss of soft tissue planes in the presence of a swollen limb, but are typically normal in the early stages of disease. Radiographic changes of osteopenia and periosteal reaction are seen beyond 10–12 days of the onset of illness [10]. MRI is also a sensitive tool and helps in detecting the presence of intramedullary and soft tissue collection and inflammation [4]. Blood cultures help in detecting the causative organism in the presence of bacteraemia.

34.5 Management

In the early stages (within 24–48 h of onset), before the formation of a subperiosteal abscess, the child is treated with IV fluids, analgesics, antipyretics, and empirical antibiotics directed against the most probable organism (Staphylococcus aureus and others, according to age). Splintage of the painful limb should be done to aid pain relief [11].

Aspiration either under USG guidance or at the site of maximum tenderness is performed to detect and obtain pus sample from subperiosteal abscess. This sample for culture and sensitivity is preferably obtained before starting empirical antibiotics. The presence of subperiosteal abscess forms an indication for surgical management [11].

Surgical management consists of drainage of the abscess, decompression of the medullary cavity by creating a cortical window and closure over a drain [11]. The samples obtained are sent for Gram staining, AFB staining, culture and sensitivity and histopathology.

34.5.1 Antibiotic Therapy

Until the availability of culture and sensitivity reports, the empirical antibiotics like cephalosporins, linezolid, vancomycin and gentamicin are commonly used as per institutional preference. Further choice of antibiotics is guided by culture and sensitivity reports. Intravenous route of administration is preferred till the child becomes afebrile and the C-reactive protein levels return to baseline levels, after which the oral route is preferred. A total antibiotic duration of six weeks is preferred [11].

34.6 Complications

Pathological fracture may occur due to weakening and destruction of bone.

Damage to physis may lead to partial or complete *growth arrest*. It may manifest as angular deformity or shortening of the limb.

Septic arthritis may occur in joints where the metaphyseal region is located intracapsular.

If treatment is delayed or inadequate, the infection may persist and progress to *chronic osteomyelitis*.

34.7 Subacute Osteomyelitis

Subacute osteomyelitis is a form of osteomyelitis characterised by a slow and indolent onset, often presenting with nonspecific symptoms such as localised pain, swelling, and low-grade fever. One particular manifestation of subacute osteomyelitis is Brodie's abscess, which is a localised, well-circumscribed abscess within the bone [12]. Brodie's abscess typically occurs in the metaphysis of long bones, particularly in the tibia and femur.

The management of subacute osteomyelitis and Brodie's abscess involves a combination of medical and surgical approaches. Initial treatment includes the use of appropriate antibiotics to target the causative bacteria, typically Staphylococcus aureus. Empirical antibiotic therapy is often started, followed by adjustment based on culture and sensitivity results. Prolonged antibiotic therapy is typically required, depending on the severity and response to treatment.

Surgical intervention may be necessary in cases where the abscess persists despite medical therapy, or when there is extensive bone destruction or the risk of pathological fracture. Surgical options include abscess drainage, debridement of infected tissues, and removal of necrotic bone. In some cases, bone grafting may be required to promote bone healing and restore structural integrity.

Multiple Choice Questions

1. Which bacterial pathogen is the most common cause of acute hematogenous osteomyelitis?
   (a) Staphylococcus aureus
   (b) Streptococcus pneumoniae
   (c) Escherichia coli
   (d) Pseudomonas aeruginosa
2. The pathogenesis of acute hematogenous osteomyelitis involves bacterial colonization in the metaphysis of long bones. Which factor contributes to this preference?
   (a) High vascularity and slower blood flow in the metaphysis
   (b) Low vascularity and rapid blood flow in the metaphysis
   (c) Greater concentration of immune cells in the metaphysis
   (d) Weaker bone structure in the metaphysis
3. The diagnostic imaging modality of choice for acute osteomyelitis is:
   (a) X-ray
   (b) Magnetic resonance imaging (MRI)

   (c) Computed tomography (CT) scan
   (d) Ultrasound
4. Intravenous (IV) antibiotics are typically administered for acute osteomyelitis for a duration of:
   (a) 1–2 days
   (b) 1–2 weeks
   (c) 4–6 weeks
   (d) 3–6 months.
5. Which of the following complications can occur in acute osteomyelitis?
   (a) Bone deformities
   (b) Septicaemia (blood infection)
   (c) Joint destruction
   (d) All of the above

Answers: 1. (a), 2. (a), 3. (b), 4. (c), 5. (d)

References

1. Peltola H, Pääkkönen M. Acute osteomyelitis in children. N Engl J Med. 2014;370(4):352–60.
2. Manz N, Krieg AH, Buettcher M, Ritz N, Heininger U. Long-term outcomes of acute osteoarticular infections in children. Front Pediatr. 2020;8:587740.
3. Whyte NSB, Bielski RJ. Acute hematogenous osteomyelitis in children. Pediatr Ann. 2016;45(6):e204–8.
4. Pugmire BS, Shailam R, Gee MS. Role of MRI in the diagnosis and treatment of osteomyelitis in pediatric patients. World J Radiol. 2014;6(8):530–7.
5. Trueta J. The three types of acute haematogenous osteomyelitis: a clinical and vascular study. J Bone Joint Surg Br. 1959;41-B(4):671–80.
6. Howard-Jones AR, Isaacs D. Systematic review of duration and choice of systemic antibiotic therapy for acute haematogenous bacterial osteomyelitis in children. J Paediatr Child Health. 2013;49(9):760–8.
7. Knudsen CJ, Hoffman EB. Neonatal osteomyelitis. J Bone Joint Surg Br. 1990;72(5):846–51.
8. Le Saux N. Diagnosis and management of acute osteoarticular infections in children. Paediatr Child Health. 2018;23(5):336–43.
9. Abernethy LJ, Lee YC, Cole WG. Ultrasound localization of subperiosteal abscesses in children with late-acute osteomyelitis. J Pediatr Orthop. 1993;13(6):766–8.
10. Pineda C, Espinosa R, Pena A. Radiographic imaging in osteomyelitis: the role of plain radiography, computed tomography, ultrasonography, magnetic resonance imaging, and scintigraphy. Semin Plast Surg. 2009;23(2):80–9.
11. Woods CR, Bradley JS, Chatterjee A, Copley LA, Robinson J, Kronman MP, et al. Clinical practice guideline by the Pediatric Infectious Diseases Society and the Infectious Diseases Society of America: 2021 guideline on diagnosis and management of acute hematogenous osteomyelitis in pediatrics. J Pediatr Infect Dis Soc. 2021;10(8):801–44.
12. Hayes CS, Heinrich SD, Craver R, MacEwen GD. Subacute osteomyelitis. Orthopedics. 1990;13(3):363–6.

Chronic and Subacute Osteomyelitis

35

Sourabh Kumar Sinha

35.1 Introduction

Chronic osteomyelitis is a serious bone infection that requires long-term management in children. In this chapter, we will discuss the aetiology, pathogenesis, clinical presentation, diagnostic criteria, treatment and possible outcomes of chronic osteomyelitis in children. It usually presents with the onset of symptoms beyond 6 weeks.

35.2 Etiopathogenesis

The most common cause of chronic osteomyelitis in children is Staphylococcus aureus. Other bacteria that can cause chronic osteomyelitis include coagulase-negative staphylococci, streptococci, Escherichia coli and Pseudomonas aeruginosa. Chronic osteomyelitis may also be caused by fungi such as Candida albicans or Aspergillus fumigatus.

Children with chronic osteomyelitis often have an underlying predisposing condition that increases their risk for developing osteomyelitis. These conditions include sickle cell disease, diabetes, immunodeficiency disorders and cancer.

Chronic osteomyelitis usually develops as a sequela of acute osteomyelitis. It can also develop following open fractures and orthopaedic surgeries. Chronic osteomyelitis is characterized by the presence of bone necrosis and sequestrum formation. Reactive new bone formation occurs around the sequestrum called 'involucrum'. The intramedullary pus drains across the bone through channels in the involucrum called 'cloaca'. This may communicate to the exterior through sinus formation. The bacteria thrive in the bone tissue that is poorly vascularized, making it difficult for antibiotics to reach the bacteria and eradicate the infection. The bacteria can remain viable and cause recurrent infections, even after several courses of antibiotic therapy.

35.3 Clinical Features

The clinical presentation of chronic osteomyelitis in children may vary depending on the child's age, type of infection, location of infection, duration of infection and underlying medical conditions.

The patient classically presents with a discharging sinus communicating with the site of osteomyelitis. The sequestrum may form part of the discharge in the form of bony spicules. Pain and tenderness may accompany periods of acute exacerbation. The bone becomes irregular to palpation. In cases of absent or healed sinuses, the acute exacerbation is accompanied by local abscess formation.

S. K. Sinha (✉)
Department of Orthopaedics, All India Institute of Medical Sciences, Bhopal, India

V. Kumar et al. (eds.), *A Quick Guide to Essential Orthopedics*,
https://doi.org/10.1007/978-981-95-2676-5_35

35.4 Investigations

Routine blood workup may show elevated total leukocyte counts, C-reactive protein levels and ESR during active infection. Radiographs reveal irregular bony cortex, sclerosis, periosteal reaction and radiodense sequestrum. Bone gaps are present in cases with pan-diaphyseal sequestration and pathological fractures (Fig. 35.1). MRI is used to detect the presence of intramedullary and soft tissue collections and inflammation. Local cultures, preferably deep tissue cultures from the site of osteomyelitis, help in detecting the causative organism and guide the choice of antibiotics.

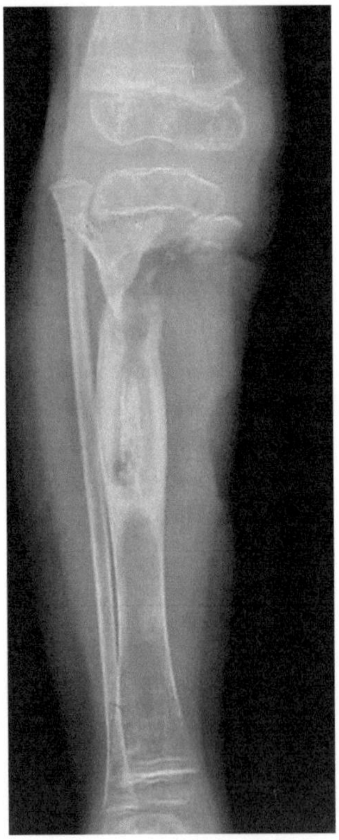

Fig. 35.1 Chronic osteomyelitis of tibia with sequestrum and bone gap

35.5 Management

The treatment of chronic osteomyelitis is usually staged and involves debridement, eradication of infection and reconstruction of bone defects.

Saucerization is a surgical procedure that involves removing the infected portion of the bone in the treatment of chronic osteomyelitis. During the procedure, the sequestrum, as well as any infected bone and surrounding tissue, is removed. The procedure results in a saucer-shaped defect in the bone, which helps to promote drainage and removal of any remaining infection. Saucerization can be done as a standalone procedure or as part of a more complex surgical treatment for chronic osteomyelitis, such as bone grafting or reconstruction. Skin grafts or fasciocutaneous flaps are commonly used for local wound management.

In addition to saucerization surgery, there are other management options for bone defects depending on the extent of the bone loss. The management of bone defects requires an individualized approach that depends on the patient's age, overall health status, the extent of the bone loss and other factors.

These options may include:

1. *Bone grafting*: Bone grafting is a procedure that involves transplanting bone tissue from other parts of the patient's body (autograft) or donor bone tissue (allograft) to the site of the bone defect to stimulate new bone growth.
2. *Bone transport*: Bone transport involves gradually moving a section of a healthy bone adjacent to the defect into the area of the defect to promote new bone growth (Ilizarov method).
3. *Masquelet technique*: The Masquelet technique is a two-stage procedure involving the placement of a bone void filler (such as cement) in the defect, followed by bone graft-

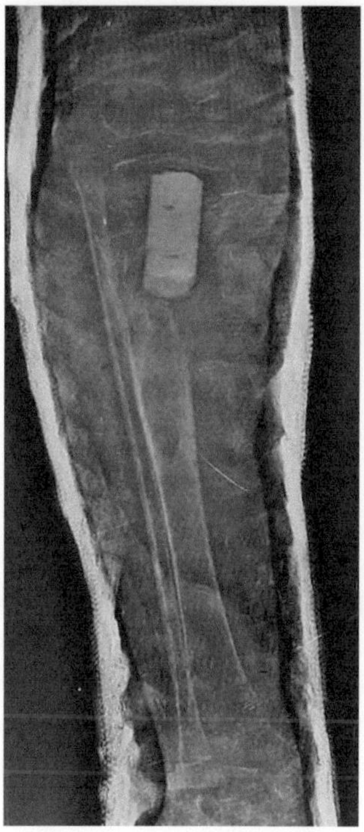

Fig. 35.2 Use of antibiotic cement spacer (Masquelet technique)

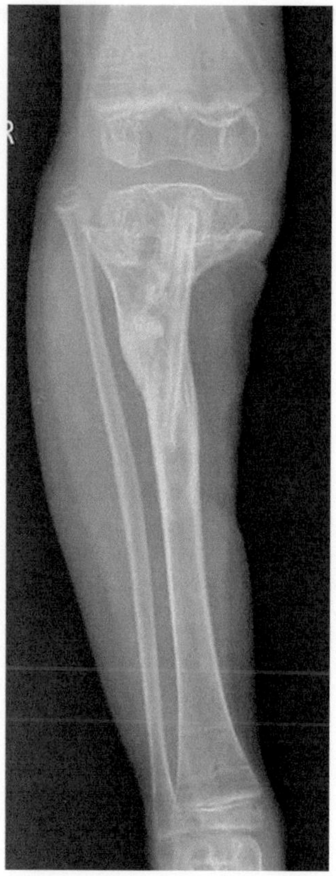

Fig. 35.3 Reconstruction with bone grafts after cement spacer removal (Masquelet technique)

ing. Bone stimulation and graft integration are enhanced by the induced membrane formed around the cement spacer, which promotes vascularization and inhibits the growth of scar tissue (Figs. 35.2 and 35.3).

4. *Artificial bone substitutes*: Artificial bone substitutes, such as biocompatible scaffolds, can be used to fill bone defects and promote new bone growth.
5. *Amputation*: In severe cases of bone loss, amputation may be necessary to prevent further complications, such as chronic infection. The decision to amputate is usually a last resort and is only considered after all other treatment options have been exhausted.

Antibiotic delivery is an important aspect of the management of chronic osteomyelitis. Antibiotics are used to control and eliminate bacterial infection in the bone tissue. However, antibiotics have limited access to the bone tissue, and the penetration of antibiotics into the affected area is often hindered by factors such as biofilm formation, reduced blood supply and the presence of necrotic tissue. To overcome these limitations, various methods have been used for antibiotic delivery in chronic osteomyelitis. These include:

1. Local Antibiotic Delivery: This involves placement of antibiotics directly into the affected bone tissue or wound, either as a powder, beads, or gel. This allows for high concentration and sustained release of antibiotics at the site of infection.
2. Systemic Antibiotic Delivery: In some cases, oral or intravenous antibiotics may be used to treat chronic osteomyelitis. The selection of antibiotics is based on the sensitivity of the bacteria causing the infection.
3. Antibiotic-Impregnated Materials: Antibiotics may be impregnated into bone substitutes,

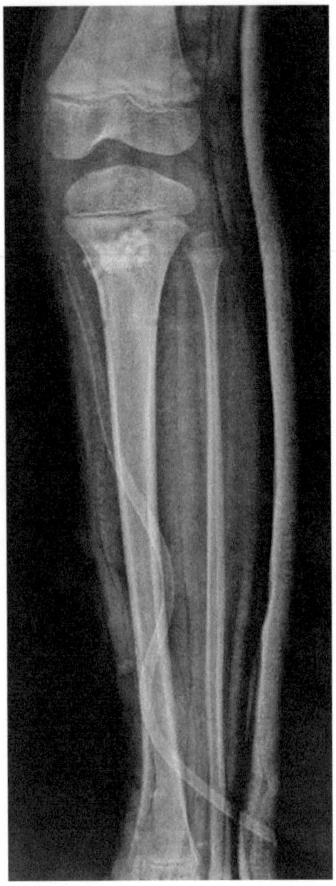

Fig. 35.4 Use of bone substitute (tricalcium phosphate) for local antibiotic delivery

such as bone cement, spacers or grafts, to deliver antibiotics locally (Fig. 35.4).

Multiple Choice Questions

1. Which of the following is a common cause of chronic osteomyelitis?
   (a) Bacterial pneumonia
   (b) Viral infection
   (c) Staphylococcus aureus
   (d) Fungal overgrowth
2. Which of the following is a key step in the management of chronic osteomyelitis?
   (a) Antibiotic therapy
   (b) Surgical debridement
   (c) Physical therapy
   (d) Pain management
3. What is the primary goal of surgical debridement in the management of chronic osteomyelitis?
   (a) Removal of infected bone and tissue
   (b) Stabilization of fractured bones
   (c) Promotion of bone healing
   (d) Reduction of pain and inflammation
4. When is the use of bone grafts or bone substitutes considered in the management of chronic osteomyelitis?
   (a) As a first-line treatment option
   (b) In cases of extensive bone loss or non-healing
   (c) Only in paediatric patients
   (d) When there is a risk of joint involvement
5. Which of the following factors should be considered when selecting the oral antibiotic for the management of chronic osteomyelitis?
   (a) Antibiotic susceptibility of the pathogen
   (b) Ability to penetrate bone tissue
   (c) Patient's renal and hepatic function
   (d) All of the above

Answers: 1. (c), 2. (b), 3. (a), 4. (b), 6. (d)

References for Further Reading

1. Sendi P, Bregenzer T, Zimmerli W. The use of antibiotics in the treatment of chronic osteomyelitis. J Antimicrob Chemother. 1999;43(6):959–69.
2. Epari DR, Bajpai J, Kumar A, et al. Role of MRI in chronic osteomyelitis: a pictorial essay. J Clin Imaging Sci. 2011;1:27.
3. Sen RK, Tripathy SK, Aggarwal S, et al. Saucerization in chronic osteomyelitis: a prospective study. Indian J Orthop. 2018;52(2):151–7.
4. Masquelet AC, Fitoussi F, Begue T, et al. Reconstruction of the long bones by the induced membrane and spongy autograft. Ann Chir Plast Esthet. 2000;45(3):346–53.
5. Hake ME, Young H, Hak DJ, et al. Local antibiotic therapy strategies in orthopaedic trauma: practical tips and tricks and review of the literature. Injury. 2015;46(8):1447–56.
6. Ostermann PA, Seligson D, Henry SL. Local antibiotic therapy for severe open fractures. A review of 1085 consecutive cases. J Bone Joint Surg Br. 1995;77(1):93–7.

36 Septic Arthritis

Sourabh Kumar Sinha

36.1 Introduction

Septic arthritis is an inflammation of a synovial joint, usually due to bacterial infection. It can also be caused by fungal, mycobacterial, and viral infections. The knee, hip, and shoulder joints are commonly affected. Due to the joint-destroying nature of the illness, it is treated as an orthopedic emergency [1].

36.2 Etiopathogenesis

The hematogenous spread of infection from a focus of infection elsewhere in the body (sinusitis, pharyngitis, otitis media, etc.) is the most common route of inoculation of infection into the synovium. Direct inoculation of infection can occur by inadvertent pricking of the hip joint capsule during femoral vascular access. In joints like the knee and hip, where the capsule covers a part of the metaphysis, infection can spread from a focus of acute osteomyelitis into the joint [2] (Fig. 36.1).

Staphylococcus aureus is the most common causative organism. Common causative organism in various age groups and underlying conditions is listed in Table 36.1.

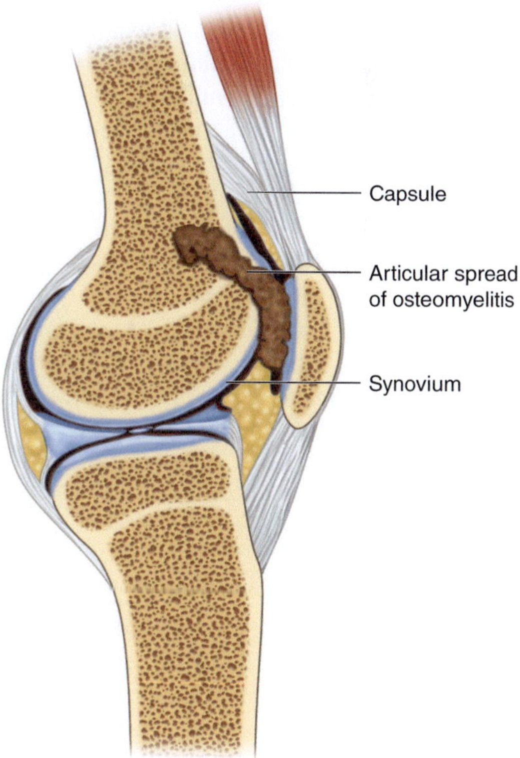

Fig. 36.1 A schematic diagram representing septic arthritis of knee as a result of contiguous spread from bone

S. K. Sinha (✉)
Department of Orthopaedics, All India Institute of Medical Sciences, Bhopal, India

V. Kumar et al. (eds.), *A Quick Guide to Essential Orthopedics*,
https://doi.org/10.1007/978-981-95-2676-5_36

Table 36.1 Common causative organism in various age groups

Patient characteristics	Causative organisms
Neonates	S. aureus, Streptococcus species, Enterobacteriaceae, Candida species
Infant	S. aureus, K. kingae, S. pneumoniae, N. meningitidis, H. influenzae type b
1–3 years	S. aureus, K. kingae, S. pneumoniae, N. meningitidis, H. influenzae type b
3–12 years	S. aureus, Group A Beta Hemolytic Streptococcus (GABHS)
12–18 years	S. aureus, GABHS, Neisseria gonorrhoeae

Once infection is established, local immune response leads to inflammation (synovitis) and exudation. The exudate containing proteolytic enzymes secreted by the activated neutrophils and synovial cells causes the degradation of hyaline cartilage, collagen, and glucosaminoglycans, leading to articular cartilage damage [3]. The distension of the capsule leads to compromised stability of joints and may predispose the joint to subluxation and dislocation, as commonly seen in the hip joint [4]. After articular cartilage damage, the joint may end with sequelae like fibrous or bony ankylosis.

36.3 Clinical Features

A child with septic arthritis presents with an acute onset of pain, redness, and swelling over the affected joint associated with systemic features of high-grade fever and malaise. There is a local rise in temperature and tenderness over the affected joint. The swelling is readily evident in superficial joints like knee and ankle, whereas in deep-seated joints like hip, it presents with fullness in Scarpa's triangle. The range of motion of the affected joint is painful and restricted. 'Pseudoparalysis' may be present, and the child may refuse to move the affected limb [5].

36.4 Investigations

Similar to other acute musculoskeletal infections, routine blood workup shows elevated total leukocyte counts, C-reactive protein levels, and ESR. Blood cultures help in detecting causative organisms in the presence of bacteremia. High-resolution ultrasound is used to detect effusion in the joint. MRI is a sensitive tool and helps in detecting the presence of even small amounts of joint effusion.

36.5 Management

In the early stages (within 24–48 h of onset), before suppuration of the joint, the child is treated with IV fluids, analgesics, antipyretics, and empirical antibiotics directed against the most probable organism (S. aureus and others, according to age). Immobilization of the painful joint should be done for pain relief.

Aspiration of the joint with aseptic precautions is performed to detect and obtain pus sample. This sample for culture and sensitivity is preferably obtained before starting empirical antibiotics. The aspiration of pus forms an indication for surgical management. Surgical management consists of evacuation of joint abscess. This may be achieved by the following methods –

- Therapeutic needle aspiration and lavage of joint
- Arthroscopic drainage and joint lavage
- Open arthrotomy of the joint

Open arthrotomy is the most commonly employed mode of treatment, and the joint is closed over a suction drain after the procedure. Pus samples and synovial biopsy are obtained and sent for Gram staining, AFB staining, culture and sensitivity, and histopathology.

36.5.1 Antibiotic Therapy

Empirical antibiotics like cephalosporins, linezolid, vancomycin, and gentamicin are commonly used as per institutional preference. Once available, culture and sensitivity reports guide further antibiotic therapy. Intravenous antibiotics are preferred till the child becomes afebrile, and the C-reactive protein levels return to baseline levels, after which oral antibiotics are preferred. A total antibiotic duration of six weeks is recommended [6].

36.6 Complications

- Subluxation/dislocation of joint
- Articular cartilage destruction and arthritis
- Partial or complete growth arrest due to nearby physeal destruction
- Damage to articular vascular supply leading to avascular necrosis (hip)

Multiple Choice Questions

1. What is the most common route of infection leading to septic arthritis?
   (a) Direct inoculation from trauma or surgery
   (b) Hematogenous spread from a distant site
   (c) Inhalation of airborne pathogens
   (d) Ingestion of contaminated food
2. What is the primary mechanism of joint damage in septic arthritis?
   (a) Direct destruction of articular cartilage by bacteria
   (b) Inflammatory response leading to erosion of cartilage
   (c) Accumulation of synovial fluid causing pressure on the joint
   (d) Autoimmune response against joint tissues
3. Which joint is most frequently affected by septic arthritis?
   (a) Knee
   (b) Hip
   (c) Shoulder
   (d) Ankle
4. What is the most important diagnostic test for confirming septic arthritis?
   (a) X-ray
   (b) Magnetic resonance imaging (MRI)
   (c) Arthrocentesis and synovial fluid analysis
   (d) Blood culture
5. Kocher's criteria are used to help diagnose septic arthritis in pediatric patients. Which of the following is NOT one of the four criteria?
   (a) Erythrocyte sedimentation rate (ESR) greater than 40 mm/hour
   (b) Fever greater than 38.5 °C (101.3 °F)
   (c) Inability to bear weight on the affected limb
   (d) Joint swelling and erythema

Answers: 1. (b), 2. (b), 3. (a), 4. (c), 5. (d)

References

1. Pediatric Septic Arthritis—ClinicalKey [Internet]. [cited 2024 May 1]. Available from: https://www.clinicalkey.com/#!/content/playContent/1-s2.0-S0030589819300835?scrollTo=%23hl0000181
2. Shirtliff ME, Mader JT. Acute septic arthritis. Clin Microbiol Rev. 2002;15(4):527–44.
3. Williams RJ, Smith RL, Schurman DJ. Septic arthritis. Staphylococcal induction of chondrocyte proteolytic activity. Arthritis Rheum. 1990;33(4):533–41.
4. Agarwal A, Rastogi P. Outcome of acute septic dislocation of hip in children reduced at arthrotomy. J Clin Orthop Trauma. 2020;13:95–8.
5. Knudsen CJ, Hoffman EB. Neonatal osteomyelitis. J Bone Joint Surg Br. 1990;72(5):846–51.
6. Shenoy B, Singhal T, Yewale V, Choudhury J, Agashe MV, Chikkamuniyappa C, et al. Indian academy of pediatrics consensus statement on diagnosis and management of bone and joint infections in children. Indian Pediatr. 2024:61.

37 Rare Infections: Salmonella, Gonococcal, Syphilis, Fungal

Vishnu R. Unnithan

37.1 Musculoskeletal Involvement in Syphilis

37.1.1 Etiopathogenesis

- Syphilis is a sexually transmitted disease caused by the spirochete Treponema pallidum
- Causes multisystemic involvement, but musculoskeletal system involvement is rare

37.1.2 Types and Stages of Syphilis

Syphilis develops in 4 stages [1]

1. Primary: Chancres
2. Secondary: Fever, rashes, lymphadenopathy
3. Latent: No signs or symptoms
4. Tertiary: Isn't contagious at this point, but the infection affects organ systems
   - Musculoskeletal syphilis can be congenital or acquired.

37.1.3 Clinical Features

37.1.3.1 Congenital Syphilis

- Can present as early congenital or late congenital
  - Congenital syphilitic arthritis is classified by D'Arcy Power into
    1. Clutton's joints
    2. Chondro-arthritis
    3. Suppurative arthritis
    4. Gummatous synovitis
    5. Hydrarthrosis
    6. Symmetrical serous synovitis
    7. Ulcerating, or Von Gie joint
- *Early Congenital Syphilis* refers to the manifestation of the disease within the first 2 years of life
  - Irritable, restless, frequently crying child. Pseudoparalysis of the limb. Skin and mucous lesions
  - "Hutchinson's triad"—The most specific sign for late congenital syphilis, which consists of Hutchinson's teeth (deformed

V. R. Unnithan (✉)
PRS Hospital, Karamana, Trivandrum, India

V. Kumar et al. (eds.), *A Quick Guide to Essential Orthopedics*,
https://doi.org/10.1007/978-981-95-2676-5_37

  - incisors), eighth cranial nerve deafness, and interstitial keratitis
  - Predominant Systemic Symptoms—Anemia, hepatosplenomegaly, skin lesions, and rhinitis
- *Late Congenital Syphilis*
  - Tertiary stage of congenital syphilis
  - Occurs after 2–3 years
  - "Parrots nodes"—Nodular thickening on outer table of skull
  - "Bull dog jaw"—prominent mandible
  - "Sabre tibia" on X-ray

37.1.3.2 Syphilitic Dactylitis Adult Acquired Syphilis

- Late stages—tertiary syphilis
- 50% have bone involvement, but only a few manifest. Periosteitis is most common

37.1.3.3 Secondary Syphilis

- Less frequently, migratory polyarthralgia or arthritis can occur in secondary syphilis, which might resemble the presentation of rheumatic fever

37.1.3.4 Tertiary Syphilis

- Axhausen described two forms of tertiary syphilitic arthritis—osseous and synovial
- Synovial form is seen mostly in children and occurs as perisynovitis
- The most involved joints are bilateral knees, hips, shoulders, and proximal interphalangeal joints, and it presents as a subacute to chronic disease
- Synovitis is the primary reason for rheumatic features in syphilis and usually presents as migratory polyarthralgia
- Osseous form, which is commonly seen in young patients, presents as epiphysitis; eroded and irregular articular surface, and cavitation in the interior of the bone, along with bony outgrowths
- Pain is usually most severe at night, aggravated by heat, and usually relieved by movement
- Pathological fractures may also occur

37.1.4 Radioological Findings

37.1.4.1 X-Ray

- Characteristic radiologic appearance is that of Bilateral symmetric involvement
- Skeletal changes in early congenital syphilis include osteitis, metaphysitis, and periosteal reaction
- "Sabre tibia"—pathognomonic feature in tibial bone. Unicortical thickening
- "Higoumenakis sign"—Thickening of inner third of clavicle
- Neonatal radiographs show periosteal reaction, diffuse or localized osteitis, and metaphysitis

Diaphysitis	Metaphysitis
Periosteal reaction or osteitis Lamellar form—Cloaking/coffin formation/"Periosteitis of Pehu"	Lucent bands Dense bands Alternating bands—Sandwich appearance "Wimberger's sign" "Wegner's sign" "Celery stalk" appearance

- Proliferative periostitis or osteolytic lesion or both
- Radiological Differential Diagnosis—Multifocal Osteitis, Rickets, Scurvy, Neuroblastoma, Battered Baby Syndrome

MRI useful in identifying the extent of involvement

- "Hot cross bun" appearance in MRI brain in cases of late congenital syphilis

37.1.5 Diagnosis

- Is by a combination of clinical and radiological manifestations of congenital syphilis with a positive family history or by therapeutic response to anti-syphilitic medications

- the nonmigratory character of arthritis and association with the characteristic mucocutaneous features of secondary syphilis can help in the diagnosis
- Congenital Syphilis
  - Serological tests: Fluorescent treponemal antibody Absorption test, VDRL, RPR
  - Generally negative in the first few months of life in congenital syphilis. Can be done by the mother
- Adult Syphilis
  - Dark field microscopy: To demonstrate the spirochete
  - Serological tests: TPHA, VDRL, PR, FTA-ABS(highly sensitive and specific)
  - Synovial fluid analysis—polymorphonuclear neutrophils and phagocytic mononuclear cells with large vacuoles. Spirochetes usually are not directly visualized in synovial fluid analysis
  - Immunofluorescent anti-treponemal antibody absorption test may reveal spirochetes in joints

37.1.6 Treatment

- Penicillin:
  - Administered in all stages of syphilis
  - IM penicillin for primary or secondary syphilis and early latent syphilis
  - IV penicillin G for late latent syphilis
- In addition to this, local management of the joints with massage and physiotherapy is also important to prevent ankylosis of the joint
- Pregnant women with syphilis should be treated to prevent congenital syphilitic arthritis. If they are allergic to penicillin, then they need to get desensitized before treatment
- Doxycycline, tetracycline, ceftriaxone—In penicillin allergy and in whom desensitization to penicillin is not feasible
- Long follow up—as relapse is common and can be asymptomatic

37.1.7 Complications

- Ankylosis is a common complication of untreated syphilitic arthritis
- Complications of tertiary syphilis—general paresis, aortic insufficiency, tabes dorsalis
- Jarisch–Herxheimer reaction: Flu-like symptoms due to toxins released by killed T. pallidum after starting treatment for syphilis

37.2 Gonococcal Musculoskeletal Infection

37.2.1 Etiology

- Bacteremic spread of Neisseria gonorrhoeae, a sexually transmitted pathogen

37.2.2 Epidemiology

- 0.5% to 3% of patients who are infected with N. gonorrhoeae develop disseminated gonococcal infection [2]

37.2.3 Pathophysiology

- Disseminated gonococcal infection causes the musculoskeletal manifestations
- Risk factors—pregnancy, complement deficiencies, history of pelvic surgery, and intrauterine devices
- Pathogenesis may be partly immune-mediated

37.2.4 Clinical Features

Two major clinical syndromes

A. Arthritis-dermatitis syndrome
   - Triad of—tenosynovitis, dermatitis, and polyarthralgia
   - Often associated with constitutional symptoms such as fever, chills, and body malaise

B. Localized septic arthritis
   - Monoarthritis or asymmetric oligo- or polyarthritis with pain and swelling of one or more joints
   - Usually, no systemic symptoms such as fever or chills

37.2.5 Investigations

- Definitive diagnosis of disseminated gonococcal infection (DGI) or gonococcal arthritis is made through
  - The identification of the etiologic pathogen in a specimen taken from a *non-mucosal site* (such as blood, synovial fluid, or skin lesions)
- Microbiologic tests, however, are not always positive, and in such cases, diagnosis is made clinically and a clinical diagnosis may be supported by
  - Evidence of N. gonorrhoeae infection from specimens obtained from mucosal sites

1. Microscopy—and Staining of blood, body fluid (mucosal, synovial) samples
2. Bacterial Culture—Thayer-Martin or modified New York City media
3. Nucleic acid amplification testing of either urine specimens in both men and women or vaginal swabs in women
4. Synovial fluid analysis

37.2.6 Management

- Ceftriaxone, as a parenteral therapy, either given intravenously or intramuscularly, is the preferred initial antibiotic of choice [2]
- Doxycycline is usually added to cover potential coinfection with Chlamydia trachomatis
- Alternative antimicrobial agents include third-generation cephalosporins such as cefotaxime and ceftizoxime
- Partners of patients diagnosed with this condition should be contacted and treated whenever possible
- Patients with recurrent DGI or gonococcal arthritis will require further evaluation for complement deficiency
- Localized purulent arthritis should undergo joint drainage, either arthroscopically or through repeated joint aspirations or Open surgical drainage

37.3 Brucella in Orthopedics

37.3.1 Etiopathogenesis

- Brucellosis (Malta fever) is the most common microbial zoonotic disease in the world, caused by Brucella, an intracellular bacterium
- Transmitted through occupational contact (veterinary, butcher, animal husbandry) or consumption of contaminated dairy products (milk, butter, and cheese)

37.3.2 Clinical Features

- Fever, sweating, musculoskeletal pains, lymphadenopathy, hepatosplenomegaly
- Back pain is the most common complaint in spinal brucellosis, can be associated with sciatic radiculopathy, and is reported by about half of the patients [3].
- Osteoarticular involvement is seen in 10–85% of patients affected [3].
  - Sacroilitis (up to 80%) and spinal brucellosis (up to 54%) are the most common manifestations.
  - Spinal brucellosis has two forms: focal and diffuse.
  - Spondylitis and spondylodiscitis are the most frequent complications.
  - Spondylodiscitis is the most severe form of osteoarticular involvement by brucellosis and can have single- or multifocal involvement.
  - Epidural abscess is a rare complication of spinal brucellosis but can lead to permanent neurological deficits or even death if not treated promptly.

  - Arthritis, osteomyelitis, bursitis, and tenosynovitis are other osteoarticular manifestations.
- Rarely Brucella infection following total joint arthroplasty (TJA) of the hip/knee are also seen.

37.3.3 Investigations

1. Serology
   - The Wright test which is a standard agglutination test (SAT)—measures the total amount of IgM and IgG antibodies
   - The 2-ME test measures IgG antibody
   - In the endemic regions, a SAT titer ≥1:160 and 2-ME titer ≥1:80 is in favor of brucellosis diagnosis
   - ELISA—has less sensitivity and specificity
   - PCR—is quick and has high sensitivity and specificity
2. Imaging
   (a) X-ray—Usually normal in early cases
   (b) USG—Peripheral arthritis
   (c) MRI—usually with contrast
      - Most valuable method to diagnose spinal brucellosis.
      - To localize spondylodiscitis, epidural abscess, or compression on the spine and spinal nerve
      - To differentiate between pyogenic spondylitis and brucellar spondylitis
      - "Pedro Pons" sign [4]—pathognomonic finding in Spondylodiscitis
   (d) Bone scintigraphy—To localize the area and to identify diffuse involvement
   (e) CT Guided Biopsy—To obtain tissue for microbiological and histopathological assessment
3. Culture—Sample from blood, bone marrow, wounds, purulent discharge, or other body tissues and fluids

37.3.4 Management

- No standard therapy exists for osteoarticular brucellosis
- Combinations of doxycycline, streptomycin, gentamicin, ciprofloxacin, ofloxacin, co-trimoxazole (trimethoprim plus sulfamethoxazole), and rifampicin are used for antibiotherapy
- long-term anti-bacterial medication (usually 3–6 months) used to prevent relapses

Surgical intervention is needed in cases of failed antibiotic therapy, progressive neurological deficit, and epidural abscess.

37.4 Fungal Infections in Orthopedics

- Musculoskeletal fungal infection is an uncommon disease with nonspecific manifestations that requires pathogen identification via tissue cultures and histopathologic studies.
- Combination of surgery and systemic antifungal therapy yields generally favorable outcomes.

37.4.1 Etiology

- The pathogens that most commonly cause musculoskeletal fungal infection include Candida spp., Aspergillus spp., Coccidioides spp., Histoplasma spp., Cryptococcus spp., and Blastomyces spp.

37.4.2 Pathogenesis

- Commonly occur in immunocompromised hosts such as those with diabetes and alcoholism

- Often associated with significant morbidity and/or mortality
- Mechanisms of musculoskeletal infection
  1. Direct inoculation
  2. Hematogenous spreading
  3. Contiguous spreading

37.4.3 Clinical Features

- Musculoskeletal fungal infection manifests as arthritis, osteomyelitis, or tenosynovitis. It usually occurs in coexistence with bacterial infection
- Fungal arthritis is usually associated with adjacent bone osteomyelitis and mostly develops in prosthetic joints
- Local symptoms—Pain and tenderness
- Other symptoms—swollen lesions, soft tissue invasion, and abscess formation

37.4.4 Investigations

1. Imaging.
   (a) X-ray—Depending on the case. Well-defined osteomyelitic lesions, narrowing of the joint space, contagious bone destruction with periarticular osteopenia, and soft tissue swelling
   (b) USG—arthritis/effusion
   (c) CT—bony destruction and ill-defined soft tissue swelling or mass with enhancement
   (d) MRI—arthritis/osteomyelitis. Details relating to soft tissue invasion, including mass, sinus tract
2. Blood Chemistry—nonspecific. ESR & CRP usually high
3. Fungal staining—of discharge, tissues, and synovial fluid
4. Culture—sample from discharge, tissues, and fluids. Needs prolonged culture time—should not be reported negative for growth until 4 weeks after incubation
5. Histopathology—of tissue
   - Acute/chronic inflammation with or without a granuloma
   - Fungi with their characteristic morphology
6. Serology—not usually performed
   - Molecular/PCR-based diagnostic tests
   - For example: serum cryptococcal antigen

37.4.5 Diagnosis

- Established via tissue biopsy—Demonstrating fungal elements or by culture

37.4.6 Differential Diagnosis

1. Bacterial arthritis
2. Tubercular arthritis
3. Sarcoidosis
4. Ewing's sarcoma
5. Osteogenic sarcoma
6. Langerhans cell histiocytosis
7. Malignant metastasis

37.4.7 Treatment

- Systemic antifungal agents—voriconazole, fluconazole, amphotericin B, itraconazole, micafungin
- Needs prolonged antifungal therapy
- Most patients need surgical debridement in addition to systemic medications for local infection control

37.4.8 Recent Advances

- Calcineurin inhibitor analogs, geldanamycin (HSP 90 Inhibitor) [5].

Multiple Choice Questions

1. Radiological sign not associated with Metaphysitis in Congenital Syphilis
   (a) Sabre tibia
   (b) Wimberger's sign
   (c) Wegner's Sign
   (d) Celery stalk appearance

2. Drug which should be given for treatment of Syphilis in patients allergic to Penicillin
   (a) Doxycycline
   (b) tetracycline
   (c) ceftriaxone
   (d) Any/all the above
3. Not true about "Arthritis-dermatitis syndrome"
   (a) Seen in Gonococcal Infection
   (b) Consists of tenosynovitis, dermatitis, and polyarthralgia
   (c) No systemic symptoms such as fever or chills
   (d) Pathogenesis may be partly immune-mediated
4. Most common osteoarticular manifestation in Brucellosis
   (a) Spondylitis
   (b) Spondylodiscitis
   (c) Epidural abscess
   (d) Sacroilitis
5. Fungal arthritis arises most commonly
   (a) Due to hematogenous spreading
   (b) From adjacent bone osteomyelitis
   (c) in prosthetic joints
   (d) (b) and (c)

Answers:

1. (a) (Sabre tibia seen due to Diaphysitis and not Metaphysitis)
2. (d)
3. (c)
4. (d)
5. (d)

References

1. French P. Syphilis. BMJ. 2007;334(7585):143–7. https://doi.org/10.1136/bmj.39085.518148.BE. Erratum in: BMJ. 2007 Sep 1;335(7617):0. PMID: 17235095; PMCID: PMC1779891
2. Tuttle CS, Van Dantzig T, Brady S, Ward J, Maguire G. The epidemiology of gonococcal arthritis in an indigenous Australian population. Sex Transm Infect. 2015;91(7):497–501.
3. Esmaeilnejad-Ganji SM, Esmaeilnejad-Ganji SMR. Osteoarticular manifestations of human brucellosis: a review. World J Orthop. 2019;10(2):54–62. https://doi.org/10.5312/wjo.v10.i2.54. PMID: 30788222; PMCID: PMC6379739
4. Eljebbouri B, El Asri AC. Pedro Pons' sign. Pan Afr Med J. 2014;17:177. https://doi.org/10.11604/pamj.2014.17.177.4003. PMID: 25392723; PMCID: PMC4225147
5. Juvvadi PR, Lee SC, Heitman J, Steinbach WJ. Calcineurin in fungal virulence and drug resistance: prospects for harnessing targeted inhibition of calcineurin for an antifungal therapeutic approach. Virulence. 2017;8(2):186–97. https://doi.org/10.1080/21505594.2016.1201250. Epub 2016 Jun 20. PMID: 27325145; PMCID: PMC5354160

Leprosy

38

Varun Garg and Sitanshu Barik

38.1 Introduction

Leprosy is an infectious disease caused by mycobacterium leprae. It is an acid-fast bacillus with a predilection for cooler places such as skin, peripheral nerves, anterior chamber of eye, upper respiratory tract and testes. Leprosy is a common problem in India with an incidence of 4.56 per 10,000 population. The prevalence rate of leprosy is 0.4 per 10,000 population in the country. Thirty per cent of the cases have an orthopaedic problem and nerve involvement at initial diagnosis [1].

38.2 Etiopathogenesis

Mycobacterium leprae has a low transmission rate. Overcrowding and contact are known risk factors for transmission. The main route of transmission of infection is through the upper respiratory tract.

Schwann cells and skin macrophages are the two main target cells of mycobacterium leprae infection. It results in demyelination and axonal conductance loss in the peripheral nerve. It damages the sensory and autonomic fibres in the skin. As a result, leprosy patients may appear with paralysis and hypo-anaesthetic skin lesions, as well as a decrease in sweating.

Lepra responses, which are acute inflammations, can occur along the course of the disease due to changes in the patient's immune condition. Chemotherapy, pregnancy, and physical stress are all established risk factors. They are of two types: type I (reversal reaction) in the BT, mid-borderline, and BL forms, and type II (Erythema Nodosum Leprosum) in the LL and BL forms [2, 3].

Primary or secondary bone changes can occur. Secondary bone changes occur more commonly. It is frequently caused by prolonged immobilisation of an extremity or by motor denervation. Motor denervation causes cancellous bone resorption and the development of concentric-type bone atrophy. The bone's length and breadth are both resorbed. This resorption at the extremity's end results in a 'licked candy stick' appearance. Distal absorption of the fingers and toes and subsequent infection result in progressive finger absorption, resulting in the "mitten hand."

Primary bone involvement is rare in leprosy. It is seen in 3–5% of the cases and usually involves the bone of face, hand and feet. Proximal and middle phalanges of hands and feet are commonly involved. Primary bone affection usually results from direct extension of the infection from the overlying skin or mucosa. Initially, the periosteum is infected, and subsequently the cortex and medulla get infected [2, 3].

V. Garg (✉)
Department of Pediatric Orthopedics, Chacha Nehru Bal Chikatsalya, New Delhi, India

S. Barik
Department of Orthopaedics, AIIMS Nagpur, Nagpur, Maharashtra, India

V. Kumar et al. (eds.), *A Quick Guide to Essential Orthopedics*,
https://doi.org/10.1007/978-981-95-2676-5_38

Table 38.1 Ridley and Jopling classification [4]

Characteristics	Tuberculoid	Borderline tuberculoid	Mid-borderline	Borderline lepromatous	Lepromatous leprosy
Number of lesions	Single or up to 3	A few (up to 10)	Several (10–30)	Numerous, asymmetrical (>30)	Innumerable, symmetrical
Size	Variable, usually large	Variable, some are large	Variable	Small, some can be large	Small
Surface changes	Hypopigmented	Dry, scaly, look bright and infiltrated	Dull or slightly shiny	Shiny	Shiny
Sensations	Absent	Markedly diminished	Moderately diminished	Slightly diminished	Minimally diminished
Hair growth	Nil	Markedly diminished	Moderately diminished	Slightly diminished	Not affected initially
Skin smear	Negative	Negative or 1+	1–3+	3–5+	Plenty, including globi (6+)
Lepromin test	Strongly positive	Weakly positive	Negative	Negative	Negative

38.3 Classification

Leprosy can be classified on the basis of number of skin patches as given by WHO. Single Skin patch as single skin lesion, patches less than or equal to 5 are classified as paucibacillary and greater than 5 as multibacillary. Leprosy can also be classified according to Ridley and Jopling scale based on clinical, histopathological and immunological criteria. It has 5 forms, with a spectrum from tuberculoid to lepromatous types (Table 38.1).

38.4 Clinical Features

- Tuberculoid form— these patients typically present with anaesthetic skin patches which are solitary papules or plaques. These lesions have asymmetric distribution over the extremities. Plaques may sometimes coalesce to form annular lesions with hypopigmented centre. There is thickening of the peripheral nerves and eye involvement.
- Lepromatous form—these patients typically present with a symmetrical distribution of nodular and papular skin lesions over the face, buttocks, wrist, elbow and knees. There is loss of the lateral part of the eyebrows (madarosis). Involvement of the nasal septum can lead to saddle nose. Nodular lesion over the face can lead to leonine facies. There is a glove and stocking pattern of anaesthesia of the limbs with involvement of major trunks of the nerves.
- Borderline forms— these patients have clinical features of both lepromatous and tuberculoid leprosy. The majority of patients present with borderline forms. They have multiple skin and nerve lesions.
- In leprosy superficial nerves such as facial, greater auricular, ulnar, median radial cutaneous, lateral popliteal and posterior tibial nerves are commonly affected due to predilection of M. leprae for the cooler places in the body. These nerves may be hypertrophied and may present with characteristic motor weakness and sensory loss that help in their diagnosis. The ulnar nerve is associated with clawing of the ring and little fingers and a loss of intrinsic hand muscle function, with sensory loss in the medial two fingers. The median nerve causes loss of thumb opposition and grasp, with sensory loss over the thumb. A radial nerve injury, though rare, can result in wrist drop and sensory loss in the first web space of the hand. The common peroneal nerve leads to foot drop and sensory loss over the lateral malleolus. Finally, injury to the posterior tibial nerve causes clawing of the

toes and sensory loss in the sole of the foot [3].

- Trophic ulceration results from repetitive trauma in the absence of protective sensation. It can secondarily lead to osteomyelitis of the underlying bone.

38.5 Diagnosis

Leprosy is a clinical diagnosis. Leprosy can be diagnosed by the presence of at least one of the three signs. These are:

1. Hypopigmented skin lesion with sensory loss.
2. Thickened peripheral nerve with definitive motor or sensory loss.
3. Presence of M. leprae in slit skin smear.

38.6 Treatment

- Antibacterial therapy: all patients with leprosy should be started on multidrug therapy as suggested by WHO. For paucibacillary leprosy, the treatment involves two 300 mg capsules of rifampicin once a month (supervised), and one 100 mg tablet of dapsone daily (self-administered), with a duration of 6 months. For multibacillary leprosy, treatment includes two 300 mg capsules of rifampicin once a month (supervised), one 100 mg tablet of dapsone daily (self-administered), three 100 mg capsules of clofazimine once a month (supervised), and one 50 mg capsule of clofazimine daily, with a duration of 12 months [5, 6].
- Steroids: the role of steroids in preventing and treating nerve damage is controversial. It is usually indicated in the presence of nerve dysfunction, which occurs during the last 6 months of treatment. Steroids should be continued for 4 to 6 months. They act by reducing the inflammation around the nerves.
- Monitoring nerve function: nerve affection can occur before, during and after the treatment. Nerve can be affected up to 2 years after the treatment has been stopped. Hence, regular clinical examination of the nerve should be done even after completion of the therapy.
- Physiotherapy: should a nerve be affected, patient should be started on regular physiotherapy, and appropriate braces should be prescribed to prevent fixed contractures.
- Surgery: surgery may be indicated in the following conditions.
  - (a) Decompression of nerve in the early stages.
  - (b) Tendon transfers for permanent deformities.
  - (c) Debridement of non-healing ulcers. Since these lesions have a good vascular supply, patients should be managed by total contact casting for complete healing of the ulcer. Patients should be counselled to use proper footwear for the prevention of secondary ulcers.
  - (d) Arthrodesis or amputation may be required in a case of Charcot joint.

References

1. Moonot P, Ashwood N, Lockwood D. Orthopaedic complications of leprosy. J Bone Joint Surg Br. 2005;87-B(10):1328–32.
2. de Macedo CS, Lara FA, Pinheiro RO, Schmitz V, de Berrêdo-Pinho M, Pereira GM, et al. New insights into the pathogenesis of leprosy: contribution of subversion of host cell metabolism to bacterial persistence, disease progression, and transmission. F1000Res. 2020;9:F1000. Faculty Rev-70
3. Bhat RM, Prakash C. Leprosy: an overview of pathophysiology. Interdiscip Perspect Infect Dis. 2012;2012:181089.
4. Ridley DS, Jopling WH. Classification of leprosy according to immunity. A five-group system. Int J Lepr Other Mycobact Dis. 1966;34(3):255–73.
5. WHO Study Group on Chemotherapy of Leprosy for Control Programmes, Organization WH. Chemotherapy of leprosy for control programmes: report of a WHO study group [meeting held in Geneva from 12 to 16 October 1981] [Internet]. World Health Organization; 1982 [cited 2023 Aug 5]. Available from: https://apps.who.int/iris/handle/10665/38984
6. World Health Organization. Guide to eliminate leprosy as a public health problem [Internet]. World Health Organization; 2000 [cited 2023 Aug 5]. Report No.: WHO/CDS/CPE/CEE/2000.14. Available from: https://apps.who.int/iris/handle/10665/66612

Tuberculosis of Spine and Pott's Paraplegia

39

Nikhil Goyal and Kumar Keshav

39.1 Introduction

Percival Pott gave the first detailed description of spinal tuberculosis, also known as 'Pott's Disease' [1]. Pott's spine is the most common form of skeletal tuberculosis. It is a slowly developing disease, characterised by pain, spinal deformity and occasionally paralysis. It is responsible for almost half of all bone and joint tuberculosis.

39.2 Relevant Anatomy

Embryology Each vertebra is formed from a pair of sclerotomes in such a way that each sclerotome is responsible for lower half of upper vertebrae, intervertebral disc and upper half of the lower vertebrae (Fig. 39.1). Each sclerotome is supplied by a single artery. This arterial supply is retained even after birth. (Fig. 39.2) Since spinal tuberculosis is predominantly haematoge-

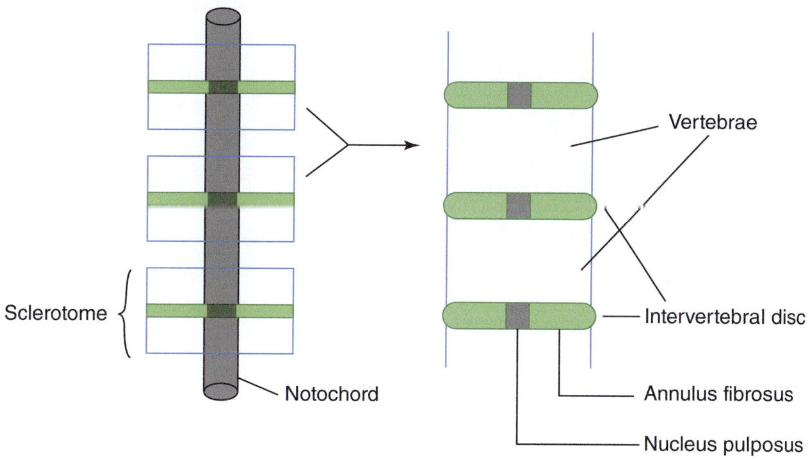

Fig. 39.1 Each vertebra is formed from two adjacent sclerotomes, which are part of somite (notochord)

N. Goyal (✉)
Department of Orthopedics, All India Institute of Medical Sciences, Rishikesh, India

K. Keshav
Department of Orthopaedics, Sanjay Gandhi Post Graduate Institute of Medical Sciences, Lucknow, Uttar Pradesh, India

V. Kumar et al. (eds.), *A Quick Guide to Essential Orthopedics*,
https://doi.org/10.1007/978-981-95-2676-5_39

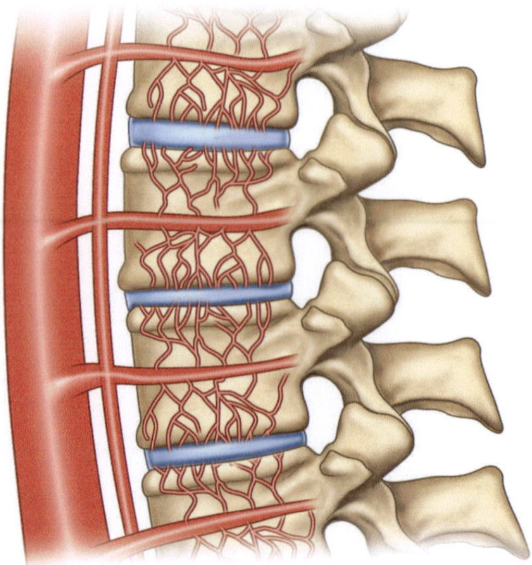

Fig. 39.2 Blood supply of adjacent parts of contiguous vertebrae, along with intervertebral disc, is from the same artery

nous in origin, paradiscal form (lower half of upper vertebra, intervening disc and upper half of lower vertebra) of involvement is the most common [2, 3].

Frequency of involvement Among all the regions of the spine, the thoracic vertebra is the most commonly involved. Reasons behind this are its proximity to the thoracic duct and cisterna chyli, increased stress of weight bearing, and presence of relatively more spongy tissue (cancellous bone), more conducive for lodgement and propagation of infection. Following the thoracic spine, the decreasing order of frequency of various regions getting affected is lumbar, dorsolumbar, cervical, cervicodorsal and lumbosacral region [3, 4].

39.2.1 Surface Anatomy

It is important to identify the vertebrae during clinical examination. The upper cervical spine can't be palpated due to the small bifid spinous process being covered with ligamentum nuchae. The seventh cervical spine is the most prominent vertebra coming from top downwards and is the first vertebra that can be felt with a reasonable level of certainty. Following this, the third and seventh thoracic vertebrae correspond to the spine and the lower angle of the scapula, respectively. The intercristal line (line joining the tops of iliac crests on both sides corresponds to intervertebral disc between fourth and fifth lumbar vertebrae. The second sacral vertebra is at the level of the posterior superior iliac spine [5].

39.2.2 Relation Between Spinal Cord Level and Vertebral Level

During embryological development and for some years after birth, the spinal cord (neurological structure) grows at a slower pace compared to the vertebral column (bone). Consequently, the spinal cord ends at L3 in children and L1 in adults. Because of this discordance between the spinal cord and vertebral column, there is usually a specific correlation between the site of affection in bone (more evident on imaging studies like X-rays and CT scans) and the level of neurological deficit (mainly elicited by clinical examination). This helps us in clinico-radiological correlation [3, 5]. The relationship has been enumerated in Table 39.1.

When the spinal cord is affected, motor function is affected before the sensory. Since the disease is predominantly from the anterior part (i.e. the vertebral bodies), pain, crude touch and temperature sensations carried by anterolateral tracts are affected before proprioception, vibration and fine touch carried by dorsal column tracts [3, 6–8].

Table 39.1 Relationship between vertebral (bony) level and spinal cord (neurological) level

Vertebral (bony) level	Spinal cord level	Example
Cervical	Add 1 to know the corresponding cord level	A lesion of 4th Cervical vertebra will affect spinal cord at C5 level
Upper Thoracic(T1–T6)	Add 2	A lesion of 3rd Thoracic vertebra will affect spinal cord at T5 level
Mid Thoracic (T7–T9)	Add 3	A lesion of 8th Thoracic vertebra will affect spinal cord at T11 level
Tenth Thoracic vertebra (T10)	L1 and L2	Cord involvement of L1 means 10th Thoracic vertebra is affected
11th Thoracic vertebra (T11)	L3 and L4	Cord involvement of L3 means 11th Thoracic vertebra is affected
12th Thoracic vertebrae (T12)	L5 and S1	Cord involvement of L5 means 12th Thoracic vertebra is affected
L1 vertebra	Rest all sacral and coccygeal segments	Cord involvement of S4 means First Lumbar vertebra is affected
Below L1	There are cauda equina- nerve roots	

39.3 Etiopathogenesis

1. *Infection:* The pathogenesis of Pott's spine begins with the inhalation of *Mycobacterium tuberculosis* (MTB) bacteria, which can enter the lungs and spread to other parts of the body. Spine is involved most commonly by hematogenous dissemination (bacillaemia) through arteries and rarely via Bateson's plexus of veins. When the bacteria reach the spine, they can infect the bone and the surrounding tissues. Usually, there is a gap of 2–3 years between primary tuberculosis and skeletal tuberculosis.
2. *Immune response:* Once the tubercle bacteria infect the spine, the immune system responds by sending immune cells to the site of infection. These immune cells can destroy the bacteria, but they can also cause inflammation and tissue damage.
3. *Formation of granulomas:* As part of the immune response, the immune cells can form small, dense structures called granulomas around the infected area. Granulomas are composed of immune cells, bacteria, and tissue debris, and they can help to contain the infection.
4. *Necrosis:* In some cases, the granulomas can become necrotic, which means that the tissue dies and breaks down. Necrosis begins as an infection of a single vertebra due to tubercular endarteritis, marrow is converted into myxomatous tissue, a tuberculous follicle develops, and caseous necrosis occurs, which can lead to the formation of a *cavity or abscess* in the spine. The bone becomes fragile and hence collapses under load, resulting in an angular deformity known as *kyphus or gibbus*. This is seen more in the thoracic spine, where the anterior part of the vertebral body may collapse like a wedge. In the lordotic cervical and lumbar region, weight is transmitted through the posterior part of the vertebral body and hence, collapse is incomplete.
5. *Cold abscess:* Due to the necrosis, there is a collection of pus and tubercular debris. This abscess lacks the usual signs of an abscess and hence is known as a cold abscess. This pus can track along bones (like ribs) and ligaments (like the anterior longitudinal ligament). Some of the common collections are prevertebral abscess (along the anterior longitudinal ligament anterior to the vertebral body), paravertebral abscess (on the lateral aspect of vertebrae) and epidural abscess (in the epidural space posterior to the vertebral body) (Fig. 39.3).
6. *Compression of the spinal cord:* As the abscess grows, it puts pressure on the spinal cord, which can cause neurological symptoms such as weakness, numbness, and pain. If left untreated, this can lead to paralysis and permanent disability. The intervertebral disc is not involved primarily because it is avascular, but involvement of the paradiscal bone affects its nutrition and hence may be involved later.

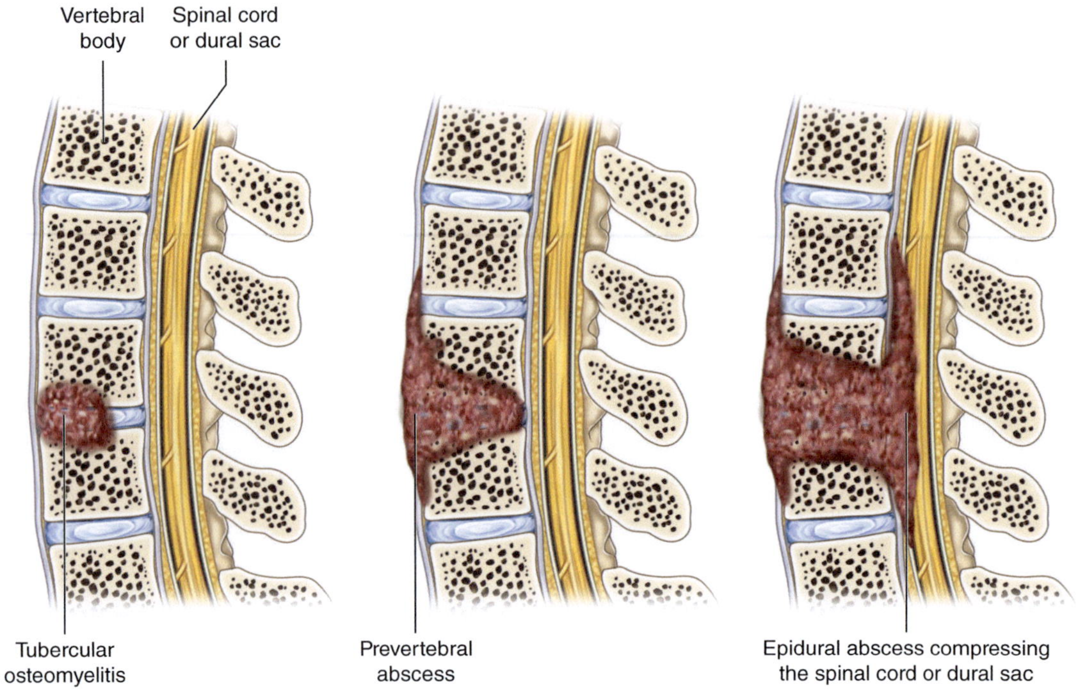

Fig. 39.3 Infection causing bone destruction and spread of pus in a vertebra

7. *Healing:* Healing in the spine following tuberculosis happens by bony ankylosis, unlike other osteoarticular tuberculosis (where there is fibrous ankylosis). There may be formation of an internal gibbus, which may further narrow down the spinal canal, leading to 'Late-onset paraplegia'.

Overall, the pathogenesis of Pott's spine involves a complex interplay between the tubercular bacteria and the host's immune system, which can lead to tissue damage, abscess formation, and compression of the spinal cord. Early detection and treatment are crucial for preventing serious complications and preserving neurological function [3, 4, 6–8].

39.3.1 Types of Vertebral Lesions (Based on Location)

Based on the part of individual vertebrae affected, spinal tuberculosis can be one of the five types (Fig. 39.4 and Table 39.2) [3, 4, 6, 8].

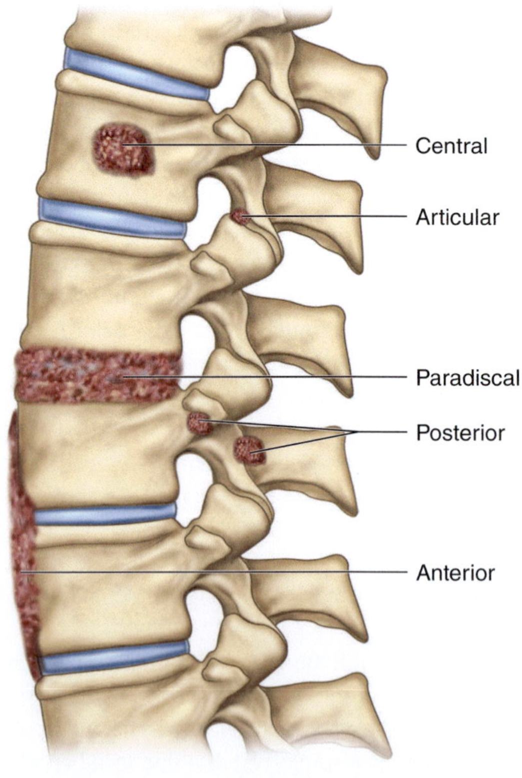

Fig. 39.4 Location of various types of spinal tuberculosis

Table 39.2 Types of vertebral lesions (based on the part of vertebra affected)

Paradiscal type	Most common type Usually found in adolescents Spread is through epiphyseal arteries There is involvement of adjacent vertebral bodies with decreased disc space
Central type	Common in children Route: Bateson's plexus or branches of the posterior vertebral artery Normal bony trabeculae lost, body may be ballooned and destroyed (lytic lesion in centre of the body) Concentric collapse resembles Vertebra Plana Minimal disc space narrowing Minimal paravertebral shadow
Anterior type	More common in thoracic region of children. Route: Bateson's plexus Skip lesions are common Infection is present in the anterior part of vertebral body It can spread superiorly and inferiorly beneath the anterior longitudinal ligament On X-ray, there may be shallow erosions on anterior surface of vertebral body which is known as aneurysmal phenomena/ saw tooth appearance At times, clinical picture resembles that of an intraspinal tumour (known as spinal tumour syndrome) Collapse of body and intervertebral space is minimal/late.
Posterior type	Posterior structures like pedicle, lamina, transverse process or spinous process are affected Lateral shift and scoliosis may occur as a result of destruction of vertebrae on one side, sparing the other half (situation similar to hemivertebra) Higher incidence of neurological deficit due to proximity to spinal canal X-ray—'Beakless owl' appearance due to destruction of spinous process
Articular type	Common in elderly Incidence <0.5% Involve facet joints. Synovitis of posterior facet joint Associated with radiculopathy due to involvement of exiting nerve root

39.4 Clinical Features

39.4.1 Symptoms

Pott's spine is most frequently encountered during the first three decades of life, with approximately 90% of cases occurring in individuals below 50 years of age. The clinical presentation varies according to the stage of the disease, the anatomical site of involvement, and the presence or absence of complications. The onset of symptoms is typically insidious, often leading to a delay in diagnosis.

Constitutional symptoms like weakness, malaise, anorexia, loss of appetite, night sweats and evening rise of temperature are often seen. Weight loss is usually of more than 10% (or 10 pounds) in six months or more than 5% (or 5 pounds) in one month. Specific symptoms pertaining to spinal tuberculosis are as follows:

(i) *Back pain* is the commonest presenting complaint which is diffuse, dull aching in early stages and localised to a specific segment in later stages. The distribution is axial/ radicular and continuous. There is diurnal variation in the form of typical night cries, where, due to muscle relaxation, movement between inflamed surfaces gives rise to severe pain at night.

(ii) *Stiffness* is also an early symptom, which occurs due to paravertebral muscle spasm. It can restrict the movement of the spine. The patient may complain of inability to do forward bending like lifting something from the ground.

(iii) *Swelling* in and around spine may be seen. This swelling is due to the cold abscess and hence lacks the signs of inflammation. For example, a psoas abscess due to tubercular involvement of the lower thoracic or upper lumbar spine may present in the Lumbar triangle of Petit or in the groin.

(iv) *Pressure symptoms* due to cold abscess, such as dyspnoea, dysphagia (cervical retropharyngeal abscess), hoarseness of voice (upper thoracic spine is usually associated with recurrent laryngeal nerve palsy) and inability to extend the hip (lumbar psoas abscess) can be among the presenting symptoms.

(v) *Deformity* can develop in the form of kyphosis (gibbus or kyphus) or scoliosis due to wedge collapse of vertebrae.

(vi) *Neurological deficits* like weakness, sensory loss and involvement of bladder and bowel due to involvement of spinal cords or nerve roots can be seen in late cases.

All of the above symptoms are seen in active spinal tuberculosis. In healed disease, all symptoms and signs disappear, except for deformity and neurological deficit [3, 4, 6, 8–10].

39.4.2 Signs

On *general examination*, there may be pallor and enlarged lymph nodes. The *Attitude* of the patient is very protective, which varies according to the region involved. If the cervical spine is involved, there may be torticollis or wry neck. In upper thoracic involvement, the patient may be stiff and have a military attitude. In lower thoracic, the patient may appear to walk with extreme caution (Alderman's gait). Tuberculosis of the lumber region may give rise to increased lordosis and prominent abdomen. On examination of the back, there is pronounced *wasting of back muscles.* On palpation, *tenderness* is present at local site. The way to assess tenderness can be one or more the following: (i) point tenderness—elicited by direct pressure over spinous process and is usually seen in posterior spinal disease (ii) rotatory tenderness—an attempt is made to move the anterior vertebral body by laterally rotating the spinous process and (iii) thrust tenderness—a crude method where we hit the spine from top to bottom by fist to elicit tenderness. *Kyphotic deformity* is commonly seen. Depending upon the number of vertebrae involved, it can be knuckle kyphosis (1 or 2 vertebra, K angle <10°) or angular kyphosis (3 or more vertebra, Mild 10–30°, Moderate 30–60°) or round kyphosis (large number of vertebra involved, K angle >60°) (Table 39.3). Other deformities that can be seen are scoliosis, lordosis, kyphosis and flattening. One may feel the cold abscess as a *paravertebral thickening/swelling.* In long standing untreated disease, there may be the presence of a *tubercular sinus*, which may be an active or a healed one. *Movements are decreased* in all directions, specially forward flexion (Coin Test). There may be *neurological deficit* in the form of paraparesis/paraplegia or quadriparesis/quadriplegia depending upon the level of lesion, sensory loss and bladder and bowel involvement. While assessing the neurological involvement, one must assess the severity of involvement (Table 39.4) and try to see for correlation between the vertebral and spinal cord level [3–10].

Table 39.3 Clinico-radiological classification of tubercular spondylitis (Kumar, 1988) [8]

Stage	Clinico-radiological feature	Duration
Pre-destructive	Straightening of curvatures, muscle spasm, MRI shows marrow oedema	<3 months
Early destructive	Decreased disc space + para discal erosions. knuckle <10° MRI—Marrow oedema & break of osseous margin CT—marginal erosion or cavitation	2–4 months
Mild kyphus	2–3 vertebra involved (K:10–30°)	4–9 months
Moderate kyphus	>3 vertebra involved (K: 30–60°)	9–24 months
Round kyphus	> 3 vertebra involved (K > 60°)	> 2 years

K = angle of kyphosis

Table 39.4 Staging of neurological deficit in Pott's Paraplegia (Goel, Tuli and Kumar) [3, 8, 12]

Stage	Clinical features
I. Negligible	Patient is unaware of neural deficit Physician detects plantar extensor or ankle clonus ±Brisk tendon reflexes
II. Mild	Patient is aware of deficit but manages to walk with support complaints of clumsiness, incoordination, spasticity or jumpiness of lower limbs while walking. Spastic Paresis signs on clinical examination: Muscles of both lower limbs in a constant state of contraction (muscles are in spasm) & exaggerated tendon reflexes.
III. Moderate	Non-ambulatory because of spastic paralysis in extension Sensory deficit <50%
IV. Severe	Stage III with flexor spasm/paralysis in flexion / flaccid paralysis sensory deficit >50% /Sphincter involved

39.5 Investigations [3, 6, 8, 9, 11]

1. *Blood Investigations*
   (a) Complete blood count with ESR and CRP.
   (b) Quantiferon gold assay—for definitive diagnosis of tuberculosis in the body. It is highly sensitive and specific test which is basically an IFN-γ release assay. But, it can't differentiate between latent infection and active tuberculosis.
   (c) ELISA—IgG and IgM against A60 antigen complex (which is a thermostable complex present in cytoplasm of exponentially growing mycobacteria).
   (d) Polymerase Chain Reaction—DNA-based PCR is more sensitive. However, mRNA-based PCR is more specific.
2. *Radiological Investigations*
   (i) *X-ray:*
   It is often the first investigation that is done. However, it's not very sensitive. Only after 30–40% of calcium has been removed from an area by osteolysis, which takes about 3–5 months after osseous infection has set in before one can see a radiolucent area on X-ray. There is rarefaction (osteopenia) present on either side of the intervertebral disc space—earliest finding (Fig. 39.5). There is localised osteoporosis, adjacent end-plate irregularity and erosion (in earlier stages) and disc space narrowing (in later stages).

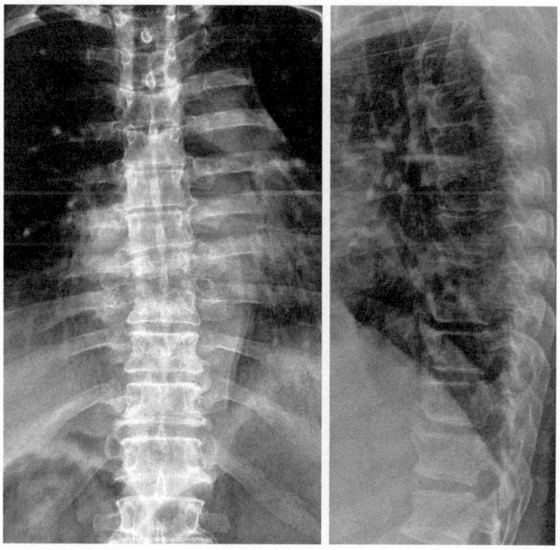

Fig. 39.5 End-plate irregularities (D8–D9) around the disc space are the first radiological sign. Narrowing of the disc space happens later when the nutrition of the disc is affected

Abscess shadows can be seen on X-ray that varies according to the region of the spine involved. In the cervical region, there is an increased prevertebral shadow. In the dorsal spine from C7 to D4, an abscess creates a V-shaped shadow on the anteroposterior view. On lateral view, there is a change in concavity of tracheal shadow, or the space between tracheal shadow increases, or the space between trachea and spine is more than 8 mm. There may be squaring of mediastinal borders. Below D_4, a typical fusiform 'Bird's

Nest' abscess is seen (Fig. 39.6a). Abscesses above the diaphragm remain in the thoracic cavity, whereas those below the diaphragm extend along the psoas muscle. In long-standing cases of cold abscess under the anterior longitudinal ligament, one may be able to see scalloping (concave erosion) along the anterior margin of the vertebral body known as aneurysmal phenomena. There may be wedge collapse (where a part of the vertebral body, usually the anterior part, collapses under load) or concertina collapse (whole vertebrae collapse, seen in the central type of tuberculosis). Deformity can be seen, such as lateral shift, scoliosis and kyphotic deformity (Fig. 39.6b). In growing children, the affected vertebrae may be even taller (tall vertebrae) compared to unaffected ones due to reactive hyperaemia [3, 6, 8, 9].

(ii) *CT scan:* It is mainly relevant for areas where there is more of cortical bone like posterior spinal disease, tuberculosis of craniovertebral and cervicodorsal region, sacroiliac joint and sacrum. It can help in delineating the shape, extent and route of spread of a cold abscess. Recently, CT-guided biopsy for obtaining tissue sample for tissue diagnosis has become more popular (Fig. 39.7) [6, 9].

(iii) *MRI:* It can help us define the extent of vertebral destruction and cold abscess. It gives a better picture of the site of cord compression and condition of the cord and can help us in identifying the cause of paraplegia (abscess, granulation tissue, sequestrum or gibbus), if present. It can also be used for diagnosing the disease in rare and difficult sites. The findings on MRI are evident before X-rays and hence are much more sensitive (Fig. 39.8) [9].

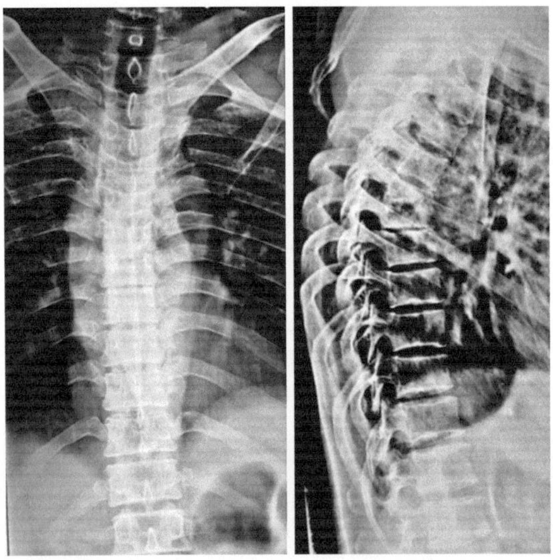

Fig. 39.6 Radiograph showing typical fusiform Bird Nest abscess (**a**) and Kyphotic deformity (**b**)

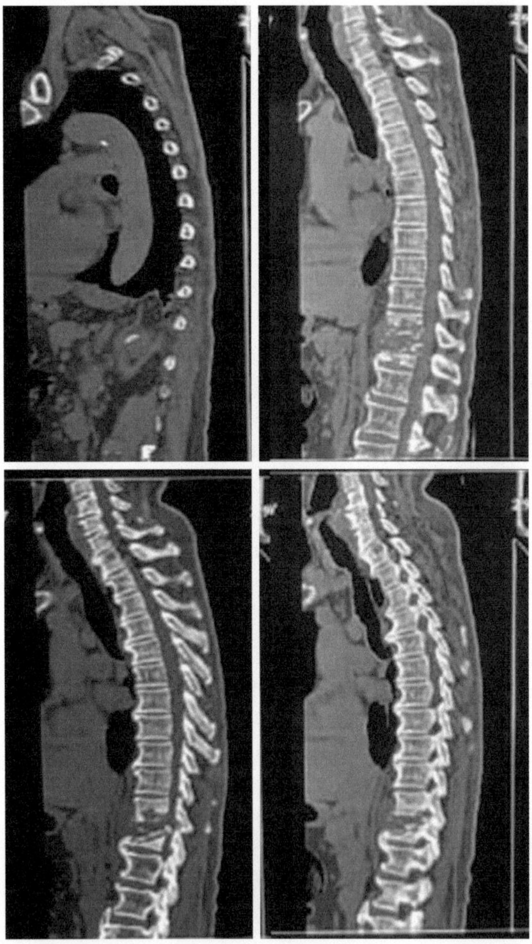

Fig. 39.7 CT scan showing osseous destruction in the affected Lumbar vertebrae

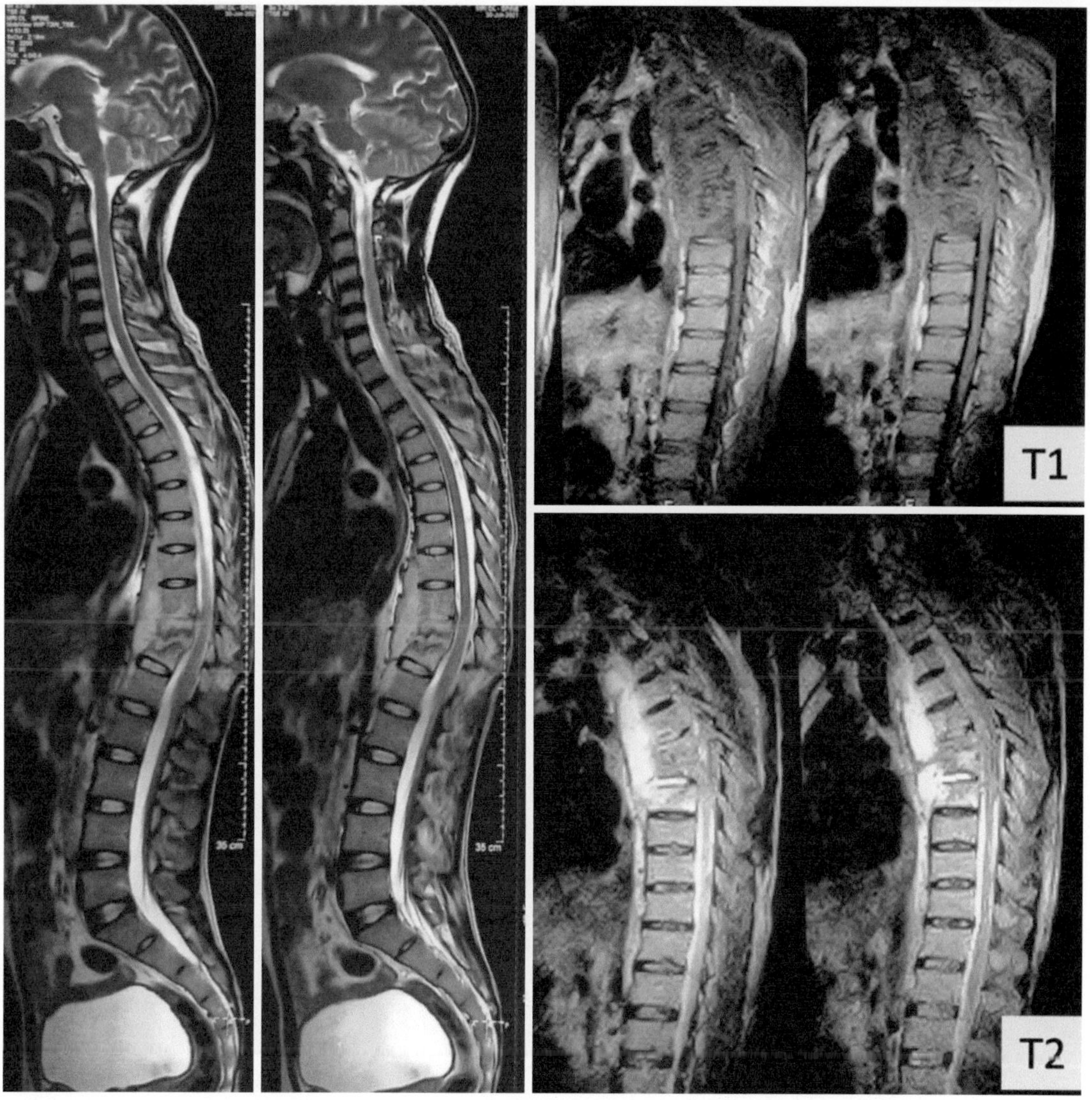

Fig. 39.8 MRI showing the extent of vertebral destruction, cold abscess and site of cord compression

(iv) *Myelography:* Indicated in paraplegia without radiological evidence of disease (spinal tumour syndrome) to know the canal status [3, 9].

3. *Tissue Diagnosis*
   This is the investigation of choice for making a conclusive/confirmatory diagnosis. The pus aspirate/ biopsied material should be sent for Gram's staining (to rule out other infections), Acid Fast Bacilli (AFB) staining, culture and sensitivity, Polymerase Chain Reaction (PCR) and histopathological examination. The culture media used for *Mycobacterium tuberculosis* are Lowenstein–Jensen media (gives results in 5–6 weeks) and BACTEC 12B (1–2 weeks). It may also be required in cases where there is no response to routine first-line drugs and hence to see the resistance pattern by GeneXpert or Line-probe Assay (gives a report within a few hours). A gene expert can detect mutations causing resistance against Rifampicin, while Line probe assay can detect resistance against Rifampicin and Isoniazid [3, 6, 9].

39.6 Differential Diagnosis [3, 5]

1. Traumatic conditions: Fracture-dislocations of spine can occur with or without neurological deficit.
2. Tumourous conditions: In the spine, secondaries are much more common compared to the primary tumour. Secondaries in spine can arise from lung, thyroid, breast, kidneys, prostate, etc. Among the primary tumours, benign lesions like Haemangioma, Aneurysmal Bone cysts or Giant cell tumours are common. Malignant spinal tumours like Ewing's Sarcoma, Osteogenic Sarcoma, Multiple myeloma and Chordoma can also mimic tuberculosis of spine.
3. Ankylosing Spondylitis: It can cause stiffness, kyphotic deformity and at times neurological deficit in young adults. The presence of sacroiliitis, positive Schober's test and chest expansion of less than 5 cm along with positive HLA-B27, is helpful in differentiating it from Pott's spine.
4. Prolapsed intervertebral disc: Symptoms of pain getting aggravated on forward bending and heavy weight lifting and clinical signs of positive straight leg raising test and Braggard's sign are diagnostic.
5. Other infectious diseases like pyogenic osteomyelitis caused by organisms like Staph. aureus, Brucella, Fungi, Typhoid, etc. can give a similar picture. However, the disease course is more dramatic, and often the patient has an immunocompromised status.
6. Developmental anomalies of the spine, like hemivertebrae, block vertebrae and synostosis of neural arches, and spinal osteochondrosis, like Scheuermann's disease, may present with a picture similar to Pott's spine.
7. Osteoporotic conditions like senile osteoporosis, rickets, osteomalacia and steroid-induced osteoporosis—Investigations like DEXA Scan (bone mineral density), and Biochemical investigations like serum levels of calcium, phosphate, Vitamin D3 and alkaline phosphatase are often helpful.

39.7 Complications Pott's Spine [3, 6, 9, 11]

1. Cold abscess
2. Paraplegia
3. Spinal deformity
4. Sinuses
5. Secondary infection
6. Amyloid disease
7. Fatality

39.8 Cold Abscess

As the vertebral body collapses, the necrotic tissue within it, comprising the granulation tissue, caseous matter and disintegrated bone lamellae and bone marrow, is squeezed outward. This is a cold abscess, which is the commonest complication of Pott's disease, which occurs in 20% of cases. It is not accompanied by inflammation and hence its signs like redness, heat, pain, etc.

It is a collection of tuberculous debris consisting of granulation tissues, serum, leucocytes, caseous matter and disintegrated bone marrow. Abscess enlarges and reaches the skin surface, leading to swelling, deformity and paravertebral thickening. A superficial abscess may burst to form a sinus or an ulcer which does not heal due to TB granulation tissue.

Treatment involves evacuation of pus, antitubercular drugs, instillation of 1gm Streptomycin after aspiration and iodoform antiseptic [3].

39.8.1 Spread of Cold Abscess [3]

- Cervical region
  - Anteriorly: Retropharyngeal or prevertebral abscess
  - On the sides: Parapharyngeal abscess
  - Along posterior border of SCM in posterior triangle of neck
  - In supraclavicular area and anterior triangle of neck
  - Down the mediastinum gravitates towards tracheas, oesophagus, pleural cavity
  - Down the brachial plexus to axilla

- Thoracic region
  - Upper thoracic (above D10)
    - Anteriorly: prevertebral or posterior mediastinal abscess
    - Laterally: paravertebral abscess (radiologically appears as Bird's nest abscess).
    - Track along intercostal nerves to:
      - Anterior end of intercostal space.
      - Abdominal wall behind rectus sheath.
      - Midaxillary line.
      - Along posterior division of the ICN lateral to the sacro-spinalis muscle
  - Lower Thoracic (D11–D12)
    - Along the 12th (subcostal), ilioinguinal and iliohypogastric nerves (bed of kidney)—present on anterior abdominal wall.
    - Behind the Lateral lumbocostal arch of the origin of diaphragm. Remains behind kidney (retro-nephritic space) on quadratus lumborum as Lumbar Abscess
    - Behind the Medial lumbocostal arch & enters the psoas sheath and presents as a psoas abscess.
      - Reaches the lesser trochanter where psoas gets inserted.
      - Palpable above the inguinal ligament or medial aspect of thigh if it traverses below the inguinal ligament
    - Behind the Median arcuate ligament along aorta and its branches and thus tracks like a lumbar cold abscess.
- Lumbar Region
  - Anteriorly: prevertebral abscess
  - Laterally: paravertebral abscess
  - Along psoas sheath—as psoas abscess—In the lumbodorsal (Petit triangle) site (Fig. 39.9)
  - Can spread along the aorta and its branches
    - To ischiorectal fossa along internal pudendal artery
    - In the buttock along superior gluteal artery
    - Along femoral vessels to femoral triangle or medial side of thigh
  - As far as back of thigh and leg via sciatic nerve and its branches

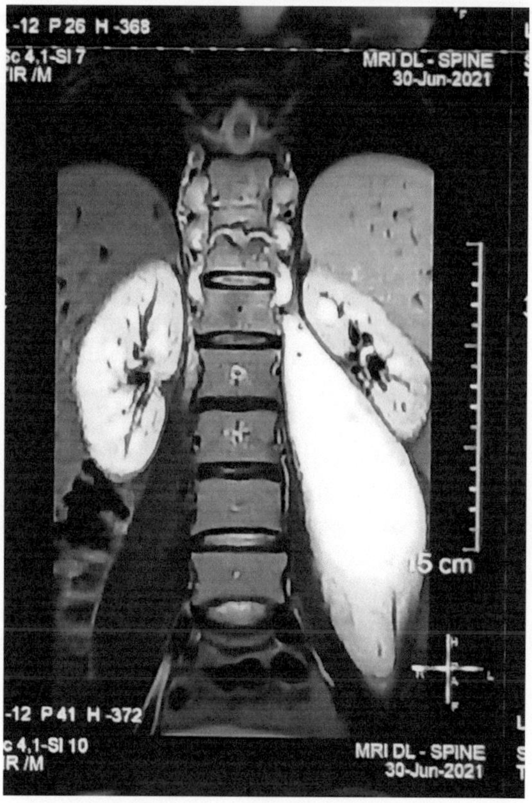

Fig. 39.9 MRI showing abscess from the dorsolumbar spine which follow along the psoas sheath

39.8.2 Management of Cold Abscess

Various methods that can be adopted for evacuation of cold abscesses are as follows:

(i) *Percutaneous aspiration* of the pus in an antigravity and Z-fashion (zig-zag tract against gravity) to avoid formation of sinus.
(ii) *Surgical drainage* depending upon the site: Like Lumbar Psoas abscess can be drained via Lumbar triangle of Petit, while an inguinal abscess or abscess on medial side of thigh may be drained by Ludloff's approach.

39.9 Pott's Paraplegia [3, 6, 9, 10]

Neurological deficit develops in 10–30% cases of Pott's spine. It is usually seen in the first three decades of life. It's the disease of lower thoracic spine which most commonly gives rise to Pott's paraplegia. Reasons behind this are—(i) Thoracic spine is the part of spine most commonly involved in tuberculosis of spine, (ii) Canal is narrowest and slightest pressure is enough to cause compression, (iii) Normal curve of dorsal spine encourages marked kyphosis, and (iv) Anterior longitudinal ligament in the dorsal area loosely confines the abscess.

Pathology of Pott's Paraplegia due to pressure on the cord by one or more of the following

1. *Inflammatory:*
   (a) Inflammatory oedema of spinal cord.
   (b) Tuberculous granulation tissue.
   (c) Tuberculous abscess—Commonest.
   (d) Tuberculous caseous tissue.
2. *Mechanical*:
   (a) Tuberculous debris (solid).
   (b) Sequestra from vertebral body and disc.
   (c) Stenosis of vertebral canal.
   (d) Internal gibbus along anterior wall of spinal canal.
3. *Intrinsic*:
   (a) Prolonged stretching of the cord over a severe deformity leading to interstitial gliosis and atrophy of cord.
   (b) Infective thrombosis/endarteritis of spinal vessels.
   (c) Pathological dislocation of vertebra.
   (d) Tuberculous meningomyelitis.
   (e) Syringomyelic changes.
4. *Spinal tumour syndrome*:
   (a) Diffuse extradural granuloma or tuberculoma (Fig. 39.10).

39.9.1 Stages of Neurological Deficit in Pott's Paraplegia

The neural deficit increases sequentially with increasing vertebral compression. Spinal tuberculosis typically affects the vertebral bodies and when compression begins in the front of the spinal cord, the first manifestation is a progressive increase in spasticity, which is not felt by the patient, but the physician elicits ankle clonus and extensor plantar response. As compression in the anterior column of the spinal cord increases, the patient begins to gradually lose motor strength, ranging from partial motor weakness to complete motor loss with signs of Upper Motor Neuron (UMN) damage. Initially, there is spastic motor paraparesis followed by spastic paraplegia in extension and subsequently spastic paraplegia in flexion. Among the sensory, anterolateral tract sensations (pain, crude touch and temperature sensations) are affected first. If the pressure is increased further, the posterior section of the spine will also be damaged, resulting in a complete loss of sensation and sphincter dysfunction. In extreme cases with continued compression, all spasticity disappears and paralysis becomes flaccid with anaesthesia and loss of sphincter control. At the time of presentation, Pott's paraplegia may be in one of the following stages as described by Goel, Tuli and Kumar. (Table 39.4) [2, 3, 5, 8, 12].

Hodgson in 1967 gave temporal classification of Pott's paraplegia as Early-onset (associated with active disease and occurring within two years of disease onset) and Late-onset paraplegia (associated with healed disease and occurring after two years of disease onset). The former is due to inflammatory oedema, granulation tissue, pus, caseous tissue and ischemia of the cord due to tubercular endarteritis and has got better prognosis. On the other hand, the cause of late-onset paraplegia is more often mechanical in nature like severe kyphotic deformity leading to internal gibbus, tubercular debris, sequestra from vertebral body and disc, stenosis of the vertebral canal and peridural fibrosis [3, 7, 13].

39.9.2 Clinical Features Specific of Pott's Paraplegia

Apart from the usual findings of Pott's spine, neurological signs that are seen in Pott's paraplegia are spontaneous twitching of muscles in lower limb, clumsiness while walking, extensor plantar response, exaggerated reflex and sustained clonus of ankle and patella. Rarely Pott's paraplegia may present as spinal tumour syndrome which is due to localised tuberculoma or diffuse granuloma or peridural fibrosis. (Fig. 39.10) [3, 5, 6].

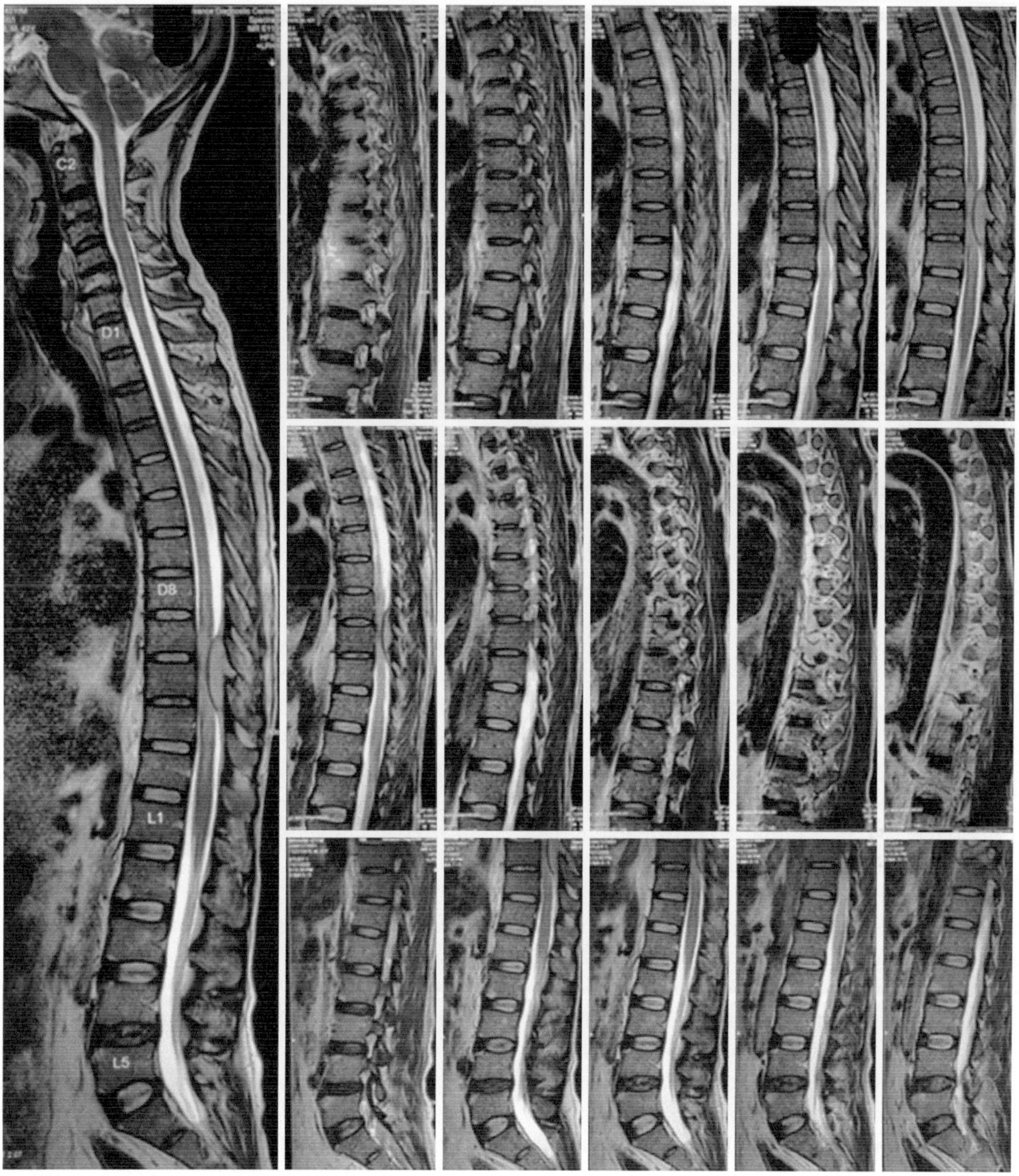

Fig. 39.10 MRI showing involvement of spinal cord at D8–D9 vertebral level by diffuse extradural granuloma (known as Tuberculoma)

39.10 Management

As the results of antitubercular multidrug treatment (ATT) have been good to excellent in most of the cases, all Pott's spine patients without neural complications and those with early neurological involvement are treated non-operatively. The goals of non-operative management are to achieve healing of the disease pathology and to avoid the possibility of any complications. A thorough evaluation by a multidisciplinary team is required to determine the best approach for each patient. The cases of Pott's spine with or without neurological involvement involve antitubercular drugs, rest (initial immobilisation), followed by gradual mobilisation. Surgery may be required only in specific scenarios and not in all. A cold abscess may require aspiration and evacuation [3, 6, 11, 14].

39.10.1 Medical Management

Antitubercular drugs are the mainstay of treatment. The first-line drugs consist of a daily dose of Isoniazid (H) (5 mg/kg), Rifampicin (R) (10–15 mg/kg of body weight), Pyrazinamide (Z) (20 mg/kg) and Ethambutol (E) (25 mg/kg). The usual regimen that is often followed by most orthopaedic surgeons in our country is HRZE for 2 months followed by HRZ for the next 4 months, and HR for 9 months to a year. The World Health Organization (WHO) recommendation is for daily HRZE for 2 months, followed by 4 months of HR or 6 months of HE. While the patient is on ATT, serial monitoring of blood parameters like complete blood count, ESR, CRP and Liver Function Tests is a must.

Absolute bed rest in a hard bed with a soft mattress is often required to avoid any possibility of further deterioration and promote healing. At times, plaster casts like Minerva Jacket for the cervical spine can be applied (for 18–24 months). Supportive therapy, like high-protein diet, multivitamins, haematinic and adequate sunlight, is given to improve the immunity of the patient. In recent years, there has been an increased incidence of drug resistance among tubercle bacteria to the first-line agents.

Multidrug resistant (MDR) tuberculosis is resistance to at least both Isoniazid and Rifampicin. Of late, resistance to any fluoroquinolone and at least one injectable second-line antibiotic in addition to Isoniazid and Rifampicin is also being seen (XDR (extremely drug-resistant) tuberculosis). One has to resort to second-line antitubercular drugs in MDR and XDR cases after consultation with a pulmonary medicine physician [3, 6, 9–11].

39.10.2 Surgical Management

The goals of surgical treatment are drainage of abscess, debridement of sequestrated bone, decompression of the spinal cord or dura and stabilisation of the spine for prevention or correction of deformity. Surgical intervention is often required in patients with neurological deficits, panvertebral lesions, severe spinal deformity (Kyphosis) or failure of conservative treatment. Advances in surgical techniques have led to more successful outcomes and improved quality of life for patients with TB spine [3, 6, 9, 15].

Indications for surgery (in patients without neurological deficit)

1. Progressive bone destruction in spite of ATT
2. Failure to respond to conservative treatment/drug-resistant TB
3. Evacuation of paravertebral abscess when it has increased in size in spite of rest and ATT (period of 3 months observation is enough)
4. Uncertainty of diagnosis
5. Mechanical instability
6. Prevention of severe kyphosis in children with extensive dorsal lesions
7. Spinal deformity
8. Childhood spine tuberculosis: spine at risk signs
   (a) Separation of the facet joints
   (b) Posterior retropulsion
   (c) Lateral translation
   (d) Toppling sign

Indications for surgery (in patients with neurological deficit)

Absolute indications for operative decompression in Pott's paraplegia, that is, Neural deficit)

1. Neurological complications (NC) do not show signs of recovery even after a fair trial (1 month) of conservative therapy.
2. NC develop during the conservative therapy.
3. NC become worse during the conservative therapy.
4. Recurrence of NC during the conservative therapy.
5. Rapid onset of paraplegia—indicates pathological subluxation or dislocation.
6. Advanced cases—Marked sensory and sphincter disturbance, flaccid paralysis or severe flexor spasm (Stage IV).
7. Patients with prevertebral cervical abscess, breathing and swallowing difficulties.
8. Cauda Equina Syndrome.

Relative indications:

1. Paraplegia with onset in old age to avoid prolonged recumbency.
2. Painful paraplegia—root compression or spasm.
3. Complications such as urinary stones or infections.
4. In posterior spinal disease with abscess, considering the risk of meningeal extension.
5. Spinal tumour syndrome.
6. Kyphosis correction.

39.10.3 Surgical Approaches

There are various approaches for tubercular spine. The decision regarding which approach to use for patients with spinal tuberculosis depends on various factors, including the location and extent of the lesions, the presence of neurological deficits, the degree of spinal instability and the patient's overall health and medical history. Generally, the surgical approaches for spinal tuberculosis can be divided into anterior, posterior, or combined approaches, and the choice depends on the specific characteristics of each patient's condition. Anterior approaches, such as a thoracotomy or retroperitoneal approach, are used to access the anterior aspect of the spinal cord and are indicated in cases where there is significant anterior compression or deformity. These approaches allow for the removal of necrotic tissue and placement of strut grafts or cages to restore the height of the affected vertebrae and prevent further collapse. Anterior debridement and strut grafting are conducted for patients with stable anterior lesions and no kyphotic deformity. Posterior approaches, such as a posterolateral or midline approach, are used to access the posterior aspect of the spinal cord and are indicated in cases where there is significant posterior compression or deformity. These approaches allow for decompression of the spinal cord, removal of necrotic tissue, and placement of pedicle screws and rods for spinal stabilisation. A posterior decompression is conducted for patients with isolated posterior lesions. Combined approaches, such as the transpedicular approach, are used to access both the anterior and posterior aspects of the spinal cord and are indicated in cases where there is significant anterior and posterior compression or deformity. These approaches allow for both decompression and stabilisation of the spine, as well as restoration of spinal alignment. Global lesions with kyphosis and instability are better treated with posterior instrumentation surgery in addition to an anterior strut graft [3, 6, 9, 10].

39.10.4 Various Surgical Procedures

Depending upon the clinico-radiological presentation, one or more of the surgical procedures may be required. Commonly done procedures are drainage of cold abscesses, decompression, debridement, fusion, anterior transposition of the cord, laminectomy and deformity correction. As discussed earlier, these can be accomplished by either an anterior, posterior, combined or minimally invasive approach. One or more of the following surgical methods may be required, depending upon the location and severity of disease [3, 6, 9, 10, 13–15].

1. *Abscess Drainage*
   A. *Cervical Spine*:
      (a) Transoral approach for C1–C2 involvement
      (b) Extraoral approach (along posterior border of Sternocleidomastoid) for Retropharyngeal abscess (Involvement of C_3–C_7)
      (c) Extraoral approach through posterior triangle of neck
   B. *Dorsal Spine*:
      Costotransversectomy—removal of 2 inches of 3 or more posterior ribs and their corresponding transverse process through an anterolateral extrapleural approach is done, which helps in drainage of tense pus (Fig. 39.11).
   C. *Lumbar Spine and Pelvis*:
      (a) Paravertebral abscess: Can be drained by a longitudinal incision given 5 cm lateral to midline and around 10 cm in length.
      (b) Psoas abscess: This abscess is extraperitoneal and along the psoas muscle. The presence of swelling depends on the size of the abscess and the area where it appears. Drainage can be done through one of the following sites: Petit triangle posteriorly, lateral incision along the crest of the ilium, anteriorly under the inguinal ligament.

2. *Decompression*
   It is done for neurological complications which fail to respond to conservative treatment and in cases where the disease is too advanced [3, 6] (Fig. 39.12).
   Anterior Cervical Decompression and Fusion (ACDF) is the most common surgical procedure used to treat cervical spine involvement in Pott's spine patients.

Anterolateral Decompression (ALD) (D_2 to L_1)
In the lateral position, a semilunar incision (convex laterally) is given. The exposure is extrapleural. Transverse processes of affected vertebrae, 2–4 ribs, pedicle and part of the body of vertebra are removed. Debridement of pus, debris, sequestrated material and disc is done (Fig. 39.13).

Transpedicular Decompression
The transpedicular approach may be used in combination with posterior instrumentation to achieve adequate decompression of the spinal cord and stabilisation of the spine. The advantages of the transpedicular approach include good visualisation of the spinal canal and anterior aspect of the spinal cord, as well as the ability to achieve both decompression and stabilisation in one procedure [15] (Fig. 39.14).

3. *Spinal Fusion*
   It is often required in cases where there is symptomatic mechanical instability. It may be done along with decompression or debride-

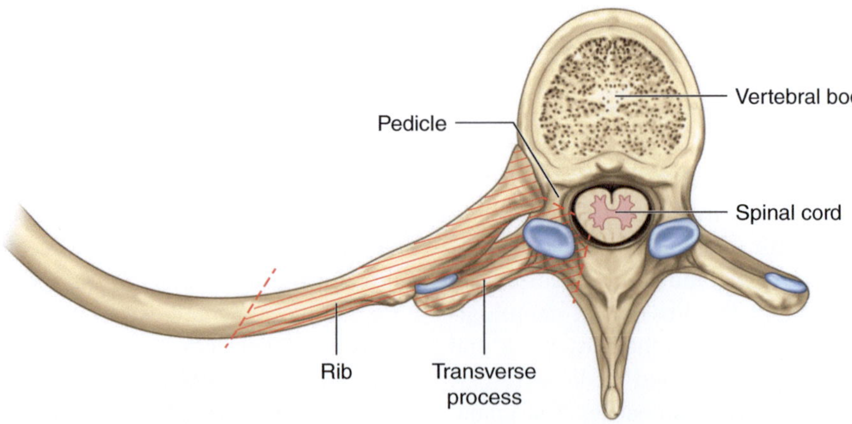

Fig. 39.11 Costotransversectomy

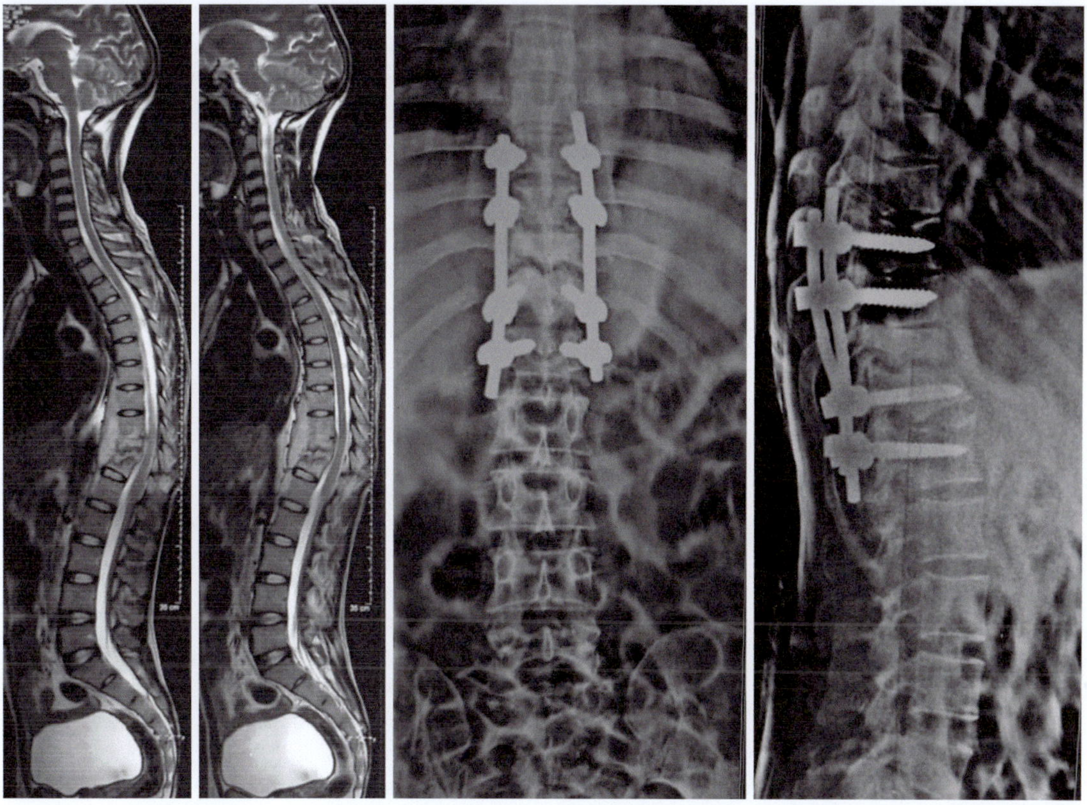

Fig. 39.12 MRI images of a 32-year-old male with Pott's paraplegia at D11– D12 vertebra with bowel and bladder involvement treated with Posterior Decompression and Instrumentation as seen on X-ray images

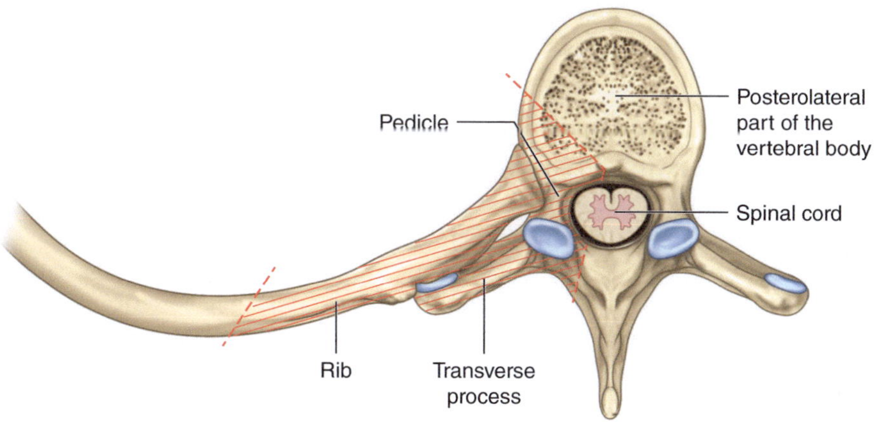

Fig. 39.13 Anterolateral Decompression

ment in the same sitting or at a later stage. It is not advisable to use anterior implants in an active Pott's spine. It's safer to use posterior implants, but if >4 vertebrae are involved, anterior instrumentation should be preferred.

Posterior Stabilisation and Posterior Spinal Arthrodesis

The posterior or posterolateral approaches have been described as the preferred surgical approach for the management of Tubercular

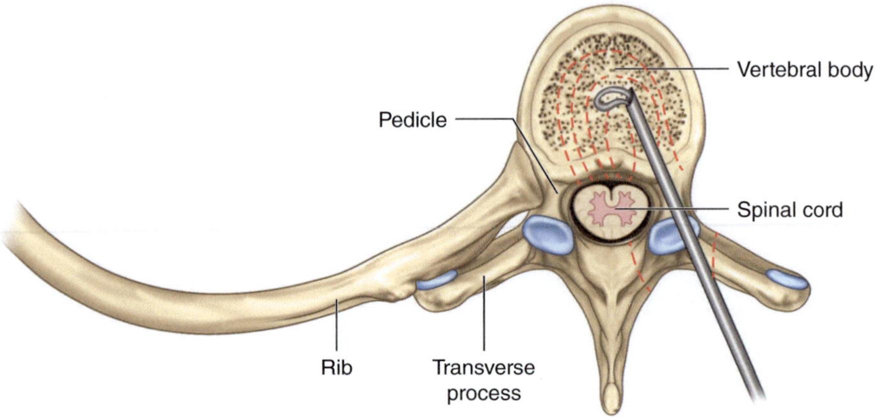

Fig. 39.14 Transpedicular approach

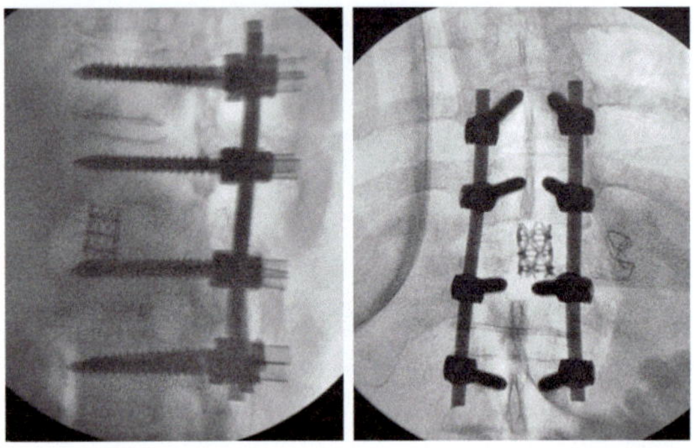

Fig. 39.15 Decompression, debridement, posterior instrumentation (T9–L2) and T11–T12 interbody fusion with titanium mesh cage. (*Courtesy: Dr. Anuj Gupta, Associate Consultant, Max Superspeciality Hospital, Vaishali, New Delhi)*

spine. These approaches offer several advantages and are associated with good outcomes. In Tubercular spine surgery, the extra-pleural space is used to gain access to the anterior and lateral columns of the spine. The use of a titanium mesh cage infused with an autograft and pedicle screw and rod fixation provides good stability and promotes bony fusion [14] (Fig. 39.15).

4. *Debridement*

   It is different from decompression in the sense that here we remove all diseased bone and infected tissue from the bleeding bone. It enhances the healing process. However, it is much more morbid compared to decompression alone, where we just evacuate the tense pus, leading to decreased pressure on the spinal cord.

   Hong Kong's Procedure (Radical Debridement and Arthrodesis)

   This technique was described by Hodgson and Stock, in which the spine is exposed from the front using a transthoracic or transperitoneal approach, and debris and pus are removed. Kyphosis is corrected partially by direct pressure, strut grafts of correct length (Iliac crest/ Rib bone graft) are inserted, and injection of Streptomycin and Isoniazid is infiltrated before closure. Anterior stabilisation led to a stable anterior column, and hence there were less chances of progression of deformity and possibility of late-onset paraplegia [13].

5. *Laminectomy* alone has no role in Pott's spine as it makes spine unstable [3].

   It is indicated only in certain scenarios, like:

   (a) Extradural granuloma/tuberculoma of spinal tumour syndrome.
   (b) Old healed disease with canal stenosis.
   (c) Non-healing posterior spinal disease.

6. *Anterior Transposition of Cord (by Extrapleural Anterolateral Approach)*: It may be required in cases with severe kyphotic deformity (>60 degrees) with or without neurological deficit [16].

7. *Recent Surgical Advancements* such as minimally invasive techniques, Lumbar Interbody Fusion surgeries, video-assisted thoracoscopic surgery (VATS) supplemented with posterior percutaneous pedicle screw fixation, Intraoperative neuromonitoring (IONM),

computer-assisted navigation, biological implants and advanced imaging techniques have improved the safety, efficacy and outcomes of TB spine surgery. These advancements have also helped to reduce the risk of complications and improve the quality of life for patients with TB spine [17].

39.10.5 Middle Path Regime

Dr. S.M. Tuli described this regimen, the rationale behind which was that all spinal tuberculosis cases do not require surgery and that only those who do not respond to conservative measures should be operated upon. This regimen is usually followed in the Indian subcontinent, because patients reach the paraplegic stage with poor health, anaemia and/or associated pulmonary tuberculosis, making them unfit for major surgery. This regime was borne out of the observation that many of the patients (38%) while waiting for their turn and fitness for surgery, start showing neurological recovery on antitubercular drugs, bed rest and nutritious diet in 4–6 weeks [3, 6, 9, 18].

The regime consists of the following:

(i) Treatment is non-operative with antitubercular drugs, rest and spinal braces

(ii) Rest in a hard bed /Plaster of Paris bed—to give rest to spine during acute phase for pain relief

(iii) Drugs: Dr. Tuli recommended the following regimen:
   - (a) Intensive phase: Isoniazid, Rifampicin and Ofloxacin (5–6 months)
   - (b) Continuation phase: Isoniazid and Pyrazinamide (3–4 months) + Isoniazid and Rifampicin (4 months)
   - (c) Prophylactic phase: Isoniazid and Ethambutol (4–5 months).

   However, it must be noted that the WHO guidelines say an intensive phase consisting of Isoniazid, Rifampicin, Pyrazinamide and Ethambutol for 2 months, followed by a continuation phase of 4 months of Isoniazid and Rifampicin or 6 months of Isoniazid and Ethambutol. The Index TB guidelines recommendation is for 10 months of continuation phase of Isoniazid, Rifampicin and Ethambutol.

(iv) Radiographs and Erythrocyte Sedimentation Rate (ESR) at 3–6 monthly intervals.

(v) Gradual mobilisation with the help of braces with spinal brace support, in the absence of any neurological deficit. Spinal Braces continued for 18–24 months and then gradually discarded.

(vi) Minor surgeries like.
   - (a) Aspiration of abscesses and instillation of 1gm Streptomycin with or without Isoniazid using zigzag tract.
   - (b) Evacuation of abscesses and debris back to healthy cancellous bone.
   - (c) Sinus Excision, if it does not heal spontaneously.

(vii) Surgery for selected cases—not responding in 4 weeks.
   - (a) Operative decompression of the cord for absolute indications like no sign of recovery after fair trial of conservative therapy, onset of neurological complications during conservative treatment, recurrence, cases showing worsening and advanced cases (bladder bowel involvement, flexor spasms, etc.)
   - (b) Excisional surgery for posterior spinal disease to avoid the possibility of meningitis.
   - (c) Operative debridement if the growth of lesions is not arrested.
   - (d) Posterior spinal arthrodesis for unstable spine when symptomatic.
   - (e) Extensive posterior decompression/ instrumented fusion and three-level posterior vertebral column resection, followed by anterior debridement/ fusion with cage reconstruction.

   Postoperatively, the patient is nursed on a hard bed/ Plaster of Paris bed for the initial few weeks, and mobilisation with spinal braces is started usually at around 3–5 months.

(viii) Supportive therapy: Haematinics, Multivitamins, High-protein diet.

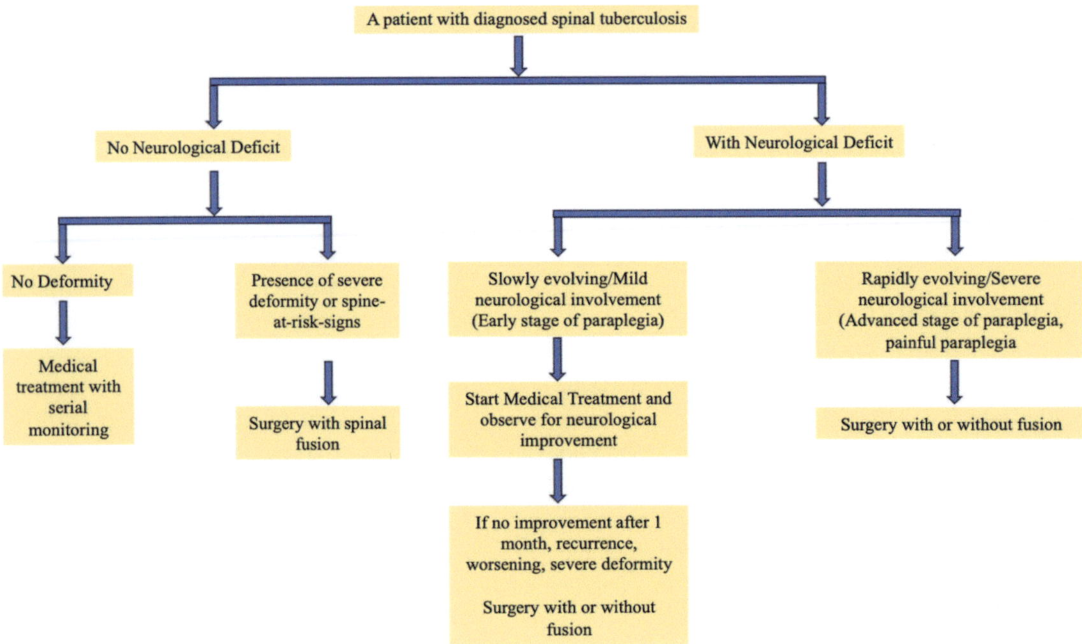

Fig. 39.16 Treatment algorithm of Pott's spine

39.11 Treatment Algorithm

Figure 39.16 summarises the treatment plan for a patient with spinal tuberculosis [9].

Multiple Choice Questions

1. In tuberculosis of spine, which of the following is not a cause of paraplegia?
   (a) Stretching of spinal cord in gibbus deformity
   (b) Spinal artery compression
   (c) Compression by granulation tissue
   (d) Oedema of spinal cord
2. Which of the following is not an absolute indication for operative decompression in Pott's paraplegia?
   (a) Neurological complications develop during the conservative therapy
   (b) Recurrence of neurological complications during the conservative therapy
   (c) Flaccid paralysis or severe flexor spasm
   (d) Kyphosis correction
3. All of the following are causes of late-onset paraplegia except:
   (a) Internal gibbus
   (b) Sequestra from vertebral body and disc
   (c) Granulation tissue
   (d) Peridural fibrosis
4. Which of the following is not a usual complication of Pott's spine?
   (a) Cold abscess
   (b) Amyloidosis
   (c) Spinal deformity
   (d) Spondylolisthesis
5. During anterolateral decompression in a case of Pott's spine, all the structures of the affected vertebrae are removed except:
   (a) Spinous process
   (b) Transverse processes of affected vertebrae
   (c) Part of vertebral body
   (d) Pedicle

Answer: 1. (b), 2. (d), 3. (c), 4. (d), 5. (a)

References

1. Dobson J. Percivall Pott. Ann R Coll Surg Engl 1972;50(1):54–65. PMID: 4550865; PMCID: PMC2388056.
2. Kumar K. Spinal tuberculosis, natural history of disease, classifications and principles of management with historical perspective. Eur J Orthop Surg Traumatol. 2016;26(6):551–558. https://doi.org/10.1007/s00590-016-1811-x. Epub 2016 Jul 19. PMID: 27435619.
3. Tuli SM, editor. Tuberculosis of the skeletal system. 5th ed. New Delhi: Jaypee Brothers Medical Publishers; 2016.
4. Jutte P, Wuite S, The B, van Altena R, Veldhuizen A. Prediction of deformity in spinal tuberculosis. Clin Orthop Relat Res. 2007;455:196–201. https://doi.org/10.1097/01.blo.0000246559.27596.33. PMID: 17091018.
5. Das S, editor. A manual on clinical surgery. 16th ed. Jaypee Brothers Medical Publishers Pvt Limited; 2022.
6. Rajasekaran S, Soundararajan DCR, Shetty AP, Kanna RM. Spinal tuberculosis: current concepts. Global Spine J. 2018;8(4 Suppl):96S–108S. https://doi.org/10.1177/2192568218769053. Epub 2018 Dec 13. PMID: 30574444; PMCID: PMC6295815.
7. Tuli SM. General principles of osteoarticular tuberculosis. Clin Orthop Relat Res. 2002;(398):11–19. https://doi.org/10.1097/00003086-200205000-00003. PMID: 11964626.
8. Kumar K. Tuberculosis of spine, natural history of disease and its judicious management. J West Pac Orthop Assoc. 1988;25:1–8.
9. Khanna K, Sabharwal S. Spinal tuberculosis: a comprehensive review for the modern spine surgeon. Spine J. 2019;19(11):1858–70. https://doi.org/10.1016/j.spinee.2019.05.002. Epub 2019 May 15. PMID: 31102727.
10. Jain AK, Kumar J. Tuberculosis of spine: neurological deficit. Eur Spine J. 2013;22 Suppl 4(Suppl 4):624–33. https://doi.org/10.1007/s00586-012-2335-7. Epub 2012 May 8. PMID: 22565802; PMCID: PMC3691413.
11. Index-TB guidelines- guidelines on extra-pulmonary tuberculosis for India. Ministry of Health and Family Welfare, Government of India. Available from: https://tbcindia.gov.in/WriteReadData/l892s/5585665076Index-TB%20Guidelines.pdf. Accessed 24 April 2024.
12. Goel MK. Treatment of Pott's paraplegia by operation. J Bone Joint Surg Br. 1967;49(4):674–81. PMID: 6073185.
13. Hodgson AR, Stock FE, Fang HS, Ong GB. Anterior spinal fusion. The operative approach and pathological findings in 412 patients with Pott's disease of the spine. Br J Surg. 1960;48:172–8. https://doi.org/10.1002/bjs.18004820819. PMID: 13714863.
14. Talu U, Gogus A, Ozturk C, Hamzaoglu A, Domanic U. The role of posterior instrumentation and fusion after anterior radical debridement and fusion in the surgical treatment of spinal tuberculosis: experience of 127 cases. J Spinal Disord Tech 2006;19(8):554–559. doi: https://doi.org/10.1097/01.bsd.0000211202.93125.c7. PMID: 17146297.
15. Lee SH, Sung JK, Park YM. Single-stage transpedicular decompression and posterior instrumentation in treatment of thoracic and thoracolumbar spinal tuberculosis: a retrospective case series. J Spinal Disord Tech. 2006;19(8):595–602. https://doi.org/10.1097/01.bsd.0000211241.06588.7b. PMID: 17146304.
16. Jain AK, Dhammi IK, Prashad B, Sinha S, Mishra P. Simultaneous anterior decompression and posterior instrumentation of the tuberculous spine using an anterolateral extrapleural approach. J Bone Joint Surg Br. 2008;90(11):1477–81. PMID: 18978269.
17. Ruparel S, Tanaka M, Mehta R, Yamauchi T, Oda Y, Sonawane S, Chaddha R. Surgical management of spinal tuberculosis-The past, present, and future. Diagnostics (Basel). 2022;12(6):1307. https://doi.org/10.3390/diagnostics12061307. PMID: 35741117; PMCID: PMC9221609.
18. Tuli SM. Results of treatment of spinal tuberculosis by "middle-path" regime. J Bone Joint Surg Br. 1975;57(1):13–23. PMID: 46867.

Tuberculosis of Hip

40

Kumar Keshav

40.1 Introduction

The hip joint is the second most frequently affected joint from tuberculosis. It mostly affects children in developing countries, where tuberculosis is still common. The clinical presentation ranges from night cries to a severe painful limp, depending upon the stage of disease. The diagnosis is made on the basis of typical clinical features and radiological findings. MRI has become the gold standard investigation, often detecting disease early in the course before X-ray changes appear. If detected early, it can be treated conservatively. However, it's not uncommon to see patients presenting late in the course of the natural history of disease which often leaves them crippled for life. The advent of total hip joint replacement is a ray of hope for such patients, allowing them to get back to a near-normal life.

40.2 Etiopathogenesis

The spread of tubercle bacteria to the hip region occurs by haematogenous route. But the bacteria reach inside the joint cavity often late in the course, which is the cause of late presentation in majority of the cases. Initial focus of infection is usually the acetabular roof. However, femoral epiphysis (which are still cartilaginous in children), proximal metaphyseal part of femur including the trochanters and synovium may be affected in several cases initially. Cold abscess may form within the joint, which may perforate the capsule. The pus and exudates may appear outside the joint in either the femoral triangle or on medial/lateral/posterior aspects of thigh or in ischio-rectal fossa.

K. Keshav (✉)
Department of Orthopaedics, Sanjay Gandhi Post Graduate Institute of Medical Sciences, Lucknow, Uttar Pradesh, India

40.3 Pathological Changes

The inflammatory process destroys the bone and cartilage due to the effect of proteolytic enzymes released either by the Mycobacterium or inflammatory cells invading the area. This leads to a few characteristic findings with special names like mortar and pestle appearance, wandering acetabulum and protrusio acetabuli (mentioned later in radiology). Based on the pathological changes, the disease can be described in four stages (Fig. 40.1):

1. *Stage of tubercular synovitis:* Due to inflammation of the synovium, there is synovial effusion, which causes the joint to go in flexion, abduction and external rotation, which is the attitude of the joint when it's maximally capacious (Fig. 40.1b).
2. *Stage of early arthritis:* This stage involves the onset of actual destruction of the articular

V. Kumar et al. (eds.), *A Quick Guide to Essential Orthopedics*,
https://doi.org/10.1007/978-981-95-2676-5_40

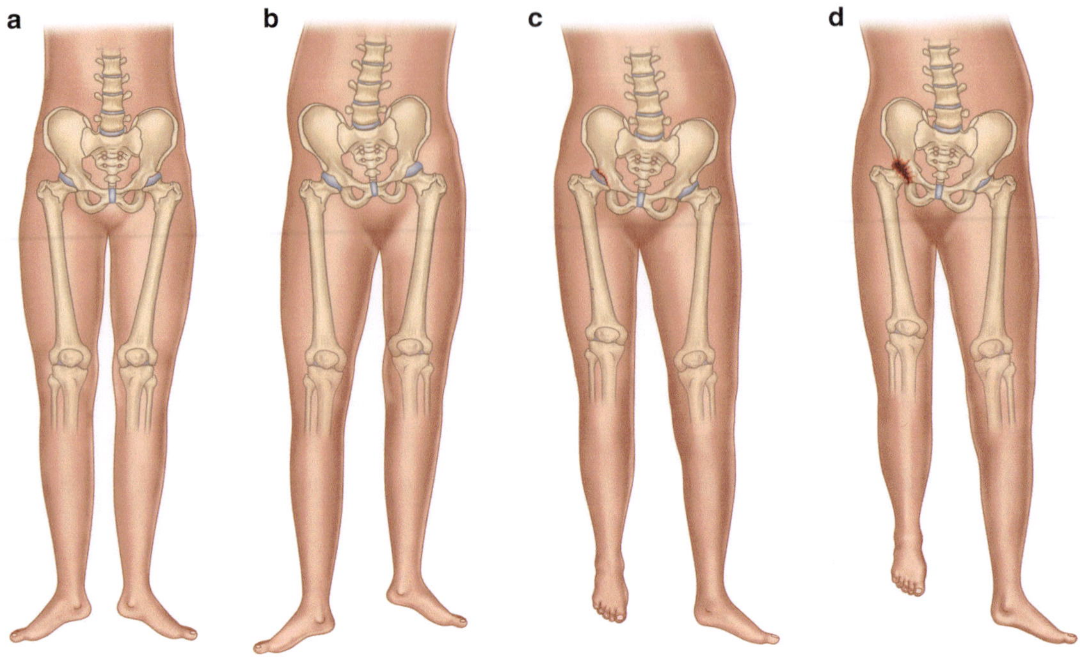

Fig. 40.1 (**a**) Normal hips, (**b**) Stage 1 (Stage of Synovitis), (**c**) Stage 2 (Stage of Early arthritis) and (**d**) Stage 3 (Stage of Advanced Arthritis)

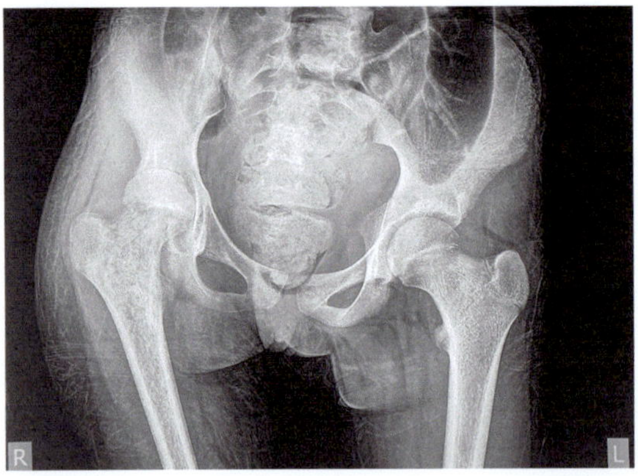

Fig. 40.2 Tuberculosis of the right hip in Stage 2, showing Phemister triad features-localized osteoporosis, slight diminution of joint space and localized erosions of articular margins

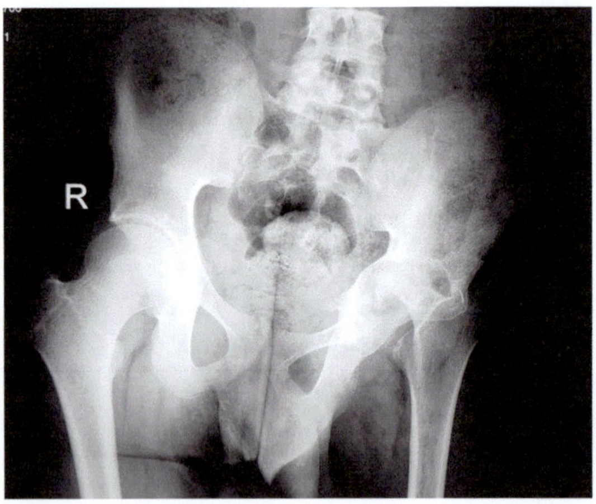

Fig. 40.3 Tuberculosis of left hip showing mortar and pestle appearance

cartilage leading to arthritis. Since arthritis leads to severe pain, the muscles go into spasm as a protective mechanism to avoid any movement of the hip. Since adductors, flexors and internal rotators are stronger compared to their antagonists, hip assumes a position of flexion, adduction and internal rotation. Bony destruction has still not set in (Figs. 40.1c, 40.2 and 40.3) and hence the shortening is an apparent one. True shortening, if present, is not more than 1 cm.

3. *Stage of advanced arthritis:* By this stage, there is gross destruction of articular cartilage, femoral head and acetabulum. Since bony destruction has happened by this stage, there is true shortening. The joint capsule may be either destroyed or thickened and contracted. (Fig. 40.1c).

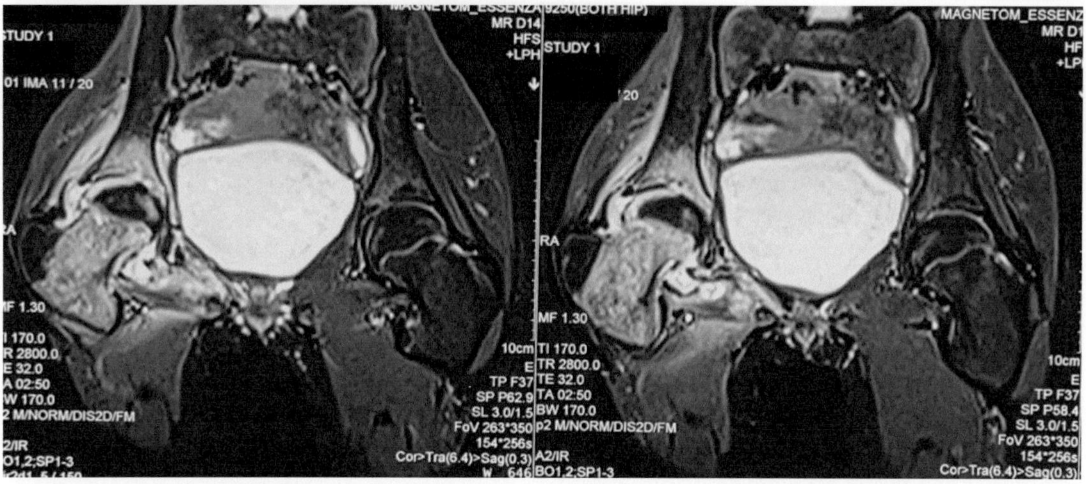

Fig. 40.4 MRI showing features of synovial effusion, osseous oedema, osteomyelitis and periarticular abscess in the right hip

4. *Stage of advanced arthritis with subluxation or dislocation:* This stage is marked by one or the other complication, like subluxation/dislocation, secondary to ongoing osteoarticular damage. A few of the pathological changes seen in this stage are: (a) protrusio acetabuli, (b) wandering acetabulum, (c) mortar and pestle appearance and (d) frank posterior hip dislocation. Protrusio acetabuli is the inward indentation of the acetabular floor in the pelvic cavity as a result of its progressive softening being thrust inside by the femoral head. Due to simultaneous damage to acetabulum and its softening, the head keeps pushing the acetabular roof. This causes the new deformed acetabulum to change its position from the natural position giving the nomenclature of 'Wandering acetabulum'. In certain cases, the acetabular cavity appears much bigger compared to the size of the femoral head which has been reduced in size due to ongoing damage, giving the appearance of 'Mortar and Pestle Appearance'. (Fig. 40.4) In a few patients, there may be a frank posterior dislocation of the hip.

40.4 Clinical Features

The disease is common among children and adolescents. It's rather uncommon beyond third decade of life. There is no specific gender predisposition. More often tuberculosis of hip is secondary to bacillaemia from other tubercular sites like lungs or lymphatic system. So, constitutional clinical features corresponding to primary foci like fever, night sweats, lymphadenopathy, dyspnoea and malaise may be present.

Symptoms

1. The most common clinical symptom is painful limp.
2. Night cries—Right from the initial stage of the disease, pain is often seen at night during sleep when the inflamed articular surfaces rub against each other, which happens when the protective and restrictive effect of spasm of hip muscles is gone.
3. Limitation of movements.
4. Shortening of the limb.
5. Swelling (due to cold abscess) or discharging sinus.
6. Pathological posterior dislocation.

Signs The clinical signs depend upon the stage of disease presentation. In Stage 1, owing to the attitude of flexion, abduction and external rotation, there is apparent lengthening. The terminal range of movements may be painful and restricted. In Stage 2, there is apparent shortening secondary to flexion, adduction and internal rotation deformity. Since there is only articular cartilage damage without obvious bony destruction, true shortening, if any, is not more than 1 cm. Muscle wasting, especially those of glutei are quite appreciable. There is global restriction of movements. Stage 3, on the other hand, is marked by true shortening, often more than 1 cm. There may, however, be some element of apparent shortening as well. Other signs are similar to those of Stage 2 but more marked. Patient who presents late in Stage 4 have all the features of Stage 3 like gross restriction of hip movements, marked shortening or at times, femoral head being felt in gluteal region due to posteriorly dislocated hip. However, there are certain conditions like protrusio acetabuli, wandering acetabulum and mortar and pestle appearance of hip, where movements are fairly preserved despite gross bony destruction.

40.5 Investigations

1. *Blood Investigations:*
   (a) Complete blood count with ESR and CRP.
   (b) Quantiferon gold assay: for definitive diagnosis of tuberculosis in the body. It is a highly sensitive and specific test which is basically IFN-γ release assay. But, it can't differentiate between latent infection and active tuberculosis.
   (c) ELISA: IgG and IgM against A60 antigen complex (which is a thermostable complex present in cytoplasm of exponentially growing mycobacteria.)
   (d) Polymerase Chain Reaction: DNA-based PCR is more sensitive. However, mRNA-based PCR is more specific.
2. *Radiological Investigations.*
   (i) *X-ray:* Before the routine use of MRI, it was the investigation which determined the stage of disease and guided treatment. Still, in the regions of the world where Tuberculosis is endemic, a clinical diagnosis supported by Koch's hip is sufficient to start the treatment. Recently, however Government of India has made it mandatory to start antitubercular treatment (ATT) only after a definitive diagnosis to avoid the development of multidrug resistant and extensive-drug resistant forms. Also, all the cases have to be notified.
   The findings on X-ray vary depending upon the stage of disease. In Stage 1, only soft-tissue swelling and some rarefaction of bones forming the hip joint are seen. Stage 2 is characterized by Phemister's triad- localized osteoporosis, slight diminution of joint space and localized erosions of articular margins (Figs. 40.2 and 40.3). Stage 3 shows more destructive changes due to the involvement of periarticular metaphyseal area (Fig. 40.4). Stage 4 often shows one of the advanced destructive features like protrusio acetabuli, wandering acetabulum, mortar and pestle appearance (Fig. 40.4) In cases presenting with pathological dislocation, the eroded femoral head may be seen out of the acetabulum.

Shanmugasundram's Radiological Types of Tuberculosis of Hip

Type 1: Normal hip
Type 2: Travelling acetabulum
Type 3: Dislocating type
Type 4: Perthe's type
Type 5: Protrusio acetabuli
Type 6: Atrophic type
Type 7: Mortar and pestle appearance

Shanmugasundaram also described that femoral head may increase in size due to chronic hyperaemia (Coxa Magna) or reduce in size due to reduced blood supply (Coxa breva). Apart from the change in size of femoral head, the neck-shaft angle can decrease (Coxa vara) owing to restricted growth of the femoral head physis or increase (Coxa valga) due to restriction in growth of the trochanteric physis. In Perthes type of tuberculosis hip, radiology is similar to Perthes disease like metaphyseal osteoporosis, decrease in height of femoral head epiphysis, increased density, fragmentation of physis, collapse of proximal fragment and coxa magna due to thrombosis or embolization of selective terminal vasculature.

(ii) *Ultrasonography*: It can detect synovial effusion and soft-tissue swelling and is thus a non-specific investigation. One may go for USG-guided aspiration for making a confirmatory microbiological diagnosis.
(iii) *MRI:* It can help in the diagnosis of the disease in earlier stages before X-ray changes appear. It is, however, a non-specific investigation as a similar kind of picture may be seen in other pathological states. MRI may reveal synovial effusion and osseous oedema. It can also show associated abnormalities like osteomyelitis, myositis, periarticular abscess and sinus tract formation (Fig. 40.4).
(iv) *CT Scan*: It can show the extent of bony destruction, if any.

3. *Tissue Diagnosis*

This is the investigation of choice for making a conclusive/confirmatory diagnosis.

(a) *Joint Aspiration* The pus aspirate/biopsied material should be sent for Gram's staining (to rule out other infections), AFB staining, culture and sensitivity, PCR and histopathological examination.
The culture media used for mycobacterium tuberculosis are:
(a) Lowenstein- Jensen media
(b) BACTEC
It may also be required in cases where there is no response to routine first-line drugs and hence to see the resistance pattern by Gene-Expert or Line-probe Assay.
(b) *Synovial Biopsy* should be done by the anterior approach to the hip and never posterior to prevent damage to the vasculature of the femoral head.

40.6 Differential Diagnosis

It's mainly in Stage 1 and early Stage 2 where there is a diagnostic dilemma when severe deformity has still not appeared.

1. Subacute Septic Arthritis: The clinical presentation is usually similar. However, constitutional symptoms of tuberculosis are usually absent. The definitive diagnosis can be made by tissue diagnosis.
2. Transient Synovitis of hip: It's self-limiting and the disease course is much milder. Ultrasound-guided aspiration may be done and the aspirate sent for differentiating between the two.
3. Proximal femoral osteomyelitis with secondary/reactive hip involvement.
4. Rheumatic disease, like Juvenile Rheumatoid arthritis or Rheumatoid arthritis, depending upon the patient's age. The involvement is usually polyarticular, but monoarticular involvement may also happen. The history of morning stiffness and blood investigations, like anti-CCP, may be done to differentiate it from Koch's hip.
5. Perthes disease: The characteristic feature is a painless/mildly painful limp in children between 6 and 9 years of age. Often, in the X-ray, there is extrusion of the femoral head, widening of femoral head and other changes. X-ray changes are much more marked compared to the clinical findings.
6. Psoas abscess: There will be pseudoflexion deformity of the hip. The differentiating feature between the two is that hip movements are painless in pseudoflexion deformity, in contrast to flexion deformity, where it is painful.
7. Inflamed Inguinal Lymph nodes.
8. Slipped Capital Femoral Epiphysis: Usually seen in an obese child around the age of onset of puberty.
9. Avascular Necrosis of Hip.
10. Osteoarthritis.

40.7 Management

Management depends upon the stage of the disease. Usually, in the early stages, antitubercular treatment (ATT) and traction followed by gradual mobilization suffice. In the later stages, one may have to go for some kind of operative intervention. Depending upon the stage, one or more of the following may be required.

1. *Multidrug Therapy*

Antitubercular treatment (ATT) is the mainstay of treatment. Usually, 4 drugs (Isoniazid, Rifampicin, Pyrazinamide and Ethambutol) are given for 3 months, 3 drugs (Isoniazid, Rifampicin and Ethambutol) for 2 months and 2 drugs (Isoniazid and Rifampicin) for the next 1–1.5 years. It must be mentioned here that the WHO regimen is different from this, which is usually for 9 months.

2. *Bed Rest, Initial Traction Followed by Progressive Movements*
   Bed rest keeps the patient non-weight-bearing and thus prevents additional damage to the hip joint and promotes healing. Plenty of fresh air and a nutritious diet should also be maintained. Traction gives/enforces rest, which is essential for healing. It relieves muscle spasm and pain, prevents or corrects deformities and maintains the length of the limb (hence preventing shortening) and joint space by keeping the acetabulum and femoral head separated from one another (hence avoiding ankylosis). Since the femoral head is not pushed against the softened acetabulum, it minimizes the possibility of the development of a wandering acetabulum. In cases of abduction deformity in the affected hip, it's important to go for bilateral traction; otherwise, abduction deformity will be exaggerated.
   Once the pain subsides, active assisted movements are started and continued for around 4–6 months. Following this, non-weight-bearing ambulation with the help of Zimmer frame/walker is initiated, and after 3 months, partial weight-bearing is started. Full unassisted weight-bearing should be started late, around 10–12 months after the initiation of ATT, depending upon healing as assessed by serial radiographs.
3. *Definitive Surgeries*
   Broadly speaking, there are two major scenarios where some kind of surgical modality is required: (i) if the response to conservative treatment is not favourable, and (ii) the outcome is unacceptable.

(a) *Synovectomy and debridement of the joint:* It may be done if the response to conservative treatment is unfavourable. It also helps in tissue diagnosis and hence confirmatory diagnosis. The tissue may be subjected to Gene-Expert test for assessment of multidrug resistant tuberculosis. For synovectomy, anterior approach to the hip like Smith-Peterson should be used to avoid damage to vascularity of femoral head.
(b) *Osteotomy:* This is usually done in the healed stage of the disease (fibrous/bony ankylosis), when there is unacceptable deformity like abduction deformity of the hip. Usually, a subtrochanteric corrective osteotomy is required.
(c) *Arthrodesis:* In patients having healed tuberculosis of hip, the joint may be arthritic, leading to pain or the hip may be ankylosed in an unacceptable position. In such cases, especially when the physical demands are high like in manual labourers, one can go for arthrodesis of the joint.
(d) *Excisional Arthroplasty:* In cases where physical demands are not that high, the patient wants mobility at the cost of stability, and is unable to afford the high cost of total hip replacement, Girdlestone excision arthroplasty is a viable option. In developing countries due to socio-cultural needs which require sitting on the floor in a cross-legged manner, this is a viable option. Also, healing of the disease is enhanced because the infected tissue gets removed in the procedure.
(e) *Replacement arthroplasty:* This surgery has completely changed the functional outcome. One can get painless, mobile and stable hip by doing total hip Replacement where diseased femoral head and acetabulum is excised and replaced by an uncemented or cemented prosthesis. Whether this procedure can be done in active disease or not is an area of controversy. Literature is quite variable regarding the timing of surgery. However, the common denominator across the studies is that there should be thorough debridement of the diseased tissues and the routine course of ATT should be given for at least 5 months.

40.8 Treatment Algorithm

40.8.1 Stage of Synovitis

ATT + Traction + Intermittent active and assisted exercises followed by ambulation with suitable braces/orthosis ± Arthrotomy/Synovectomy.

40.8.2 Stage of Early Arthritis

ATT + Traction + Intermittent active and assisted exercises followed by ambulation with suitable braces/orthosis ± Synovectomy/Joint Debridement.

Usually, analgesics are required for mitigating pain and muscular spasm.

40.8.3 Stage of Advanced Arthritis

ATT + Traction + Intermittent active and assisted exercises followed by ambulation with suitable braces/orthosis ± Arthrolysis.

Arthrolysis, wherein pathological and fibrous tissues are excised without compromising the proximal femoral vascularity, helps to achieve a range of movements.

40.8.4 Stage of Advanced Arthritis with or Without Dislocation/Subluxation:

When ankylosis is the aim or expected result: ATT + Immobilization of hip in slight abduction (10–15^0), external rotation (5–10^0) and flexion depending upon age (10^0 in children to 30^0 in adults) with the help of a hip spica.

In the healed stage of the disease: Corrective osteotomy/Conversion of painful ankylosis to painless arthrodesis (painless immobile hip) / Conversion of ankylosed hip to mobile hip by Girdlestone excision arthroplasty (mobile unstable hip) or to total hip replacement (mobile stable hip).

Multiple Choice Questions

1. In a patient with tuberculosis of the hip joint, which of the following deformities is not seen in stage of early arthritis?
   (a) Flexion deformity of hip
   (b) Adduction deformity of hip
   (c) External rotation of hip
   (d) True Shortening of less than 1 cm
2. Which of the following is not a component of the Phemister triad?
   (a) Osteophyte formation
   (b) Localized osteoporosis
   (c) Joint space narrowing
   (d) Localized erosions of articular margins
3. Which of the following is not a surgical option in a hip joint that has ankylosed following tuberculosis of the hip?
   (a) Corrective osteotomy
   (b) Arthrolysis
   (c) Arthrodesis
   (d) Girdlestone excision arthroplasty
4. All of the following are seen in the stage of advanced tubercular arthritis of the hip except:
   (a) Frank anterior hip dislocation
   (b) Protrusio acetabuli
   (c) Wandering acetabulum
   (d) Mortar and pestle appearance
5. The earliest change of tubercular arthritis on X-ray is:
   (a) Wandering acetabulum
   (b) Increased bone density
   (c) Rarefaction of bones adjacent to the joint
   (d) Narrowing of joint space

Answers: 1. (c), 2 (a), 3. (b), 4. (a), 5. (d)

Tuberculosis of Knee and Other Joints

41

Kumar Keshav and Siddhartha Singh

41.1 Introduction

Tuberculosis (TB) of knee is the third most common site (accounting for around one-tenth) of osteoarticular tuberculosis. Unlike spine and hip, one can make an early diagnosis because knee is located superficially and gives rise to obvious swelling and limitation of movements early in the course of the disease. Anti-tubercular treatment (ATT) is the mainstay of treatment. If treatment is not initiated on time, it can lead to triple dislocation (deformity) of knee. If diagnosed late along the course of disease, some kind of surgical intervention like synovectomy, joint debridement, arthrodesis, or arthroplasty may be required, depending upon the stage of the disease [1–3].

41.2 Etiopathogenesis

As with other forms of musculoskeletal tuberculosis, the tubercle bacilli travel through the bloodstream from a site of primary focus, such as lungs, kidneys, and lymph nodes, to affect the axial and appendicular skeletal system. The most common sites involved in the knee are the synovium (Synovial tuberculosis) or the subchondral bone or any juxta-articular area (Osseous tuberculosis). The bacilli at these sites initiate a series of events which can lead to the formation of caseating granulomas, thickening of the synovium, pannus formation resulting in the destruction of articular cartilage and abscess formation. The articular cartilage becomes detached from the parent bone and may lie freely as flakes within the joint. In advanced stages, there may be gross bony destruction over weight-bearing areas. The soft tissue structures, like joint capsule and ligaments, are stretched and disrupted, leading to triple deformity- Knee joint flexion, posterolateral subluxation, and external rotation with abduction of tibia. Due to the buildup of pus, the joint may burst open to give rise to a subcutaneous cold abscess or even a sinus [1–4].

41.3 Pathological Changes

Pathological changes depend upon the part of knee joint (synovium or bone) that is affected first [5–7] (Table 41.1)

K. Keshav (✉)
Department of Orthopaedics, Sanjay Gandhi Post Graduate Institute of Medical Sciences, Lucknow, Uttar Pradesh, India

S. Singh
SGPGIMS, Lucknow, Uttar Pradesh, India

V. Kumar et al. (eds.), *A Quick Guide to Essential Orthopedics*,
https://doi.org/10.1007/978-981-95-2676-5_41

Table 41.1 Pathological changes seen in the tuberculosis of knee joint

	Osseous tuberculosis	
Synovial tuberculosis	Primary Metaphyseal involvement	Primary Epiphyseal involvement
Majority of tuberculosis of knee starts from synovium.	Second most common site	Only a small proportion of cases have involvement of epiphysis as the initial focus of infection
The tubercle bacilli can produce marked changes in the synovium in the form of hyperemia and inflammation. This will cause the synovial membrane to become swollen and congested due to granulation tissue. There is effusion within the joint, leading to clinical appearance of swollen joint. Many times, tubercular synovitis may continue for months without any damage to the articular cartilage or underlying bone. Hence, this stage is often painless. However, the swelling within the joint can cause stretching of the inflamed synovial membrane lining the capsule and ligaments, giving rise to pain. In the later stages, tubercular granulation tissue, like the pannus, erodes the articular cartilage and the sequestrated cartilages may lie freely within the joint cavity. This is clinically apparent as arthritis with reduction of joint space. From the ulcerated cartilage, the infection progresses to bone, which causes further reduction in joint space and osseous lesions in the subchondral bone. The granulation tissue may destroy the ligaments and capsule, giving rise to pathological dislocation, which is clinically apparent as triple deformity of knee.	In these cases, the lesion remains localized for some time following which there is sympathetic effusion within the joint. The lesion may cross the physis and involve the epiphysis. From here, it may ulcerate through the articular cartilage within the joint. Large areas of bony destruction are seen radiologically because of the abscesses, leading to bony destruction.	In such cases, primary focus may be just underneath the articular cartilage or close to physis. Gradually, it works its way through the articular cartilage to the joint.

41.4 Stages of Tuberculosis of Knee

Based on the natural history of disease, tuberculosis of knee when untreated, goes through the following stages [1, 2, 5–7].

1. Stage of synovitis: The tubercle bacilli can produce marked changes in the synovium in the form of hyperemia and inflammation. This will cause the synovial membrane to become swollen, and in most cases, congestion will be present in the synovium due to granulation tissue.
2. Stage of early arthritis: As the disease process ensues, synovium attempts to heal itself by fibrosis, resulting in thickening of its membrane. The granulation tissue starts spreading over the articular cartilage.
3. Stage of late arthritis: The erosion of the articular cartilage is more evident in this stage. Caseous lesions may be present in the subchondral bone. The surrounding bone will show features of decalcification. Joint space will be increasingly diminished in this stage.
4. Stage of advanced arthritis: The granulation tissue in the form of pannus will cause complete erosion of the articular cartilage. There will be destruction of the bony architecture of the subchondral and metaphyseal regions. Joint space obliteration will be seen due to involvement of the periarticular tissues, capsule, and various ligaments. Triple deformity will be most evident in this stage.
5. Stage of terminal arthritis: The joint space is completely reduced in this stage. The destruction and healing process in the periarticular,

subchondral, and metaphyseal regions will result in ankylosis of the knee joint.

41.5 Clinical Presentation

Tuberculosis of knee can affect people of any age group. However, this is a disease more commonly found in children. The clinician must have a high index of suspicion to diagnose the onset of disease at an early stage. Evening rise of temperature, loss of appetite, weight loss, night cries/sweats are the systemic symptoms, like in any other kind of osteoarticular tuberculosis.

The classical symptoms of knee joint pain (gradual onset) as well as swelling can be seen in majority of the patients. As the disease continues to spread, there will be marked limitation of movement of the affected joint. A combination of the above symptoms will start bringing about changes of wasting in the surrounding muscle groups. This can result in increased stiffness combined with deformities which occur at a later stage [1–3, 8, 9].

Clinical signs Depending upon the stage, one or more of the following may be found [1, 5, 6].

1. Knee joint swelling- More often, it is the first clinical sign to appear. Initially, the swelling is evident in the medial parapatellar fossa, which gradually involves all aspects of joint, like suprapatellar area and even in popliteal fossa. The skin may be stretched and give a whitish look—referred to as tumor alba (white swelling).
2. Tenderness is most marked at the joint line and at synovial reflections.
3. Raised temperature- The swollen knee is often warm on palpation due to hyperemia within the joint.
4. Synovitis- The synovial hypertrophy gives a doughy feel of the synovium on palpation. It is felt best on the medial aspect of knee.
5. Limitation of joint movements—In the initial synovitis and early arthritis stages, there will be only terminal restriction. Later, it may increase due to pain and spasm of muscles. In the advanced arthritis stage, there may be fibrous ankylosis leading to almost completely stiff joint.
6. Muscle wasting- Quadriceps wasting is quite apparent even in early stages.
7. Deformity- In the advanced stages, due to the spasm and contracture of hamstring muscles (especially biceps femoris), there may be pathological dislocations giving rise to a classical deformity known as triple deformity. As the name mentions, it has three components: (i) Flexion of knee, (ii) External rotation and valgus at the knee, and (c) Posterior subluxation of tibia. While the deformity has set in, there is a stage where beyond a certain degree of flexion, tensor fascia lata starts acting as a flexor leading to further accentuation of deformity.
8. Shortening or lengthening of limb—Usually due to bony destruction and damage to the epiphysis or premature physeal closure, there may be shortening. Premature physeal closure was seen earlier in cases where the lower limb is kept in high groin cast or hip-spica and was referred to as "Frame Knee". However, at times, due to hyperemia leading to increased activity of the physis, lengthening may be seen.

41.6 Investigations

1. *Blood Investigations*: They are like the ones described earlier and include the following:
   (a) *Complete Blood Count*: Lymphocytic leukocytosis with raised ESR
   (b) *Interferon Gamma Release Assays (IGRAs)*: The patient's blood cells are stimulated with M. tuberculosis-specific antigens which will result in the formation of gamma interferon which is measured in this test. These T-cell assays have a drawback of not being able to differentiate active form of the disease from latent infection.
   (c) *Polymerase Chain Reaction (PCR) Testing*: TB-PCR tests, although highly specific, lack the required amount of sen-

sitivity. The test can be performed with tissue specimens, synovial fluid, blood, and bone marrow aspirate. This test is unable to distinguish a living bacillus from a dead bacillus. However, it can be employed for the diagnosis in a shorter duration of time when compared to the gold standard test [1, 3].

2. *Synovial Fluid examination and synovial biopsy*: The synovial fluid in TB knee has a turbid and non-hemorrhagic appearance. It will demonstrate an increased white blood cell count (polymorphonuclear leukocytosis). Synovial biopsy can be used to confirm the diagnosis microscopically with the presence of increased lymphocytes, caseating granulomas, and giant cells [3].
3. *Tissue Diagnosis* [1–3]
   (a) *Microscopy*: Traditionally, microscopy and culture for confirming the presence of acid-fast bacilli (AFB) in the tissue has been considered the gold standard investigation to establish the diagnosis of tuberculosis.
   (b) *Culture*: The biopsied tissue (usually synovium) or the tissue taken after thorough debridement may be subjected to culture in one of the specific culture media for tuberculosis.
4. *Imaging Studies*
   (a) *X-ray*: Initial stage of synovitis may reveal increased soft-tissue swelling and osteoporosis. The stage of early arthritis is marked with the appearance of Phemister's triad (Fig. 41.1)—peripheral osseous erosions, joint space narrowing, and juxta-articular osteopenia/ osteoporosis. In late arthritis, marginal erosions and osseous destruction may be evident. In advanced arthritis stage, there may be gross diminution of joint space, marked osteolysis due to bony destruction, and presence of triple deformity [1–3].

   Based on X-rays, Kerri and Martini staged the radiological changes seen in tuberculosis of knee in the order of increasing severity [9] (Table 41.2)

   (b) *CT scan*: CT helps to identify the changes in the bony architecture, and it provides a broader perspective in assessing deformity of the involved region. The findings which can be seen on CT scans are the presence of a kissing sequestrum (wedge-shaped necrotic areas near the involved area) and widespread areas of bony destruction.
   (c) *MRI*: MRI has an upper hand in delineating the changes occurring in the soft tis-

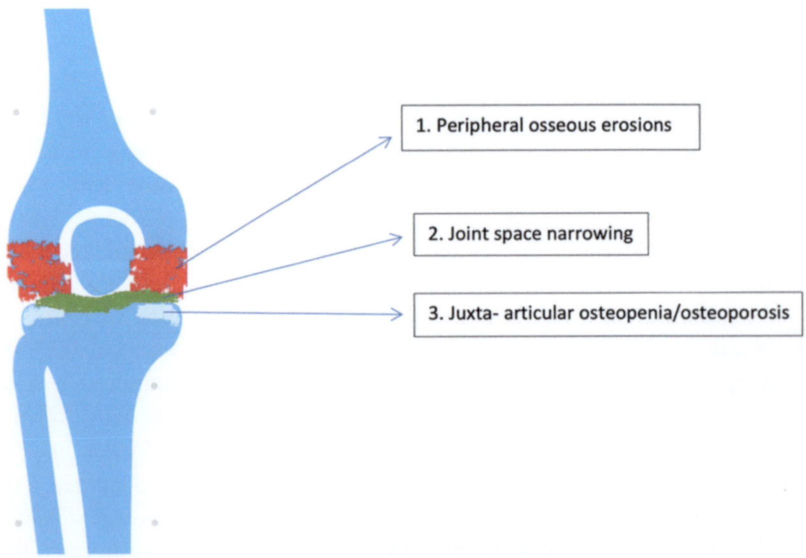

Fig. 41.1 Phemister triad

Table 41.2 Kerri and Martini classification

Stage	Radiographic findings
1	Localized osteopenia, no bone lesions, +/− soft tissue swelling
2	One or more areas of osseous erosion, without narrowing of the joint space
3	Narrowing of the joint space without gross anatomical disorganization
4	Narrowing of the joint space with gross anatomical disorganization

sues of the affected area. MRI findings can demonstrate chronic pannus, synovial changes (decreased signal intensity in synovium), effusion, presence of abscess, as well as peripheral/central bony erosions. It has increased sensitivity in determining the area and amount of joint capsule, cartilage, and subchondral bone involvement [8].

41.7 Differential Diagnosis

Various arthritic conditions of the body may have similar kind of presentation as Tuberculosis of knee, especially in the initial stages [4]. Some of them are as follows:

1. Rheumatoid arthritis/ Juvenile Rheumatoid Arthritis
2. Subacute pyogenic arthritis/synovitis
3. Villonodular synovitis
4. Synovial chondromatosis
5. Hemarthrosis
6. Hemophilic arthropathy
7. Osteomyelitis

41.8 Management

Achieving a painless, mobile joint is the ultimate aim of treatment. However, it may not always be possible, especially if the patient presents late in the natural course of the disease. The treatment is usually started conservatively by starting anti-tubercular treatment (ATT) and application of splintage/traction. Care should also be taken to improve the general well-being of the patient, like clean air, adequate sunshine, and nutritious diet. In late cases and nonresponders, surgical intervention may be required [1, 3, 4].

41.9 Conservative Treatment

41.9.1 Antimicrobial Therapy

The duration for which multidrug anti-tubercular treatment (ATT) can be given to the patient is controversial. Usually, the most common routine practice is (a) An Intensive phase for a period of 2 months consisting of four drugs—Isoniazid, Rifampicin, Pyrazinamide, and Ethambutol followed by a maintenance phase of two drugs—Isoniazid and Rifampicin for a period of 7 to 16 months, depending upon the resolution of the disease. Since the antitubercular drugs come with surplus side effects, regular monitoring of the hematological parameters must be done (preferably 2–3 months) [1–5, 7, 9].

41.9.2 Splintage, Traction, and Progressive Mobilization

Splinting the involved area results in a relief of symptoms as it can prevent excess movements at the knee joint. Traction plays an important in relieving the muscle spasm. It also prevents the diseased and damaged articular surfaces to come in contact with each other, resulting in a decreased amount of pain, delay in the development of deformities, and maintenance of the joint space. In children presenting with triple deformity, double traction is required, wherein there is an additional traction in the anterior direction to combat the posterior subluxation.

Once the pain and swelling have subsided a bit, gradual knee mobilization has to be started. Initially, gentle active and active-assisted movements are started. Usually, by the end of three months, partial weight-bearing ambulation on crutches or orthosis may be started. Depending upon the healing, full-weight-bearing may be started around 6–9 months after the onset of disease treatment [1].

41.10 Surgical Treatment Options

Depending upon the stage and severity of the disease, one or more of the following surgeries may be done [1–4, 8, 10].

1. *Synovectomy*: In cases where the diagnosis is still uncertain, or in cases where the response to conservative treatment is not favorable, removal of the synovium may help in tissue diagnosis, reduce the disease burden and lead to a faster response to ATT. Usually, a medial or lateral parapatellar approach is required for getting synovectomy done. One should make an attempt to remove as much as of synovium as possible. Nowadays, this can be done by arthroscopic means.
2. *Abscess drainage, Debridement*: The site of the abscess can be incised and drained if required. Arthroscopy can aid in the debridement of the knee joint, synovectomy and adhesion release. It has the advantage of being minimally invasive. However, a radical debridement is often missed in arthroscopic procedure for which an open procedure may be preferred. Tissue biopsy can be sent along with these procedures for a definite diagnosis.
3. *Arthrodesis*: Arthrodesis can be considered in patients where extensive destruction of the articular surface has occurred. It should be performed in the functional position of the knee joint. Charnley's compression arthrodesis of knee is the most commonly done procedure. Other methods, like Crossed K-wires or Steinmann pins, Ilizarov apparatus, Kuntscher's nail, and angled plates, may be used. Although arthrodesis serves its purpose of alleviation of pain, it renders the joint completely motionless, resulting in functional limitation for the patient. Proper counseling and consent of the patient are a must before performing the procedure.
4. *Joint Replacement Surgery*: A Total Knee Replacement can be considered in patients with severe deformities and in those who want a good pain-free range of motion. Although there can be a risk of reactivation of tuberculosis, several studies are showing promising results with effective antitubercular therapy pre- and post-surgery. A duration of 3 months of ATT must be given to such patients before as well as after surgery.

41.11 Simplified Treatment Algorithm

Figure 41.2 summarizes the treatment plan for tuberculosis of knee

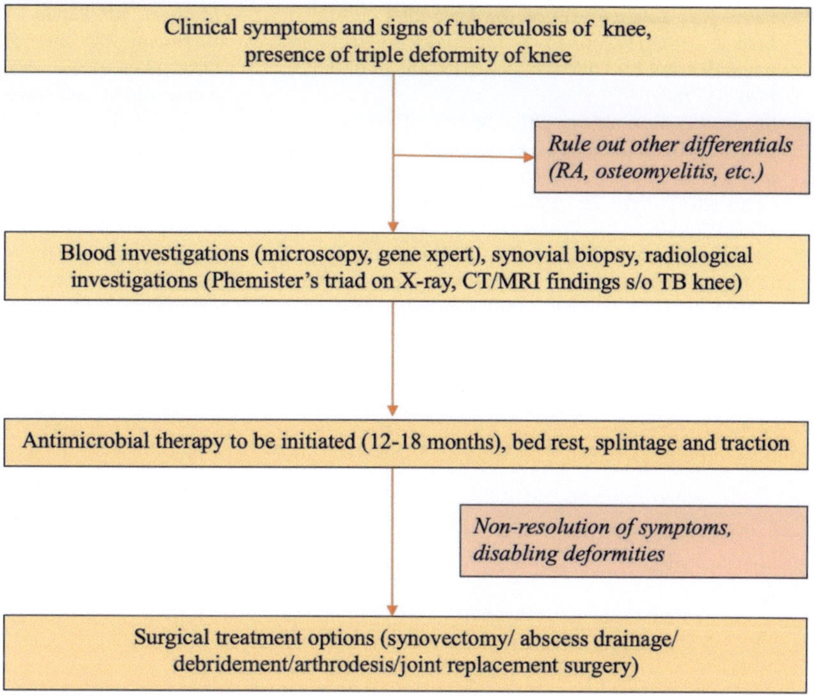

Fig. 41.2 Treatment algorithm for tuberculosis of knee

Multiple Choice Questions

1. Which of the following is not a feature of triple deformity of knee?
   (a) Flexion of knee
   (b) External rotation of tibia
   (c) Varus deformity at the knee
   (d) Posterior subluxation of tibia
2. Tubercular arthritis of knee in advanced stages leads to:
   (a) Fibrous ankylosis
   (b) Bony ankylosis
   (c) Charcot's joint
   (d) Loose joint
3. What is the functional position of knee in which arthrodesis of knee is done?
   (a) Full extension
   (b) 5–10 degrees of flexion
   (c) 10–20 degrees of internal rotation
   (d) 20–30 degrees of external rotation
4. Which of the following is not a clinical finding in tubercular arthritis of knee?
   (a) Joint tenderness
   (b) Limitation of joint movements
   (c) Raised temperature
   (d) Quadriceps hypertrophy
5. Which of the following is not a treatment modality for synovitis stage of tubercular arthritis of knee?
   (a) Anti-tubercular drugs
   (b) Traction
   (c) Arthrodesis
   (d) Splintage

Answers: 1. (c), 2. (a), 3. (b), 4. (d), 5. (c)

References

1. Tuli SM, editor. Tuberculosis of the skeletal system. 5th ed. New Delhi: Jaypee Brothers Medical Publishers; 2016.
2. Lee AS, Campbell JA, Hoffman EB. Tuberculosis of the knee in children. J Bone Joint Surg Br. 1995;77(2):313–8. PMID: 7706356.
3. Hoffman EB, Allin J, Campbell JA, Leisegang FM. Tuberculosis of the knee. Clin Orthop Relat Res. 2002;398:100–6. https://doi.org/10.1097/00003086-200205000-00014. PMID: 11964637.
4. Chow SP, Yau A. Tuberculosis of the knee -- a long term follow-up. Int Orthop. 1980;4(2):87–92. https://doi.org/10.1007/BF00271090. PMID: 7429686.

5. Paton RY. Tuberculosis of the knee-joint. Postgrad Med J. 1943;19(206):11–7. https://doi.org/10.1136/pgmj.19.206.11. PMID: 21313285; PMCID: PMC2477887.
6. Scanzello CR, Goldring SR. The role of synovitis in osteoarthritis pathogenesis. Bone. 2012;51(2):249–57. https://doi.org/10.1016/j.bone.2012.02.012. Epub 2012 Feb 22. PMID: 22387238; PMCID: PMC3372675.
7. Vankayalapati R, Barnes PF. Innate and adaptive immune responses to human Mycobacterium tuberculosis infection. Tuberculosis (Edinb). 2009;89 Suppl 1:S77–S80. https://doi.org/10.1016/S1472-9792(09)70018-6. PMID: 20006312.
8. Mahajan NP, Pande KP, Dadhaniya RR, Talukder P, Bagimani PK. Surgical management of aggressive knee tuberculosis with open subtotal synovectomy - a case report and review of literature. J Orthop Case Rep. 2022;12(3):48–51. https://doi.org/10.13107/jocr.2022.v12.i03.2712. PMID: 36199929; PMCID: PMC9499057.
9. Kerri O, Martini M. Tuberculosis of the knee. Int Orthop 1985;9(3):153–157. https://doi.org/10.1007/BF00268165. PMID: 4077334.
10. Tan SM, Chin PL. Total hip arthroplasty for surgical management of advanced tuberculous hip arthritis: case report. World J Orthop. 2015;6(2):316–21. https://doi.org/10.5312/wjo.v6.i2.316. PMID: 25793173; PMCID: PMC4363815.

42 Tubercular Osteomyelitis

Varun Garg and Manuj Jain

42.1 Introduction

Tubercular osteomyelitis accounts for around 2–3% of all TB osteoarticular manifestations. The tibia is the most often affected long bone, followed by the ulna, radius, femur, fibula and humerus.

42.2 Etiopathogenesis

Tuberculosis of the bone occurs due to hematogenous dissemination after primary infection in the lung. Because of the abundant vascular supply, the initial focus becomes lodged in the metaphyseal region. Following this exudative inflammatory reaction of the bone occurs. Decalcification of the bone is caused by localized hyperaemia. This reaction, however, is frequently restricted by a fibroblastic response. When this healing response cannot control the damage, the infection travels along the route of least resistance, up and down the shaft of the bone and the periphery of the bone, to the subperiosteal space before breaking into the soft tissue. This could appear like a cold abscess for several months before developing into sinus formation.

It is vital to understand how a child's bone differs from an adult's bone. The physis in children acts as a natural barrier to prevent infection from spreading into the epiphysis and joints. However, there is a lack of anastomosis of the intra-osseous vascular supply. As a result, thrombosis caused by the inflammatory response might result in severe diaphyseal sequestration.

42.3 Clinical Features

Tubercular infection of the bone has an insidious onset. Usually, there is mono-osseous involvement, but it may involve other visceral organs (lungs, intestine and kidneys). Family history is usually positive with the presence of constitutional symptoms such as low-grade evening rise of temperature, anorexia, weight loss, night sweats, malaise, tachycardia and anaemia.

The patient presents with complaints of pain and swelling of the bone involved. On examination, there is a local rise of temperature, tenderness and thickening of the underlying bone. Movements of the adjacent joints may be restricted due to muscle spasm. An accompanying cold abscess, discharging sinus, and swelling of the regional lymph nodes may be present.

V. Garg (✉)
Department of Pediatric Orthopedics, Chacha Nehru Bal Chikatsalya, New Delhi, India

M. Jain
Department of Orthopaedics, 166 Military Hospital, Jammu, Jammu and Kashmir, India

V. Kumar et al. (eds.), *A Quick Guide to Essential Orthopedics*,
https://doi.org/10.1007/978-981-95-2676-5_42

42.4 Investigations

- Complete blood count—it shows anaemia and lymphocytosis.
- ESR and CRP—these are markers of inflammation and are elevated in tuberculosis.
- X-ray—Radiographs of the affected part show irregular cavities (caseating necrosis) surrounded by incomplete sclerosis (healing response) (Fig. 42.1). Cavities may contain dense coke-like sequestrum due to the deposition of calcium in the central caseation. Periosteal reaction is usually seen when the lesion is superficial. In children, there may be a presence of sitting a stride lesion across the growth plate (Fig. 42.2).
- Ultrasonography—it is useful for detecting soft tissue swelling especially when the abscess is deep-seated. It may help in guided aspiration of the pus.
- Computerized tomography—the role of CT is limited in tubercular osteomyelitis. However, it is useful in certain areas where radiographs are difficult to interpret such as ribs and sternum.
- MRI—it is a very sensitive investigation and can diagnose the disease in the pre-destructive stage of the disease. Moreover, it shows abscesses in multiple planes.
- Diagnosis of tubercular osteomyelitis should be confirmed by microbiological evidence of mycobacterium before starting ATT. A biopsy should be done after all the radiological investigations have been done. The specimen obtained should be sent for culture, ZN stain, CBNAAT and histopathological examination.

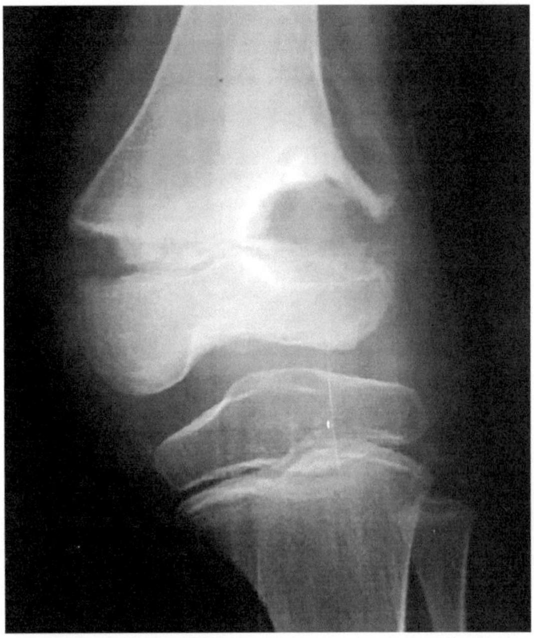

Fig. 42.2 Sitting-stride lesion in a 9-year-old child

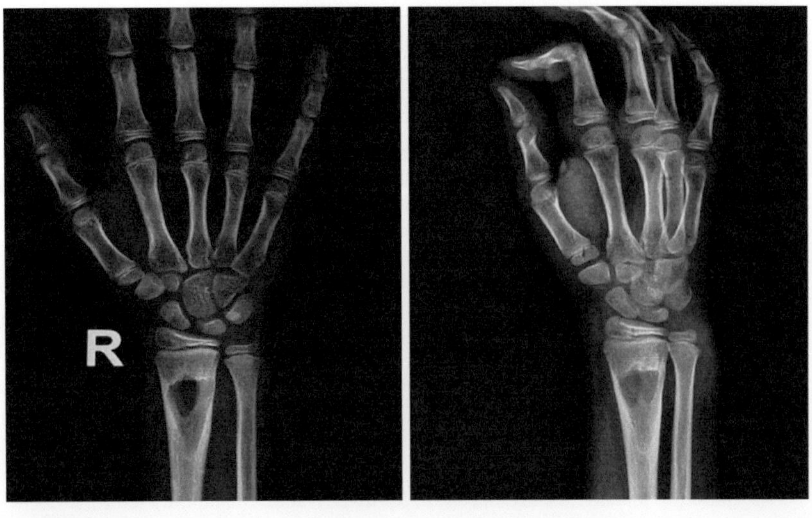

Fig. 42.1 Lytic lesion in the metaphysis of the distal radius surrounded by incomplete sclerosis

42.5 Differential Diagnosis

- Chronic pyogenic osteomyelitis
- Brodie's abscess
- Tumours

42.6 Treatment

- General care—High-protein diet and vitamins should be started to improve the general condition of the patient. Limb should be immobilized in a slab to prevent pathological fracture and reduce pain.
- Chemotherapy—Response to ATT is usually favourable with resolution of the radiographic lesion by 6 months (Fig. 42.3). ATT should be continued for 12–18 months.

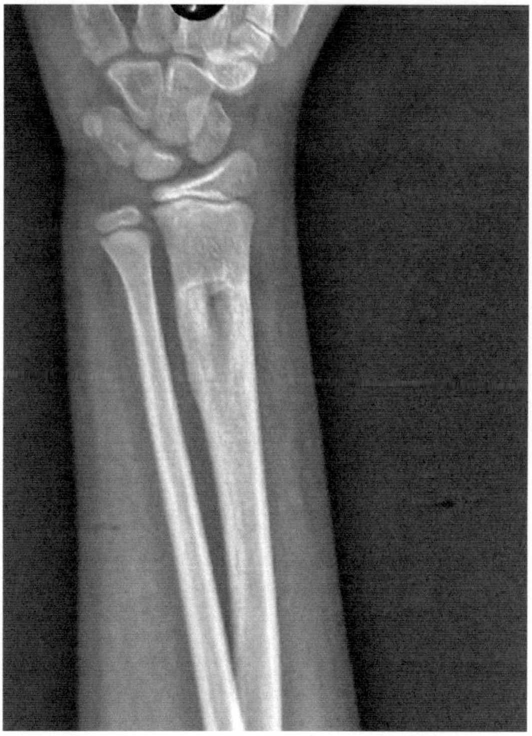

Fig. 42.3 Near-complete healing of the lesion after 7 months of ATT in the same patient

- Surgical intervention—it is indicated when the abscess is very large or in refractory cases.

References

1. Tuli SM. Tuberculosis of the skeletal system (Bones, joints, spine and bursal sheaths). 4th ed. New Delhi: Jaypee Brothers Medical Publishers Pvt. Ltd; 2010. pp. 4, 69–110.
2. Jain AK. Tuberculosis of bones, joints, and spine: evidence-based management guide. 1st ed. New Delhi: CBS Publishers and Distributors Pvt. LTD; 2017. pp. 4, 44–69.
3. Index-TB guidelines- guidelines on extra-pulmonary tuberculosis for India. Ministry of Health and Family Welfare, Government of India.

Tuberculous Infections of the Hand

43

Varun Garg

43.1 Introduction

Tuberculosis of the hand and wrist can have a varied presentation. The disease can present as tenosynovitis, dactylitis, arthritis, bursitis, carpal tunnel syndrome, and paronychia. There is usually a delay in diagnosis, leading to poor outcomes in these patients.

43.2 Tubercular tenosynovitis

It is the most common tubercular affection of the hand. The flexor side is more affected than the extensor, and the ulnar side is more affected than the radial side. Tendon rupture may occur as a result of a delay in diagnosis. A compound palmar ganglion is an uncommon symptom caused by chronic tenosynovitis of long flexor tendons at the wrist or palm. This mass can occasionally compress the median nerve, resulting in carpal tunnel syndrome [1].

43.3 Etiopathogenesis

The disease is considered to spread to the synovial sheaths by direct hematogenous dissemination or through underlying bone/joint disease. The infected synovium becomes edematous and is filled with granulations. With time, these granulations become hyperplastic, thickened, and villous. With movement and friction, the villi get broken and resemble rice bodies/melon seeds. They are similar to the rice bodies/melon seeds of rheumatoid arthritis.

43.4 Tubercular Dactylitis

Tuberculous infection of the metacarpals, metatarsals, and phalanges of the hands and feet is known as tuberculous dactylitis. It is usually seen in children less than 5 years of age. The hand is involved more commonly than the foot. Tuberculous infection of the hand leads to spindle-shaped enlargement of the bone known as *spina ventosa*. Spina ventosa is a Latin word with "Spina" meaning short bones and "Ventosa" meaning filled with air [1].

43.5 Etiopathogenesis

During early childhood, a single nutrient artery enters the center of the bones. Hence, the initial focus gets trapped in the center of marrow cavity of the short tubular bone, leading to destruction of internal lamellae and endosteal bone. This leads to the formation of *spina ventosa*. Over a period of time, repeated layers of subperiosteal new bone are deposited over the involved bone [1].

V. Garg (✉)
Department of Pediatric Orthopedics, Chacha Nehru Bal Chikatsalya, New Delhi, India

V. Kumar et al. (eds.), *A Quick Guide to Essential Orthopedics*,
https://doi.org/10.1007/978-981-95-2676-5_43

43.6 Clinical Features

Like other tubercular infections of the bone, it has an insidious onset. Family history is usually positive with the presence of constitutional symptoms such as low-grade evening rise of temperature, anorexia, weight loss, night sweats, malaise, tachycardia, and anemia.

The patient presents with complaints of pain and swelling of the hand. On examination, there is a local rise of temperature, tenderness, and thickening of the underlying bone (spina ventosa). Movements of the interphalangeal/ MCP joints may be restricted. It may be associated with boggy swelling of the synovium, discharging sinus, and swelling of the regional lymph nodes (axillary and supratrochlear). Rarely, signs of medial nerve palsy can also be seen. Other findings on examination are wasting of the forearm, thenar, and hypothenar eminences [2].

43.7 Investigations

- Complete blood count—it shows anemia and lymphocytosis.
- ESR and CRP—these are markers of inflammation and are elevated in tuberculosis.
- X-ray—Radiographs shows localized osteoporosis, increased soft tissue shadows, decreased joint space, marginal erosions, ballooning of cortex of metacarpals (spina ventosa), and irregular cavities surrounded by incomplete sclerosis. Cavities may contain dense coke-like sequestrum. Periosteal reaction can also be seen.
- Ultrasonography—There are no pathognomonic findings on USG. It may show cold abscess, collection in bursae, hyperechoic bodies (rice bodies), and synovial hypertrophy. It may also be helpful for aspiration of collection for microbiological and histopathological confirmation.
- Computerized tomography—The role of CT is limited, and findings are nonspecific.
- MRI—It is a very sensitive investigation, but findings are usually nonspecific. These findings include high signal on T-2-weighted images and low signal on T-1-weighted images, which is suggestive of marrow edema, tenosynovitis, joint effusion, or cold abscess. Rice bodies are usually represented by low signal dots scattered in the synovial fluid on T-2-weighted images.
- Diagnosis of tubercular osteomyelitis should be confirmed by microbiological evidence of *Mycobacterium tuberculosis* before starting ATT. A biopsy should be done after all the radiological investigations have been completed. The specimen obtained should be sent for culture, ZN stain, CBNAAT, and histopathological examination.

43.8 Differential Diagnosis

- Pyogenic arthritis
- Fungal arthritis
- Gout
- Pigmented villo-nodular synovitis
- Rheumatoid arthritis
- Hemophilic arthropathy
- Sarcoidosis
- Tumors (giant cell tumor, Ewing's sarcoma, enchondroma)

43.9 Treatment

- General care—High-protein diet and vitamins should be started to improve the general condition of the patient. The limb should be immobilized in a functional position to relieve the patient from pain and spasm. After the pain has subsided, physiotherapy should be instituted to prevent stiffness of the fingers.
- Chemotherapy—ATT should be instituted for 12–18 months [3].
- Surgical intervention—most of the patients usually heal with good clinico-radiological outcomes after instituting chemotherapy and physiotherapy. Surgery is rarely required in cases where there is entrapment of the median nerve, deformity of the joints, impending collapse of the bone, or healed disease with fibrous ankylosis of the joints. Sometimes, surgery may also be required to obtain tissue for histopathological and microbiological confirmation (Figs. 43.1 and 43.2).

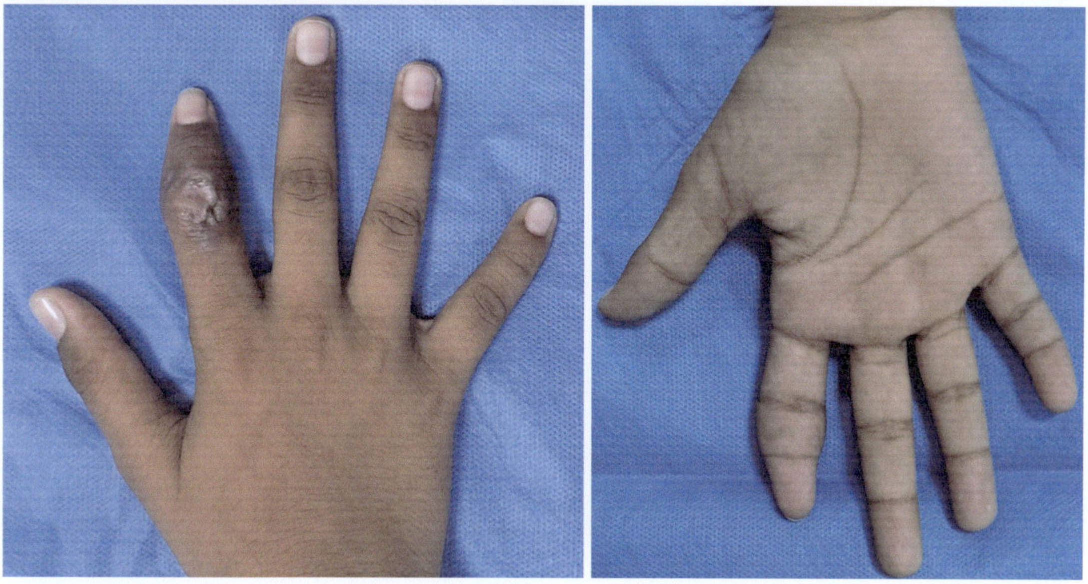

Fig. 43.1 Diffuse swelling of the right index finger at MCP joint (sausage finger)

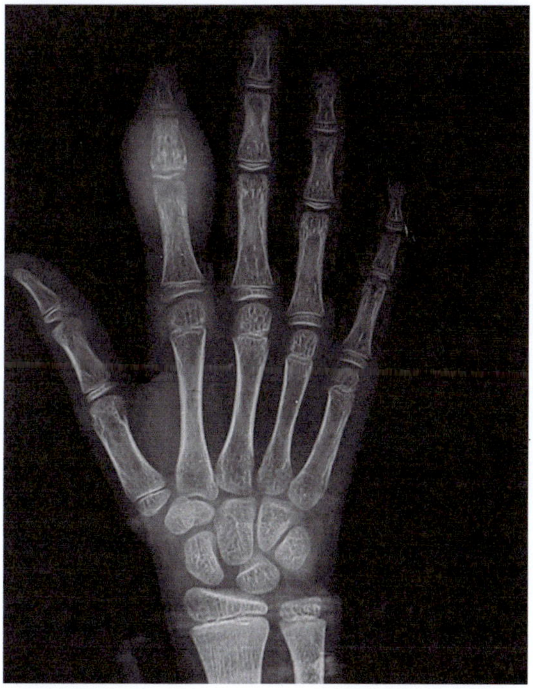

Fig. 43.2 Radiograph of the same patient showing ballooning of the middle phalanx of the right index finger with increased soft tissue collection

References

1. Tuli SM. Tuberculosis of the skeletal system (Bones, joints, spine and bursal sheaths). 4th ed. New Delhi: Jaypee Brothers Medical Publishers Pvt. Ltd; 2010. pp. 4, 69–110.
2. Jain AK. Tuberculosis of bones, joints, and spine: evidence-based management guide. 1st ed. New Delhi: CBS Publishers and Distributors Pvt. LTD; 2017. pp. 4, 44–69.
3. Index-TB guidelines- guidelines on extra-pulmonary tuberculosis for India. Ministry of Health and Family Welfare, Government of India.

Part V

Pediatric Orthopedics

44 Congenital Talipes Equinovarus

Kumar Suprashant and Vishal Kumar

Congenital clubfoot is the commonest foot deformity which presents at birth.

In India, of all the birth defects that are seen in children, this is the most common after Spina Bifida. It is estimated that clubfoot is seen in 0.8–1 per 1000 live births

44.1 Aetiology

The exact reason for development of clubfoot is not clearly understood. However, after the unravelling of the Genome sequence, many associations and key developmental pathways have been identified. Clubfoot is associated with intrauterine packaging issues such as primiparous mother, oligohydramnios, breech delivery, twin delivery and early amniocentesis. Most cases are idiopathic clubfeet, that is, they have no other associated anomalies.

Many cases are associated with spinal problems like myelomeningocele and spina bifida, while many others are associated with syndromes. Multiple congenital contracture (Arthrogryposis Multiplex Congenita) can also present as equinovarus deformity at birth. Several syndromes have clubfoot associated with their phenotype like Freeman–Sheldon Syndrome, TARP Syndrome and many others.

Acquired causes of equinovarus deformity may be in paralytic disorders like poliomyelitis and Charcot-Marie-Tooth Disease. With the eradication of paralytic poliomyelitis, Cerebral palsy with spastic paralysis has become a common cause of acquired equinovarus. It can also be acquired from traumatic paralysis of lateral popliteal nerve. In absence of any identifiable cause, clubfoot is idiopathic in the majority of cases.

While there is a clear male predilection, a positive family history in a first-degree relative may be associated, and a history of a sibling or relative should be sought at the first examination. A careful and thorough head-to-toe examination should be done to exclude any associated problems, as the outcome of treatment of Idiopathic clubfoot is different from that of non-idiopathic clubfoot. About 40% of cases are unilateral while 60% are bilateral.

K. Suprashant (✉)
Department of Orthopaedics, St Stephen's Hospital
New Delhi, New Delhi, India

V. Kumar
Department of Orthopaedics, PGIMER,
Chandigarh, Chandigarh, India

V. Kumar et al. (eds.), *A Quick Guide to Essential Orthopedics*,
https://doi.org/10.1007/978-981-95-2676-5_44

44.2 Deformities of Clubfoot

The acronym CAVE identifies the key deformities of clubfoot.

C	Cavus (increased arch of foot due to plantarflexion of first metatarsal and pronation of forefoot)
A	Adductus (bending of forefoot inside toward midline of body)
V	Varus (turning of foot mainly hindfoot medially)
E	Equinus (plantarflexion of foot)

The deformity is complex when seen in three dimensions with a complex and multiple axes of deformity. The forefoot is adducted, the whole foot is supinated with the sole of the foot turned medially, and the arch of the foot is exaggerated (cavus) because of the relative pronation of the forefoot in relation to the hind foot. The ankle is in severe equinus. The key to understanding the deformities and the correction sequence by the Ponseti method is that the calcaneum and the rest of the bones of the foot move as one unit beneath the talus that remains fixed in the ankle mortice. The talonavicular joint, therefore, becomes the fulcrum beneath which the calcaneum and the rest of the foot are manipulated to achieve correction of the deformity. In a typical clubfoot, the foot appears small compared to a normal foot, with the sole turned inward, the medial aspect hidden, and the lateral aspect prominent. Heel is small and turned inward. Inner side of foot is concave whereas the outer side is convex. Overall, the foot looks like a Golf Club.

44.3 Pathology of Clubfoot

There is considerable debate on the primary problem of clubfoot, whether it is the ligament capsule complex or the musculotendinous structures. The cartilaginous anlage of the osseous bones of the foot does show deformities, but if corrected before weight-bearing of the foot develops normally suggesting that possibly these are not primarily abnormal. The master of the evolution of the current gold standard of treatment of clubfoot believed that the primary problem is the presence of an abnormal, retracting fibrosis on the postero-medial joints of the foot in a child with clubfoot. Achilles tendon along with the posterior capsule of ankle joint are contracted contributing to the equinus at the ankle

44.4 Diagnosis

The typical deformities of cavus, adductus, varus and equinus present from birth in a child without any associated neuromuscular abnormalities suggest the diagnosis of idiopathic Clubfoot. However, a careful head-to-toe examination should be carried out to rule out other congenital anomalies of spine, hip, other joint contracture or associated syndromes before labelling a child as having idiopathic clubfoot.

44.5 Differential Diagnosis

A similar condition that has forefoot adduction but characteristically no equinus is a metatarsus adductus.

Postural clubfoot is exactly similar, but is different in that the deformities are very mild and are corrected in two or three casts.

Secondary, syndromic and acquired clubfeet are easily identified based on a careful history and physical examination.

44.6 Scoring

Several scoring systems have been designed to score the degree of severity of the deformity in a given child. Of these, the simplest and the most popular is the 6-point Pirani's Scoring system (Figs. 44.1, 44.2, and 44.3). In Pirani scoring system, we,

Look for two components, the crease on the medial side of the foot (medial crease) and on the posterior side of the foot (posterior crease).

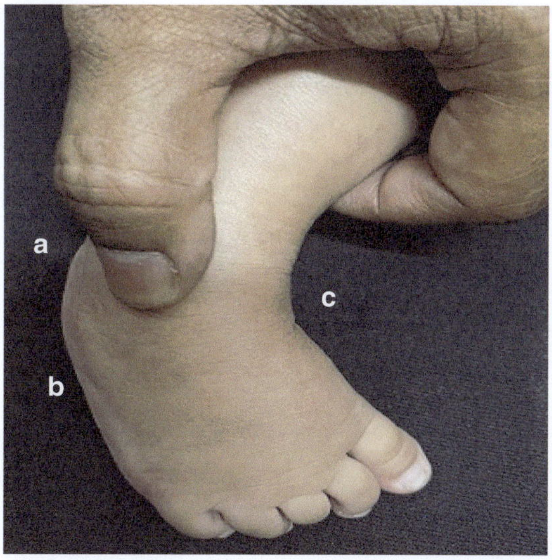

Fig. 44.1 (**a**) Thumb depicting position of talar head; (**b**) convex lateral border and (**c**) concave medial border

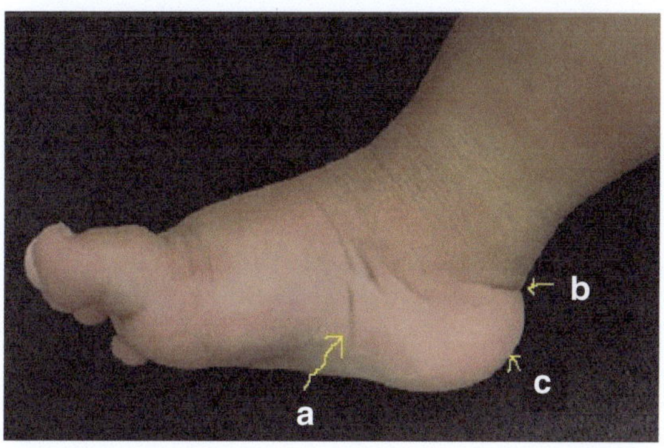

Fig. 44.2 (**a**) Medial crease; (**b**) posterior crease and (**c**) empty heel

Feel for two components, the softness of the edge of the back of the heel—soft, semisoft and hard (empty heel) and reducibility talar head (unreducible, partially reducible, completely reducible)

Measure for two components, the severity of equinus and how severely the lateral border is curved.

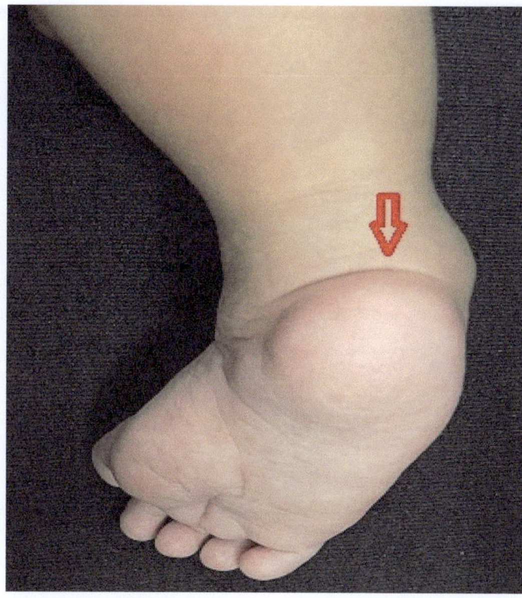

Fig. 44.3 Arrow depicting heel varus and posterior crease

Each of these is scored on a 3-point scoring system: 0, 0.5 and 1, with 0 being the best while 1 is the worst.

So, the best corrected foot score is "Zero," while the worst score is 6.

During the course of clubfoot treatment using the Ponseti method, a small subset of typically chubby children with severe deformities—despite showing initial correction—may develop cast slippage, leading to recurrence of equinus, shortening of the foot, a short and dorsiflexed great toe, and the appearance of a deep plantar crease across the sole (known as the plantaris crease). This iatrogenic condition is called a complex clubfoot (earlier called as atypical clubfeet). These feet cannot be corrected by the Ponseti method of manipulation but need a modified manipulation method where the forefoot is dorsiflexed with the fulcrum at the tarsometatarsal joint (Fig. 44.4).

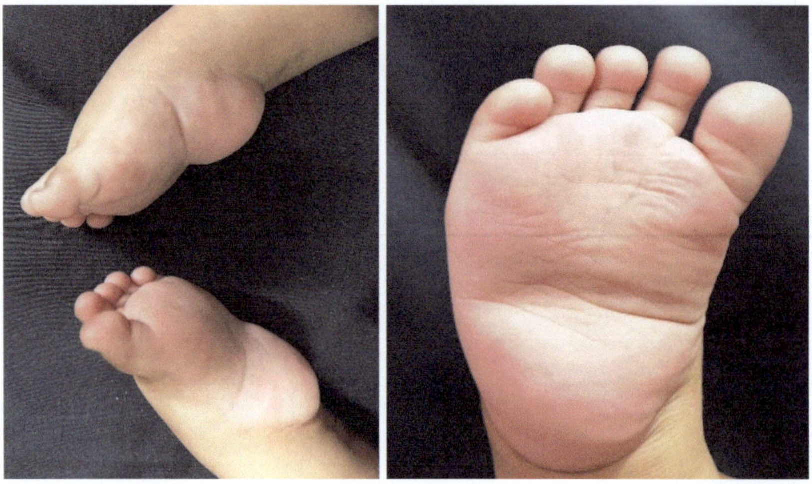

Fig. 44.4 Complex clubfoot—deep plantaris crease running from medial to lateral border of sole with severe plantarflexion of forefoot

44.7 Investigations

The diagnosis of clubfoot is essentially clinical, and no investigations are required in treatment of a case of idiopathic clubfoot. If it is a case of secondary or syndromic clubfoot, then the investigations relevant to the primary condition and or Syndrome may be essential.

In a syndromic foot or a foot with resistant or recurrent deformities, dorsiflexion lateral and antero-posterior views are taken. In the antero-posterior view, the plantar surface of the foot is kept on the cassette, and a 30-degree antero-posterior tilted view is taken. But most of the time radiographs are not essential.

44.8 Treatment

The aim of treatment is to provide a plantigrade foot which looks cosmetically and functionally normal, rests flat on the ground so that weight is evenly distributed over the foot, joints of the foot should be supple and painless throughout and after the treatment, and the foot should achieve a near normal function without the need for a permanent orthosis.

The current Gold standard of treatment is Ponseti method of manipulation. The method has a manipulation phase and correction phase followed by a maintenance phase. Both phases are equally important. This method is essentially a manipulation and serial casting method to correct cavus, adductus and varus. The rigid equinus at the ankle is corrected by a total tenotomy of the Tendoachilles at the level of the ankle. The manipulation is based on the principle that movements of the calcaneum and the rest of the foot occur beneath the talus in a kinematically coupled manner. The manipulation is done with the thumb on the fulcrum that is the head of the Talus and abducting the supinated foot. Every cast starts with the thumb on the head of the Talus, supinating the forefoot to bring it in line with the hindfoot and then abducting the foot. With each manipulative cast, the varus corrects as the foot goes from varus and adduction to valgus and abduction. The final correction is achieved by tenotomizing the Tendoachilles using a closed tenotomy under local anaesthesia. Usually, the manipulation requires 5 or 6 serial casts given weekly, a tenotomy followed by a 3-week casting. The maintenance phase entails wearing of a foot abduction brace for 23 hours a day for the first 3 months followed by night-time and nap-time for 5 years.

At final correction, the foot is in 40–70 degree of abduction with 10–20 degree of dorsiflexion.

Complications of casting can be pressure sores or compromised neurovascular status of foot due to inappropriate casting. To avoid complications, casting should be done by gentle manipulation with changing the pressure point by thumb over the time when cast is being moulded to the shape of the foot. Circulation of toes should be observed after casting and parents should be counselled to observe for any swelling, disappearance of toes within cast or decreased circulation of toes and remove cast if required. Slipping of cast can lead to complex clubfoot with similar picture to atypical clubfoot which need to be identified by history of slippage and clinical examination and corrected by modified Ponseti technique.

Most feet today in the younger child with Idiopathic clubfoot can be corrected by Ponseti method. However, depending on the age of the child and associated conditions, a few children may require surgical intervention. But unlike yesteryears, most children are benefitted by Ponseti's method (Figs. 44.5, 44.6, 44.7, 44.8, 44.9, and 44.10).

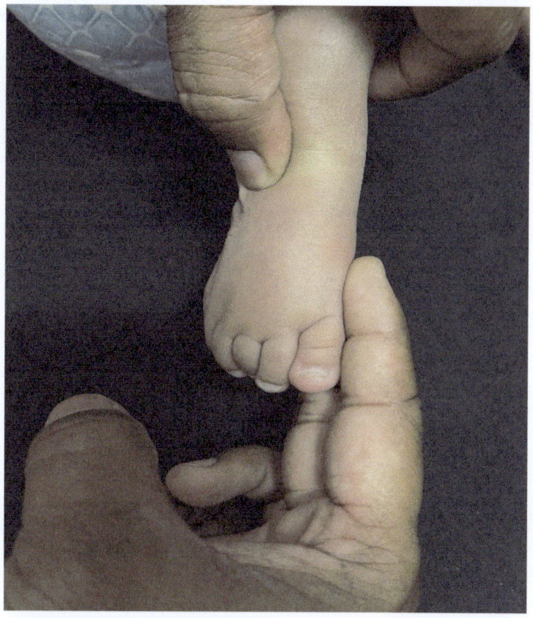

Fig. 44.6 Ponseti manipulation—with thumb over the head of talus which acts as fulcrum, the whole foot is abducted underneath the talus

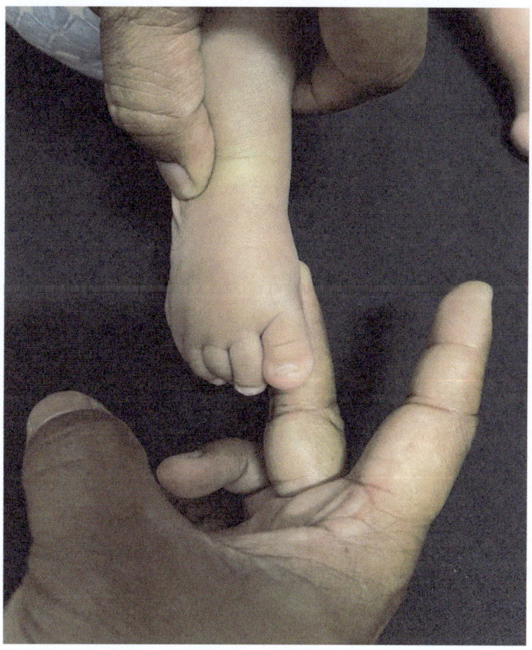

Fig. 44.5 Ponseti manipulation—supinating the forefoot to bring forefoot in line with hindfoot

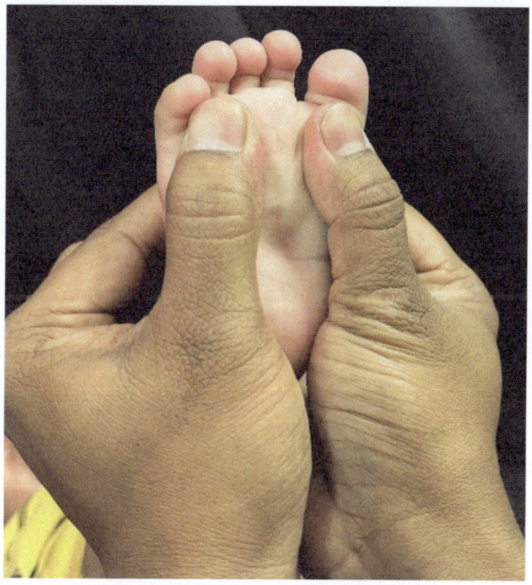

Fig. 44.7 Complex clubfoot—modified Ponseti manipulation (dorsiflexing the metatarsals by both thumbs with counter-pressure by index fingers on the dorsum of foot at tarsometatarsal joints (tarsometatarsal joints act as a fulcrum)

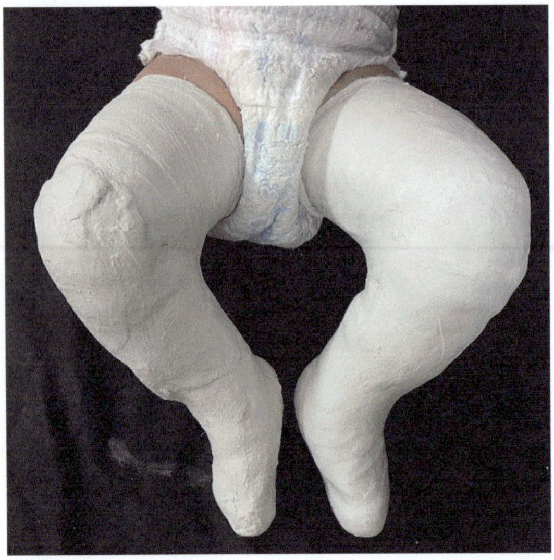

Fig. 44.8 Ponseti cast

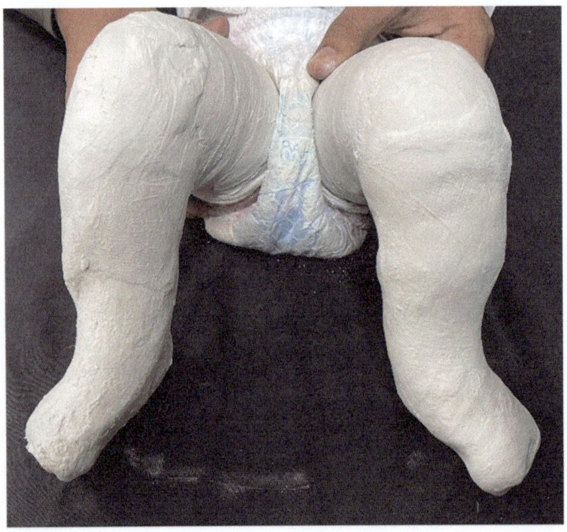

Fig. 44.9 Ponseti cast—with each serial cast abduction of foot is increased

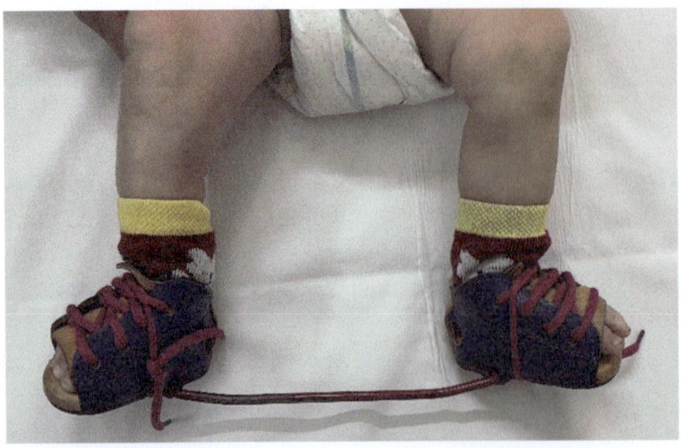

Fig. 44.10 Steenbeek foot abduction brace

44.9 Other Methods of Conservative Treatment

Kite's method J. H. Kite advocated serial manipulation and casting by treating each component separately, starting with forefoot adduction with fulcrum at calcaneocuboid joint, followed by heel varus (inversion) and finally equinus. One cannot proceed to the next deformity until the previous one was corrected. The correction took a long time of 7–8 months, and his results could not be reproduced by others and are rarely used now.

French physiotherapy (functional) method This method uses regular manipulation of newborn's foot, stimulation of muscles around the foot and temporary stabilization by strapping. The manipulation and strapping is done by the physical therapist who works closely with orthopaedist. An orthopaedist makes the initial diagnosis, assesses the severity according to Dimeglio score, refers to a physical therapist for manipulation and does monthly follow-ups.

44.10 Surgery

Surgery is rarely required for idiopathic clubfoot that presents in infancy.

Other techniques of correction are reserved for feet which do not respond to treatment by Ponseti method. These are usually neglected, resistant or relapsed cases especially in older and syndromic children.

Soft tissue release Usually in children after 1 years of age. Postero-medial soft tissue release, isolated posterior release, complete circumferential subtalar release can be done depending on which structure is tight or contracted. Access to the involved structures is through Turco (postero-medial incision), Cincinatti (transverse circumferential incision) and Caroll (postero-lateral and postero-medial incision)

Gradual distraction Gradual distraction by means of JESS or circular Ilizarov fixator is used in case of intractable and resistant cases of deformity. It can be combined with osteotomies to treat adults and adolescents with severe deformity, in which gradual correction initially provides soft tissue stretching and some correction of deformity, followed by osteotomy to treat the rest of deformity and stabilize the foot.

44.11 Tendon Transfers

Tibialis anterior tendon transfer is done to treat residual forefoot dynamic supination deformity where it is detached from its original insertion (medial cuneiform and first metatarsal) and rerouted to lateral cuneiform. It is done after 3 years of age.

44.12 Osteotomies

Open wedge osteotomy of the medial cuneiform to lengthen the medial column of foot.

Closed wedge osteotomy of cuboid to shorten the lateral column of foot.

Dwyer osteotomy (lateral closing wedge osteotomy of calcaneum to correct heel varus), Lichtblau procedure (lateral closing wedge osteotomy of calcaneum or cuboid enucleation to correct heel varus and shorten long lateral column of foot) and lateral displacement osteotomy of the calcaneum to correct heel varus. Dilwyn Evan's procedure—fusion of the calcaneocuboid joint along with PMSTR, fusion of calcaneocuboid joints leads to gradual correction of deformity by ongoing growth of medial side and decreased growth of fused lateral side.

Talectomy is reserved for severe cases of very stiff clubfeet with little or no ankle movement. It refers to complete surgical removal of talus and gives satisfactory results when performed between 1 and 6 years of age.

Triple arthrodesis (Arthrodesis of talonavicular, calcaneocuboid and talocalcaneal joint) is done in a skeletally mature foot (over 9–10 years of age). Lambrinudi's triple arthrodesis is done for isolated fixed equinus deformity.

Multiple Choice Questions

1. Which of the following is not a cause of clubfoot in a newborn?
   (a) Idiopathic
   (b) Arthrogryposis Multiplex Congenita
   (c) Rickets
   (d) Cerebral Palsy
2. What is the most common deformity seen in clubfoot?
   (a) Equinovalgus
   (b) Equinovarus
   (c) Calcaneovalgus
   (d) Calcaneovarus
3. What is the sequence of correction for a clubfoot deformity?
   (a) Equinus, Varus, Adduction, Cavus
   (b) Varus, Adduction, Cavus, Equinus
   (c) Adduction, Cavus, Equinus, Varus
   (d) Cavus, Adduction, Varus, Equinus
4. What is the best age to start the correction of clubfoot deformity in a newborn?
   (a) At 3 months of age
   (b) At 6 months of age
   (c) As early as possible, depending on skin condition
   (d) At 1 year of age
5. The Ponseti method of correction of CTEV involves:
   (a) Observation till 6 months of age
   (b) Splinting followed by correction
   (c) Sequential manipulation and casting followed by bracing
   (d) Postero-medial soft tissue release

Answers: 1. (c), 2. (b), 3. (d), 4. (c), 5. (c)

Developmental Dysplasia of Hip 45

Ritesh Arvind Pandey
and Alapati Hari Venkata Bramesh

45.1 Introduction

Developmental Dysplasia of Hip (DDH) was earlier known as congenital dislocation of hip (CDH). As some hips are not dislocated at birth and develop dysplastic changes in later life, the term CDH was replaced with DDH. It includes a wide spectrum of pathology, ranging from mild acetabular dysplasia presenting in adulthood to irreducible hip dislocation at birth. A considerable knowledge regarding pathology, diagnosis and management is essential in treating the patient. The incidence of hip dysplasia in India is reported to be 0–75 per 1000 live births, and that of frank dislocation is between 0 and 2.6/1000 live births. Late-presenting DDH is common in India, with most studies reporting a mean age of >20 months for children presenting for treatment.

45.2 Aetiology

The cause of DDH is multifactorial and includes genetic, intra-uterine and environmental factors [1]. The risk factors can be remembered as 5Fs:

1. **F**irst born—uterus in primigravida mother is tighter and elastic
2. **F**emale—lax foetal ligaments due to influence of maternal hormones
3. **F**amily history—genetic predisposition
4. **F**oetal malposition—breech presentation
5. **F**oetal packaging defects—oligohydramnios, twins

Left hip is involved in approximately 60% of cases due to foetal position, causing left hip adduction against maternal sacrum. Affection of right hip occurs in 20%, and 20% have involvement of both hips. DDH is more common in Europeans than in Asians or Africans. This is due to usage of cradle boards for infant care in these countries which limits hip mobility and positions the hip in adduction and extension. Whereas in India and other Asian countries, mother carries child on the side of her waist with the hips of the child abducted (Fig. 45.1).

R. A. Pandey (✉) · A. H. V. Bramesh
Department of Orthopedics, All India Institute of Medical Sciences, Patna, India

V. Kumar et al. (eds.), *A Quick Guide to Essential Orthopedics*,
https://doi.org/10.1007/978-981-95-2676-5_45

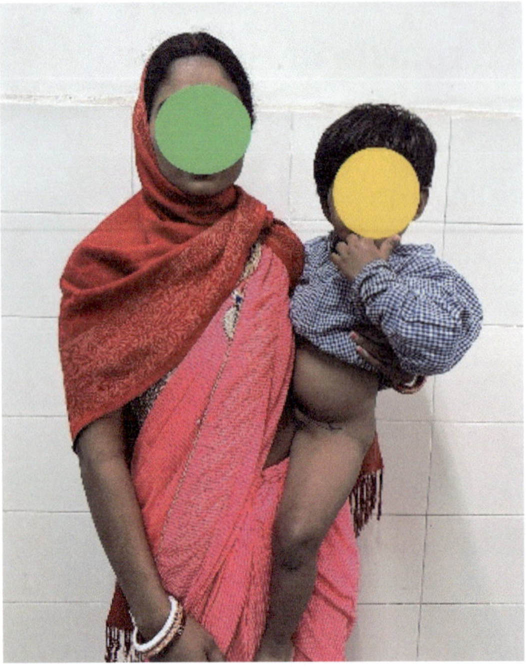

Fig. 45.1 The Asian way of carrying a child

45.3 Pathology

The distinct pathologic features are reversible in the initial stages. The affected hip spontaneously slides in and out at or after birth, leading to presentation of a dislocated or dislocatable hip. The underlying hereditary causes lead to dislocated hip at birth, whereas joint laxity along with precipitating causes leads to dislocatable hip.

The sliding movement of femoral head over acetabulum leads to flattening of postero-superior rim of hyaline cartilage. The deforming forces result in pathological changes such as inverted or everted acetabular rim. Around 90% of hips become stable by 6–8 weeks of life spontaneously without any secondary pathological changes. In some hips, fibrofatty tissue known as the pulvinar may fill acetabulum and impede reduction (Fig. 45.2). The ligamentum teres and transverse acetabular ligament get hypertrophied and make hip irreducible. With age, joint capsule in a dislocated hip assumes an hourglass shape with a constriction smaller than femoral head due to pull of iliopsoas, making hip irreducible. This

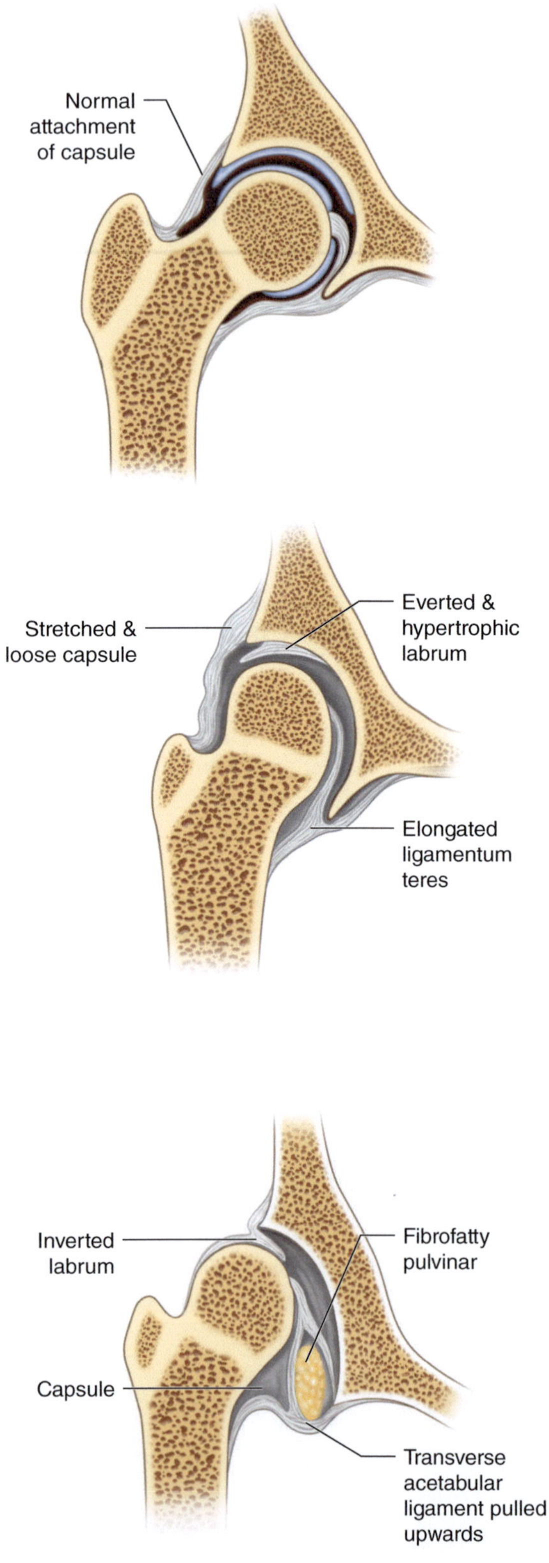

Fig. 45.2 Pathological changes in DDH

results in flattening of femoral head and increased femoral anteversion.

45.4 Clinical Presentation

The clinical features depend on age of presentation.

45.4.1 Neonates

Most cases at this age are asymptomatic. Routine clinical hip examination of all newborns is advisable for early detection of DDH in neonates [2]. Child may be brought occasionally to the physician due to asymmetric creases in the groin and thigh (Fig. 45.3). The only positive signs of hip instability in neonates are positive Ortolani and Barlow test, and these should be performed meticulously by an experienced physician. The Ortolani test identifies a dislocated hip that can be reduced back into the acetabulum. The hips and knees of an infant are flexed to 90 degrees, and thigh is abducted gently while fingers lying over the trochanter push the femoral head inwards. A soft click can be appreciated when the femoral head is reduced. The Barlow test is an attempt to dislocate the femoral head out of acetabulum. In this manoeuvre, thighs are adducted and the thumb over upper medial thigh gently pushes the femoral head laterally (Fig. 45.4). Ortolani and Barlow tests together have a sensitivity of 60% and specificity of 96%.

45.4.2 Infants

The neonatal signs of hip instability are difficult to appreciate after 10 weeks of life. Around 90% of unstable hips in neonates become stable spontaneously by 8–10 weeks. In those still remaining unstable, typical clinical features of DDH appear. The involved hip shows limited abduction movement, and thigh can't be abducted enough to touch the bed as happens with the normal hip (Fig. 45.5). The hip instability gradually progresses into dislocation, and one can elicit shortening of thigh, proximal migration of greater trochanter and a positive telescopy test (Fig. 45.6). Galeazzi test, also known as Allis sign or Skyline test, identifies limb shortening (Fig. 45.5). The child lies supine with both hips flexed to 45° and both knees flexed to 90° with both feet lying flat on examining surface. The positive sign is indicated by unequal height of the knees.

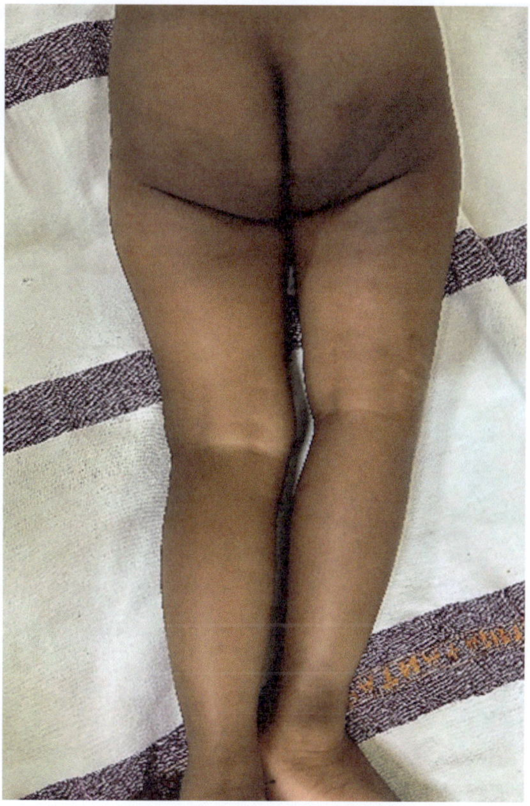

Fig. 45.3 Asymmetric thigh folds

Telescopy test is performed with child lying supine with hip and knee flexed to 90°. The pelvis is supported with one hand by placing thumb over anterior superior iliac spine and fingers over the greater trochanter. The other hand holds ipsilateral distal thigh and knee to exert a gentle push and pull force along the long axis of thigh. Positive test is indicated by an appreciation of up and down trochanteric excursion under the fingers. Detection of bilateral dislocated hip is difficult, as changes are symmetrical and hence don't attract attention of the caregivers.

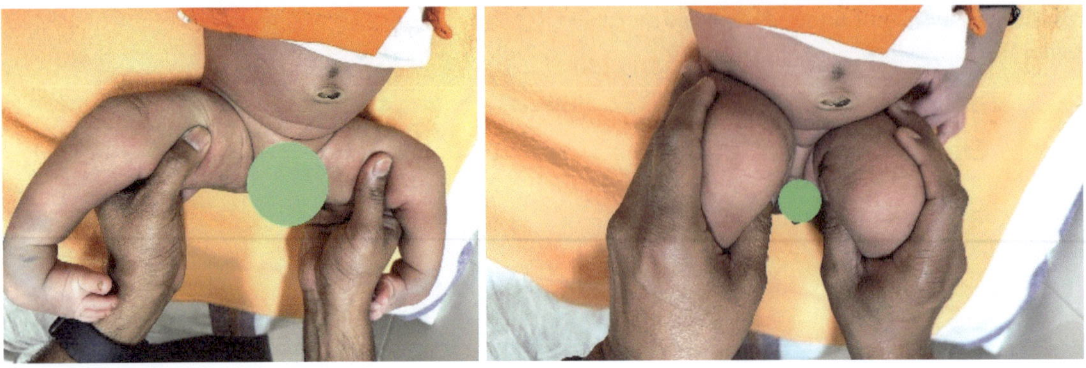

Fig. 45.4 Evaluation for DDH using Ortolani and Barlow manoeuvre in a child with DDH

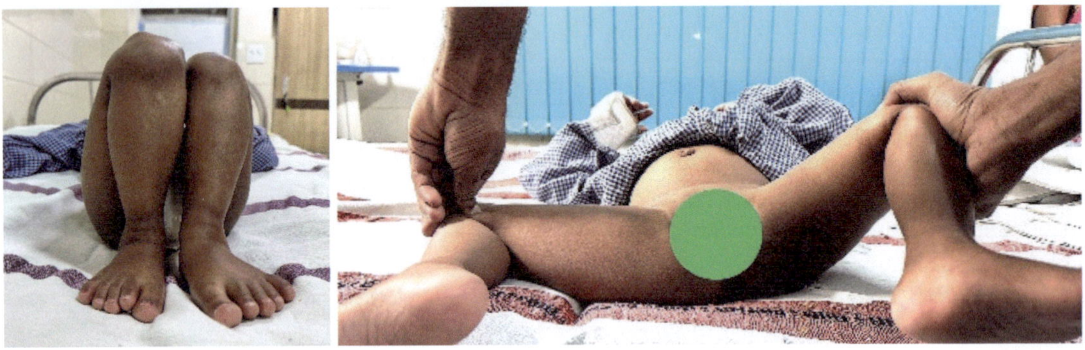

Fig. 45.5 Galeazzi sign and decreased hip abduction in DDH

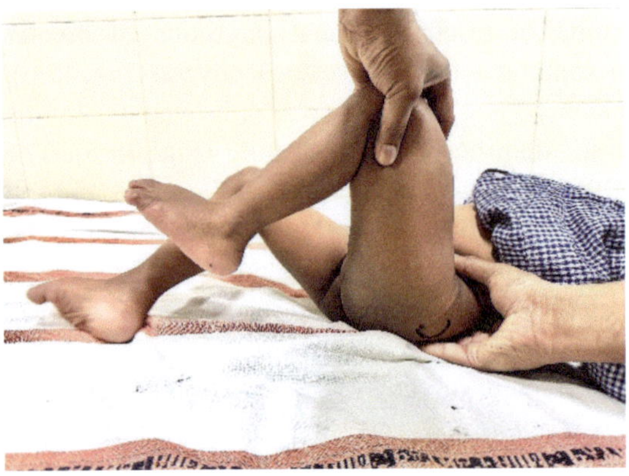

Fig. 45.6 Telescopy test in DDH

45.4.3 Walking Child

Some children with DDH may skip the early diagnosis and present late for evaluation and treatment [3]. The affected limb appears shortened (Fig. 45.7) and abnormally positioned. Shortening at this age is appreciated by unequal levels of knee and ankle in supine position and a positive Galeazzi test. The child walks with a Trendelenburg gait or abductor lurch. With each step, the pelvis drops on the contralateral side as the affected hip remains adducted. When a child attempts to stand on the involved side with other foot off the ground, he leans towards the affected

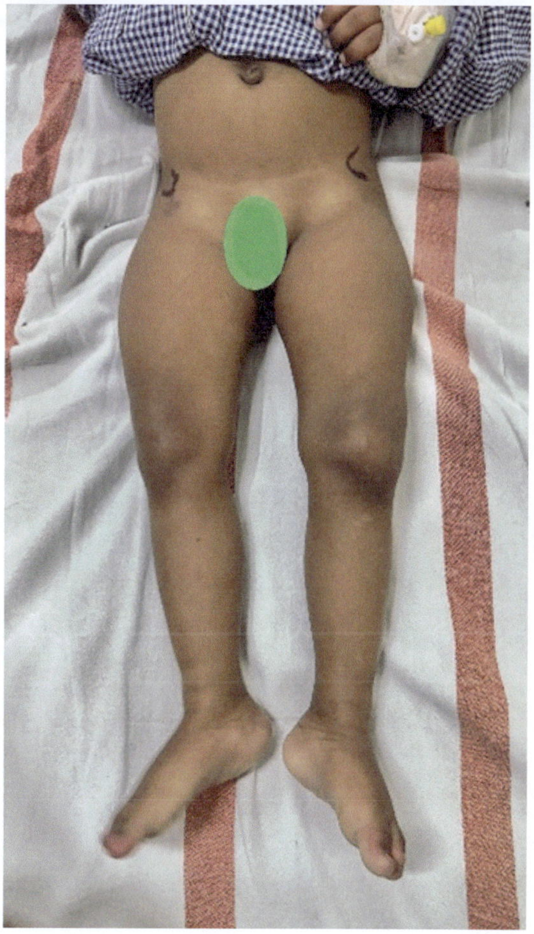

Fig. 45.7 Limb length discrepancy in a child with right-sided DDH

side (Trendelenburg sign). Abduction of involved hip is limited. The children with bilateral dislocation show a typical waddling gait (bilateral Trendelenburg gait) and increased lumbar lordosis. With further growth, children may complain of difficulty in sitting and squatting and may face frequent falls. If left untreated, the condition eventually leads to painful degeneration of hip and spine [4, 5].

45.5 Radiographic Findings

The femoral head does not ossify until 6 months, and hence it is difficult to identify DDH on plain radiographs in early months of life. Ultrasound of hip is the investigation of choice to identify an unstable hip at this age.

45.5.1 Ultrasonography

It shows the soft anatomy of the hip and the relationship of femoral head with the acetabulum (Fig. 45.8). Graf proposed a classification system based on the angles formed between the structures. Alpha angle represents the depth of bony acetabular roof and is formed by the intersection of baseline (iliac wing) and bony acetabular roof line. Its value is greater than 60° in a normal hip. Beta angle reflects cartilaginous coverage and is formed by intersection of baseline with acetabular labrum line. In a normal hip, value of beta angle is less than 55°. A smaller alpha angle and bigger beta angle are suggestive of hip dysplasia.

45.5.2 Plain Radiograph

In children over 6 months of age, a frankly dislocated hip is appreciable on plain radiograph. The classic radiographic lines are helpful in doubtful situations. The Hilgenreiner line is a line through the triradiate cartilage (Fig. 45.10). The Perkin line is a perpendicular line to Hilgenreiner line that passes through the lateral margin of acetabulum (Fig. 45.10). The intersection of these lines forms four quadrants in hip region. In a normal hip, the femoral head lies in the lower and inner quadrant, whereas in dysplastic hip, it lies lateral to Perkin line. In children younger than 6 months where femoral head has not ossified, radiographs can still be helpful in diagnosing and grading the severity by using the International Hip Dysplasia Institute (IHDI) classification for DDH (Fig. 45.9). The IHDI grading is:

Grade I—H point lies medial to P line
Grade II—H point lies lateral to P line and medial to D line
Grade III—H point lies lateral to D line but below H line
Grade IV—H point lies above the H line

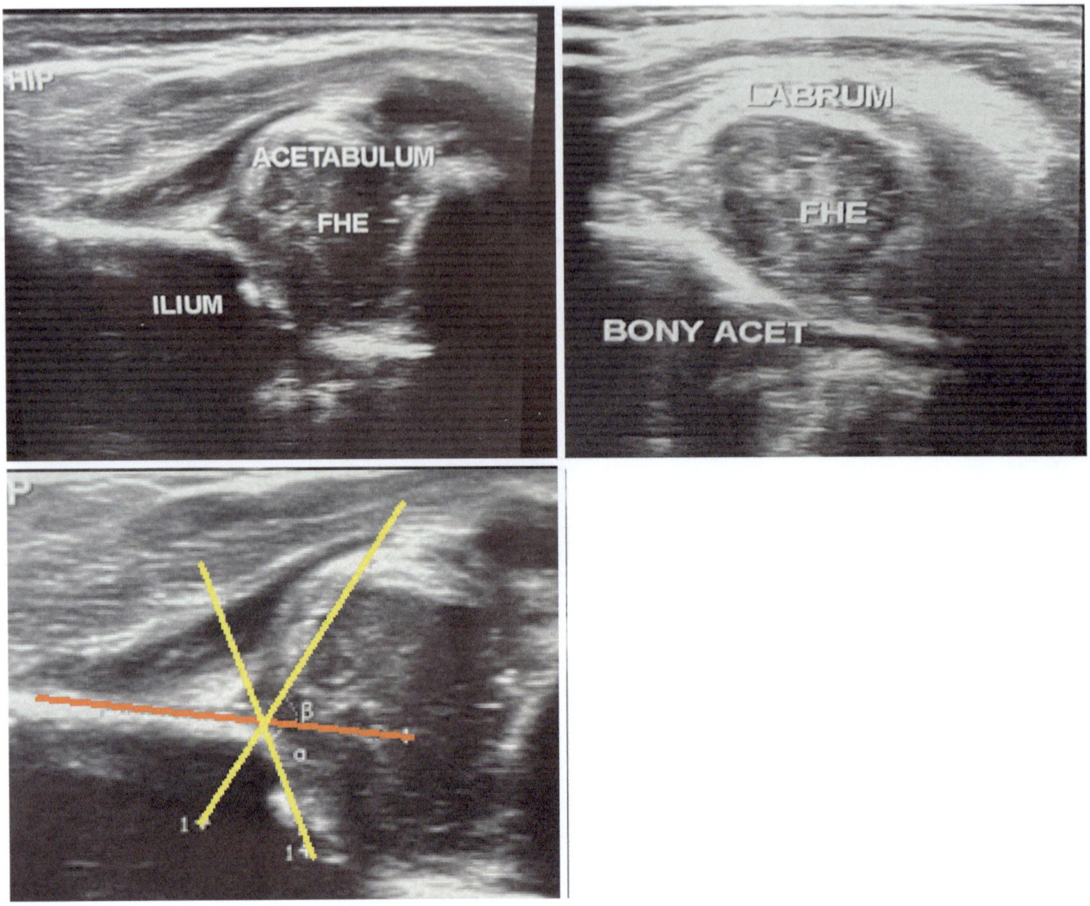

Fig. 45.8 Ultrasonic evaluation of DDH in an infant

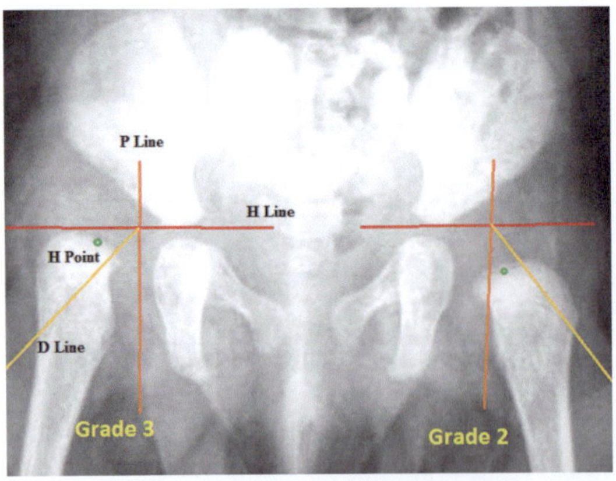

Fig. 45.9 The IHDI classification for DDH. H Line—Hilgenreiner's line, P line—Perkin's line, D line—Diagonal line at 45° from intersection of H line and P line, H point—Midpoint of superior margin of metaphysis

Similarly, Tonnis has classified the DDH into four types based on the position of ossification centre of femoral head (Table 45.1).

The Shenton arc is a curved line that begins at the lesser trochanter, goes up along the inferior border of femoral neck and continues along the inferior border of superior pubic rami (Fig. 45.10). This arc is disrupted in abnormal hips. The shape of the femoral head may be distorted with aspherical head, short neck, coxa valga and exaggerated anteversion of neck.

Acetabular index is an angle formed by the junction of the Hilgenreiner line and a line drawn along the acetabular surface. It shows measurement of femoral head bony coverage by the acetabulum.

Table 45.1 Tonnis classification for DDH

Grade	Description
I	Ossification Centre is medial to Perkin's line
II	Ossification Centre is lateral to P line but below H line
III	Ossification Centre is at the level of H line
IV	Ossification Centre is above H line

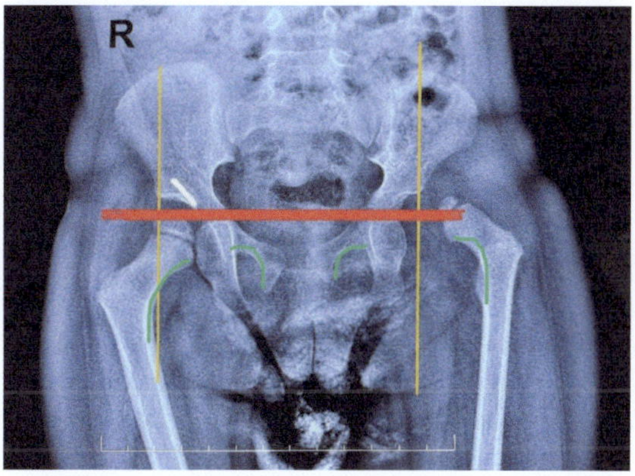

Fig. 45.10 Radiographic lines on pelvis X-ray. Red: Hilgenreiner's line, yellow: Perkin line and green: Shenton arc

In normal newborns, the acetabular index averages 27.5 degrees and decreases with age. Thirty degrees is considered the upper limit of normal.

Lateral centre-edge angle/angle of Wiberg is an angle between Perkin line and line joining centre of femoral head with lateral edge of acetabulum. It assesses superolateral coverage. The normal angle ranges between 25 and 40°. An angle of <20° suggests dysplasia.

45.5.3 Arthrography

Arthrography is useful in evaluating the congruency and stability of hip joint. It also demonstrates cartilaginous anatomy of acetabulum and femoral head. It is useful intra-operatively while doing closed reduction and for identifying barriers to reduction.

45.5.4 Magnetic Resonance Imaging (MRI)

MRI provides excellent visualization of hip and reveals all relevant details about unossified femoral head and soft tissue structures which are not visualized on plain radiograph. However, it is not routinely used due to the expense and need for sedation in children.

45.6 Treatment

The treatment of DDH depends on the age of child at diagnosis [6, 7]. The aim of the treatment is to achieve and maintain concentric reduction of femoral head in the acetabulum, thereby allowing proper moulding with time (principle of containment). As the remodelling potential of bone decreases with increasing age, the earliest possible treatment is recommended to have the best outcome.

45.6.1 Neonates (0–1 Month)

As around 90% of DDH detected at birth resolve spontaneously, these can be observed and reevaluated after 6 weeks. Those still remaining unstable are treated in an orthosis. However, many surgeons prefer to treat the dislocated and dislocatable hips right from the beginning and prefer to observe the subluxable hips. Pavlik harness is the orthosis of choice (Fig. 45.11).

45.6.2 1- to 6-Month-Old Child

Pavlik harness is the first choice of treatment in this age group. The hip is reduced by closed manoeuvre, and Pavlik harness is applied with hips in 90° of flexion and 40–60° of abduction. Straps are secured loosely to allow for active limb movements. Position of excessive flexion and abduction should be discouraged to avoid inferior dislocation of femoral head and the incidence of

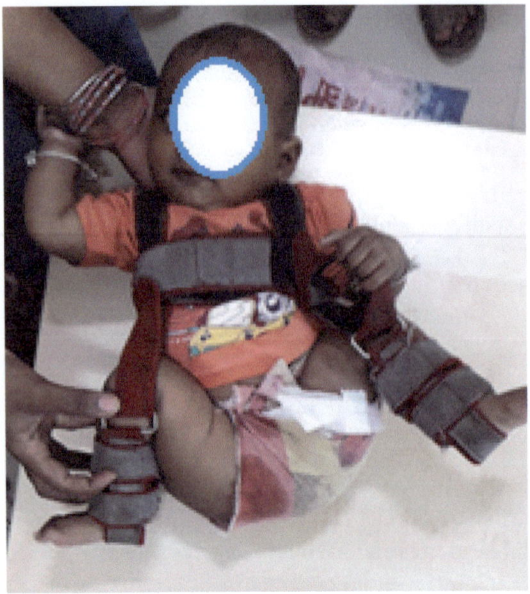

Fig. 45.11 Usage of Pavlik harness in treatment of DDH

AVN. After 6 weeks, child is assessed clinically, and harness is discontinued if hip is stable. If hip still remains dislocated, it should be evaluated further and treated with an abduction brace.

45.6.3 6-Month to 2-Year-Old Child

The treatment at this age consists of both closed and open reduction under anaesthesia and immobilization in a hip spica cast. Close reduction is usually successful for children under one year of age. The reduced position is maintained in a hip spica cast for 3 months. An adductor tenotomy is frequently added to facilitate reduction and to increase the safe zone of stability. If the attempt at closed reduction fails, then open reduction of hip is recommended.

45.6.4 2-Year to 6-Year-Old Child

Femoral head at this age lies at a more proximal location and hence close reduction is not successful in majority of cases. Treatment invariably consists of open reduction to remove possible anatomic blocks such as iliopsoas contracture, capsular constriction, inverted labrum, pulvinar and hypertrophied ligamentum teres. Femoral shortening aids in reduction and reduces pressure on femoral head after reduction, thereby avoiding the risk of AVN. Femoral osteotomy is fixed in internal rotation and varus, depending on the amount of deformity, to achieve concentric reduction and stability. Pelvic osteotomies are indicated for acetabular dysplasia to increase anterolateral coverage over the femoral head. The type of pelvic osteotomy depends on the age of child at presentation and may differ from case to case.

Innominate Salter osteotomy is done to redirect the acetabulum and improve anterolateral coverage once concentric reduction has been achieved. A single transverse cut is made above the acetabulum. It starts above the anterior inferior iliac spine and is directed posteriorly and medially into the ilium to end in greater sciatic notch. Acetabulum hinges through the pubic symphysis to improve the anterolateral coverage. It is recommended for children between 2 and 4 years of age.

Pemberton and Degas osteotomies (Fig. 45.12) reposition the acetabulum to improve anterior and lateral coverage. Osteotomy starts above the anterior inferior iliac spine and is directed towards triradiate cartilage. The posteromedial bone near the greater sciatic notch remains intact. This osteotomy reduces the volume of acetabulum and can be successful up to 8 years of age.

Reconstructive pelvis osteotomies such as Ganz, Triple and Dega osteotomies are also employed in DDH depending on the case scenario. Salvage pelvic osteotomies, such as Shelf and Chiari osteotomies, are performed in case of late presentation with inadequate femoral head coverage and when concentric reduction is not achieved.

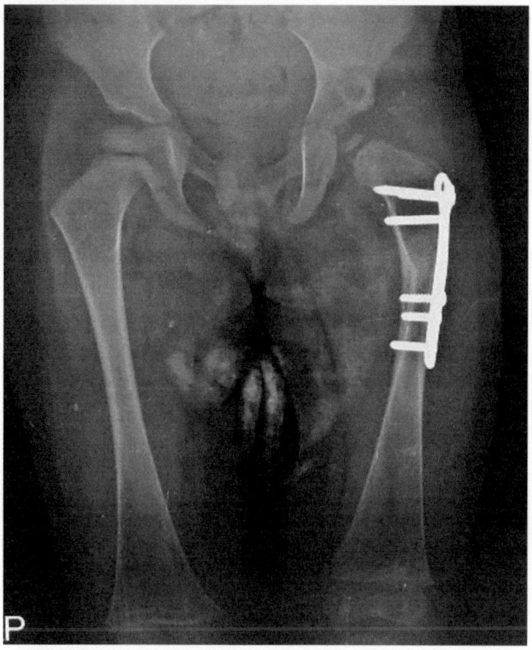

Fig. 45.12 Radiographic image of postoperative case of open reduction, Dega osteotomy and varus derotation osteotomy

Multiple Choice Questions

1. Which one of the following is not a risk factor for DDH?
   (a) Female child
   (b) Breech presentation
   (c) Prematurity
   (d) Home delivery
2. The investigation of choice to detect DDH before 6 months of age is:
   (a) Radiograph
   (b) MRI
   (c) Ultrasound
   (d) CT scan
3. Which is the preferred screening test for DDH in a newborn?
   (a) Barlow and Ortolani test
   (b) Asymmetry of thigh folds
   (c) Limited hip abduction test
   (d) Galeazzi test
4. In a normal hip, position of femoral head is:
   (a) Lateral to Perkin's line and inferior to Hilgenreiner line
   (b) Medial to Perkin's line and inferior to Hilgenreiner line
   (c) Lateral to Perkin's line and superior to Hilgenreiner line
   (d) Medial to Perkin's line and superior to Hilgenreiner line
5. Treatment of choice for DDH after 2 years of age is:
   (a) Pavlik harness
   (b) Closed reduction and spica casting
   (c) Open reduction alone
   (d) Open reduction and osteotomies

Answers: 1. (d), 2. (c), 3. (a), 4. (b), 5. (d)

References

1. de Hundt M, Vlemmix F, Bais JM, Hutton EK, de Groot CJ, Mol BW, Kok M. Risk factors for developmental dysplasia of the hip: a meta-analysis. Eur J Obstet Gynecol Reprod Biol. 2012;165(1):8–17. https://doi.org/10.1016/j.ejogrb.2012.06.030. Epub 2012 Jul 21. PMID: 22824571
2. Pandey RA, Johari AN. Screening of newborns and infants for developmental dysplasia of the hip: a systematic review. Indian J Orthop. 2021;55(6):1388–401. https://doi.org/10.1007/s43465-021-00409-2. PMID: 35003532; PMCID: PMC8688670
3. Johari AN, Pandey RA, Mahapatra SK, John B. Causes of late-presenting developmental dislocation of the hip beyond 12 months of age: a pilot study. Indian J Med Res. 2023;157:403–11. https://doi.org/10.4103/ijmr.IJMR_3569_20.
4. Chen J, Zhang WB, He JZ, Zhang R, Cao YQ, Liu X. Developmental dysplasia of the hip: a special pathology. Chin J Traumatol. 2018;21(4):238–42. https://doi.org/10.1016/j.cjtee.2018.02.001. Epub 2018 Mar 26. PMID: 30007532; PMCID: PMC6085197
5. Nandhagopal T, De Cicco FL. Developmental Dysplasia of the Hip. [Updated 2022 Oct 3]. In: StatPearls [Internet]. Treasure Island (FL): StatPearls Publishing; 2023 Jan-. Available from: https://www.ncbi.nlm.nih.gov/books/NBK563157/
6. Johari AN, Pandey RA, Chand S, Aroojis A. The evolution of DDH Management in India. Indian J Orthop. 2021;55(6):1440–55. https://doi.org/10.1007/s43465-021-00537-9. PMID: 35003535; PMCID: PMC8688609
7. Alves C, Truong WH, Thompson MV, Suryavanshi JR, Penny CL, Do HT, Dodwell ER. Diagnostic and treatment preferences for developmental dysplasia of the hip: a survey of EPOS and POSNA members. J Child Orthop. 2018;12(3):236–44. https://doi.org/10.1302/1863-2548.12.180034. PMID: 29951123; PMCID: PMC6005222

Cerebral Palsy

46

Anil Agarwal

46.1 Introduction

Cerebral palsy (CP) has been described as a group of disorders of the development of movement and posture that are attributed to nonprogressive disturbances that occurred in the developing fetal or infant brain. Diseases of the peripheral nerves/ spinal cord (e.g., spinal muscular atrophy, myelomeningocele) or muscles (e.g., muscular dystrophies), although they may cause early motor abnormalities, are typically not considered CP.

CP is related to brain damage, so there are several associated problems in such individuals. Intellectual disabilities, learning difficulties, visual, hearing or speech impairment, and imperfect sensory prehension may additionally impair their physical and functional capabilities. Although considered nonprogressive, the clinical manifestations may change over time with interplay of brain maturity, muscle strength and coordination, bone length, formation of secondary deformities and contractures as the child grows older.

The true prevalence of CP is not well established, but estimates are between 1.5 and 5.6 cases per 1000 live births [1]. The disorder is substantially higher among preterm and very preterm infants. The approximate incidence of comorbidities in children with CP is mental retardation (IQ < 50): 30%; seizures: 20% and being nonambulatory: 20%.

A. Agarwal (✉)
Department of Pediatric Orthopedics, Chacha Nehru Bal Chikitsalaya, New Delhi, India

46.2 Causes

The causes of cerebral palsy are not fully understood. The following events happening during child's neural development due to maternal, gestational, fetal, or postnatal factors may be responsible in some children (Table 46.1):

1. Brain injury or abnormal brain development: injury to the developing brain can occur anytime from gestation to early childhood. However, fewer than 10% of injuries occurring during the birth process result in CP.
2. Prematurity and postmaturity: children born preterm or postterm may be at higher risk for developing CP.
3. Cerebral leukomalacia especially periventricular leukomalacia (PVL) is a condition resulting in death of small areas of brain tissue around ventricles. The cause of cerebral leukomalacia can be intracranial hemorrhage, hypoperfusion injuries in the distribution of the middle cerebral artery, basal ganglia, or other regions of brain.
4. Cerebral infections or inflammations can sometimes be responsible for CP.

V. Kumar et al. (eds.), *A Quick Guide to Essential Orthopedics*,
https://doi.org/10.1007/978-981-95-2676-5_46

Table 46.1 Risk factors for cerebral palsy [2]

Gestational and maternal	Fetal and postnatal
Prematurity (gestational age <36 weeks) or postmaturity	Abnormal brain development, injury or hemorrhage
Low birth weight (<2.5 kg)	Cerebral infections or toxemia
Maternal diseases, e.g., epilepsy, hyperthyroidism, drug abuse, infection, eclampsia	Hypoxia, bradycardia, seizures, hyperbilirubinemia, altered coagulation profile
Trauma	
Incompetent cervix	
Multiple pregnancies or breech presentation	
Complications during pregnancy, e.g., bleeding in last trimester or during labor, placental insufficiency, premature rupture of membranes, prolonged or difficult labor	

46.3 Classification

46.3.1 Geographical Classification (Table 46.2)

Based on involvement of appendicular skeleton.

46.3.2 Physiological Classification (Table 46.3)

Physiologically, CP can be divided into a spastic type, which affects the corticospinal (pyramidal) tracts, and an extrapyramidal type, which affects other regions of the developing brain. The extrapyramidal CP includes athetoid, choreiform, rigid, ataxic, and hypotonic types.

46.3.3 Gross Motor Function Classification System (GMFC System) (Table 46.4)

The Gross Motor Function Classification System (GMFCS) is a five-level classification used for functional evaluation in CP-affected individuals. It is based on self-initiated movements, with emphasis on mobility, transfers, and use of assistive devices. The levels make possible to identify meaningful ambulation in daily life. Individuals categorized under "Level I" can generally walk without restrictions but may be limited in some of the more advanced motor skills. Individuals categorized under "Level V" have more severe forms of motor affection. They are generally very limited in their ability to move themselves around, even with the use of assistive technology. GMFCS often provides insights into a child's overall motor capabilities and ambulatory ability prediction for CP.

Table 46.2 Geographical classification of cerebral palsy

Major types	Description
Monoplegia	One extremity involved, usually lower
Hemiplegia	Both extremities on same side involved. Usually, upper extremity involved more than lower extremity
Paraplegia	Both lower extremities equally involved
Diplegia	Lower extremities more involved than upper extremities
Quadriplegia	All extremities involved equally. Normal head/neck control present
Double hemiplegia	All extremities involved, upper more than lower
Total body	All extremities severely involved. No head/neck control

Table 46.3 Physiological classification of cerebral palsy

Major types	Description
Spastic (80%)	Velocity-dependent increase in muscle tone with passive stretch. Joint contractures are common
Athetoid	Dyskinetic, purposeless movements. Joint contractures are uncommon. Dystonia or hypotonia can be associated
Choreiform	Continual purposeless movements
Rigid	Hypertonicity occurs in the absence of hyperreflexia, spasticity, and clonus. "Cogwheel" or "lead pipe" muscle stiffness
Ataxic	Disturbance of coordinated movement, most commonly walking. Normal head/neck control
Hypotonic	Low muscle tone and normal deep tendon reflexes
Mixed	Features of more than one type

Table 46.4 Gross motor function classification system (GMFCS)[a]

Level I
Can walk indoors and outdoors and climb stairs without using hands for support Can perform usual activities such as running and jumping Has decreased speed, balance and coordination
Level II
Can climb stairs with a railing Has difficulty with uneven surfaces, inclines or in crowds Has only minimal ability to run or jump
Level III
Walks with assistive mobility devices indoors and outdoors on level surfaces May be able to climb stairs using a railing May propel a manual wheelchair and need assistance for long distances or uneven surfaces
Level IV
Walking ability severely limited even with assistive devices Uses wheelchairs most of the time and may propel power wheelchair Standing transfers, with or without assistance
Level V
Has physical impairments that restrict voluntary control of movement Ability to maintain head and neck position against gravity restricted Impaired in all areas of motor function Cannot sit or stand independently, even with adaptive equipment Cannot independently walk but may be able to use powered mobility

[a]Based on Palisano, Robert; Rosenbaum, Peter; Walter, Stephen; Russell, Dianne; Wood, Ellen; Galuppi, Barbara (2008). "Development and reliability of a system to classify gross motor function in children with cerebral palsy." Developmental Medicine & Child Neurology. 39: 214–223. Relevant illustrations can be viewed at https://canchild.ca/system/tenon/assets/attachments/000/004/470/original/GMFCS_English_Illustrations_V2_-May1-2023-ACCESS.pdf

46.4 Clinical Features

There is a wide spectrum of CP symptoms and their severity. They can vary from very mild affections to severe impairment and inability to live independently. Manifestations in CP depend upon the part of brain affected and also the age of the individual. The main symptoms include alteration in muscle tone, impairment of gross and fine motor functions, loss of balance, sensory processing difficulties, and lack of coordination. There can be several associated problems such as presence of seizures or epilepsy, visual or hearing impairments, learning, and intellectual difficulties. There can be a variable degree of communication abnormalities, poor posture, gait impairments, and oral issues (e.g., drooling of saliva and dysphagia). Specific CP types, such as athetoid and ataxic, have symptoms accordingly.

46.5 Management

The diagnosis of CP is established clinically supplemented with careful history taking and supportive imaging. In general, birth history, review/evaluation of developmental milestones, muscle tone, coordination, posture, balance, and gait provide clues to the diagnosis. Sometimes, associated problems such as speech abnormalities, visual/ hearing impairments, and oral manifestations corroborate the diagnosis. Imaging methods like Computed tomography (CT) and Magnetic resonance imaging (MRI) may be required to look for lesions in the brain. An electroencephalogram (EEG) test may be necessary if seizure or epilepsy is associated. Advanced treatment planning sometimes mandates the use of specialized gait laboratories [1, 3].

In view of the complex body involvement, individuals with cerebral palsy should be supported by a multidisciplinary team (health professionals of different specialties including pediatrician, neurologist, orthopedic surgeon, physiotherapists, occupational therapists, speech therapists, psychologists, etc.). The associated conditions require direct medical and therapeutic interventions from other medical specialties. Over the years, the approach to cerebral palsy has shifted away from tackling individual physical problems alone to a broader, comprehensive goal of maximizing a person's independence, self-reliability, and community engagement. Recent research also supports interventions in early childhood when the developing brain is far more capable of receiving, interpreting, and responding to external stimuli.

Overall, the management in CP is aimed to develop and maintain the motor and mental capabilities of the child. Pharmacological and non-pharmacological interventions are used for CP.

46.5.1 Pharmacological Interventions

Numerous medications help control symptoms such as muscle spasms, abnormal movements, and seizures. The common medications utilized for the purpose are spasticity-lowering drugs, anti-seizure drugs, anti-inflammatory drugs, and anti- depressants. Baclofen, administered either orally or intrathecally, is often helpful in reducing spasticity. Use of botulinum toxin injections, once in popular use for control of localized or segmental spasticity, has become controversial following reports of muscle weakness and atrophy following their long-term use. Benzodiazepines such as diazepam, valproic acid, and barbiturates have been useful in the management of myoclonus.

46.5.2 Non-pharmacological Interventions

1. Surgical interventions: Orthopedic and neurosurgical interventions help improve the overall mobility, joint range of motion, and gait in CP individuals. The common interventions are osteotomies (correction of bone deformities and restoring alignment), enhancing joint range of motion (release of contractures, muscle/ tendon transfers, muscle/ tendon lengthening), and reducing spasticity (selective dorsal rhizotomy spinal surgery). The judicious use of a variety of orthotic splints and assistive devices can also help improve function.
2. Physiotherapy and occupational therapy interventions: They take into account the age of patient, existing motor abilities and cognitive maturity, his/her adaptation to the environment, and they bring out the best possible functional performance. The interventions can be gait and balance training, muscle strengthening and stretching, functional positioning and posture correction, etc. Occupational therapists use specific techniques such as constraint-induced manual therapy (promote use of the affected part by restraining the unaffected part) and sensory integration therapy (ability to receive, interpret, and act on stimulations or inputs received through sensory receptors) to improve function.
3. Interventions for other problems: Speech and language interventions, and psychological support may also be required. Special educators use individualized teaching methods to suit the physical and learning abilities of the individuals with CP.

Multiple Choice Questions

1. The most common type of cerebral palsy is
   (a) Spastic
   (b) Ataxic
   (c) Dystonic
   (d) Mixed
2. The most common deformity of the upper limb in cerebral palsy is
   (a) Swan neck deformity
   (b) Boutonniere deformity
   (c) Pronation contracture of the forearm
   (d) Wrist drop
3. Which of the following joints need regular surveillance in a child with cerebral palsy?
   (a) Knee
   (b) Hip
   (c) Shoulder
   (d) Elbow
4. The commonest site of involvement of brain in cerebral palsy is
   (a) Motor cortex
   (b) Sensory cortex
   (c) Hypothalamus
   (d) Pons

5. The deformities noticed in cerebral palsy are
   (a) Static
   (b) Progressive
   (c) Dynamic
   (d) Dynamic and progressive

Answers: 1. (a), 2. (c), 3. (b), 4. (a), 5. (d)

References

1. Patel DR, Neelakantan M, Pandher K, Merrick J. Cerebral palsy in children: a clinical overview. Transl Pediatr. 2020;9(Suppl 1):S125–35. https://doi.org/10.21037/tp.2020.01.01. PMID: 32206590; PMCID: PMC7082248
2. Mohanty T, Joseph SD, Gunasekaran PK, Doreswamy SM, Saini L. Predictors of risk for cerebral palsy: a review. Pediatr Phys Ther. 2023;35(3):347–57. https://doi.org/10.1097/PEP.0000000000001020. Epub 2023 Apr 28. PMID: 37126801
3. Paneth N. Establishing the diagnosis of cerebral palsy. Clin Obstet Gynecol. 2008;51(4):742–8. https://doi.org/10.1097/GRF.0b013e318187081a. PMID: 18981799

Poliomyelitis

47

Prateek Behera

Poliomyelitis is an infectious disease caused by an enterovirus. The polio virus is of high infectivity, with the route of infection being via the human gastrointestinal tract. Before the introduction of vaccines, type 1 poliovirus accounted for 85% of paralytic disease.

After entering by oral route, the virus multiplies in the pharynx and intestine for 1–3 weeks. It is either contained by the local immune response or results in a viraemic phase. The virus continues to be excreted in the saliva for two or three days, and in the faeces for two to three weeks. The infection rate is extremely high, but it is probable that 95% of all infections are either asymptomatic or characterized by an abortive flu-like illness. In the temperate climates of the northern hemisphere, epidemics of polio occurred commonly during the summer months, and the incidence was greatest where children bathed together.

At present, acute poliomyelitis has been eradicated from most of the countries due to extensive vaccination campaign. The national immunization program of India at present incorporates the use of both oral and intramuscular polio vaccines.

P. Behera (✉)
Department of Orthopaedics, All India Institute of Medical Sciences Bhopal, Saket Nagar, Bhopal, Madhya Pradesh, India
e-mail: prateek.ortho@aiimsbhopal.edu.in

47.1 Acute Phase

The natural history of polio infection ranges from asymptomatic infection to severe disease. In most individuals, the response is in the form of a mild viral illness with symptoms like sore throat and fever, and it tends to improve by 1–2 weeks. In a group of patients, after the minor flu-like illness, meningitic phase develops when the virus reaches the central nervous system. Fever with pharyngitis, myalgia, anorexia, nausea, vomiting, headache and neck stiffness are the common manifestations of this phase. Further, a group of patients tends to develop spinal poliomyelitis. Its presentation is in the form of myalgia and muscle spasms. Subsequently, an asymmetrical, predominantly lower limb flaccid weakness tends to develop. The flaccid paralysis is at its peak by 48 h of onset. Earlier, a bulbar form of polio was found to be common in children, too.

47.2 Treatment of Acute Phase

In the acute phase, the aim of treatment is primarily to support the patient till the phase is over. This is done in the form of strict bed rest to prevent aggravation and spread of the paralysis. Analgesics primarily NSAIDs are used for pain relief. Acute respiratory failure may develop in cases where the thoracic musculature and the diaphragm are involved, and these patients end up requiring intubation and intermittent positive

V. Kumar et al. (eds.), *A Quick Guide to Essential Orthopedics*,
https://doi.org/10.1007/978-981-95-2676-5_47

pressure ventilation. As the patient is paralyzed, the joints are often positioned in abnormal position. Appropriate positioning, splinting and frequent passive movements are helpful in preventing contractures and joint ankylosis. After the acute phase is over, during the first few weeks of rehabilitation, the main aim is to prevent deformity by stretching and splinting of affected limbs. Intensive physiotherapy is recommended to regain strength and function. Appropriate orthotic devices and splints are essential to compensate for loss of function and to facilitate mobility. In most cases, the paralysis is often temporary. Nerve impulses tend to return to the paralyzed muscle within a month, and frequently the recovery is complete in six to eight months' time. The muscles can retain normal strength even if half the original motor neurons have been lost. Any residual paralysis after one year of the acute disease tends to be permanent, although there are reports mention about the probable recovery of muscle strength up to 18 months after infection.

47.3 Post-polio Syndrome

Many patients who have had paralytic poliomyelitis and have residual impairments develop new disabilities after a period of stability. These late changes were recognized and defined as progressive muscular atrophy, weakness, pain and fatigue. However, most patients were more particularly aware of late functional deterioration manifesting as impairment of activities of daily living, mobility, upper limb function and respiratory capacity. This phenomenon of developing new impairments later after the acute phase is labelled as post-polio syndrome.

While the exact definition is not well elucidated, most reports indicate that the new symptoms and signs should be unrelated to any orthopaedic, neurological, respiratory, or systemic medical illness. Studies have suggested that these new-onset wasting and weakness may be due to distal degeneration of motor units that had been previously affected by poliomyelitis and are believed to be associated with age and overuse or disuse. It has also been postulated that the new impairments occur because of prolonged stress on an exixting skeletal deformity and on the previously weakened muscles. Thus, this type of Progressive wasting and weakness occurs in already affected limbs. The contralateral limb usually has compensatory hypertrophy because of weight bearing or distorted mechanics.

47.4 Orthopaedic Manifestations in the Post-paralytic Period

Once the recovery phase after the acute paralytic phase is over, residual paralysis can be present in several patients. This residual paralysis influences not only the muscle but also the bones and joints. The flaccid paralysis results in the joints continuing to stay flail. If the involvement of one group of muscles is more than the opposing group, then the pull by the stronger group of muscles can result in development of contractures. Deformities occur due to an imbalance of muscle power and poor posture. There can be disuse atrophy of muscles and shortening of the leg due to interference with growth. In neglected cases, gross fixed deformities of the hip, knee and foot occur with severe wasting of muscles. The disuse of the limb results in underdevelopment of the bones as a result of which they can be deformed and weak. These result in two major issues in such patients:

1. The limb is practically non-functional If the lower limb is involved, then the individual might not be able to bear weight on the affected limb and thus it is not possible for the person to walk unaided. They require the use of an orthotic device with or without the support of crutches for ambulation. If the upper limb is involved, then the ability to grip and position the hand in space for various day-to-day activities might be affected and such a limb can not independently be used for perfroming meaningful tasks.
2. If the bones fracture, then they need special strategies for fracture management - The bones are underdeveloped, weak and often deformed. Consequently, the standard

implants especially the anatomically contoured ones cannot be used for fracture fixation and the surgeon has to improvise for management of fractures.

The orthopaedic surgeon comes into picture for the management of both the above conditions. The flail joints are often initially managed using orthotic devices with the type decided by the muscles paralyzed and the deformity arising out of that paralysis. The international nomenclature for orthotic appliances describes the joints that are stabilized by the appliance, for example, Ankle Foot Orthosis stabilizes the ankle. While these orthotic devices are useful for stabilization of joints, they have the limitations of being difficult to use if the joints have severe contractures. In such cases, the limb needs to be made braceable by doing contracture release surgeries. Usually, the deformities around the hip and knee that are more than 30 degrees in magnitude need to be operated upon.

In case there is availability of a suitable expendable tendon around a joint, a tendon transfer surgery can be considered. In selecting a tendon to transfer, the muscle should be sufficiently strong to supplement the power of a paralyzed muscle. The nerve and blood supply of the transferred muscle should be preserved in order to avoid iatrogenic weakness. The joint across which the muscle acts must be in a satisfactory position; all contracted structures must be released before the tendon transfer.

Stabilization of flail joints by surgical procedures is often needed to provide enough stability to make a joint bear weight. Several options are available for achieving this objective. Tenodesis, fixation of ligaments and construction of artificial check ligaments have been used in the past to restrict the range of movement or to eliminate abnormal motion of a joint. However, most of these procedures are not used at present, as deformity in the opposite direction may occur, and the tendon or artificial check ligaments may stretch with time resulting in a failure of the procedure after an early success. Finally, a flail joint might be stabilized definitively by fusion of the joints—a procedure called arthrodesis. Arthrodesis involves clearing out the cartilage from the opposing surfaces of the joint, bringing the joint's two surfaces to an acceptable functional position and then providing compression across the two surfaces using implants.

The joints that have developed osteoarthritis in otherwise normal individuals are managed by joint replacement surgeries. However, these are tricky in patients with post-polio residual paralysis. The issues are twofold—primarily related to the strength of the muscles to retain the hip and knee prosthesis while maintaining its longevity, and the second being related to the availability of appropriately sized implants for replacement. Often, the armamentarium that needs to be made available in the operating room needs to be extensive.

In conclusion, management of the residual weakness of poliomyelitis and post-polio syndrome necessitates an understanding of the pathological process in poliomyelitis as well as the variations in the pattern of the disease in different parts of the body. Poliomyelitis causes a lower motor neuron disease that is quite different from other types of neuromuscular paralysis, like those resulting from spinal cord trauma and spinal cord tumours. The paralysis from these conditions is upper motor neuron type and tends to be spastic rather than flaccid. Knowledge of pathoanatomy before embarking on surgery is necessary.

Further Reading

1. Quarleri J. Poliomyelitis is a current challenge: long-term sequelae and circulating vaccine-derived poliovirus. Geroscience. 2023;45(2):707–17. https://doi.org/10.1007/s11357-022-00672-7. Epub 2022 Oct 19. PMID: 36260265; PMCID: PMC9886775
2. Howard RS. Poliomyelitis and the postpolio syndrome. BMJ. 2005;330(7503):1314–8. https://doi.org/10.1136/bmj.330.7503.1314. PMID: 15933355; PMCID: PMC558211
3. Trojan DA, Cashman NR. Post-poliomyelitis syndrome. Muscle Nerve. 2005;31(1):6–19. https://doi.org/10.1002/mus.20259. PMID: 15599928
4. Faraj AA. Poliomyelitis: orthopaedic management. Curr Orthop. 2006;20(1):41–6.
5. Gupta M, Jain VK, Upadhyaya GK, Arya RK. Comprehensive review of challenges associated with management of lower limb fractures in poliomyelitis patients. J Clin Orthop Trauma. 2016;7(4):276–81. https://doi.org/10.1016/j.jcot.2016.08.007. Epub 2016 Sep 6. PMID: 27857503; PMCID: PMC5106482

Spina Bifida

48

Prateek Behera and Sourabh Kumar Sinha

48.1 Introduction

Spina bifida is a congenital condition characterized by the incomplete development of the spinal cord, spinal column, or both during early fetal development. "Spina bifida" is a Latin term which literally means "split spine," and it encompasses a spectrum of neural tube defects that can vary widely in severity. This chapter aims to provide a comprehensive understanding of spina bifida, including its causes, types, symptoms, diagnosis, treatment options, and the impact on individuals and their families.

48.2 Development of the Neural Tube

The neural tube, a crucial structure in embryonic development, forms the foundation for the central nervous system, including the brain and spinal cord. In a healthy pregnancy, the neural tube closes completely by the end of the first month. However, in cases of spina bifida, this closure is incomplete, leading to several manifestations that span from being benign to severely disablings.

48.3 Types of Spina Bifida

There are three main types of spina bifida: occulta, meningocele, and myelomeningocele. Figure 48.1).

Occulta There is a bony defect in the closure of posterior spine. This is the mildest form, often asymptomatic, with the spinal cord and nerves usually unaffected. It may go undetected for years or throughout an individual's life.

Meningocele In this form, the protective covering of the spinal cord (meninges) pushes through the opening in the spine, forming a sac filled with cerebrospinal fluid. However, the spinal cord remains relatively unaffected and does not form the content of the sac.

Myelomeningocele This is the most severe form, involving the protrusion of both the spinal cord and meninges through the open part of the spine. It can result in serious neurological complications and functional impairments.

P. Behera (✉) · S. K. Sinha
Department of Orthopedics, All India Institute of Medical Sciences Bhopal, Saket Nagar, Bhopal, Madhya Pradesh, India
e-mail: prateek.ortho@aiimsbhopal.edu.in

V. Kumar et al. (eds.), *A Quick Guide to Essential Orthopedics*,
https://doi.org/10.1007/978-981-95-2676-5_48

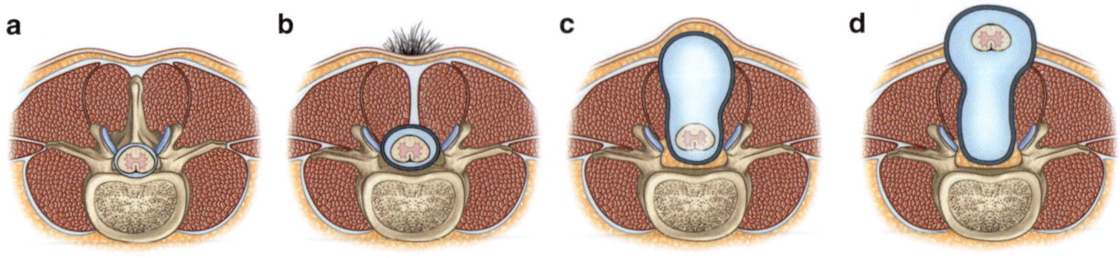

Fig. 48.1 (**a**) Normal, (**b**) spina bifida occulta, (**c**) meningocele, and (**d**) myelomeningocele

48.4 Causes and Risk Factors

The exact cause of spina bifida is not entirely understood, but both genetic and environmental factors play a role. Folic acid deficiency during early pregnancy has been identified as a significant risk factor. Other factors include a family history of neural tube defects, certain medications like valproate, carbamazepine, and maternal conditions such as diabetes.

48.5 Prenatal Diagnosis and Screening

Advancements in medical technology have allowed for the early detection of spina bifida during pregnancy. Prenatal screening, including ultrasound and maternal blood tests especially the ones done in the second trimester, can help identify potential neural tube defects. While these tests provide valuable information, it's important to note that they are not always conclusive, and further diagnostic procedures, such as amniocentesis, may be recommended.

48.5.1 Ultrasound Imaging

Spina bifida may be visible on ultrasound as an open area in the spine, especially during the second trimester. The severity and location of the defect can be evaluated, providing important information for decision-making.

48.5.2 Maternal Serum Alpha-Fetoprotein (AFP) Test

The maternal serum alpha-fetoprotein test measures the levels of AFP in the mother's blood. Elevated AFP levels may indicate a neural tube defect, including spina bifida. However, increased AFP levels can also be associated with other conditions, so further diagnostic testing is typically recommended to confirm the diagnosis.

48.5.3 Multiple Marker Screening

In addition to AFP, multiple marker screening may include the measurement of other substances in the mother's blood, such as human chorionic gonadotropin (hCG) and unconjugated estriol.

Abnormal levels of these markers may suggest an increased risk of neural tube defects, prompting further investigation.

48.5.4 Amniocentesis

If prenatal screening indicates an elevated risk of spina bifida or other neural tube defects, amniocentesis may be recommended. Amniotic fluid contains cells shed by the developing fetus, and examining these cells can provide a more definitive diagnosis.

48.5.5 Non-invasive Prenatal Testing (NIPT)

NIPT, which analyzes cell-free DNA in the mother's blood, is primarily used for screening common chromosomal abnormalities. While it is not specifically designed for spina bifida, it may provide some additional information.

48.6 Clinical Features

Myelomeningocele and meningoceles appear as sac-like lesions over the back and are obvious at birth. The sac may be covered with meningeal membrane only or with membrane and skin. In open myeloceles, the neural elements form the floor of the cyst, and CSF leaks continuously from the open cord. The baby's posture may suggest some type of paralysis or even the neurological level of the lesion. Deformities of the lower limbs, such as equinovarus or calcaneovalgus of the feet, recurvatum of the knee, and hip dislocation, are common and probably due to a combination of factors such as muscle imbalance, lack of movement, and abnormal limb position in utero, or to associated anomalies that are independent of the paralysis. The symptoms and complications associated with spina bifida vary depending on the type and severity of the condition. Common issues include motor and sensory deficits, orthopedic problems, bowel and bladder dysfunction, and, in more severe cases, hydrocephalus. Individuals with spina bifida may also face challenges related to mobility, learning, and social interactions.

48.7 Multidisciplinary Approach to Treatment

Treatment for spina bifida is often multidisciplinary, involving a team of healthcare professionals such as pediatric surgeons, neurosurgeons, orthopedic surgeons, urologists, physical therapists, and social workers. Parental education and counselling forms the cornerstone of effective management. Early intervention is crucial to address the specific needs of individuals with spina bifida and optimize their quality of life.

Surgical Interventions: In cases of myelomeningocele, surgery is typically performed shortly after birth to repair the spinal defect and minimize the risk of infection. Additional surgeries may be required as the individual grows to address orthopedic and neurological issues.

Therapeutic Interventions: Physical therapy, occupational therapy, and speech therapy play essential roles in managing the challenges associated with spina bifida. These interventions aim to enhance mobility, promote independence, and improve overall function.

Management of Associated Conditions: Addressing complications such as hydrocephalus, bowel and bladder dysfunction, and orthopedic issues is integral to the comprehensive care of individuals with spina bifida.

48.7.1 Prevention

Folic acid supplementation with a dose of 400 mcg/day is recommended before conception and continued throughout the first trimester of pregnancy. This has been shown to reduce the risk of neural tube defects.

48.8 Assistive Devices and Adaptive Technology

Assistive devices and adaptive technology can significantly improve the daily lives of individuals with spina bifida. Wheelchairs, braces, and other mobility aids enhance independence, while technology, such as voice recognition software and computer adaptations, facilitates communication and education.

48.9 Psychosocial Impact and Family Support

Living with spina bifida can present emotional and social challenges for individuals and their families. Psychosocial support, including counseling and support groups, can be invaluable in helping individuals cope with the emotional aspects of the condition. Additionally, family support and education are crucial in navigating the complexities of caring for a child with spina bifida.

48.10 Educational and Employment Opportunities

Despite the challenges posed by spina bifida, individuals with the condition can lead fulfilling lives, pursue education, and engage in meaningful employment. Inclusive educational environments, reasonable accommodations, and workplace support contribute to the success of individuals with spina bifida.

48.11 Research and Future Perspectives

Ongoing research continues to advance our understanding of spina bifida, with a focus on preventive measures, improved treatment options, and enhanced quality of life for affected individuals. Genetic studies, stem cell research, and innovative surgical techniques offer hope for further progress in the field.

48.12 Key Points

Spina bifida is a complex and challenging condition that requires a comprehensive and multidisciplinary approach to care. Advances in medical science, coupled with increased awareness and support, contribute to improved outcomes for individuals with spina bifida. By addressing the physical, emotional, and social aspects of the condition, healthcare professionals, families, and communities can work together to enhance the lives of those affected by spina bifida.

Spina bifida, particularly the more severe form known as myelomeningocele, can give rise to various orthopedic manifestations due to the impact on the spine, nerves, and musculoskeletal system. The orthopedic issues associated with spina bifida often require ongoing management and intervention. Below are some common orthopedic manifestations:

48.12.1 Muscle Weakness and Imbalance

Cause: The incomplete closure of the spinal column can result in damage to the nerves that control the muscles below the affected area.

Manifestation: Muscle weakness and imbalance, particularly in the lower limbs, are common. This can lead to difficulties with standing, walking, and maintaining proper posture.

48.12.2 Joint Contractures

Cause: Imbalance in muscle strength and tone, coupled with reduced mobility, can lead to joint contractures.

Manifestation: Contractures, which involve the shortening of muscles and tendons, can affect the flexibility and range of motion in joints. Commonly affected areas include the hips, knees, and ankles.

48.12.3 Scoliosis

Cause: Weakness in the muscles supporting the spine and the uneven pull of muscles can contribute to the development of scoliosis.

Manifestation: Scoliosis, an abnormal curvature of the spine, is a common orthopedic issue in individuals with spina bifida. Regular monitoring and, in some cases, bracing or surgical intervention may be necessary.

48.12.4 Hip Dysplasia and Dislocation

Cause: Muscle imbalances and weakness can lead to abnormal forces on the hip joint during development.

Manifestation: Hip dysplasia (abnormal development of the hip joint) and dislocation are common, requiring early detection and intervention, often through the use of orthopedic devices or surgery.

48.12.5 Foot Deformities

Cause: Nerve damage and muscle weakness can result in foot deformities.

Manifestation: Clubfoot and other foot deformities may occur, affecting mobility. Orthopedic interventions, such as braces or corrective surgery, may be employed to address these issues.

48.12.6 Orthopedic Surgeries

Cause: Progressive orthopedic issues may necessitate surgical interventions.

Manifestation: Orthopedic surgeries, such as those to correct scoliosis, address joint contractures, or manage hip dysplasia, may be required to improve function and quality of life.

48.12.7 Pressure Sores and Skin Issues

Cause: Limited mobility and sensation can lead to increased pressure on certain areas of the body.

Manifestation: Pressure sores, particularly in areas where bones are close to the skin surface, are common. Proper skin care, regular repositioning, and pressure-relief devices are crucial in preventing and managing these issues.

48.12.8 Osteoporosis

Cause: Reduced weight-bearing activities and muscle weakness can contribute to decreased bone density.

Manifestation: Individuals with spina bifida may be at an increased risk of developing osteoporosis. Adequate nutritional support, weight-bearing exercises, and medical interventions may be necessary to address this concern.

48.12.9 Functional Limitations

Cause: Cumulative effects of orthopedic manifestations can result in functional limitations.

Manifestation: Reduced mobility, challenges with activities of daily living, and the need for assistive devices are common functional limitations. Rehabilitation and assistive technology can help individuals maximize their independence.

48.12.10 Long-Term Management

Cause: Orthopedic manifestations often require lifelong management and monitoring.

Manifestation: Regular follow-ups with orthopedic specialists, physical therapists, and other healthcare professionals are essential to address the evolving needs of individuals with spina bifida.

In conclusion, the orthopedic manifestations of spina bifida are diverse and can significantly impact the musculoskeletal system. A multidisciplinary approach involving orthopedic specialists, physical therapists, and other healthcare professionals is crucial in providing comprehensive care and improving the overall quality of life for individuals with spina bifida.

Muscle Dystrophies and Myopathies

49

Bhaskar Sarkar

Myopathies are a heterogeneous group of disorders primarily affecting the skeletal muscle structure, metabolism, or channel function. Common signs and symptoms of myopathies include weakness, stiffness, cramps, and spasms in activities of daily living.

49.1 Aetiology

Myopathies are generally caused by disruption in the muscle tissue integrity, and the metabolic stability which may be due to inherited genetic diseases or metabolic errors, certain drugs and toxins, bacterial or viral infections, inflammation, or minerals, electrolytes and hormonal irregularities.

B. Sarkar (✉)
Department of Orthopaedics, All India Institute of Medical Sciences, Rishikesh, India

V. Kumar et al. (eds.), *A Quick Guide to Essential Orthopedics*,
https://doi.org/10.1007/978-981-95-2676-5_49

49.1.1 Inherited Myopathies [1]

Congenital
- Nemaline myopathy
- Core mypthies
- Centronuclear myopathies

Mitochondrial
- MELAS
- Kearns-Sayre syndrome
- Others

Metabiloc
- Lipid myopathies
- Glycogen storage disease myopathy

Muscular dystrophies
- Dystrophinopathies (Duchene muscular dystrophy, Beckers muscular dystrophy)
- Myotonic muscular dystrophy
- Fascioscapulohumeral muscular dystrophies (type 1 and 2)
- Emery-Dreifuss muscular dystrophy
- Limb-girdle muscular dystrophies
- Congenital muscular dystrophy (most common being LAMA2-related, collagen VI-related and alfa-dystroglycan-related)

Channelopathies
- Periodic paralysis (Hypokalemic, hyperkalemic, Andersen-Tawil syndrome)
- Nondystrophic myotonias (p.e. paramyotonia congenita, Thomsen disease)

49.1.2 Congenital Myopathies [2]

Congenital myopathy involves a variety of clinicopathological features, typically involving a patient with early-onset weakness together with characteristic histopathological findings on muscle biopsy and normal to slightly elevated creatine phosphokinase levels.

Abnormal excitation-contraction coupling is a common pathology in the congenital myopathies, either as a result of malformed contractile filaments in the case of the nemaline myopathy or disruption of calcium homeostasis at the level of the triad (the smallest functional component of the myofiber that includes the T-tubule and sarcoplasmic reticulum [SR]) in the case of the centronuclear/myotubular and core myopathies.

49.1.3 Mitochondrial Myopathy [3]

Mitochondrial myopathies can occur due to mutations in both mitochondrial DNA (mtDNA) and nuclear DNA (nDNA). Defects in the mitochondrial respiratory chain affect energy production and almost invariably involve skeletal muscle, causing exercise intolerance, cramps, recurrent myoglobinuria or fixed weakness, which often affects extraocular muscles and results in droopy eyelids (ptosis) and progressive external ophthalmoplegia.

49.1.4 Metabolic Myopathies [4]

The metabolic myopathies are a heterogeneous group of disorders that share the common feature of decreased production of cellular energy in the muscle. It is characterised by transient or fixed weakness, exercise-induced fatigue, muscle cramping and rhabdomyolysis.

Most of the fuel for muscle is provided by carbohydrates in the form of glycogen and by lipids in the form of free fatty acids. Glycogen is metabolised to pyruvate inside the muscle cells. Pyruvate is then decarboxylated into acetyl-coenzyme A (acetyl-CoA) inside the mitochondria. Similarly, b-oxidation of free fatty acids (fatty acid oxidation; FAO) inside mitochondria provides another source of acetyl-CoA. Acetyl-CoA then enters the Krebs cycle, generating ATP. Defects in any one of the steps involved in this complex metabolic pathway can lead to an insufficient supply of ATP and an inability to sustain normal muscle function in times of increased metabolic demand. Common aetiology of metabolic myopathies are:

- Lipid myopathies (most common are carnitine palmitoyl transferase II deficiency, very-long-chain-acyl-CoA dehydrogenase deficiency and trifunctional protein deficiency).
- Glycogen storage disease myopathy (Acid maltase deficiency—Pompe disease, Debrancher deficiency—Cori disease—and muscle phosphorylase deficiency—McArdle disease—are the most frequently encountered).

49.1.5 Muscular Dystrophies [5]

Muscular dystrophies are genetic, progressive, degenerative disorders with the primary symptom of muscle weakness. Duchenne, Becker, facioscapulohumeral, and myotonic muscular dystrophies are most prevalent. The limb-girdle, Emery–Dreifuss, and oculopharyngeal muscular dystrophies are less common.

(a) Dystrophinopathies:
  - Most common mutation in dystrophin gene present as DMD, but other phenotypic manifestations are Becker muscular dystrophy; isolated quadriceps myopathy; asymptomatic or minimally symptomatic hyperkalaemia; aches, pains, cramps, and rhabdomyolysis, dilated cardiomyopathy; and cognitive disorders.
  - DMD is an X-linked recessive disorder leading to complete absence of dystrophin protein which leads to poor muscle fibre regeneration and progressive replacement of muscle tissue with fibro-fatty tissue. DMD is most often present in boys between 3 and 5 years of age because of delayed motor milestones and falls, along with difficulty running and jumping. Boys with DMD also have head lag when pulled to sitting from supine and a Gower manoeuvre when rising from the floor. Cognitive involvement is common in DMD. Of patients with DMD, 30% have intellectual disability.

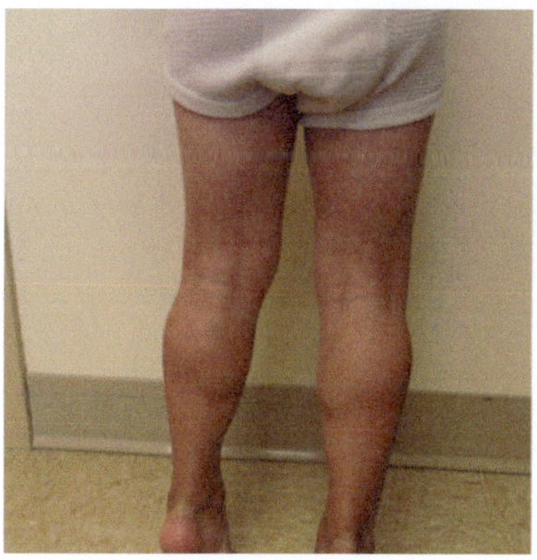

Calf muscles pseudohypertrophy

Calf muscles pseudohypertrophy

- Becker's dystrophy is similar to DMD; it differs in that dystrophin protein is decreased instead of absent, has a later onset, slower progression and longer life expectancy. The severity of weakness varies substantially in patients with BMD. Weakness may begin as early as 5–6 years of age or may start in the fifth or sixth decade. Patients are more prone to cardiomyopathy irrespective of skeletal muscle involvement. The intellectual function is generally normal.

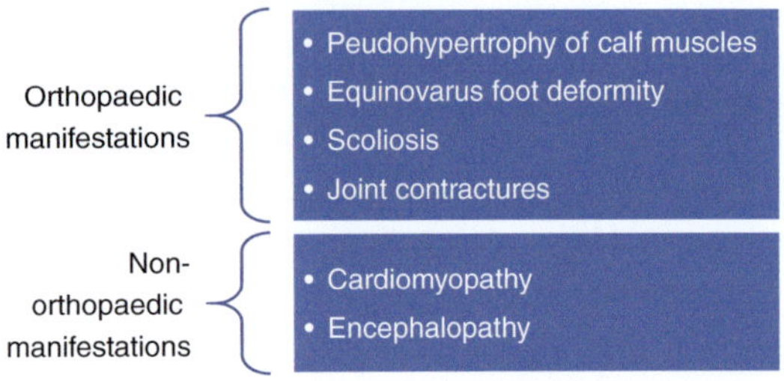

(b) Facioscapulohumeral muscular dystrophy
- Autosomal dominant disorder with predominant involvement of fascial, periscapular, biceps and triceps muscles. Weakness spreads asymmetrically and cranio-caudally with onset in the face, then the scapular region, followed by the proximal arms, then the legs.
- Symptoms appear in the patient's teens. Facial weakness appears first with perioral and periocular weakness. Extraocular and bulbar muscles remain unaffected. In shoulder girdle, scapular winging is prominent. Wasting of pectorals leads to reversal of axillary folds (the fold exits inwards towards neck). Periscapular wasting leads to triple hump deformity (prominent deltoid, AC joint and overriding scapula).

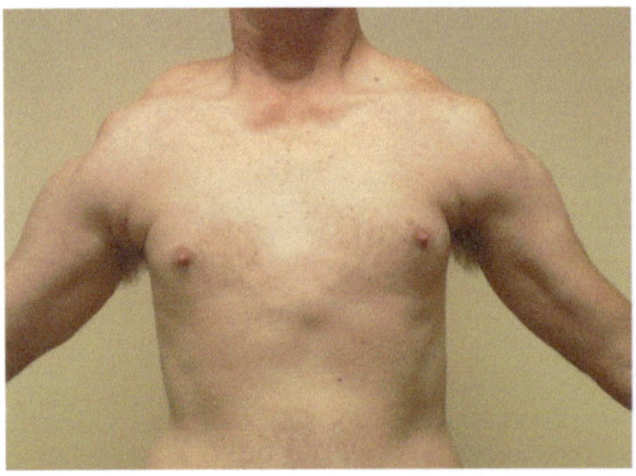

Triple hump deformity, pectoral wasting and reversal of axillary

Triple hump deformity, pectoral wasting and reversal of axillary

(c) Myotonic dystrophy [6]

- Myotonia is the most common muscular dystrophy in adults. It has autosomal dominant inheritance. Two major forms are recognised based on clinical and molecular presentation: Myotonic dystrophy type I (DM1), known as Steinert disease, and myotonic dystrophy type II (DM2), or proximal myotonic myopathy which is a milder variety of DM1. Clinical presentation is diverse and can range from asymptomatic electrical myotonia to severe weakness and disability, including cardiac conduction defects, infertility, cataracts, and insulin resistance. Myotonia is characterised by impaired relaxation of muscles after voluntary contraction due to repetitive depolarisation of the muscle membrane.
- DM1 is caused by expansion of cytosine-thymine-guanine (CTG) repeat in the 3′-untranslated region of the DM1 protein kinase (DMPK) gene on chromosome 19q13.3. The more the CTG repeats, the more severe the disease.
- The cardinal feature of adult-onset DM1 includes myotonia, weakness and cataract. The patients present with typical facial features ("Hatchet-facies") such as temporalis and masseter muscle wasting, male pattern baldness, and facial weakness (ptosis and a "fish-mouth" look). The patient's inability to release a weak introductory handshake (reflecting grip myotonia and flexor digitorum profundus weakness) gives an early clue for diagnosis. Other systems' involvement is outlined in the table below.

> Hatchet facies: Temporalis and masseter wasting, ptosis and fish mouth appearance dur to perioral weakness.

Eye	Cataract (Christmas tree cataract)
Cardiac involvement	Arrhythmias and conduction blocks
Respiratory system	Respiratory muscle weakness and pneumonias
Endocrine system	DM, thyroid deficiencies, testosterone deficiency
Higher function	Avoidant personality, depression, apathy, and mild cognitive impairment

- DM2 most often presents in middle age. Myalgia and stiffness are the predominant symptoms; myotonia may be minimal or even absent. Contrary to DM1, weakness occurs mainly in the proximal muscles, and facial muscles are not involved. In most patients, the systemic manifestations in DM2 are less frequent and milder than in DM1.

(d) Limb-girdle muscular dystrophy:

- Limb-girdle muscular dystrophies are genetic muscle diseases with postnatal onset of progressive weakness and muscle atrophy affecting proximal upper and lower extremity muscles. Autosomal dominant limb-girdle muscular dystrophies occur less frequently, have lower creatine kinase rates, and account for only around 10% to 15% of cases. Autosomal recessive limb-girdle muscular dystrophies tend to have much higher creatine kinase levels and comprise the majority of cases.

(e) Emery–Dreifuss muscular dystrophy.

- Disease starts in the first or second decade of life with early features of inability to extend elbow. Cardinal triad includes (1) contractures of the elbow flexors, ankle plantar flexors, and cervical spine early in disease; (2) childhood onset of humeroperoneal weakness and (3) cardiac disease with arrhythmias, conduction block, and cardiomyopathy.

49.2 Acquired Myopathies

(a) Toxic / Drug induced myopathies: [7]

- The major symptoms in drug-induced myopathies are proximal muscle weakness, increased muscle enzyme levels, electromyographic changes and histological lesions.
- Drugs which can lead to myopathies are: statins, fibrates, propofol, alcohol, corti-

costeroids, neuromuscular blockers, TNF alpha inhibitors, diuretics, etc.

(b) Inflammatory myopathies: [8]
- Idiopathic inflammatory myopathies are rare conditions that can affect multiple organs apart from muscle and often lead to a severe impairment of the quality of life. Major symptoms include weakness of arms and legs, problems in walking and climbing stairs or lifting an object above the head. Pain is often an accompanying symptom and, except for inclusion body myositis (IBM) cases.
- Patients with dermatomyositis presents with skin manifestations like Gottron papules on the dorsal sides of the hands and fingers, a periorbital oedema and erythema of the face (heliotrope rash), the anterior upper chest (V-sign) or the posterior neck (shawl sign). Periungual erythema and telangiectasia as well as cracked, thickened skin of the ventral and dorsal parts of the fingers and hands occur ("mechanic's hands").
- Myopathy can also be acquired through bacterial infections (Lyme disease, pyomyositis—Staphylococcus aureus), viral infections (Human immunodeficiency virus (HIV), Coxsackie A and B viruses, Influenza), parasitic infections (trichinosis, toxoplasmosis, cysticercosis) and fungal infections (Candida, Coccidiomycosis). Other causes of acquired myopathy are outlined in the chart above.

49.3 History and Clinical Examination

Muscle weakness is a common complaint among patients with myopathy. Diagnosis begins with patient history, distinguishing weakness from fatigue and asthenia. Positive points in history includes:

- Motor involvement with no sensory symptoms.
- Proximal muscle weakness- pelvic and shoulder girdle. Patients usually complain of difficulty in rising from a sitting position, climbing stairs or practicing overhead activities.
- Some myopathies may present with involvement of different groups of muscles like thigh, back, facial and bulbar muscles.

Polymyositis and dermatomyositis both affect women more than men and involve proximal muscles. Polymyositis is associated with arthralgia, and dermatomyositis with skin lesions discussed earlier. Similarly, classical clinical findings of myopathies have been discussed under individual topics above.

49.3.1 Evaluation

A. Blood parameters
1. Complete blood count: Anaemia and increased leucocyte count may be associated with infectious myopathy and inflammatory myopathy.
2. BUN and serum creatinine.
3. Electrolytes: Dyselectrolytaemia is frequently associated with myopathy.
4. Liver enzymes (AST, ALT, GGT): Abnormal liver enzymes are frequently associated with rhabdomyolysis. AST is found in the cytosolic and mitochondrial isoenzymes of skeletal muscles. ALT is specific to liver but also found in skeletal muscles in low concentrations [9].
5. Creatine kinase: CK is elevated in myopathies with muscle degeneration and rhabdomyolysis. It is significantly elevated in IIM, muscular dystrophies, drugs, or infections associated myopathies.
6. Thyroid function test.
7. Specific antibody tests for myositis.
8. Urine analysis for myoglobinuria.

B. EMG & NCS
These are helpful to distinguish myopathy from neurologic diseases. EMG findings of short, small, low-amplitude polyphasic motor unit potentials, fibrillation potentials even at rest, and bizarre high-frequency repetitive discharges support findings of myopathic disease.

C. MRI
Useful to detect the location, extent of the disease and fatty replacement of muscle tissue. It guides the site to perform muscle biopsy.

D. Muscle Biopsy [10]
Muscle biopsy can be very useful to define the aetiology of muscle disease. Histologic features specific to the myopathies are listed below.

Myopathy	Histopathological features
Nemaline myopathy	Rod inclusions
Core myopathy (central and multi-minicore)	Cores and/or multi-minicores inclusions
Centronuclear myopathy/ myotubular myopathy	Nuclei centralisationnecklace fibres
Mitochondrial myopathy	Sub-sarcolemmal and intermyofibrillar accumulation of mitochondria: "ragged blue/red fibers"
Metabolic myopathy (glycogen storage disease)	Basophilic/PAS-positive vacuolescytosolic inclusions
Metabolic myopathy (lipid storage disease)	Increased number and size of lipid droplets and neutral-lipid containing vacuoles inside muscle fibers
Muscular dystrophy	Muscle fibre necrosis, regeneration, fibrosis and atrophy, nuclei internalisation
Idiopathic inflammatory myopathy	Lymphocytic infiltration with endomysial inflammation, necrosis and atrophy

49.4 Management

Treatment of congenital myopathies is generally supportive. The care includes physical exercise, nutrition, physical and occupational therapies, genetic analysis and counselling [11].

Muscular dystrophies are treated with corticosteroids [5]. Common corticosteroid regimens include (1) prednisone 0.75 mg/kg/d; (2) deflazacort 0.9 mg/kg/d; (3) prednisolone 0.75 mg/kg/d for 10 days alternating with 10 days off corticosteroids and (4) prednisone 2.5 mg/kg to 5 mg/kg every Friday and Saturday. In patients with mitochondrial myopathies, creatine monohydrate 5–10 g/day may benefit in improving the symptoms.

Acquired myopathies are managed by treating the causing disease. Inflammatory myopathy is treated by immunomodulators [12]. Corticosteroids, methotrexate, azathioprine, cyclosporin, and cyclophosphamide are the commonly used drugs. In myopathies with rhabdomyolysis, acute kidney injury prevention by adequate hydration and monitoring renal parameters is important.

Multiple Choice Questions

1. Which of the following describes the inheritance pattern of Duchenne's muscular dystrophy?
   (a) Autosomal dominant
   (b) X-linked dominant
   (c) Autosomal recessive
   (d) X-linked recessive

Ans: Autosomal recessive

2. Emery–Dreifuss muscular dystrophy is unique among the dystrophies because of the development of which deformity?
   (a) Neck extension contracture
   (b) Knee flexion

(c) Hip abduction
(d) Equinus contracture

Ans: Emery–Dreifuss muscular dystrophy is an X-linked disorder of emerin, which is a cell-membrane protein. Symptoms and signs develop within the first decade in most cases. A unique deformity, neck extension contracture, develops, in addition to elbow flexion contractures and peroneal wasting. The other deformities listed above are common in many dystrophies. Correct Answer: Neck extension contracture

3. Which of the following muscles is first affected in facioscapulohumeral dystrophy?
(a) Orbicularis oris
(b) Deltoid
(c) Serratus anterior
(d) Supraspinatus

Ans: In facioscapulohumeral dystrophy, the facial muscles are affected first, commonly presenting with an inability to whistle. The serratus muscles and scapular stabilisers are affected next. The deltoid, supraspinatus, and infraspinatus are typically not affected in this disease. Correct Answer: Orbicularis oris

4. A 15-year-old girl is experiencing progressive weakness. She is unable to abduct her arms above 100Â° (Slide). She has a progressive lordosis. Her facial expression is flat, and she cannot smile. Her mother has the same constellation of findings. No scoliosis is present. She and her mother are able to walk independently. The most likely diagnosis is:
(a) Parsonage-Turner syndrome
(b) Facioscapulohumeral dystrophy
(c) Friedreich ataxia
(d) Nemaline rod myopathy

Ans: This patient most likely has facioscapulohumeral dystrophy. With a frequency of 1:20,000, it is a rare disorder inherited in an autosomal-dominant fashion. The genetic abnormality is found on chromosome 4, with a decreased number of D4Z4 tandem repeats, but this does not appear to code for a protein product. Scoliosis is not present. In this condition, selective weakness of the serratus anterior, trapezius, and rhomboid muscles is present. Therefore, the scapula is not effectively stabilised against the trunk during use. Correct Answer: Facioscapulohumeral dystrophy.

5. Emery–Dreifuss syndrome is manifest by all of the following except:
(a) Heel cord contractures
(b) Limited cervical flexion
(c) Elbow contractures
(d) Cardiomyopathy
(e) Scoliosis

Ans: Emery–Dreifuss syndrome is due to an encoding error in emerin, which may be a stabiliser of the nuclear membrane. Emery–Dreifuss syndrome is characterised by a triad of contractures of the heel cord, elbow, and cervical spine. Cardiomyopathy may cause heart block or other arrhythmias. Scoliosis is not commonly found in this condition. Correct answer: Scoliosis

6. A 20-year-old boy presents with weakness and difficulty in relaxing his hands and feet. Muscle biopsy reveals centrally located nuclei, chains of nuclei and disorganised sarcoplasmic masses. The mutation is most likely on which chromosome?
(a) 19
(b) X
(c) 11
(d) 9

Ans: The long arm of chromosome 19 carries the gene for myotonic dystrophy type 1. The gene for myotonic dystrophy type 2 is found on chromosome. Correct answer: 19.

References

1. Nagy H, Veerapaneni KD. Myopathy. [Updated 2023 Aug 14]. In: StatPearls [Internet]. Treasure Island: StatPearls Publishing; 2023. Available from: https://www.ncbi.nlm.nih.gov/books/NBK562290/.
2. Nance JR, Dowling JJ, Gibbs EM, Bönnemann CG. Congenital myopathies: an update. Curr Neurol Neurosci Rep 2012;12(2):165–174. https://doi.org/10.1007/s11910-012-0255-x. PMID: 22392505; PMCID: PMC4491488.

3. DiMauro S. Mitochondrial myopathies. Curr Opin Rheumatol. 2006;18(6):636–41. https://doi.org/10.1097/01.bor.0000245729.17759.f2. PMID: 17053512
4. Smith EC, El-Gharbawy A, Koeberl DD. Metabolic myopathies: clinical features and diagnostic approach. Rheum Dis Clin N Am. 2011;37(2):201–17. https://doi.org/10.1016/j.rdc.2011.01.004. PMID: 21444020
5. Wicklund MP. The muscular dystrophies. Continuum (Minneap Minn). Muscle Dis. 2013;19(6):1535–70. https://doi.org/10.1212/01.CON.0000440659.41675.8b. Erratum in: Continuum (Minneap Minn). 2014 Jun;20(3 Neurology of Systemic Disease):520. PMID: 24305447
6. Vydra DG, Rayi A. Myotonic Dystrophy. [Updated 2023 Jun 26]. In: StatPearls [Internet]. Treasure Island: StatPearls Publishing; 2023 Jan-. Available from: https://www.ncbi.nlm.nih.gov/books/NBK557446/
7. Le Quintrec JS, Le Quintrec JL. Drug-induced myopathies. Baillieres Clin Rheumatol. 1991;5(1):21–38. https://doi.org/10.1016/s0950-3579(05)80294-8. PMID: 2070426
8. Schmidt J. Current classification and management of inflammatory myopathies. J Neuromuscul Dis. 2018;5(2):109–29. https://doi.org/10.3233/JND-180308. PMID: 29865091; PMCID: PMC6004913
9. Lim AK. Abnormal liver function tests associated with severe rhabdomyolysis. World J Gastroenterol. 2020;26(10):1020–8. https://doi.org/10.3748/wjg.v26.i10.1020. PMID: 32205993; PMCID: PMC7081005
10. González-Jamett AM, Bevilacqua JA, Díaz AMC, Hereditary Myopathies [Internet]. Muscle cell and tissue—current status of research field. InTech. 2018; https://doi.org/10.5772/intechopen.76076.
11. Voet NB, van der Kooi EL, Riphagen II, Lindeman E, van Engelen BG, Geurts AC. Strength training and aerobic exercise training for muscle disease. In: Cochrane Database Syst Rev, vol. 1; 2010. p. CD003907.
12. Castro C, Gourley M. Diagnosis and treatment of inflammatory myopathy: issues and management. Ther Adv Musculoskelet Dis. 2012;4(2):111–20. https://doi.org/10.1177/1759720X11425092. PMID: 22870499; PMCID: PMC3383519

50 Perthes Disease

Ritesh Arvind Pandey, Anand Bhushan, and Lakshay Garg

50.1 Introduction

Legg–Calvé–Perthes disease is a self-limiting avascular necrosis of capital femoral epiphysis in children which frequently leads to deformation of femoral head. The name was derived as this pathology was discovered independently and simultaneously by Arthur Legg in USA (February), Jacques Calvé in France (July) and George Perthes in Germany (October) in 1910 [1, 2]. It is also known by different synonyms like Osteochondritis deformans juvenilis, coxa plana, pseudocoxalgia, arthritis deformans juvenilis, precoxalgia, coxa vara capitalis and quiet hip disease.

50.2 Epidemiology

Legg–Calvé–Perthes disease is fairly common with an incidence of 0.4–29/lakh children. The incidence varies among different regions and races. Caucasians are affected more than Asian or black population. Children between the age of 5 and 7 years are most commonly affected, though cases of early and late onset are possible. It is more frequently seen in boys with a male: female ratio of 4:1. Bilateral affection is seen in 10–20% of children and around 10% children have genetic inheritance.

50.3 Aetiology

The exact aetiology of LCPD is still unknown. The cause could be multifactorial and includes a combination of environmental, metabolic and genetic factors [3]. The most common risk factors for LCPD include;

- Genetic inheritance: The most common mode of inheritance is autosomal dominant. However, patterns ranging from autosomal recessive to polygenic inheritance have been observed.
- Trauma: Lateral epiphyseal artery in growing proximal femur is susceptible to disruption even with mild trauma, and it may compromise the vascularity of femoral head.
- Coagulopathies: Factor V Leiden coagulopathy, protein C or S deficiency
- Thrombophilias: This is present in about 50% of cases.
- Hypofibrinolysis: The ability to dissolve clots is reduced.
- Exposure to smoke: Both active and passive exposure have been associated with LCPD
- Low socioeconomic status: Malnourished children are at greater risk of developing LCPD

R. A. Pandey (✉) · L. Garg
All India Institute of Medical Sciences Patna, Patna, Bihar, India

A. Bhushan
Big Apollo Spectra Hospital, Patna, India

V. Kumar et al. (eds.), *A Quick Guide to Essential Orthopedics*,
https://doi.org/10.1007/978-981-95-2676-5_50

- Maturation disorder: Children with LCPD commonly have a delayed bone age and short stature.

50.4 Pathogenesis

The key event in the pathogenesis of LCPD is ischemia of the femoral head. Necrosis softens the femoral head, and its ability to resist deformation is compromised (Fig. 50.1). The necrotic femoral head passes through different stages as mentioned below:

1. *Stage of necrosis:* The normal turnover of calcium in the femoral head is reduced. This results in accumulation of calcium in necrotic bone, thereby compromising its mechanical properties and making it more prone to microfractures. As a result of degeneration of bone cells, these microfractures remain unrepaired.
2. *Stage of revascularisation (fragmentation):* the necrotic bone is resorbed, causing further compromise in mechanical properties of femoral head.
3. *Stage of reossification (healing):* The femoral epiphysis starts re-establishing as osteoblastic activity takes over.
4. *Stage of remodelling:* The newly formed femoral head may be deformed. Reshaping takes place to some extent as the child grows further.

Usually, the stage of necrosis and fragmentation lasts for six months, the reossification stage lasts for 18–36 months and stage of remodelling continues thereafter till maturity. It is crucial to identify different stages as it helps in decision-making in management of Perthes disease. Primarily, the disease does not involve the acetabulum, but it may be secondarily involved due to degenerative changes or remodelling of the deformed femoral head.

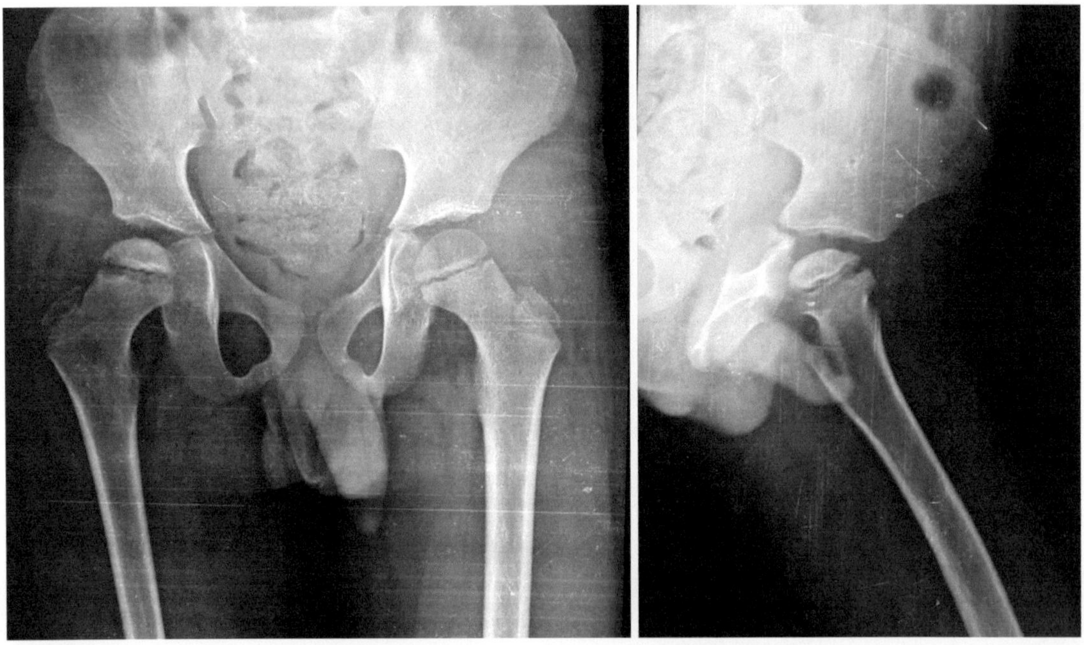

Fig. 50.1 Legg–Calvé–Perthes disease on right side. Stage of necrosis is characterised by sclerosis of epiphysis and widening of joint space

50.5 Clinical Features

- The children typically present with a painless limp of acute or insidious onset.
- Some patients may complain of pain which is localised to hip or may be referred to thigh, knee or abdomen. The pain worsens with progression of disease. The systemic symptoms are typically absent.

50.6 Clinical Examination

- The extremes of all movements are diminished and painful at a very early stage.
- Later, the movements improve, but abduction and internal rotation are almost always limited.
- In most of the cases the earliest clinical sign is limitation of abduction in flexion. When the hip is flexed it may go into obligatory external rotation and knee points towards ipsilateral axilla (normally it goes towards mid clavicular region). This is called *Catterall's sign*.
- In advanced stages, the leg-length discrepancy may be observed and Trendelenburg test is usually positive.
- Mild to moderate disuse atrophy of the thigh and buttocks may be present as a result of pain.
- Gait is initially antalgic in cases of acute onset. As the disease becomes chronic, children develop Trendelenburg and waddling gait in unilateral and bilateral affection, respectively.

50.7 Classification

Several classifications for LCPD have been suggested. Most of them are based on the area of femoral head involvement and help in predicting the prognosis and deciding appropriate management [4].

1. *Waldenstrom classification (1922):* After the initial reporting of condition in 1910, Waldenstrom described the detailed interpretation and stages of LCPD in 1922. Based on the microscopic and gross pathology, four stages were described.
    - *Incipient or stage of synovitis*: The synovium is inflamed, and joint fluid is increased. It lasts for about 1–3 weeks.
    - *Stage of avascular necrosis*: There is significant necrosis of bone, and trabeculae are crushed into minute fragments without any evidence of regeneration. However, gross contour of femoral head is maintained. This stage lasts for 6–12 months
    - *Stage of fragmentation / regeneration*: The dead bone is invaded with vascular connective tissue and is actively resorbed by the osteoclast. The necrotic bone is replaced by newly formed immature bone. It is marked by loss of epiphyseal height as a result of collapse of bony trabeculae and bone resorption and lasts for 2–3 years.
    - *Healed or residual stage*: In this stage, maturation of the newly formed bone takes place. Ossific nucleus is permanently deformed. The femoral head is enlarged, flattened and subluxates laterally.
2. *Catterall classification (1971)*: This is a prognostic classification based on the extent of involvement of femoral head. Accordingly, four groups were suggested (Fig. 50.2)
    - Group I: 25% involvement
    - Group II: 50% involvement
    - Group III: 75% involvement
    - Group IV: 100% involvement

A greater extent of femoral head involvement is associated with poorer prognosis. Additionally, radiographic head at-risk signs were described indicating a poor prognosis. These are lateral epiphyseal calcification (cage sign), lateral subluxation, small osteoporotic segment forming a translucent V-shaped trough in lateral epiphysis (Gage's sign), metaphyseal cyst, subchondral fracture in anterolateral part of epiphysis (crescent sign / Caffey's sign / Salter's sign) and horizontal growth plate.

3. *Stulberg classification (1981):* It predicts the onset of degenerative disease following LCPD

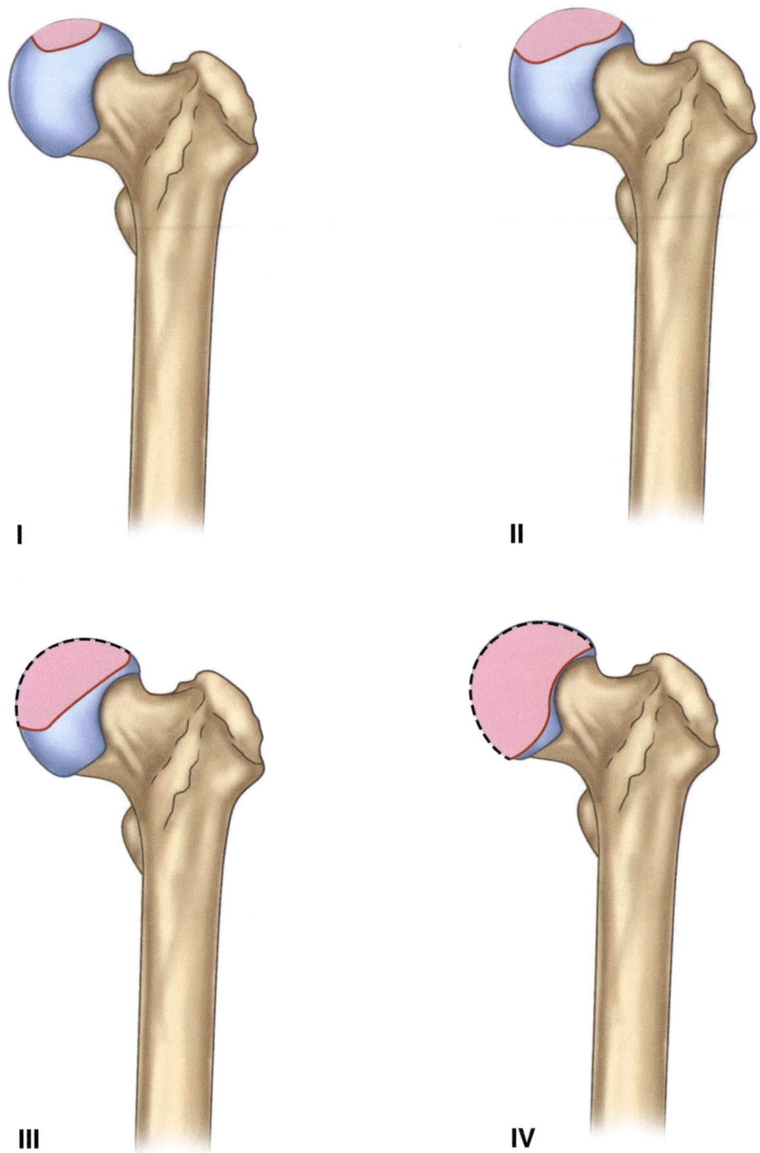

Fig. 50.2 Catterall classification

and is based on the size and shape of femoral head.

- I: Spherical congruency
- II: Spherical congruency with one or more of the following: coxa magna, coxa vara, oblique acetabulum
- III: Aspherical congruency but head is not flat
- IV: Aspherical congruency with flat head and acetabulum
- V: Aspherical incongruency

Type I and II carry a good prognosis, while type III, IV and V have a worse prognosis in order of increasing severity.

4. *Salter and Thompson classification (1984):* This classification is based on the size of subchondral fracture and identifies two subgroups (Fig. 50.3)
    - Group A: Subchondral fracture involving <50% of femoral dome
    - Group B: subchondral fracture involving >50% of femoral dome

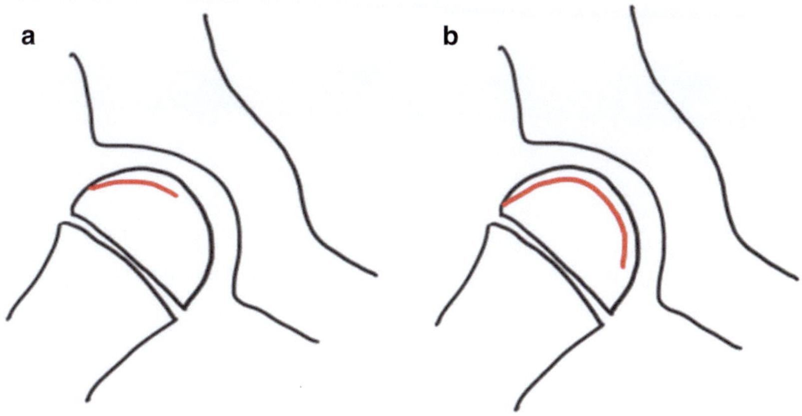

Fig. 50.3 Salter and Thompson classification

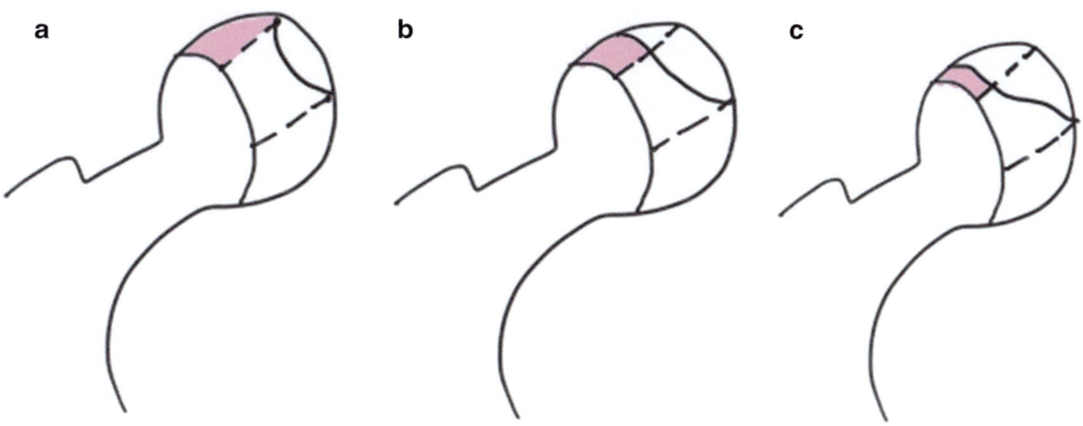

Fig. 50.4 Herring classification

Group A is claimed to have a better prognosis than group B.

5. *Herring classification (1992):* This uses the height of lateral pillar of epiphysis on an anteroposterior (AP) radiograph. The changes are specifically noted in the fragmentation stage of disease. Accordingly, three subgroups have been described (Fig. 50.4).
   - Group A: Normal height of lateral pillar
   - Group B: >50% of lateral pillar height is maintained
   - Group C: <50% of lateral pillar height is maintained

As per this classification, group A has good outcome and doesn't need any intervention. Group B benefits from intervention and has good to intermediate outcome, whereas group C has poor outcome despite a surgical intervention.

6. *Modified Elizabethtown Classification (2003):* This is the most commonly used classification as of now. It describes various stages of LCPD on an AP and lateral radiograph and aids in deciding the time and type of intervention (Fig. 50.5).
   - I: Stage of necrosis
     Ia: (early) sclerosis of epiphysis without any loss of epiphyseal height
     Ib: (late) sclerosis of epiphysis with some loss of epiphyseal height
   - II: Stage of fragmentation
     IIa: (early) fragmentation with one or two fissures in the epiphysis
     IIb: (late) advanced fragmentation without evidence of new bone formation
   - III: Stage of new bone formation

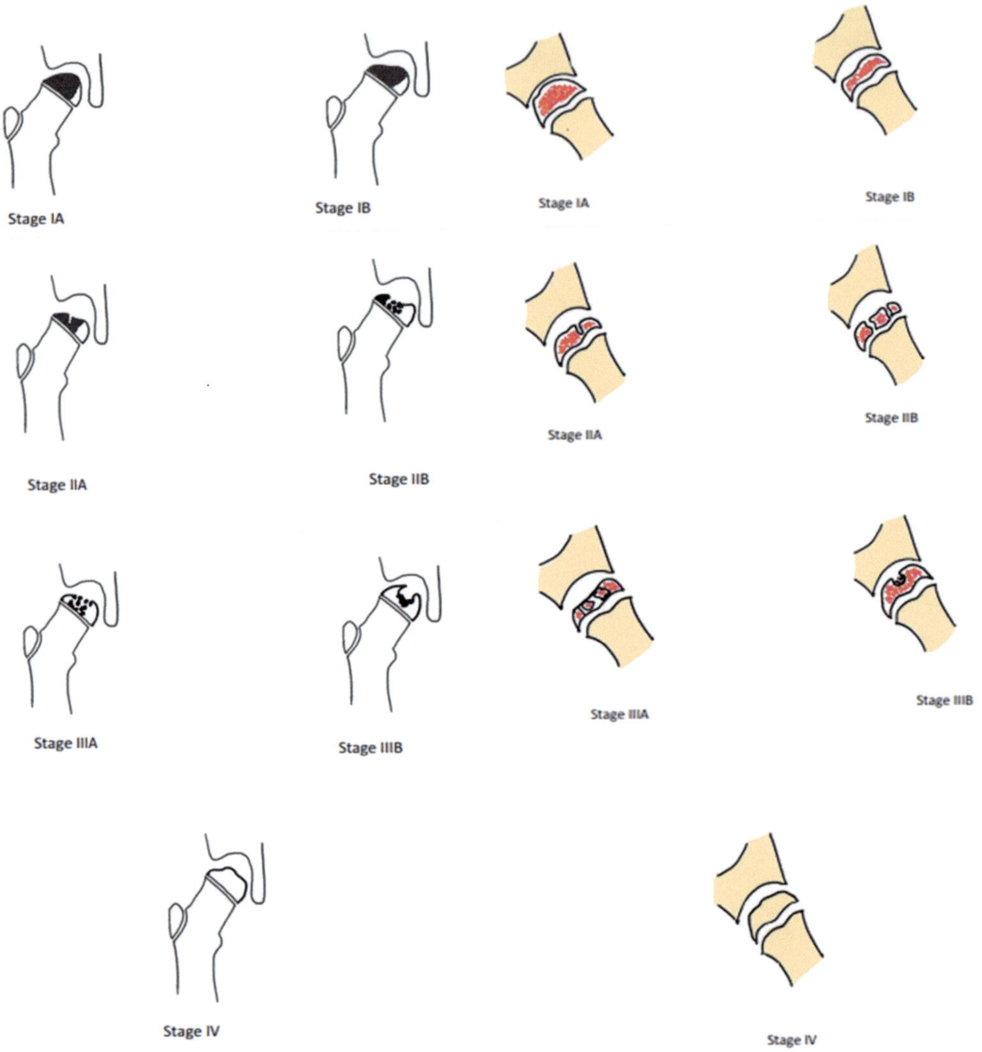

Fig. 50.5 Modified Elizabethtown classification AP and lateral views

IIIa: (early) new bone formation at the periphery involving <1/3 of the circumference of epiphysis
IIIb: (late) new bone formation at the periphery involving >1/3 of the circumference of epiphysis
- IV: Complete healing

50.8 Diagnosis

Diagnosis of LCPD can be difficult. The important diagnostic criteria that can be helpful are;

- *Clinical*: Pain is primarily localised in the hip. Most of the patients show limited hip internal rotation. Patients often have a history of practice of high-impact sports, smoke exposure and deprivation.
- *Radiological*: Typical radiographic features such as osteosclerosis, cystic change, and a "crescent sign" are apparent in earlier stages. After collapse, there is a loss of sphericity of the femoral head and degenerative arthritis in the late stages.
- *CT scan*: It shows zone of osteosclerosis surrounding the necrotic bone and shows subchondral bone fracture much earlier.

- *MRI*: It is the investigation of choice for evaluation of suspected Perthes disease. MRI may show abnormalities in femoral head much before radiography. It also assesses for revascularisation, healing and complications in the course of disease. MRI findings are variable and depend on the stage of disease.

50.9 Differential Diagnosis

1. Transient synovitis and septic arthritis: The early symptoms of the condition should be differentiated if they are of short duration and should undergo laboratory analysis.
2. Slipped capital femoral epiphysis SCFE and osteomyelitis / pyomyositis may also be included in the differential diagnosis.
3. Synchronous bilateral involvement should be differentiated from systemic skeletal dysplasia including multiple epiphyseal dysplasia, spondyloepiphyseal dysplasia, conditions with mucopolysaccharidosis or endocrine abnormalities like hypothyroidism.
4. Meyer's dysplasia: It is commonly bilateral, with very early mild involvement. It is characterised by delayed ossification or diffuse granular fragmentation as compared to conspicuous condensation and fragmentation seen in LCPD.

50.10 Management

LCPD is a self-healing local disease. Since the amount of femoral head deformity is variable, treatment is decided on a patient-to-patient basis [5, 6]. The goals of treatment include pain and symptom management, preservation of hip movements, and containment of femoral head in the acetabulum.

A variety of treatment options ranging from simple observation to invasive surgical procedures have been suggested [7]. The aim is to prevent deformity of femoral head, thereby avoiding hip incongruity and secondary osteoarthritis.

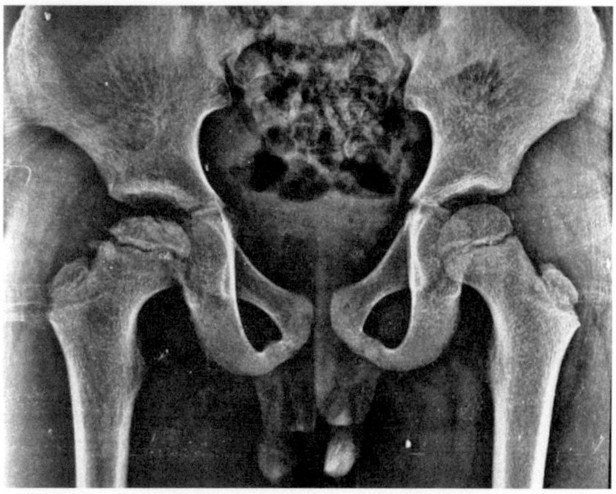

Fig. 50.6 Stage of early fragmentation on the right side. Surgical containment after this stage has a poor prognosis

Surgical or non-surgical containment is needed if a child is less than 8 years of age and there is extrusion of femoral head, or if a child is over 8 years of age regardless of head extrusion. The treatment has a better outcome if started before early fragmentation stage, whereas containment does not help if the disease is in reossification stage or if age is more than 12 years (Fig. 50.6).

50.10.1 Non-surgical Treatment

Close observation is sufficient in most children below 6 years of age with no limitation of range of motion or no lateral extrusion of the femoral head. Regular follow-up at every 3 months with clinical examination and radiographs is needed. Activity restriction and protective weight-bearing are suggested till complete ossification is evident on radiographs.

The use of orthotics, braces or casts is not recommended anymore as it needs prolonged immobilisation and leads to joint stiffness. It also causes anxiety in parents and has compliance issues. Instead, active physiotherapy is recommended to avoid disuse atrophy and to preserve range of hip movements.

50.10.2 Surgical Treatment

A variety of surgical procedures have been suggested depending on the age of patient, stage of disease and status of hip movement. The selection of appropriate surgical intervention requires meticulous clinical and radiological evaluation of patient [8].

- *Surgical containment*: This can be achieved either by proximal femoral (varus derotation) osteotomy or by a pelvic osteotomy (Fig. 50.7). It is indicated in presence of lateral extrusion of femoral head regardless of patient's age. It is also indicated as a prophylactic surgery in children over 8 years of age regardless of the epiphyseal extrusion.

  The prerequisites for doing so are a normal range of hip movements and a disease earlier or in the stage of early fragmentation. The containment of femoral head offers an opportunity for its satisfactory remodelling while it is going through advanced stages of LCPD.

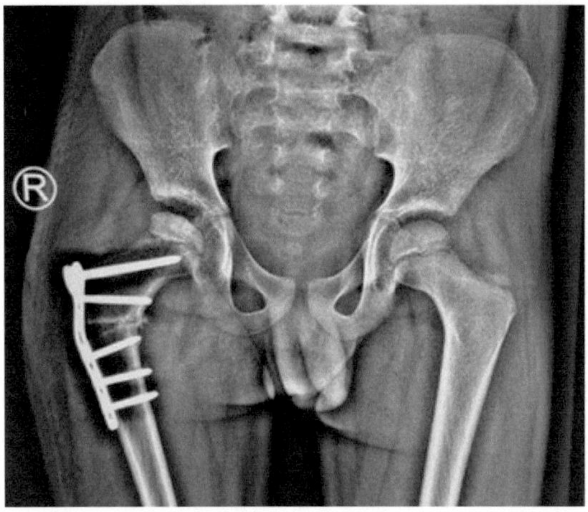

Fig. 50.7 Varus Derotation Osteotomy (VDRO) for surgical containment of femoral head

- *Valgus osteotomy*: It is indicated in the presence of hinged abduction and coxa vara. It overcomes the hinging and brings a more congruent surface of the femoral head under the acetabulum. It also brings the trochanter down and improves hip mechanics (Fig. 50.8).
- *Arthrodiastasis*: It refers to distracting the hip joint using an external fixator in an attempt to unload the femoral head and facilitate remodelling.
- *Shelf acetabuloplasty and Chiari's osteotomy*: These procedures are indicated in late stages of disease where femoral head is significantly uncovered and a surgical containment procedure is not possible. They offer extended coverage to the femoral head anterolaterally and may be helpful in delaying the onset of osteoarthritis.
- *Surgeries for treating sequelae of LCPD*: These surgeries attempt to reshape the

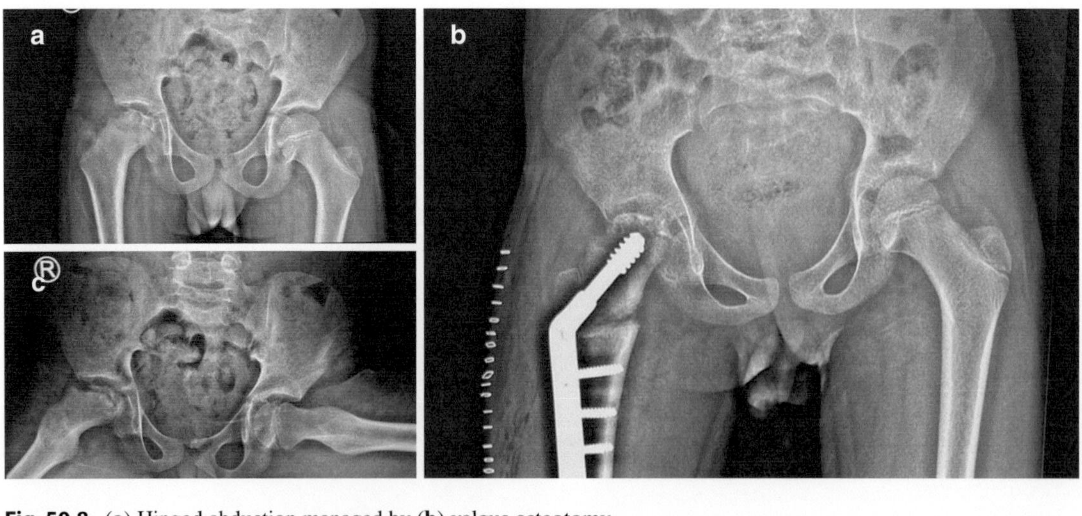

Fig. 50.8 (**a**) Hinged abduction managed by (**b**) valgus osteotomy

deformed femoral head by performing safe surgical dislocation of hip or by arthroscopy. Any labral tears can be repaired, and femoroacetabular impingement can be treated simultaneously. Even though the early results are encouraging, long-term outcomes need validation.

- *Salvage surgeries for advanced arthritis*: a painful and arthritic hip will not benefit from any of the above-mentioned surgeries. Such cases may be treated by pelvic support osteotomy or may undergo total hip replacement after maturity.

Multiple Choice Questions

1. All of the following are true about Perthes disease except
   (a) More common in boys
   (b) More common between 5 and 7 years of age
   (c) Genetic inheritance in all cases
   (d) Key event is the ischemia of femoral head
2. Which of the following is a head at-risk sign for Perthes disease?
   (a) Lateral epiphyseal calcification
   (b) Lateral subluxation of femoral head
   (c) Gage sign
   (d) All of the above
3. Investigation of choice for evaluation of suspected Perthes disease is;
   (a) Radiograph
   (b) Ultrasound
   (c) MRI
   (d) CT scan
4. All are indications for varus derotation osteotomy in Perthes disease except;
   (a) Age more than 7 years
   (b) Early fragmentation stage
   (c) Lateral subluxation of femoral head
   (d) Stiffness of hip joint
5. Which of the following is a poor prognostic factor for Perthes disease?
   (a) Late fragmentation stage
   (b) Lateral pillar collapse of more than 50%
   (c) Arthritic changes in hip joint
   (d) All of the above

Answers: 1. (c), 2. (d), 3. (c), 4. (d), 5. (d)

References

1. Rodríguez-Olivas AO, Hernández-Zamora E, Reyes-Maldonado E. Legg-Calvé-Perthes disease overview. Orphanet J Rare Dis. 2022;17(1):125. https://doi.org/10.1186/s13023-022-02275-z. PMID: 35292045; PMCID: PMC8922924.
2. Padilla-Santamaría F, Maya-Franco L, Bolaños-Méndez GZ, Guerrero-Gómez DA. El posible origen de la enfermedad de Legg-Calvé-Perthes [The possible origin of Legg-Calvé-Perthes disease]. Rev Med Inst Mex Seguro Soc. 2019;57(1):36–41. Spanish. PMID: 31071253.
3. Pavone V, Chisari E, Vescio A, Lizzio C, Sessa G, Testa G. Aetiology of Legg-Calvé-Perthes disease: a systematic review. World J Orthop. 2019;10(3):145–65. https://doi.org/10.5312/wjo.v10.i3.145. PMID: 30918798; PMCID: PMC6429000.
4. Rampal V, Clément JL, Solla F. Legg-Calvé-Perthes disease: classifications and prognostic factors. Clin Cases Miner Bone Metab. 2017;14(1):74–82. https://doi.org/10.11138/ccmbm/2017.14.1.074. Epub 2017 May 30. PMID: 28740529; PMCID: PMC5505718.
5. Joseph B. Management of Perthes' disease. Indian J Orthop. 2015;49(1):10–6. https://doi.org/10.4103/0019-5413.143906. PMID: 25593353; PMCID: PMC4292319.
6. Nelitz M, Lippacher S, Krauspe R, Reichel H. Perthes disease: current principles of diagnosis and treatment. Dtsch Arztebl Int. 2009;106(31–32):517–23. https://doi.org/10.3238/arztebl.2009.0517. Epub 2009 Aug 3. PMID: 19730720; PMCID: PMC2735835.
7. Mazloumi SM, Ebrahimzadeh MH, Kachooei AR. Evolution in diagnosis and treatment of Legg-Calve-Perthes disease. Arch Bone Jt Surg. 2014;2(2):86–92. Epub 2014 Jun 15. PMID: 25207324; PMCID: PMC4151449.
8. Caldaci A, Testa G, Dell'Agli E, Sapienza M, Vescio A, Lucenti L, Pavone V. Mid-long-term outcomes of surgical treatment of Legg-Calvè-Perthes disease: a systematic review. Children (Basel) 2022;9(8):1121. https://doi.org/10.3390/children9081121. PMID: 36010012; PMCID: PMC9406809.

Torticollis

51

Anil Agarwal

51.1 Introduction

Torticollis (wry neck) is the tilting of head to one side with concomitant rotation of the chin to the opposite direction. When long standing, the deformity is often associated with facial asymmetry.

51.2 Types [1, 2]

1. Acute torticollis: It is usually seen after trauma or acute respiratory tract infection. Muscle spasm is mostly present.
2. Torticollis due to congenital anomalies: Numerous developmental anomalies of the occipitocervical junction or upper cervical vertebrae may manifest as torticollis. They are present since birth. There is no muscle spasm.
3. Ocular torticollis: Sometimes, the cause of torticollis is an ocular pathology rather than neck or vertebral structures.
4. Neurogenic torticollis: Lesions of the brain, like Arnold-Chiari malformation, may sometimes cause torticollis. The sternomastoid muscle is seldom contracted in this type.
5. Congenital muscular torticollis: It is the classical variety resulting from sternocleidomastoid muscle contracture (described below).

The diagnosis of the congenital muscular torticollis is mainly clinical. Besides local examination, a careful ocular and neurological examination is often necessary to rule out other causes of torticollis. Sometimes radiographs and higher imaging are required to investigate the cervical spine and occipitocervical junction, if their involvement is suspected.

51.3 Relevant Pathoanatomy

Although birth trauma and ischemic aetiology are postulated, the definitive cause of congenital muscular torticollis remains unknown [3]. There is a variable degree of fibrosis in the sternocleidomastoid muscle. The short and contracted muscle results in neck tilt.

A. Agarwal (✉)
Department of Pediatric Orthopedics, Chacha Nehru Bal Chikitsalaya, New Delhi, India

V. Kumar et al. (eds.), *A Quick Guide to Essential Orthopedics*,
https://doi.org/10.1007/978-981-95-2676-5_51

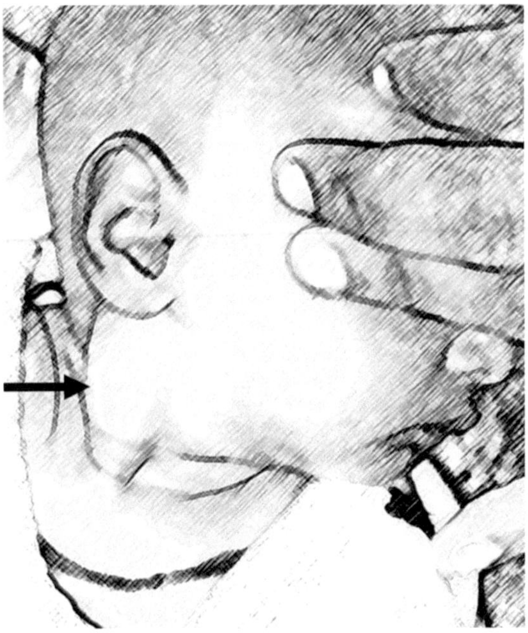

Fig. 51.1 'Sternomastoid' tumour: A non-tender soft to firm swelling over the sternocleidomastoid muscle seen in the postnatal period. The swelling subsides in a few weeks. In some children, the underlying muscle becomes fibrotic and results in congenital muscular torticollis

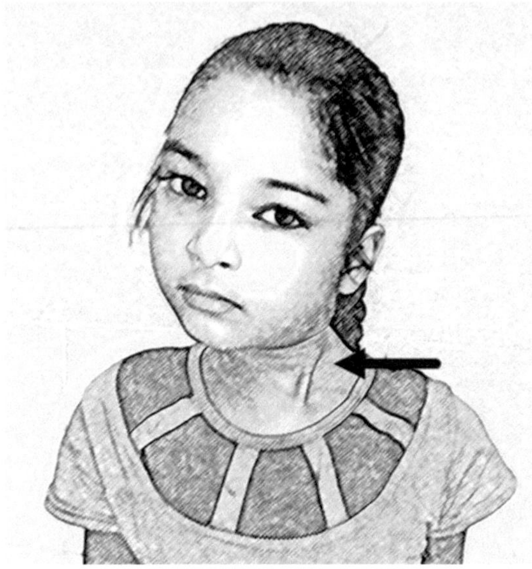

Fig. 51.2 The neck is tilted to one side and the chin to the opposite side in congenital muscular torticollis. In long-standing cases, facial asymmetry of the same side is associated

51.4 Clinical Features

When the child presents in infancy, the only finding may be a 'sternomastoid tumour' (Fig. 51.1). The same is a non-tender firm swelling in the neck region over one of the sternocleidomastoid muscles, seen a few weeks post birth. This swelling gradually resolves, resulting in fibrosis of the involved sternocleidomastoid muscle and subsequent torticollis (Fig. 51.2). As the child grows older, facial asymmetry (plagiocephaly) develops on the ipsilateral side.

51.5 Treatment

When the deformity is seen early, manual stretching of the contracted muscle and active positioning of the head can treat most of the children [3]. Facial asymmetry also improves once torticollis deformity is corrected. When the child presents late, release/lengthening of the fibrotic sternocleidomastoid muscle is required to correct the deformity. The lengthening of the contracted muscle can be performed either by its division in the mid-substance region (for mild deformity) or using the bipolar release procedure (for severe deformity). This procedure entails the release of both proximal and distal ends of sternocleidomastoid muscle near the mastoid process and just above the clavicle, respectively.

Multiple Choice Questions

1. The most common cause of torticollis in a child is ________________.
   (a) Cervical spine anomaly
   (b) Congenital muscular torticollis
   (c) Posterior fossa tumour
   (d) Basal invagination
2. Which of the following is not a bony aetiology for torticollis?
   (a) Klippel–Feil Syndrome
   (b) Sternocleidomastoid tumour
   (c) Hemivertebra
   (d) Os odontoideum
3. Which muscle is commonly involved in torticollis?
   (a) Omohyoid
   (b) Trapezius
   (c) Sternocleidomastoid
   (d) Levator scapulae
4. A 2-month-old child presents with fever and torticollis. Which of the following differentials in this condition is potentially life-threatening?
   (a) Sternocleidomastoid tumour
   (b) Grisel syndrome
   (c) Klippel–Feil Syndrome
   (d) Gastroesophageal reflux
5. The treatment of choice in a 6-year-old child with congenital muscular torticollis is ______________.
   (a) Unipolar release of sternocleidomastoid
   (b) Bipolar release of sternocleidomastoid
   (c) Manual stretching of sternocleidomastoid
   (d) Resection of sternocleidomastoid

Answers: 1. (b), 2. (b), 3. (c), 4. (b), 5. (b)

References

1. Herman MJ. Torticollis in infants and children: common and unusual causes. Instr Course Lect. 2006;55:647–53.
2. Gross PW, Chipman DE, Doyle SM. The tilts, twists, and turns of torticollis. Curr Opin Pediatr. 2023;35(1):118–23. https://doi.org/10.1097/MOP.0000000000001194.
3. Nilesh K, Mukherji S. Congenital muscular torticollis. Ann Maxillofac Surg. 2013;3(2):198–200. https://doi.org/10.4103/2231-0746.119222.

52 Slipped Capital Femoral Epiphysis

Ritesh Arvind Pandey and Lakshay Garg

52.1 Introduction

Slipped capital femoral epiphysis (SCFE) is a disorder of adolescents in which the proximal femoral epiphysis is displaced inferiorly and posteriorly. The physis is weakened due to an underlying pathology and is predisposed to a slip. The term SCFE is a misnomer because the epiphysis remains within its position in the acetabulum, while the metaphysis moves upward and anteriorly. The slip commonly occurs through the zone of maturing hypertrophied cartilage in the physis.

52.2 Epidemiology

The incidence of SCFE varies between 1 and 10 per 100,000 population [1]. Males are affected more than females with a ratio of 2:1.4. The affected age group for males is 12–17 years (averages 13.5 years), whereas it is 10–15 years for females (averages 12 years). The left hip is more commonly involved as compared to right, but bilateral involvement is seen in 20–50%. Blacks, Africans, Polynesians and Hispanics have reportedly higher rates of SCFE.

52.3 Etiology

The exact cause of SCFE is not known, and it remains idiopathic in the majority of cases [2]. The most common proposed theories include overloading of normal physis and physeal instability due to an underlying metabolic disorder. Genetic inheritance in the form of autosomal dominant with variable penetrance is found in 2–7% of cases and is associated with human leukocyte antigen (HLA-DR4).

Increased weight for age (obesity) is a common risk factor. Often, there is no history of trauma before the onset of symptoms. The common endocrinopathies associated with SCFE are hypothyroidism (most common), hypogonadism, hypopituitarism, an increase in the level of growth hormone and a decreased level of sex hormones.

An association with an abnormally high level of the leptin hormone has also been reported. Other less common responsible factors include radiation therapy, renal osteodystrophy and Down syndrome. Recently, an association with low levels of vitamin D has been reported, but its role as an etiological factor is not clearly established.

R. A. Pandey (✉) · L. Garg
All India Institute of Medical Sciences Patna,
Patna, Bihar, India

V. Kumar et al. (eds.), *A Quick Guide to Essential Orthopedics*,
https://doi.org/10.1007/978-981-95-2676-5_52

52.4 Natural History

The natural history of SCFE is related to the degree of slip [3]. Mild slips are well tolerated and are known to have a low rate of disability in the absence of avascular necrosis or chondrolysis. Progression to a more severe degree and hence the appearance of arthritic changes in the hip can be seen in 10% of cases with mild slip. On the contrary, almost all moderate and severe cases develop arthritic changes eventually. The onset of hip pain in these cases causes significant deterioration of the hip mobility score and overall functional capacity.

52.5 Pathogenesis

The physeal slip leads to a varus and external rotation deformity at the hip, thereby restricting abduction and internal rotation. Slip typically occurs through the hypertrophied zone of physis, and the resulting gap is filled by a combination of fibrous tissue and callus. The posterior periosteum containing blood vessels to the epiphysis remains intact. The early stages are marked by synovitis and hypervascularity, whereas in later stages, the synovium is atrophied and fibrosed.

Healing of the slip occurs over time with the formation of callus and fibrocartilage, leading to early closure of the physis. Early damage to the anterior acetabular labrum and acetabular rim leads to osteoarthritic changes in the long run and necessitates early hip arthroplasty.

52.6 Classification

SCFE can be classified into different subtypes based on the duration of symptoms, the status of stability of physis and the severity of slip.

52.6.1 Duration of Symptoms

Acute—duration of symptoms <3 weeks
Chronic—duration of symptoms >3 weeks
Acute on chronic—duration >3 weeks with acute exacerbation of symptoms within 3 weeks

52.6.2 Physeal Stability (Loder's Classification)

Stable SCFE—patient is able to bear weight while walking.
Unstable SCFE—patient is not able to bear weight while walking.

Ziebarth et al. suggested another classification based on intraoperative stability of the physis. The slip was considered stable if the periosteum around the physis was found intact and separation of the epiphysis seemed difficult without cutting through the physis. On the other hand, it was considered unstable if the epiphysis was mobile and easily separable without any added effort.

52.6.3 Morphological Classification (Fig. 52.1)

This is based on the severity of the slip as seen on anteroposterior and lateral radiographs. The possible types are:

Pre-slip—widening of the physis without any displacement
Mild slip—displacement up to 1/3 of physeal width or slip angle up to 30°.
Moderate slip—displacement between 1/3–2/3 of physeal width or slip angle between 30° and 60°.
Severe slip—more than 2/3 displacement or slip angle more than 60°.

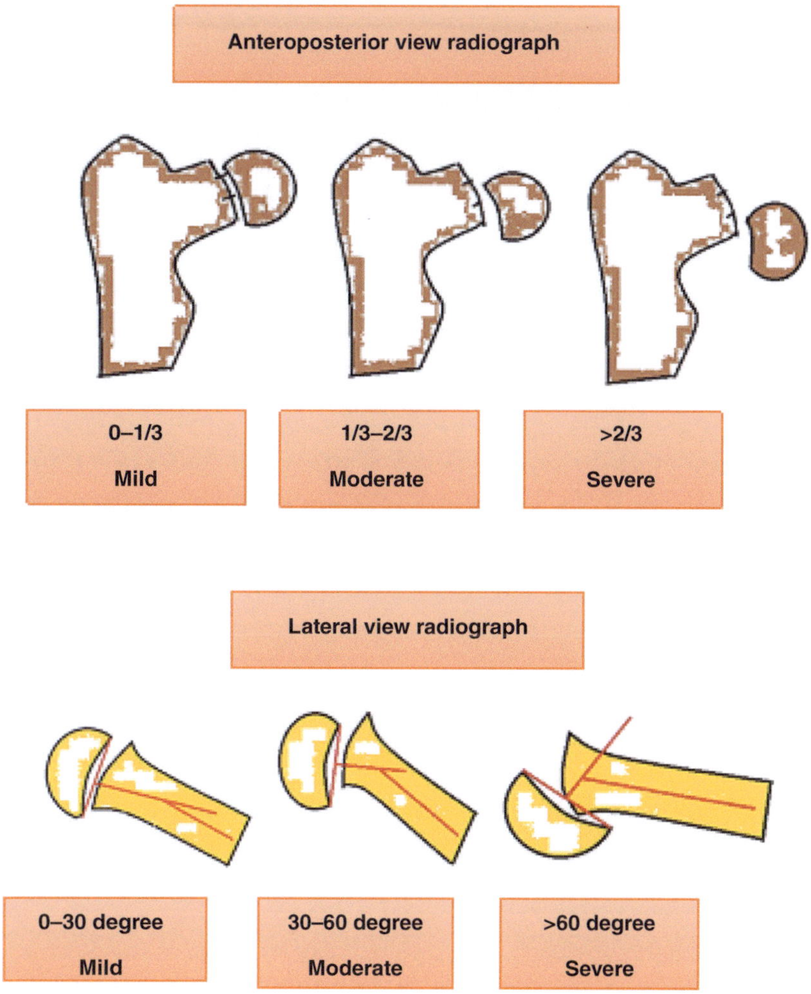

Fig. 52.1 Classification of SCFE based on severity of slip

52.7 Clinical Features

Clinical presentation in SCFE may vary according to the stage and type of slip. The onset of pain is gradual and is usually present for weeks or months before diagnosis is made.

- Child is obese, short and sexually immature due to the underlying endocrinopathy.
- *In the stage of pre-slip*, children have vague symptoms in the groin and thigh without any apparent slip on radiographs. The pain may radiate along the anterior division of the obturator nerve to anteromedial thigh and knee.
- *An acute slip* typically occurs after trivial trauma, and a history of prodromal symptoms preceding the episode can be interrogated. Pain is significant in intensity, and the child is unable to bear weight on the affected limb. The movements of the hip are painful.
- *In chronic slip*, the onset of pain is insidious and increases gradually in intensity. Patients are able to walk with an antalgic limp.
  On clinical examination, the abduction, flexion and internal rotation movements are limited. With further flexion, the thigh goes into external rotation and the knee moves to the ipsilateral axilla (obligatory external rotation).

The limb gradually develops shortening and a combination of adduction and external rotation deformity.

- The child walks with a Trendelenburg gait with an increased foot progression angle, and one can elicit a positive Trendelenburg test. A condition affecting both hips results in a Trendelenburg gait on both sides, which is known as a waddling gait.

52.8 Imaging Findings (Fig. 52.2)

Radiographic findings in the pre-slip stage are very subtle in the form of:

- Irregular widening of the physis. The typical inferior and posterior displacement of epiphysis is more apparent in later stages.
- Shenton's line is disrupted.

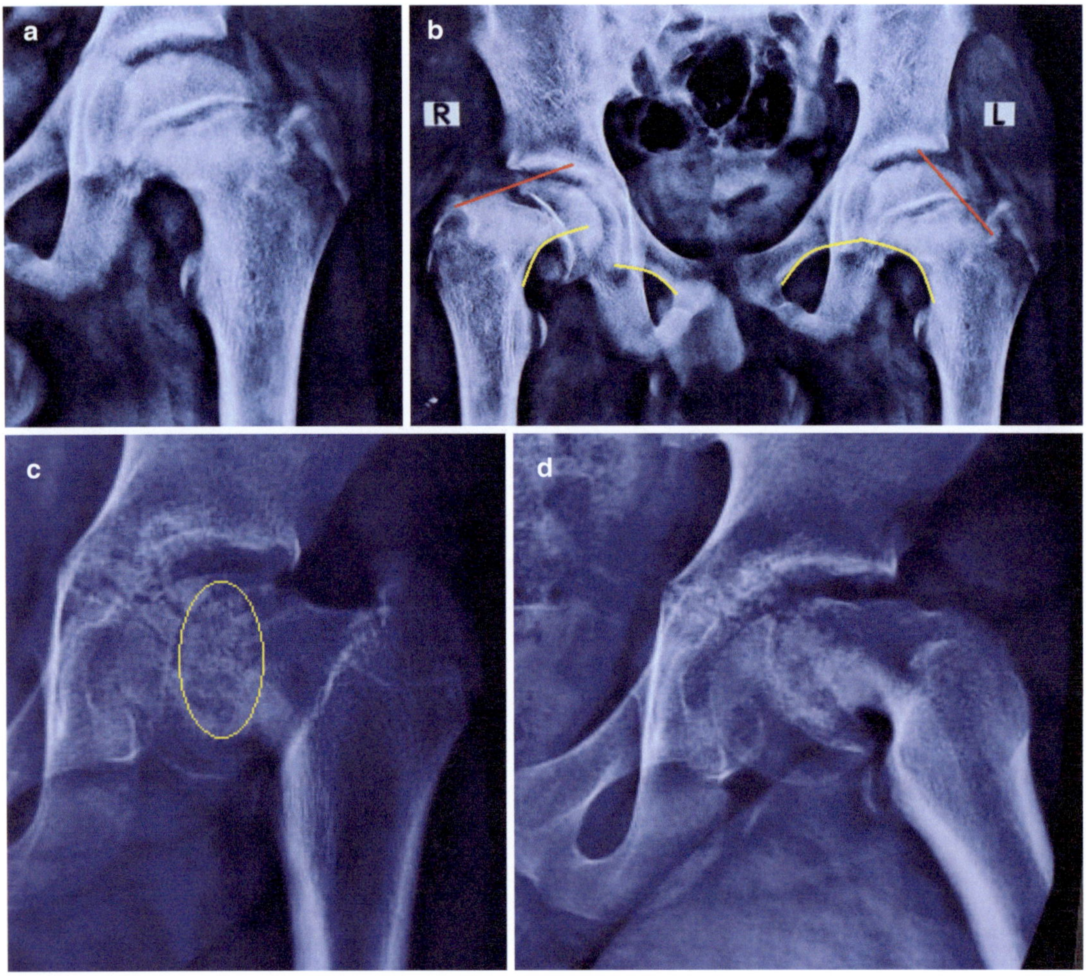

Fig. 52.2 Radiographic signs of SCFE: (**a**) wide and irregular physis in pre-slip stage, (**b**) disruption of Shenton's line and Trethowan's sign, (**c**) metaphyseal blanch sign and (**d**) Herndon hump

- A line drawn tangential to the upper border of the femoral neck (Klein's line) should intersect the epiphysis in normal hips. However, in SCFE, the epiphysis remains inferior to this line (*Trethowan's sign*).
- A crescent-shaped area of increased density appears due to the overlapping of the femoral neck and posteriorly displaced capital epiphysis (*metaphyseal blanch sign*).
- The anterior angulation and hump of bone growth around the physis is evident on the lateral view and is known as *Herndon hump*.
  With time, the gap between epiphysis and metaphysis is gradually filled with callus and fibrous tissue, and with final healing, only deformity in the neck is visible.

52.9 CT Scan

A CT scan of the hip may be done to evaluate the details of neck deformity and to assess the severity of the slip more precisely (Fig. 52.3). Additionally, it helps to rule out the presence of complications like screw penetration and avascular necrosis (AVN) after surgical intervention.

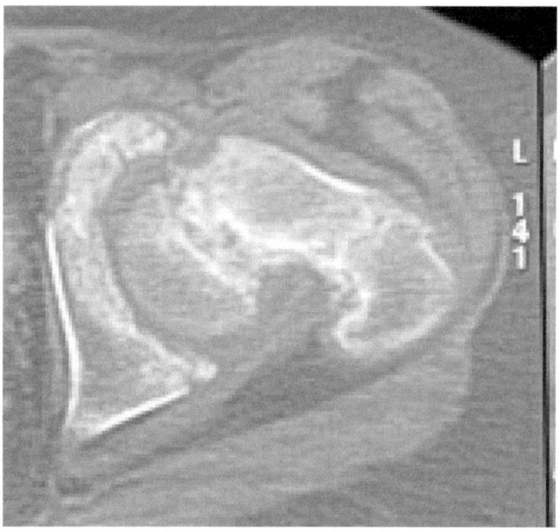

Fig. 52.3 Transverse section CT scan showing details of severity in SCFE

52.10 MRI

MRI is the investigation of choice for early diagnosis in the pre-slip stage when radiographic findings are absent. It shows widening of growth plate and marrow oedema in the metaphysis. It also reveals the amount of cartilage and labral damage and picks up the findings of AVN much earlier.

52.11 Treatment

The treatment of SCFE is primarily surgical [4–6]. The goals of treatment are to prevent progression of the slip by achieving early closure of the physis, to correct severe deformities and to avoid complications. Conservative treatment by means of rest, crutches, cast and brace has a role only while the patient waits for surgical intervention.

- *Mild stable slip*—mild stable slips are treated by in situ fixation using pins or screws (Fig. 52.4). The slip is fixed in a displaced position without any attempt to reduce. This avoids any further damage to the vascularity of the femoral head, thereby avoiding the onset of AVN. The aim is to stabilize the epiphysis and to prevent further slippage by achieving early fusion of the physis.
  The mild neck deformity is anticipated to remodel with time without creating any significant problem [7]. A single large-diameter pin or screw is used, which is placed in the centre of the epiphysis and remains perpendicular to the growth plate. Care should be taken not to penetrate the articular cartilage of the femoral head to avoid chondrolysis.
- *Moderate stable slip*—the treatment of moderate slips remains debatable. Most of the surgeons prefer to treat them like a mild slip by doing in situ fixation, while others suggest a more aggressive approach and recommend corrective osteotomy of the proximal femur.
- *Severe stable slip*—severe slips are treated by corrective osteotomy to restore alignment between head and neck, thereby avoiding fem-

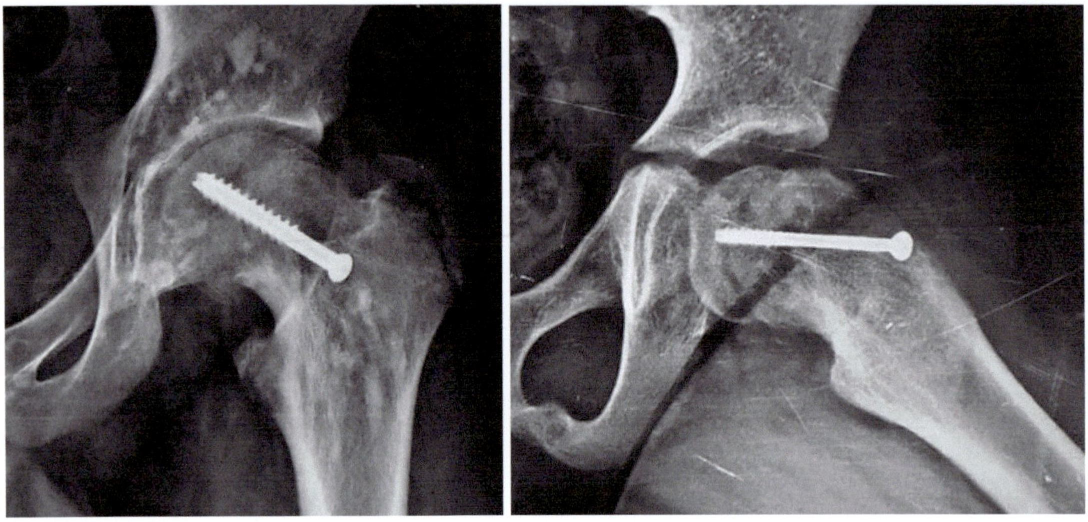

Fig. 52.4 Anteroposterior and lateral view radiograph showing in situ pinning of SCFE

oroacetabular impingement (FAI) and subsequent osteoarthritis of the hip.

Different types of corrective osteotomies have been described. These include:

1. Fish and Dunn osteotomy in the subcapital region
2. Kramer osteotomy at the base of the neck
3. Southwick osteotomy in subtrochanteric region

More proximal osteotomies in the neck of the femur restore the alignment but carry the risk of developing AVN of femoral head. Distal osteotomies in the trochanteric or subtrochanteric region have a lower risk for AVN but fail to restore the alignment.

The use of safe surgical dislocation of the hip for doing neck osteotomy (modified Dunn procedure) has been reported to serve both the purpose of minimizing the incidence of AVN and restoring the alignment and is now an accepted technique for management of SCFE (Figs. 52.5 and 52.6).

- *Acute unstable slip*—an acute unstable slip presenting within 24 hours is often reduced by longitudinal traction. If this fails, a very gentle Leadbetter manoeuvre just prior to surgical invasion may be permitted. Once a satisfactory reduction is achieved, it is stabilized by in situ screw fixation. The use of two screws has been recommended for the unstable slips. Late presentations are managed in a way similar to stable slips.

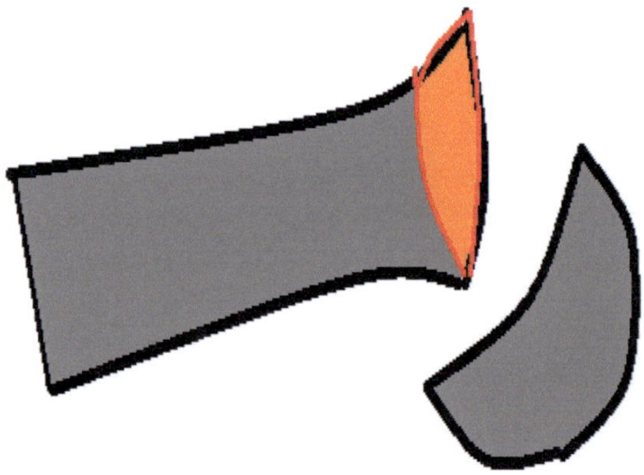

Fig. 52.5 Anterosuperior wedge resection from the medial part of the femoral neck

Bone peg epiphysiodesis (Fig. 52.7) In this procedure, a bone graft is inserted through an opening in the neck of the femur and across the epiphyseal plate, thereby achieving early physeal fusion and avoiding further progression of slip.

Open bone graft epiphysiodesis is best indicated for severe chronic slips where percutaneous pinning may not be possible. However, since the

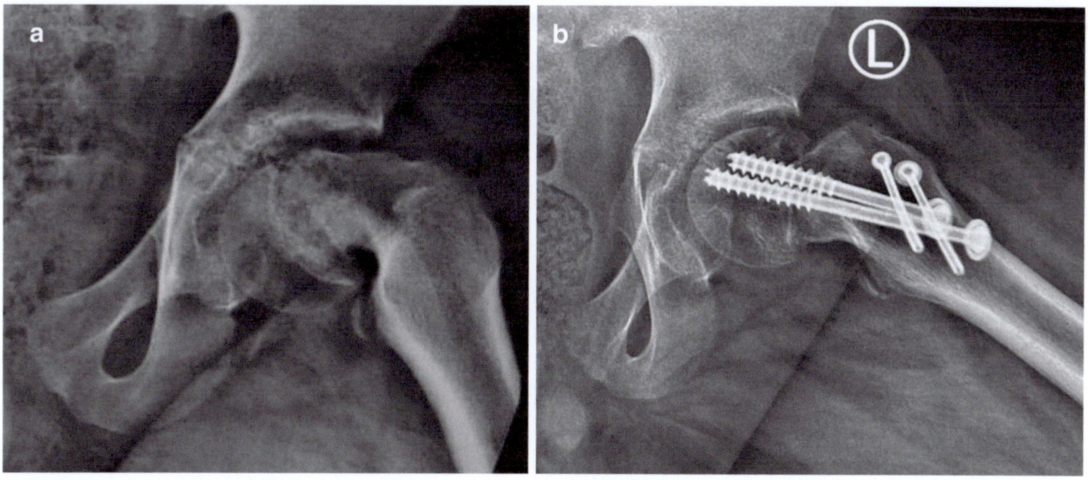

Fig. 52.6 Radiographs before and after modified Dunn osteotomy

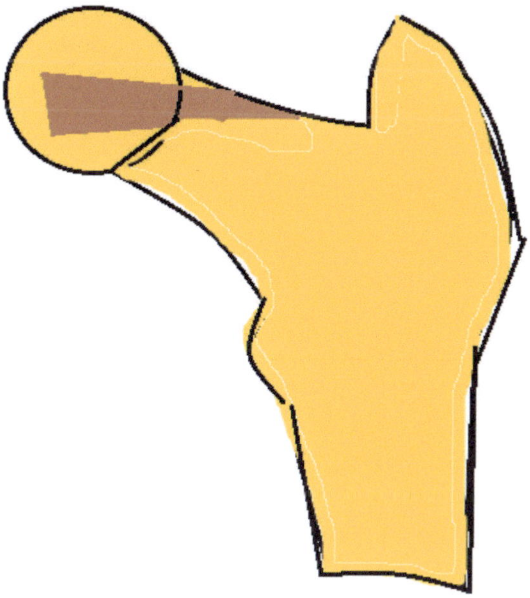

Fig. 52.7 Epiphysiodesis with bone graft

advent of the modified Dunn osteotomy, bone peg epiphysiodesis is rarely used.

52.11.1 Prophylactic Treatment of Contralateral Normal Hip

As the normal contralateral hip may subsequently develop a slip, prophylactic pinning of normal hip is advocated (Fig. 52.8). However, this remains debatable as it may lead to unnecessary

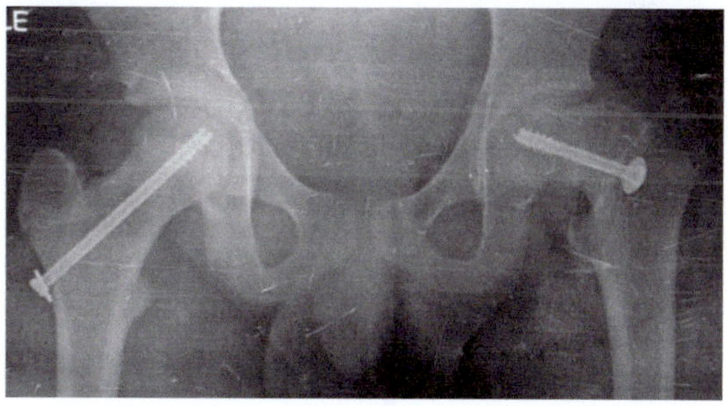

Fig. 52.8 Anteroposterior radiograph showing in situ pinning of SCFE on left side and prophylactic pinning on right side

procedures and overtreatment in many patients. Some indications of prophylactic pinning are obesity, underlying endocrine disorders and doubtful regular follow-up of patients.

52.12 Post-operative Care

Following in situ fixation for a chronic slip, the patient may be allowed to walk with crutches, while for an acute slip, partial weight bearing should be delayed. For those undergoing corrective osteotomy, only toe-touch weight bearing is allowed for 6 weeks.

Thereafter, partial weight bearing is allowed, and full weight bearing is encouraged after 12 weeks once satisfactory healing is seen on the radiograph.

52.13 Complications

1. *Osteoarthritis of hip joint*—untreated SCFE is known to cause femoroacetabular impingement, which in turn leads to osteoarthritis of the hip joint in the long run. The risk increases with increased severity of slip and necessitates early hip arthroplasty.
2. *Avascular necrosis of femoral head*—avascular necrosis of the femoral head can occur with treatment of both stable and unstable slips, though the risk is higher for unstable variants [8]. Forceful attempts to reduce the slip is strongly discouraged as it destroys the remaining vascularity of the femoral head.

The risk is more with proximal neck osteotomies; however, the technique of safe surgical dislocation of the hip before corrective osteotomy has proved to reduce the risk of AVN.

3. *Chondrolysis*—this refers to the acute loss of femoral head cartilage and is characterized by a painful and stiff hip. The incidence in SCFE varies from 1% to 7% and may develop due to forceful closed manipulation.

Prolonged immobilization of the hip in a spica cast and screws penetrating the cartilage of the femoral head may be other significant contributing factors. Radiologically, it is marked by concentric reduction of the joint space and eventually by arthritic changes in the hip joint.

52.13.1 Treatment of Healed SCFE

Healed SCFE refers to the situation where physeal closure has occurred in a case of SCFE with the femoral head lying displaced posteriorly and inferiorly. It is commonly seen in the absence of treatment and after in situ pinning. The resulting deformity is known to cause femoroacetabular impingement (FAI) and ultimately arthritis of the hip joint.

Treatment of healed SCFE is primarily aimed to treat the symptoms and sequelae of FAI. Surgical options for healed SCFE are reorientation osteotomy, open osteochondroplasty, arthroscopic osteochondroplasty and periacetabular osteotomy.

Multiple Choice Questions

1. Which of the following is a wrong statement about SCFE?
   (a) Common in adolescence
   (b) It can have an underlying hormonal disorder
   (c) More common in females
   (d) Obesity can be a cause
2. All are radiological features of SCFE except:
   (a) Fragmentation of epiphysis
   (b) Trethowan's sign
   (c) Disrupted Shenton's line
   (d) Herndon hump
3. The treatment of choice for a mild stable SCFE is:
   (a) Skin traction
   (b) In situ pinning
   (c) Closed reduction and internal fixation
   (d) Open reduction and internal fixation
4. Which of the following is not a feature of SCFE?
   (a) Limited external rotation
   (b) Trendelenburg gait
   (c) Out-toeing gait
   (d) Pain in knee
5. The usual displacement of the femoral head in SCFE is:
   (a) Anterior and superior
   (b) Anterior and inferior
   (c) Posterior and superior
   (d) Posterior and inferior

Answers: 1. (c), 2. (a), 3. (b), 4. (a), 5. (d)

References

1. Novais EN, Millis MB. Slipped capital femoral epiphysis: prevalence, pathogenesis, and natural history. Clin Orthop Relat Res. 2012;470(12):3432–8. https://doi.org/10.1007/s11999-012-2452-y. PMID: 23054509; PMCID: PMC3492592.
2. Millis MB. SCFE: clinical aspects, diagnosis, and classification. J Child Orthop. 2017;11(2):93–8. https://doi.org/10.1302/1863-2548-11-170025. PMID: 28529655; PMCID: PMC5421350.
3. Carney BT, Weinstein SL. Natural history of untreated chronic slipped capital femoral epiphysis. Clin Orthop Relat Res. 1996;(322):43–7. PMID: 8542712.

4. Haider S, Podeszwa DA, Morris WZ. The etiology and management of slipped capital femoral epiphysis: current concept review J Pediatr Orthop Soc North Am. 2022;4(4). https://doi.org/10.55275/JPOSNA-2022-589.
5. Johari AN, Pandey RA. Controversies in management of slipped capital femoral epiphysis. World J Orthop. 2016;7(2):78–81. https://doi.org/10.5312/wjo.v7.i2.78. PMID: 26925378; PMCID: PMC4757661.
6. Johns K, Mabrouk A, Tavarez MM. Slipped capital femoral epiphysis. [Updated 2023 Apr 22]. In: StatPearls [Internet]. Treasure Island (FL): StatPearls Publishing; 2023. Available from: https://www.ncbi.nlm.nih.gov/books/NBK538302/
7. de Poorter JJ, Beunder TJ, Gareb B, Oostenbroek HJ, Bessems GH, van der Lugt JC, Maathuis PG, van der Sande MA. Long-term outcomes of slipped capital femoral epiphysis treated with in situ pinning. J Child Orthop. 2016;10(5):371–9. https://doi.org/10.1007/s11832-016-0759-z. Epub 2016 Jul 20. PMID: 27438268; PMCID: PMC5033778.
8. Lubicky JP. Chondrolysis and avascular necrosis: complications of slipped capital femoral epiphysis. J Pediatr Orthop B. 1996;5(3):162–7. https://doi.org/10.1097/01202412-199605030-00005. PMID: 8866280.

53 Deformities Around Knee

Sunny Chaudhary and Vivek Singh

53.1 Normal Mechanical Alignment of Knee

To understand the malalignment of the mechanical axis and deformity at knee, we must first understand the normal alignment of the knee.

Mechanical malalignment not only results in poor cosmesis, but it also predisposes the joint to early damage. It may alter the patellar mechanics and tracking.

A full-length standing anteroposterior (AP) radiograph with the patella facing forward is needed to analyse the mechanical alignment of knee. The knee should be in a neutral position, and the patella should be central on femoral condyles.

The mechanical axis of lower limb is an imaginary line joining the centre of femoral head and the centre of ankle joint. Normally, the line should pass just medial to the centre of the knee. The mechanical axis may be deviated medially or laterally, and the deviation is called the mechanical axis deviation (MAD). It is measured in millimetres (mm) (Fig. 53.1).

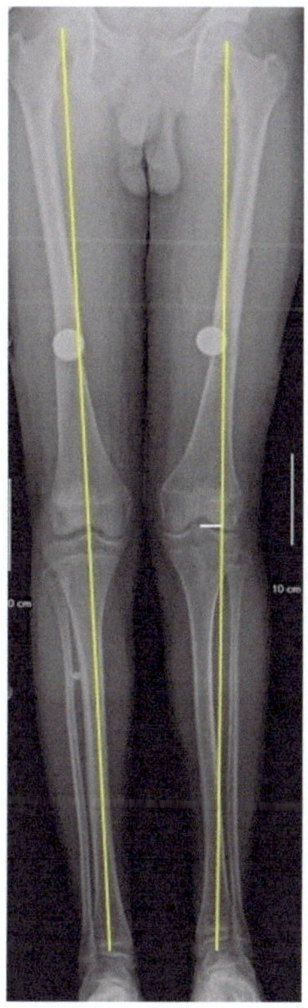

Fig. 53.1 Standing scanogram of a patient with mild genu valgum deformity on the left side. The yellow line represents the Mechanical axis. The white line on the left side denotes (mechanical axis deviation (MAD)

S. Chaudhary (✉)
Department of Spine Surgery, Alberta Children's Hospital, Calgary, AB, Canada
e-mail: sunny.chaudhary@albertahealthservices.ca

V. Singh
Department of Orthopedics, All India Institute of Medical Sciences, Rishikesh,
Rishikesh, Uttarakhand, India

V. Kumar et al. (eds.), *A Quick Guide to Essential Orthopedics*,
https://doi.org/10.1007/978-981-95-2676-5_53

53.2 Genu Varum

53.2.1 Definition

Genu varum, also known as bowlegs, is a condition in which the legs appear bowed outward when standing upright. The apex of the angle formed between the femur and tibia is away from the midline (Fig. 53.2).

53.2.2 Aetiology

- Physiological factors
- Rickets (vitamin D deficiency)
- Blount's disease (tibia vara)
- Congenital abnormalities (tibia hemimelia)
- Genetic factors (osteogenesis imperfecta)
- Endocrine disorders (such as hypothyroidism)
- Skeletal dysplasia (such as achondroplasia and focal fibrocartilaginous dysplasia)
- Trauma to physis/infection (bony bar formation)
- Osteoarthritis of the knee joint (adults)
- Overweight or obesity

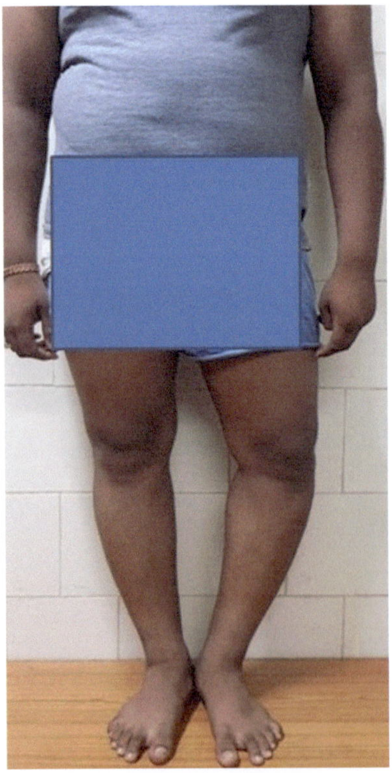

Fig. 53.2 Clinical image of a patient with genu varum deformity of the left lower limb. On further evaluation, it was found that mild deformity was also noted on the right side

53.2.3 Physiological Genu Varum

The normal angle formed between the femur and tibia changes with growth. At birth, there is varus, which gradually changes to valgus by the age of 2 years. The physiological varus is typically symmetrical (Fig. 53.3).

53.2.4 Pathological Genu Varum

The bowing is considered pathological under the following circumstances:

- Unilateral deformity
- Persistence beyond the age of 2 years.
- Presence of leg shortening along with bowing.
- The angular deformity exceeds the normal physiological range for the given age.

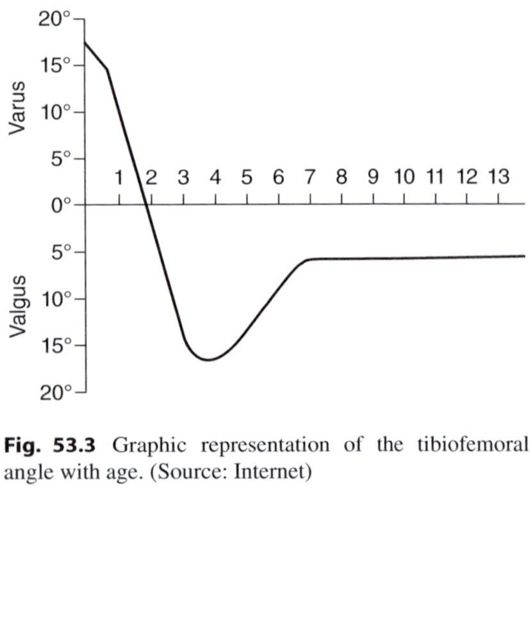

Fig. 53.3 Graphic representation of the tibiofemoral angle with age. (Source: Internet)

In *Blount's disease*, the medial aspect of proximal tibial physis demonstrates abnormal growth. It has been further classified into early onset (infantile, 2–5 years) and late onset (adolescent >10 years). It is more common in African Americans and Hispanics.

Early-onset Blount's disease (infantile) is associated with obesity and early walking age. It is bilateral in most cases.

It has been classified by Langenskiold based on the involvement of physis, the increase in slope and the presence of beaking.

Late-onset Blount's disease (adolescent) is more common in obese children and is usually unilateral. The deformity is less severe as compared to infantile type. It may present with internal tibial torsion and limb length discrepancy.

53.2.5 Clinical Evaluation

Family history is present in cases with hereditary multiple exostosis, hypophosphataemic rickets or dysplasia.

The knee is examined in the straight position without flexion as this may conceal the deformity or decrease its perceived magnitude. The origin of deformity is assessed by the 'cover test', and it helps us to differentiate between tibial shaft deformity of true genu varum.

The child should be evaluated in the standing position with knee fully extended and patella facing forward. The distance between the medial aspects of two knees can be measured with both ankles together. The angle between thigh axis and leg axis gives an idea of the amount of deformity.

The gait of the child is also noted, and it may show lateral thrust of the knee while the limb is taking weight in the stance phase of gait cycle.

53.2.6 Radiology

Dedicated knee radiographs are needed to understand the pathology and to classify the deformity (Fig. 53.4).

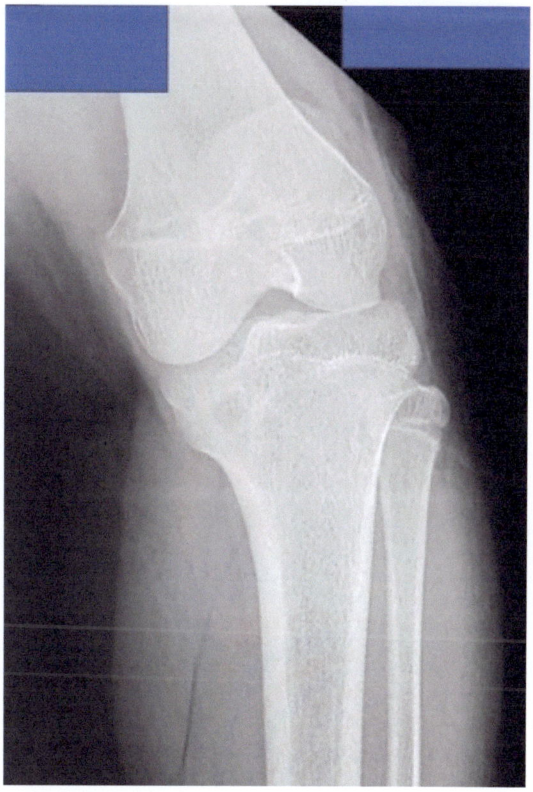

Fig. 53.4 Anteroposterior radiograph of the left knee of the patient with genu varum. The deformity is present in both femur and tibia. It is more pronounced in proximal tibia

Drennan's metaphyseal–diaphyseal angle (MDA) helps us to differentiate between physiological and pathological variants of early-onset deformity. An angle of <11 degrees is regarded as physiological, and it resolves. An angle of >11 degrees is considered pathological, and it usually progresses without intervention.

To assess the magnitude of deformity, standing long-cassette hip–knee–ankle anteroposterior radiographs are recommended, with the patella facing forward (scanogram). Mechanical axis deviation is measured in millimetres of distance from the centre of the knee and the line joining the centre of the femoral head and centre of the ankle joint (mechanical axis line) (Fig. 53.5).

Rarely, magnetic resonance imaging (MRI) is needed to study the bony bar if there is a history of any trauma or infection. Bony bar is mapped,

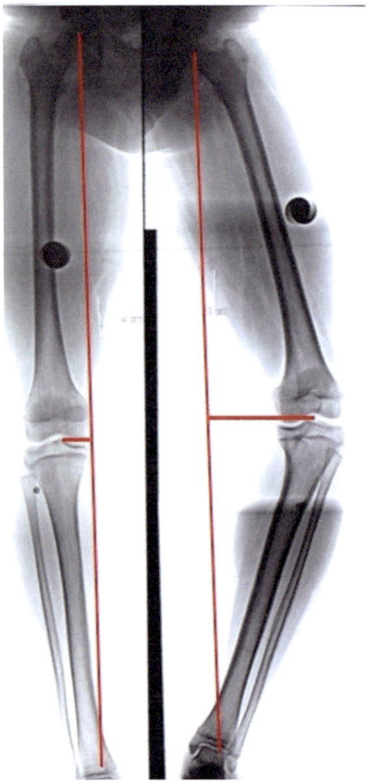

Fig. 53.5 Standing scanogram of the same patient with bilateral genu varum (more on the left side). The vertical red line is the mechanical axis. The horizontal red line represents mechanical axis deviation (MAD)

and treatment is based on the percentage of the area of physis involved.

53.2.7 Treatment

The aim of the treatment is to restore the mechanical alignment and to maintain it. The various factors to be considered while deciding the management are the age of the patient, severity of deformity, presence of underlying bony bar, tendency of deformity progression and associated shortening of limb.

Medical management of rickets helps to decrease the deformity, and usually it resolves fully without the need for orthotics or surgery.

Observation for improvement is advocated in mild deformity of less than 11 degrees in a young child.

Orthotic management is advised only in a child of less than 4 years of age with mild disease (Langenskiold stage I and II) and deformity (11–16 degrees) without any bony bar. About 90% of cases improve within 18 months of bracing. Bracing has a better outcome in unilateral disease. Obesity and bilateral disease have a poor outcome.

Surgery is usually needed when the deformity is progressive or severe. It is also needed with advanced age. Various surgical options available are as follows:

- Growth modulation by hemiepiphysiodesis (not if bony bar is present)
- Acute corrective osteotomy
- Gradual correction by osteotomy +/– lengthening (Figs. 53.6 and 53.7)

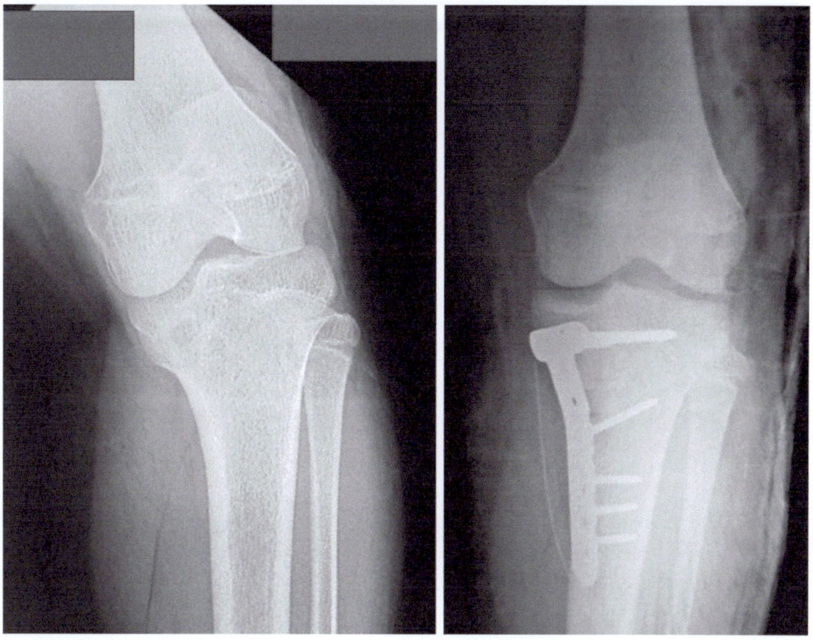

Fig. 53.6 Preoperative and postoperative radiographs of knee. The patient underwent medial hemi plateau elevation of tibia on the left side as the first stage

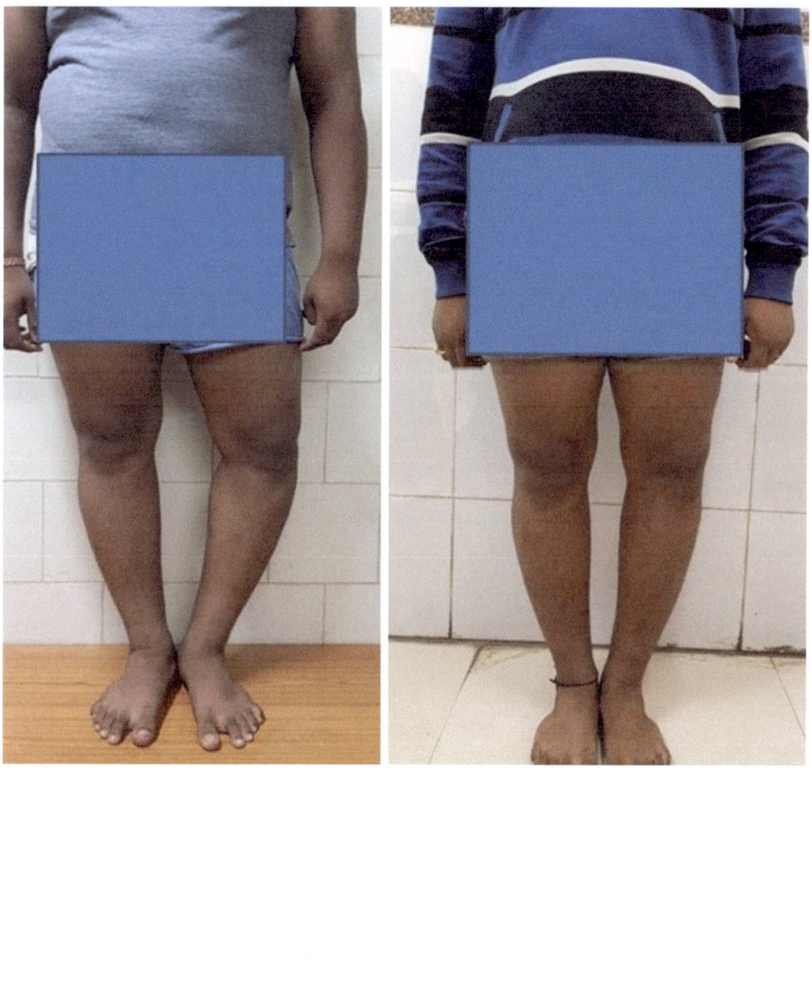

Fig. 53.7 Preoperative and postoperative clinical images of the patient. Note the improvement in the axis of left limb

53.3 Genu Valgum

53.3.1 Definition

The normal alignment of the tibia with femur is a valgus angle after the age of 2 years. Usually, it is more from 2 to 7 years of age as compared to adults. The adult value of the tibiofemoral angle is usually attained by the age of 7 years.

Genu valgum or knock knees is a type of deformity in which the knee is closer to the midline when compared to the normal population at that age. The angle formed between the tibia and femur should not be more than 12 degrees after the age of 7 years.

It is considered pathological if

- It progressively increases after the age of 7.
- It is more than 12 degrees after the age of 7.
- Intermalleolar distance is more than 8 cm after the age of 7. It is the distance between the two medial malleoli of tibia when the patient is standing with the knee extended and touching each other.

53.3.2 Aetiology

Bilateral

- Physiological genu valgum
- Idiopathic
- Metabolic bone diseases (renal rickets)
- Skeletal dysplasias (Morquio syndrome, chondroectodermal dysplasia, spondyloepiphyseal dysplasia [SED])
- Obesity

Unilateral

- Physeal injury (infection/trauma)
- Cozen phenomenon (overgrowth after proximal tibia fractures)
- Tumours (exostosis and fibrous dysplasia)
- Fibula hemimelia
- Hypoplasia of lateral femoral condyle

53.3.3 Clinical Examination

Abnormal alignment and cosmesis are usually the causes of clinical opinion. Parents may also give a history of frequent falls while running. Few patients may present with medial side knee pain or anterior knee pain.

- Abnormal alignment between thigh and leg is observed in the standing and supine position with knee extended and the patella facing forward.
- Circumduction gait is seen if the deformity is more, and the patient tries to clear the knee from the other.
- Patellofemoral instability should be assessed, and patellar tracking should be noted.
- Deformity of knee disappears on flexion in true genu valgum.
- The measurement of intermalleolar distance is done in the standing position.
- Rotational profile of the tibia and femur should be checked (Fig. 53.8).

53.3.4 Radiology

Dedicated knee radiographs are needed to understand the pathology (Fig. 53.9).

To assess the magnitude of deformity, standing long-cassette hip–knee–ankle anteroposterior radiographs are recommended, with the patella facing forward (scanogram). Mechanical axis deviation is measured.

53.3.5 Treatment

The aim of treatment is to restore the mechanical alignment and to maintain it.

Observation is the mainstay of treatment in young patients (age <7 years) with bilateral genu valgum and mild deformity (<15 degrees). It is also advised that the intermalleolar distance is

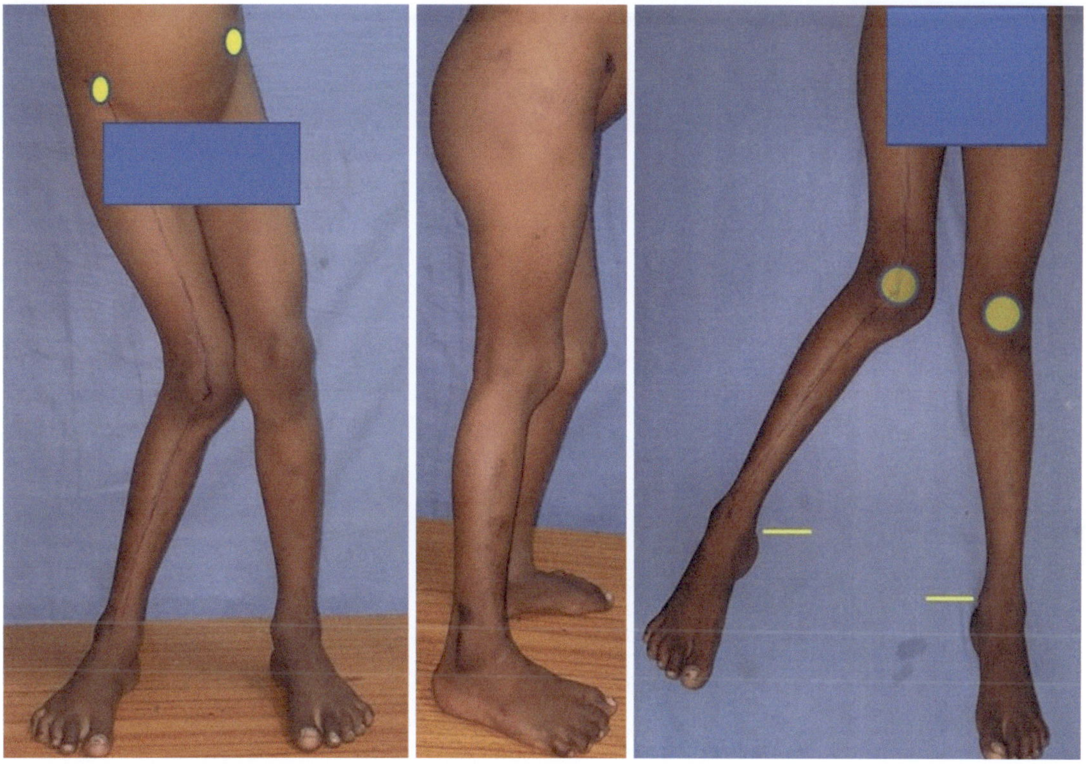

Fig. 53.8 Clinical images of a patient with right-sided genu valgum deformity

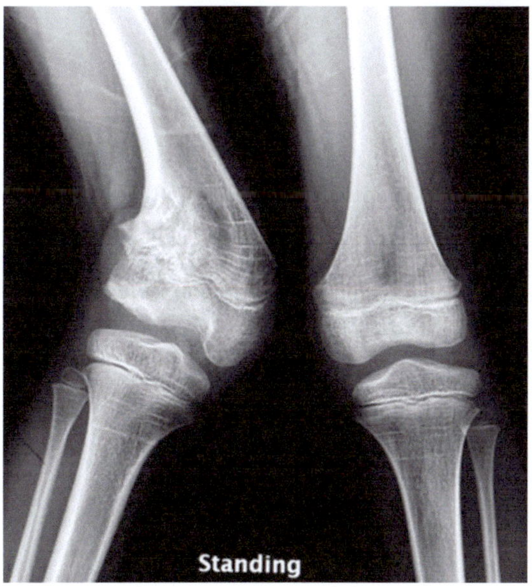

Fig. 53.9 The AP radiograph of both knees of the patient with right-sided genu valgum deformity. Note the converging growth arrest lines and distortion of physis on lateral aspect of the femur

less than 15 cm in a young child. Clinically, the intermalleolar distance can be measured and used as a guide on follow-up.

Medical management is given in cases with metabolic diseases. Bracing is usually ineffective.

Surgery is usually needed in older patients with severe deformity. It is indicated in patients with an intermalleolar distance of more than 10 cm after the age of 10 years. It is also indicated when tibiofemoral angle is more than 15 degrees.

The various factors that affect the management are the severity of deformity, residual age, the presence of local lesion/physeal bar and associated limb length discrepancy.

Various surgical modalities are as follows:

- Medial hemiepiphysiodesis
- Acute corrective osteotomy +/− common peroneal nerve decompression
- Gradual corrective osteotomy (Figs. 53.10 and 53.11)

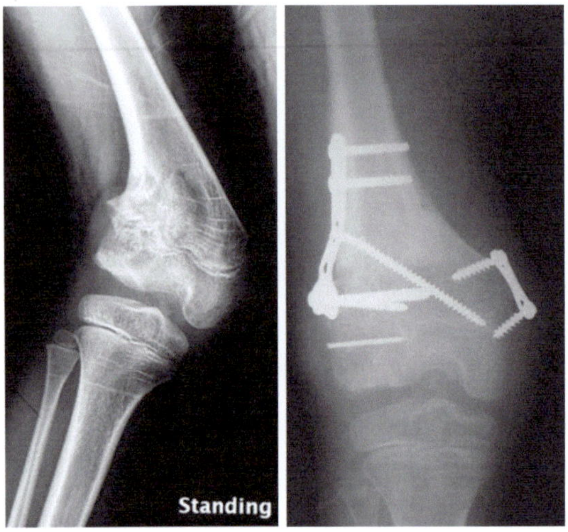

Fig. 53.10 Preoperative and postoperative radiographs of knee. The patient underwent acute osteotomy and physeal bar excision on lateral side. Medial hemiepiphysiodesis was done to prevent the recurrence of deformity. A titanium wire is inserted in epiphysis and cut flushing the bone surface to monitor the start of lateral side growth

Multiple Choice Questions

1. Which radiographic view is needed to analyse the mechanical alignment of the knee?
   (a) Lateral radiograph
   (b) Supine radiograph
   (c) Anteroposterior radiograph with patella facing backwards
   (d) Full-length standing anteroposterior radiograph with patella facing forward
2. In physiological genu varum, the normal angle between the femur and tibia:
   (a) Increases with growth
   (b) Decreases with growth
   (c) Remains constant throughout growth
   (d) Fluctuates during growth
3. Which surgical option is NOT mentioned as a treatment for genu varum?
   (a) Growth modulation by hemiepiphysiodesis
   (b) Acute corrective osteotomy
   (c) Gradual correction by osteotomy +/− lengthening
   (d) Supramalleolar osteotomy

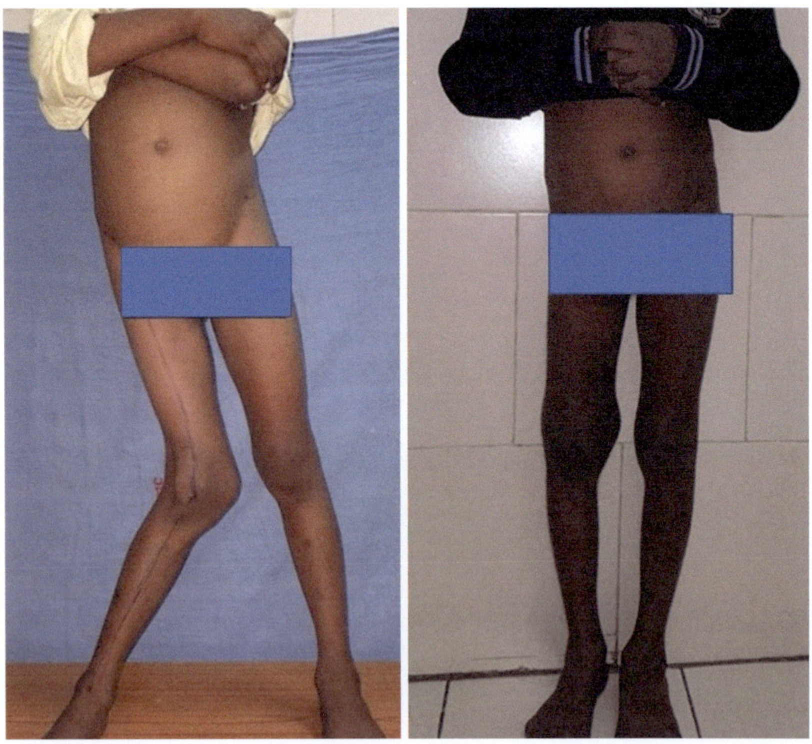

Fig. 53.11 Preoperative and postoperative clinical images of the patients. The patients will need serial surgeries to keep the limb length equal.

4. At what age is the adult value of the tibiofemoral angle usually attained?
   (a) 2 years
   (b) 5 years
   (c) 7 years
   (d) 10 years
5. In true genu valgum, what happens to the deformity on knee flexion?
   (a) It remains unchanged.
   (b) It becomes more pronounced.
   (c) It disappears.
   (d) It becomes asymmetrical.
6. When is surgery usually indicated for genu valgum?
   (a) In young patients with mild deformity
   (b) When intermalleolar distance is less than 15 cm in a young child
   (c) When the intermalleolar distance is more than 10 cm after the age of 10 years
   (d) When the tibiofemoral angle is less than 15 degrees
7. Which surgical modality is NOT mentioned as a treatment for genu valgum?
   (a) Medial hemiepiphysiodesis
   (b) Acute corrective osteotomy
   (c) Gradual corrective osteotomy
   (d) Lateral decompression

Answers: 1. (d), 2. (b), 3. (d), 4. (c), 5. (c), 6. (c), 7. (d)

54 Pes Planus

Pratik Shahare and Pratik Kotangale

54.1 Introduction

Pes planus or flatfoot is a complex deformity seen in pediatric, adolescent, and adult populations. The medial arch of the foot collapses such that the foot is in near-complete or complete contact with the ground (Fig. 54.1). These arches are stabilized by static stabilizers (bones and ligaments) and the dynamic stabilizers (muscles and tendons). The function of the arches is to support the weight of the body, to act as shock absorption at heel strike, and to facilitate forward propulsion in the pre-swing phase of the gait cycle. The most important static and dynamic stabilizers are the talocalcaneonavicular ligament (spring ligament) and the tibialis posterior (TB).

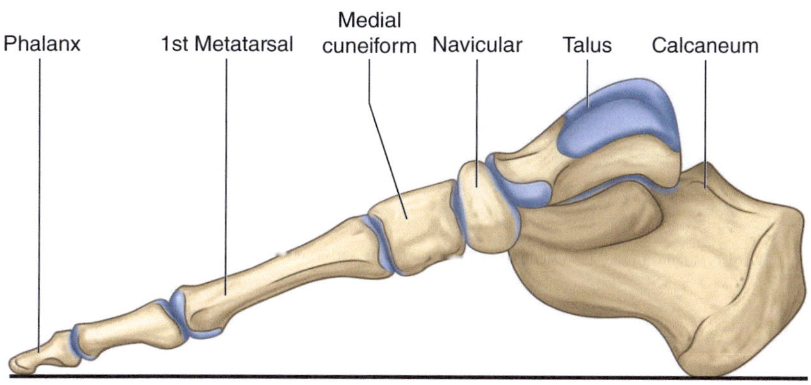

Fig. 54.1 Medial longitudinal arch

P. Shahare (✉) · P. Kotangale
All India Institute of Medical Sciences, Nagpur, Nagpur, Maharashtra, India

V. Kumar et al. (eds.), *A Quick Guide to Essential Orthopedics*,
https://doi.org/10.1007/978-981-95-2676-5_54

54.2 Types

Pediatric:

1. Flexible flatfoot—(a) physiological and (b) postural
2. Rigid flatfoot—congenital vertical talus

Adolescent flatfoot:

1. Tarsal coalition (most common)
2. Accessory navicular

Adult:

1. Tibialis posterior insufficiency

54.3 Radiology

Longitudinal Arch (Sagittal Plane): Lateral View

1. Meary's angle (talus–first metatarsal angle): normal 0 degrees, increased in flatfoot (Fig. 54.2)
2. Calcaneal pitch: angle between the line along the inferior border of the calcaneum and line along the plantar surface of the foot, normal 20–45 degrees, decreased in flatfoot (Fig. 54.2)

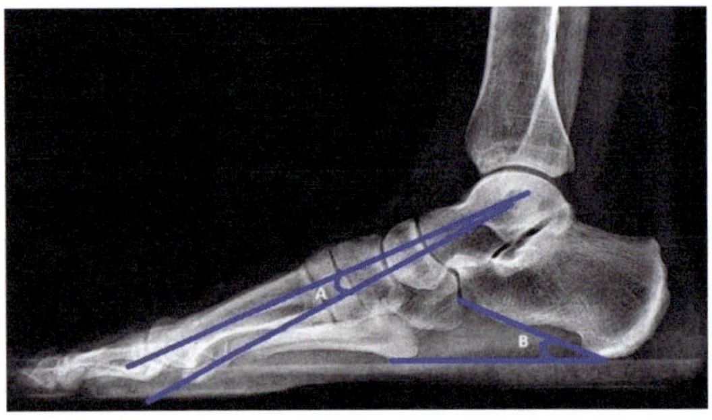

Fig. 54.2 A Meary's angle and B calcaneal pitch

Hindfoot Valgus (Frontal)

Talocalcaneal angle: normal 25–45 degrees, increased in foot valgus and decreased in foot varus

Forefoot Abduction (Transverse): In Anteroposterior (AP) Weight-Bearing Images

Talus–first metatarsal angle: normal 0–3 degrees, increased in flatfoot

Talonavicular coverage angle: normal 0–3 degrees, increased in flatfoot

54.4 Pediatric Flatfoot

Physiological flatfoot is a type of flatfoot in which the arch is absent from birth. This may take up to a decade to develop. It is usually bilateral, painless, and associated with heel valgus and forefoot abduction (too many toes sign). It may persist in 3% of adults.

Examination/screening: Arch is absent on weight-bearing (Fig. 54.3).

1. Arch appears on sitting (non-weight bearing) (Fig. 54.4)
2. Standing on toes—arch appears
3. Standing on the inner and outer borders of the foot

Jack's test: When the great toe is dorsiflexed, the plantar fascia tightens, resulting in the appearance of the medial arch.

Sometimes it may be symptomatic and present with pain. Common causes of pain include heel cord (tendo Achilles [TA]) tightening, hindfoot or midfoot stiffness, and hindfoot valgus

Fig. 54.3 Arch absent on weight-bearing

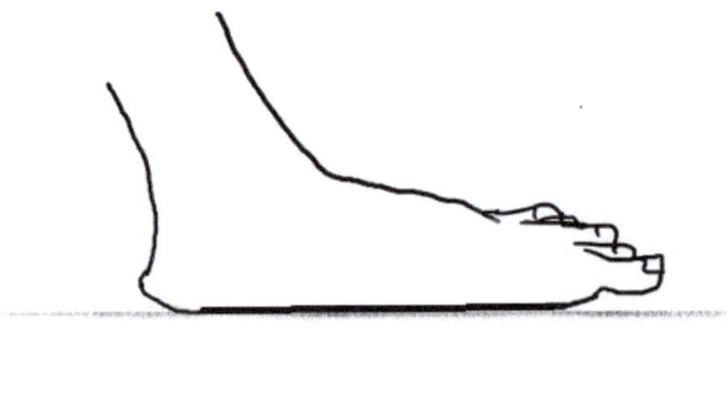

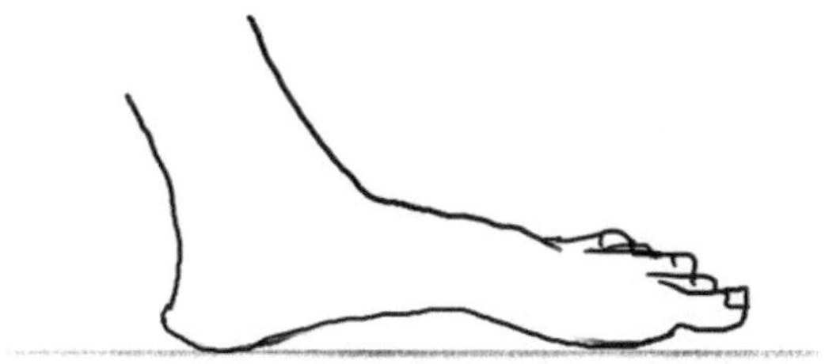

Fig. 54.4 Arch present on non-weight bearing

(sinus tarsi pain) due to talocalcaneal impingement.

Management

Asymptomatic: reassure the patient

Symptomatic: physiotherapy in the form of tendo Achilles stretching and tibialis posterior strengthening. Orthotics in the form of insoles/ shoe modification and ankle foot orthosis

Surgical intervention may be rarely required. It includes:

Bony: lateral column lengthening (lateral calcaneal open-wedge osteotomy)

Soft tissue: tendo Achilles lengthening, peroneal lengthening, tibialis posterior advancement (navicular to cuneiform)

Arthroereisis: sinus tarsi implant

Postural flexible flatfoot is a congenital, flexible, and painless type of flatfoot with calcaneovalgus and dorsiflexion of the foot. It is usually asymptomatic and associated with other packaging disorders such as developmental dysplasia of the hip, torticollis, metatarsus adductus, etc. Both dorsiflexion and heel valgus are correctable.

Management

- Responds to manipulation

Corrective casting (rarely required)

Pediatric Fixed Flatfoot (Congenital Vertical Talus)

It is also called a rocker-bottom foot. It may be genetic (autosomal dominant) or associated with neurological disorders such as meningomyelocele, arthrogryposis, spinal muscular atrophy, or neurofibromatosis. It may also be associated with genetic syndromes (trisomy 13, 15, and 18).

Pathoanatomy

1. Fixed hindfoot valgus: os calcis and talus in equinus, Achilles tendon contracture
2. Fixed midfoot dorsiflexion: dorsal dislocation of navicular, foot dorsiflexor contracture
3. Fixed forefoot abduction
4. Plantar surface: convex/rounded (rocker-bottom foot)

Management

Conservative: serial casting/reverse Ponseti casting to correct the talonavicular joint, followed by Achilles tendon tenotomy

Surgical: may be done in one or two stages. Requires multiple bony and soft tissue releases

54.5 Adolescent Flatfoot

Tarsal coalition: most common cause in adolescent flatfoot. It is due to failure of segmentation (autosomal dominant). It may be bilateral in 50% cases. It is also called peroneal spastic flatfoot, which is a misnomer as the peronei are actually shortened. The most common sites are calcaneonavicular (Fig. 54.5) and talocalcaneal (most common—middle facet of calcaneum). Depending on the ossification of the coalition bar, it may be divided into synostosis (fully ossified bar), synchondrosis (partially ossified bar), and syndesmosis (non-ossified bar). Synostosis may be associated with other conditions such as fibular hemimelia or proximal femoral focal deficiency (PFFD).

Pain usually corresponds to the age of ossification of the bar. Calcaneonavicular and talonavicular coalitions usually become symptomatic at 9–13 years of age and in late adolescence, respectively. Heel valgus and flatfoot do not get corrected on toe standing.

A 45-degree oblique view is useful to see calcaneonavicular coalition (anteater sign), and a lateral view of the foot demonstrates talocalcaneal coalition (C sign). MRI scan will be required for cartilaginous coalition.

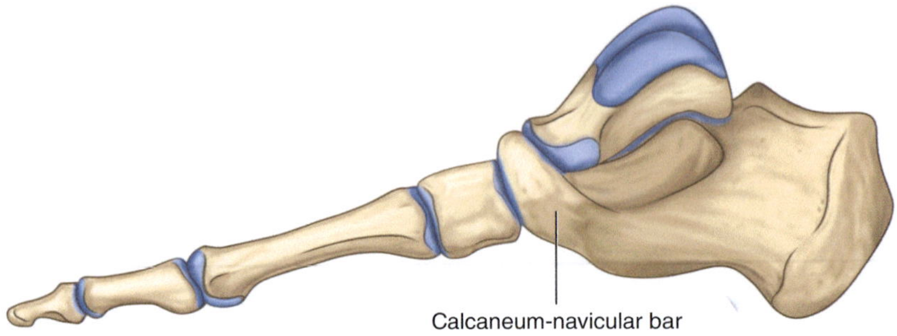

Fig. 54.5 Calcaneonavicular coalition

Management

Incidental finding: long-term follow-up and observation.

Conservative management: medial arch support and heel cups (moderate pain) and below-knee (BK) cast (severe pain).

Surgical management: Calcaneonavicular coalition in early age may be managed by excision and extensor digitorum brevis (EDB) interposition with calcaneal osteotomy, and in older adults by subtalar triple arthrodesis. Talocalcaneal coalition may be managed by excision with fat graft placement (middle facet) and triple fusion or subtalar arthrodesis (posterior facet).

Accessory navicular: Usually asymptomatic and presents as a bulge on the medial side of the foot. It is often bilateral. Depending on the degree of ossification, it is classified as type 1 (small ossicle in the substance of tibialis posterior, not connected to navicular), type 2 (larger ossification connected to navicular via cartilaginous joint), and type 3 (completely fused with navicular bone). It becomes symptomatic after a history of trauma.

A lateral oblique X-ray view of the foot can demonstrate accessory navicular, and MRI scan may be used to see cartilaginous union.

Management

Asymptomatic: no management

Symptomatic: managed conservatively by rest, nonsteroidal anti-inflammatory drugs (NSAIDs), and BK cast

In case of painful nonunion, surgical management via excision may be done.

54.6 Adult Flatfoot

Tibialis Posterior Insufficiency

Tibialis posterior muscle has multiple attachments in the foot. This results in multiple functions of the muscle:

Insertion on navicular: elevates the medial margin of the foot

Insertion on the os sustentaculum tali: holds the talar head in the proper position

Insertion on the base of the third to fifth metatarsals: supination of the foot

Pathogenesis: Chronic tibialis posterior insufficiency due to overload, microtrauma, and inflammation leads to a tear (watershed area), and along with failure of static stabilizers, it ultimately results in arch collapse and arthritis.

Multiplanar deformity: hindfoot valgus, forefoot abduction, forefoot supination, and medial column instability

Risk factors include obesity, preexisting flatfoot, diabetes, increasing age, corticosteroid use, and systemic inflammatory disorders.

Classification: (1) Johnson and Strom, (2) Myerson, and (3) Bluman and Myerson

Bluman and Myerson Classification

Stage 1: impairment of tibialis posterior (TP) tendon

Stage 2: impairment of TP + hindfoot and forefoot deformity (flexible deformity)

Stage 3: impairment of TP + hindfoot and forefoot deformity (rigid deformity)

Stage 4: impairment of the ankle joint

Management

Stage 1: rest, NSAIDs, orthosis, physiotherapy, tenosynovectomy (rarely)

Stage 2: medial calcaneal shift (extra-articular osteotomy of calcaneum) + flexor digitorum longus (FDL) tendon augmentation for hindfoot valgus, lateral column lengthening for forefoot abduction and talar head uncoverage, Cotton osteotomy (dorsal opening wedge osteotomy), and first tarsometatarsal (TMT) joint fusion for first TMT joint hypermobility

Stage 3 and Stage 4: Triple arthrodesis

Multiple Choice Questions

1. Jack's test is positive in?
   (a) Fixed flatfoot
   (b) Flexible flatfoot
   (c) Calcaneonavicular coalition
   (d) Talocalcaneal coalition
2. Anteater sign is seen in?
   (a) Calcaneonavicular coalition
   (b) Talocalcaneal coalition
   (c) Tibialis posterior dysfunction
   (d) Physiological flatfoot
3. Medial longitudinal arch is formed by all except?
   (a) First metatarsal
   (b) Medial cuneiform
   (c) Cuboid
   (d) Navicular
4. Normal Meary's angle on lateral foot X-ray is?
   (a) 0–3 degrees
   (b) 15–20 degrees
   (c) 25–45 degrees
   (d) 40–60 degrees
5. Most common cause of adolescent fixed flatfoot is?
   (a) Physiological flatfoot
   (b) Accessory navicular
   (c) Tibialis posterior dysfunction
   (d) Tarsal coalition

Answers: 1. (b), 2. (a), 3. (c), 4. (a), 5. (d)

55 Pes Cavus

Pradeep Meena

55.1 Introduction

Pes cavus is a foot deformity characterized by an excessively high medial longitudinal arch (Fig. 55.1). It is usually fixed (i.e., inflexible), meaning that it does not flatten on weight-bearing. The components of pes cavus are a varus hindfoot, plantar-flexed first metatarsal (MT), adducted forefoot, and clawed toes. It has been reported as bilateral in 8–15% of the population worldwide.

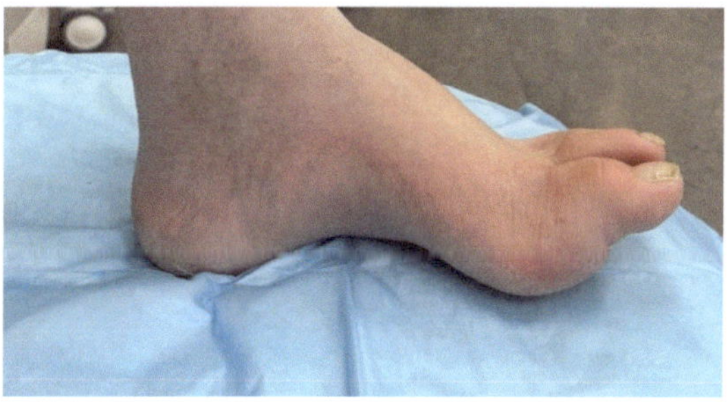

Fig. 55.1 Image showing pes cavus

55.2 Causes

Neuromuscular diseases are the most common causes of pes cavus, followed by idiopathic causes. In Charcot-Marie-Tooth disease (CMT; hereditary peripheral neuropathy), the imbalance between foot intrinsic muscles and leg muscles leads to pes cavus. Patients with CMT typically have a weak tibialis anterior and a weak peroneus brevis. These are overpowered by preservation of the posterior tibialis and peroneus longus, which results in hindfoot varus, forefoot equinus, and pronation. Spinal cord anomalies (e.g., myelodysplasia, syringomyelia, tethered cord, etc.) should be ruled out by a thorough examination of the spine as they are among the common causes leading to pes cavus. Various causes of pes cavus can be summarized below (Table 55.1)

P. Meena (✉)
AIIMS, Rishikesh, Rishikesh, Uttarakhand, India

V. Kumar et al. (eds.), *A Quick Guide to Essential Orthopedics*,
https://doi.org/10.1007/978-981-95-2676-5_55

Table 55.1 Summary of causes resulting in pes cavus

Unilateral cavus	Bilateral cavus
Volkmann ischemic contracture, scarring of the deep posterior compartment of the leg	Charcot-Marie-Tooth disease
Post-traumatic: calcaneal or talar fractures	Friedrich's ataxia
Spinal cord tumor	Myelodysplasia
Tethered cord	Syringomyelia
Peroneal nerve injury	Cerebral palsy
Poliomyelitis	Muscular dystrophy
Iatrogenic	Idiopathic/familial

55.3 Clinical Features

Foot pain is a common complaint in patients with pes cavus. Pes cavus has been associated with callosities over metatarsal heads and the lateral foot due to an altered tripod of the foot, plantar heel pain, Achilles tendinopathies, ankle and knee arthritis, fractures, and stress injuries. In later stages, it is associated with heel varus and claw toes.

There are two tests that may be used to diagnose pes cavus clinically and determine if it is a fixed deformity: the peek-a-boo sign and the Coleman block test (Fig. 55.2).

The Coleman block test is helpful in determining the flexibility of the subtalar joint, and thus helping to differentiate between a forefoot-driven flexible pes cavus and a hindfoot-driven rigid pes cavus. For performing this test, the patient is asked to stand on a 1-in. block of wood or a book while leaving the great toe and first metatarsal head to drop off. In a high-arched foot, if valgus correction of the heel occurs (i.e., mobile subtalar joint), it signifies that the deformity is caused by a plantar-flexed first ray; this is referred to as a forefoot-driven hindfoot varus. If the hindfoot does not correct and stays in varus, the deformity is rigid.

Radiologically, on the anteroposterior (AP) view, the talo–first metatarsal angle and Kite's angle (talocalcaneal angle) are decreased, and on the lateral view, calcaneal pitch, navicular height, Meary's angle (lateral talo–metatarsal angle), and Hibbs angle (lateral calcaneo–first metatarsal angle) are increased (Fig. 55.3).

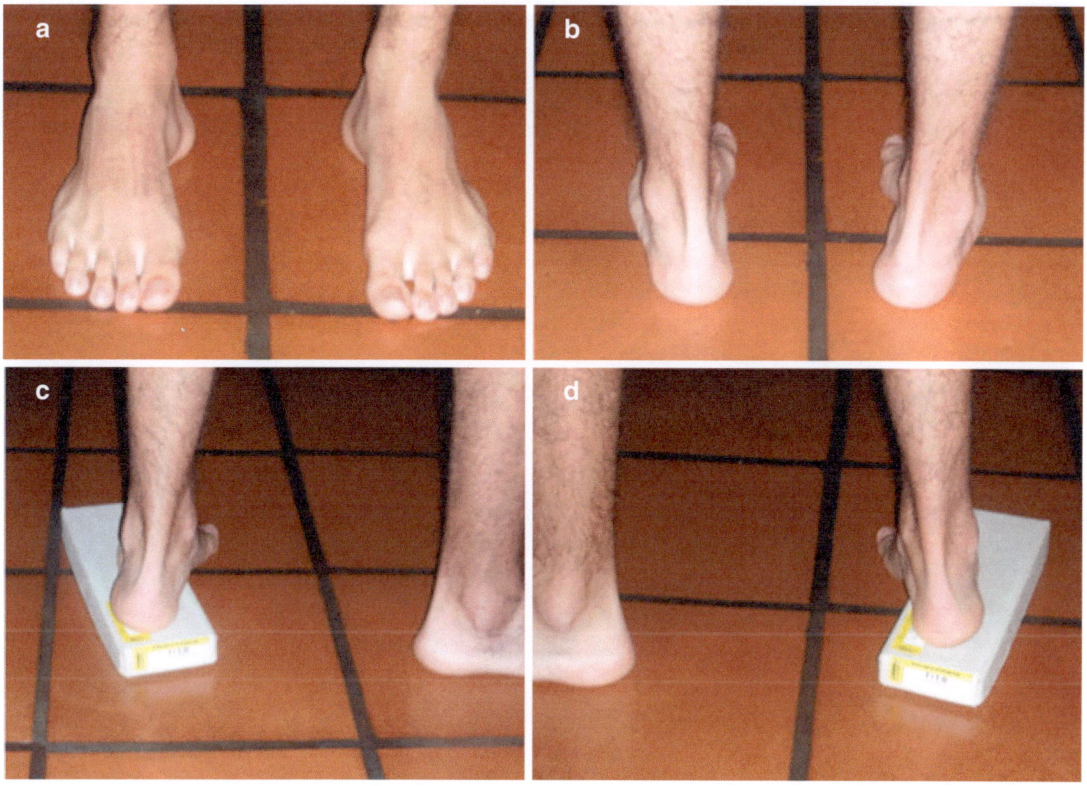

Fig. 55.2 (**a**) Peek-a-boo heel, (**b**) bilateral heel varus, and (**c**) Coleman block test

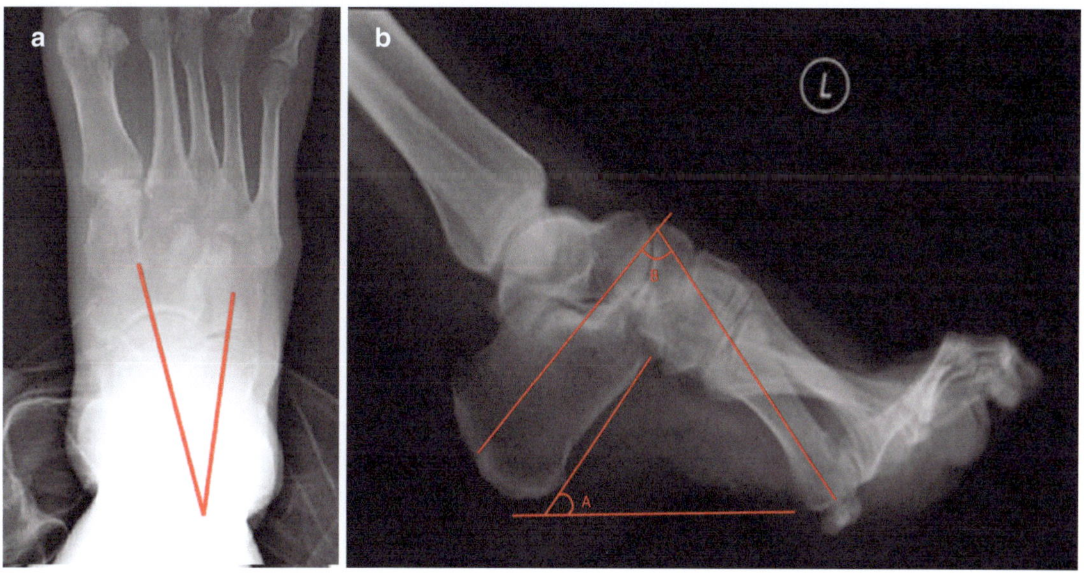

Fig. 55.3 Foot AP X-ray showing Kite's (talocalcaneal) angle; lateral X-ray showing increased (A) calcaneal pitch, navicular height, and (B) Hibbs angle

55.4 Management

55.4.1 Conservative

In earlier stages, where the deformity is flexible, pes cavus can be managed with conservative management, which includes physical therapy, tendo Achilles stretching, plantar fascia stretching, strengthening of the lateral compartment muscles of the foot, and splinting. Offloading casts and modified shoewear are helpful in managing pressure sores over metatarsal heads, lateral foot, etc.

55.4.2 Surgical

Soft tissue reconstruction surgeries such as plantar fascia release, Steindler procedure, tendo Achilles lengthening, and gastrocnemius recession are helpful in early stages of deformity when the foot is supple and bony anatomy is maintained.

Tendon transfers, such as peroneus longus to Peroneus brevis, tibialis posterior to tibialis anterior/cuneiforms, long toe extensors to the cuboid or lateral cuneiform (modified Hibbs procedure), and split tibialis anterior tendon transfer to the cuboid or peroneus tertius, are most commonly used and are helpful in managing cases where pes cavus is due to muscle imbalance and altered foot biomechanics in a supple foot.

Bony reconstructions are often required in patients with rigid deformity and a positive Coleman block test. First metatarsal closing-wedge and cuneiform plantar open-wedge osteotomies are used to manage predominantly forefoot equinus, often in isolation or in combination with midfoot osteotomies such as naviculectomies or cuboid closing-wedge osteotomy [1, 2].

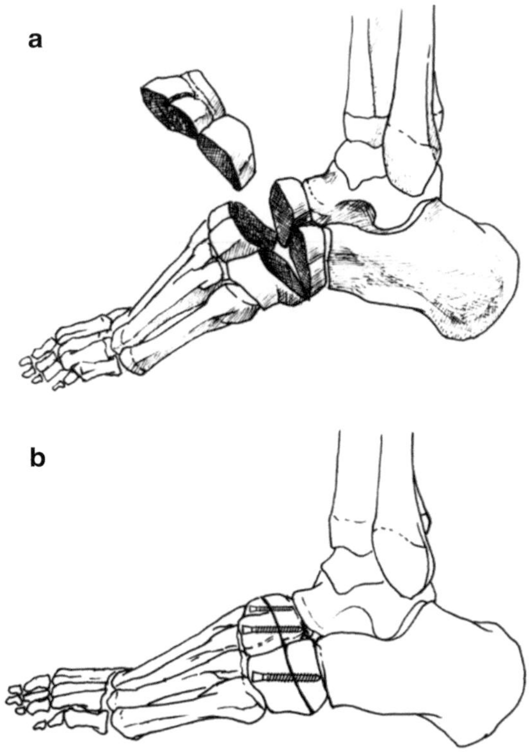

Fig. 55.4 Image showing deformity correction using Japas midfoot osteotomy

Japas osteotomy, Cole osteotomy, and Meary osteotomy are the best-known osteotomies at the level of midfoot for the correction of rigid pes cavus. Japas osteotomy is a large osteotomy in which a dorsal closing wedge is taken through the entire midfoot with the apex at the navicular bone and extending medially and laterally, ending just proximal to the first and fifth tarsometatarsal joints (Fig. 55.4).

Hindfoot osteotomies such as calcaneal lateral sliding osteotomy and Dwyer calcaneal lateral closing-wedge osteotomy (Fig. 55.5) are also required when pes cavus is associated with rigid hindfoot deformities (increased calcaneal pitch, heel varus).

In patients with more rigid deformities or arthritis of the midfoot and hindfoot joints, salvage procedures such as triple arthrodesis (fusion of talocalcaneal, talonavicular, and calcaneocuboid joints) are often considered (Fig. 55.6).

To summarize, treatment in a patient with pes cavus is based on factors such as rigidity of deformity, apex of deformity, whether it is forefoot driven or hindfoot driven, associated arthritis, etc. [3] (Fig. 55.7).

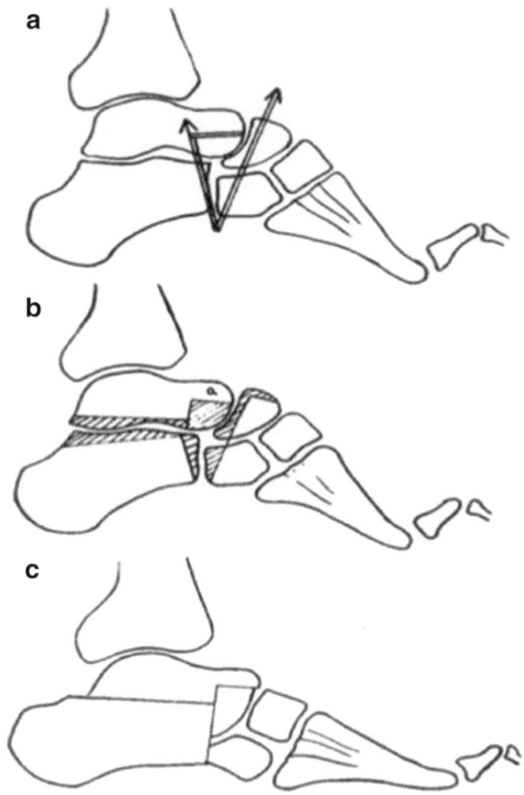

Fig. 55.5 Dwyer lateral calcaneal closing-wedge osteotomy

Fig. 55.6 Deformity correction in pes cavus with beak triple arthrodesis

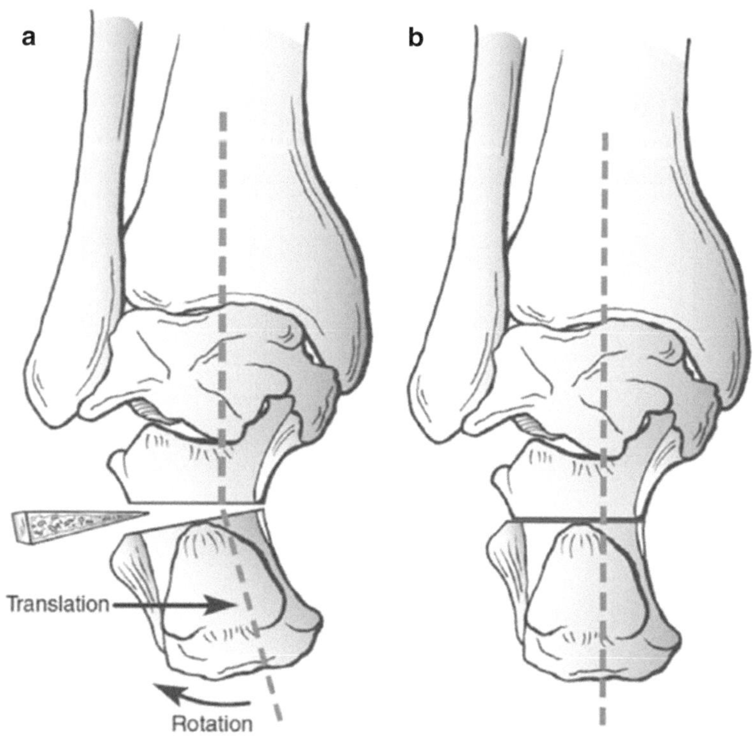

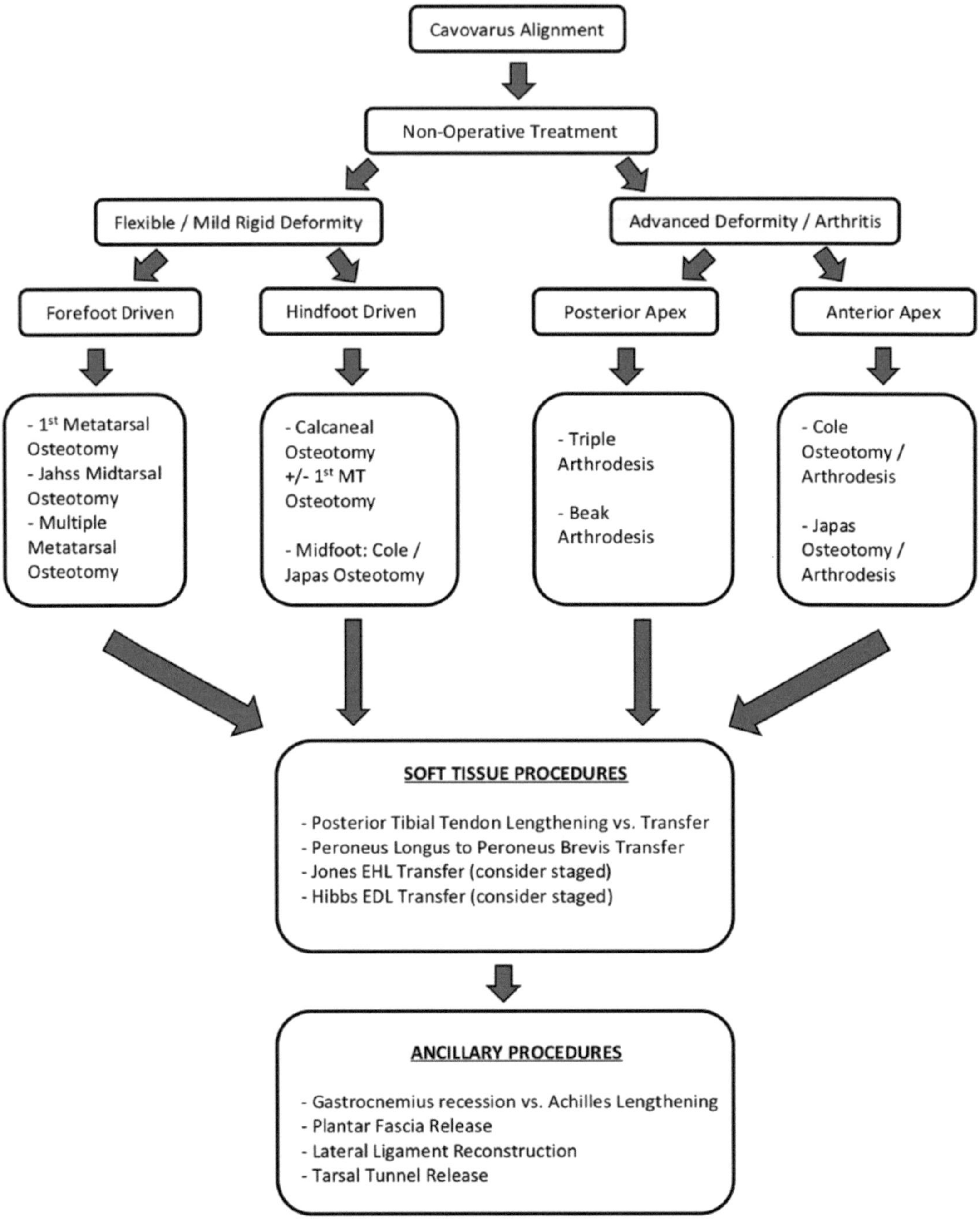

Fig. 55.7 Treatment algorithm in pes cavus

Multiple Choice Questions

1. In pes cavus, which of the following is decreased?
   (a) Kite's angle
   (b) Meary's angle
   (c) Calcaneal pitch
   (d) Hibbs angle
2. Which osteotomy is a hindfoot osteotomy?
   (a) Japas osteotomy
   (b) Cole osteotomy
   (c) Dwyer osteotomy
   (d) Meary osteotomy
3. A patient with pes cavus on clinical examination has a positive Coleman block test. What does it signify?
   (a) Forefoot-driven deformity
   (b) Hindfoot-driven deformity
   (c) Midfoot-driven deformity
   (d) Global deformity
4. Which of the following is weak in a patient with Charcot-Marie-Tooth disease presenting with pes cavus?
   (a) Peroneus longus
   (b) Peroneus brevis
   (c) Peroneus tertius
   (d) Tibialis posterior
5. Which of the following is not seen in pes cavus?
   (a) Peek-a-boo sign
   (b) Too many toes sign
   (c) Painful callosities over metatarsal heads
   (d) Claw toes

Answers: 1. (a), 2. (c), 3. (a), 4. (b), 5. (b)

References

1. Zhou Y, Zhou B, Liu J, et al. A prospective study of midfoot osteotomy combined with adjacent joint sparing internal fixation in treatment of rigid pes cavus deformity. J Orthop Surg Res. 2014;9:44. https://doi.org/10.1186/1749-799X-9-44.
2. Jastifer JR, Coughlin MJ. Hindfoot deformity and calcaneal tuberosity osteotomies. Foot Ankle Spec. 2015;8(1):50–8.
3. Rosenwasser KA, Judd H, Hyman JE. Evidence-based management strategies for pediatric pes cavus: current concept review. J Pediatr Orthop Soc N Am. 2022;4(2)

Part VI

Musculoskeletal Oncology

Classification of Bone Tumors

56

Mohit Dhingra and Anil Regmi

56.1 Dedicated to "Naina"Introduction

Classification of any pathology is important to know about its origin, pathogenesis, and prognosis in the long run. Bone tumors need classification and staging in order to prognosticate and decide about their treatment.

The rarity of primary bone tumors has probably lead to limited data collection about their relative frequency and inadequate understanding of their risk factors. Consistent classification of tumors helps to understand their intrinsic biology necessary for their reproducibility. It is widely accepted that histopathologic classifications are necessary for reproducibility of diagnostic criteria, which is a prerequisite for predicting the biological potential of a tumor and, therefore, for treating it.

Bone tumors are classified based on the differentiation line of neoplastic cells and their similarity to normal cells. Tumors that form cartilage or bone can easily be assessed using these criteria. Because benign lesions are often asymptomatic and not clinically recognized, they are likely underestimated despite having a higher incidence than primary malignant tumors. Moreover, primary bone tumors are outnumbered by metastases from carcinomas, melanoma, or hematologic malignancies, including plasmacytomas.

56.2 World Health Organization (WHO) Classification of Bone Tumors

- Providing updated classification schemes and essential diagnostic criteria for bone tumors, the 2020 World Health Organization (WHO) classification of tumors of soft tissue and bone provides an updated classification scheme.
- It is essential to conduct a thorough histologic examination in order to determine the appropriate treatment and prognosis.
- The diversity and considerable morphologic overlap of bone tumors with other mesenchymal and non-mesenchymal bone lesions can complicate diagnosis.

M. Dhingra (✉) · A. Regmi
Department of Orthopedics, All India Institute of Medical Sciences, Rishikesh, Uttarakhand, India

V. Kumar et al. (eds.), *A Quick Guide to Essential Orthopedics*,
https://doi.org/10.1007/978-981-95-2676-5_56

56.3 2020 WHO Classification [1]

	Benign	Intermediate (locally aggressive)	Malignant
Chondrogenic tumors	Subungual exostosis Bizarre parosteal osteochondromatous proliferation Periosteal chondroma Enchondroma Osteochondroma Chondroblastoma Chondromyxoid fibroma Osteochondromyxoma	Chondromatosis Atypical cartilaginous tumor	Chondrosarcoma, grades 1 Chondrosarcoma, grades 2 Chondrosarcoma, grades 3 Periosteal chondrosarcoma Clear cell chondrosarcoma Mesenchymal chondrosarcoma Dedifferentiated chondrosarcoma
Osteogenic tumors	Osteoma Osteoid osteoma	Osteoblastoma	Low-grade central osteosarcoma Osteosarcoma Conventional osteosarcoma Telangiectatic osteosarcoma Small cell osteosarcoma Parosteal osteosarcoma Periosteal osteosarcoma High-grade surface osteosarcoma Secondary osteosarcoma
Fibrogenic tumors		Desmoplastic fibroma	Fibrosarcoma
Vascular tumors of bone	Hemangioma	Epithelioid hemangioma	Epithelioid hemangioendothelioma Angiosarcoma
Osteoclastic giant cell-rich tumors	Aneurysmal bone cyst Non-ossifying fibroma	Giant cell tumor of bone	Giant cell tumor of bone, malignant
Notochordal tumors	Benign notochordal cell tumor		Chordoma Chondroid chordoma Poorly differentiated chordoma Dedifferentiated chordoma
Other mesenchymal tumors of bone	Chondromesenchymal hamartoma of chest wall Simple bone cyst Fibrous dysplasia Osteofibrous dysplasia Lipoma-like hibernoma	Osteofibrous dysplasia-like adamantinoma Mesenchymoma	Adamantinoma of long bones Dedifferentiated adamantinoma Leiomyosarcoma Pleomorphic sarcoma, undifferentiated Bone metastases

The above classification system shows tumors according to the cell of origin histologically. Tumors that are benign are suffix by -oma and the malignant ones are suffix by -sarcoma except in cases of adamantinoma which is regarded as malignant tumors.

All the tumors, be it benign or malignant, need staging in order to prognosticate them. The different staging systems used for benign and malignant tumors are described as follows:

56.4 Enneking Staging [2]

- The Enneking surgical staging system is reliable, reproducible, and of prognostic importance for musculoskeletal sarcomas, especially for those originating in the axial skeleton.
- It has been used widely for classification by orthopedic oncologic surgeons around the world. However, this classification system is applicable only to mesenchymal malignancies.

Enneking staging for benign musculoskeletal tumors:

Based on radiographic characteristics of the tumor host margin.

Stage	Definition	Description
1	Latent	Well-demarcated margins, e.g., non-ossifying fibroma (Fig. 56.1a)
2	Active	Demarcated margins but expands thinning of cortex, e.g., ABC (Fig. 56.1b)
3	Aggressive	Indistinct margins, not limited by natural barriers, e.g., GCT (Fig. 56.1c)

Enneking staging for malignant musculoskeletal tumors:

Based on surgical grade, local extent, and presence or absence of metastasis (Fig. 56.2).

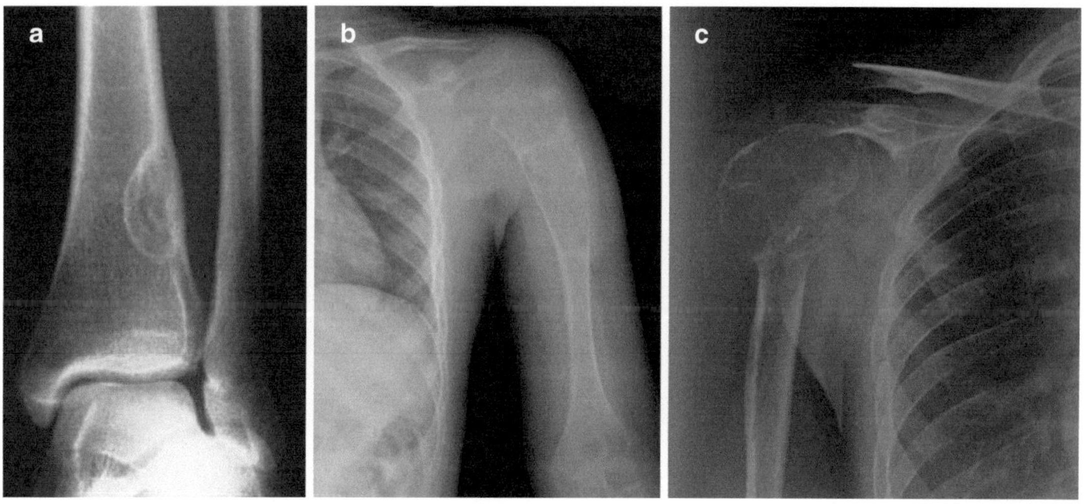

Fig. 56.1 Benign tumor of appendicular skeleton; (**a**) 15-year-old female with non-ossifying fibroma of right distal tibia with well-demarcated margins (Enneking stage 1: latent); (**b**) 8-year-old male with aneurysmal bone cyst of left proximal humerus with demarcated margins and thinning of cortex (Enneking stage 2: active); (**c**) 27-year-old male with giant cell tumor of the right proximal humerus with indistinct margins and cortical breach (Enneking stage 3: aggressive)

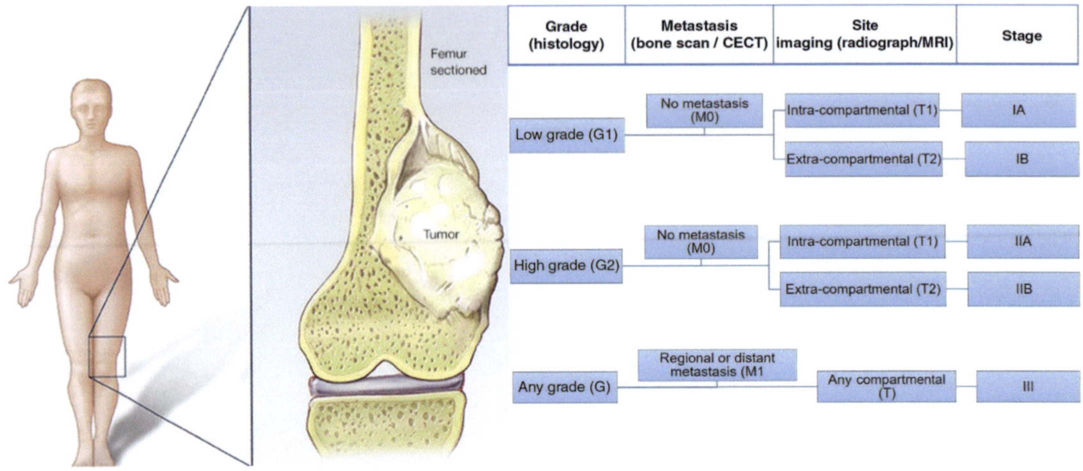

Fig. 56.2 The grades of malignant bone tumors—Enneking staging

56.5 AJCC Grading [3]

Another grading which is being used for malignant bone tumors is by American Joint Committee of Cancer (AJCC)

It is based on TNM system which stands for

T—depth of tumor infiltration and the greatest diameter of the tumor

N—lymph node metastasis

M—distant metastasis

In addition to TNM, fourth parameter known as G factor (grade of histology) is being used for the staging as well (Fig. 56.3).

To conclude,

- The imaging, lymph node status, metastasis, and histologic grading make a complete diagnosis and staging of any tumor.
- Imaging helps to determine the anatomic confines of the primary tumor and the presence of metastasis.
- Local extent for any neoplasm refers to its containment in the anatomic boundaries of a compartment.
- Anatomic compartments have inherent barriers to tumor spread, including fascial planes and bone structures.
- Local extent determines the approach for surgical procedure and feasibility for desired surgical margins.
- In general, a high-grade lesion is more likely to invade the surrounding host tissue.
- This places the patient at greater risk of local recurrence and metastasis.
- The use of adjuvant therapies then is indicated to eradicate tumor cells that would remain after surgical resection.

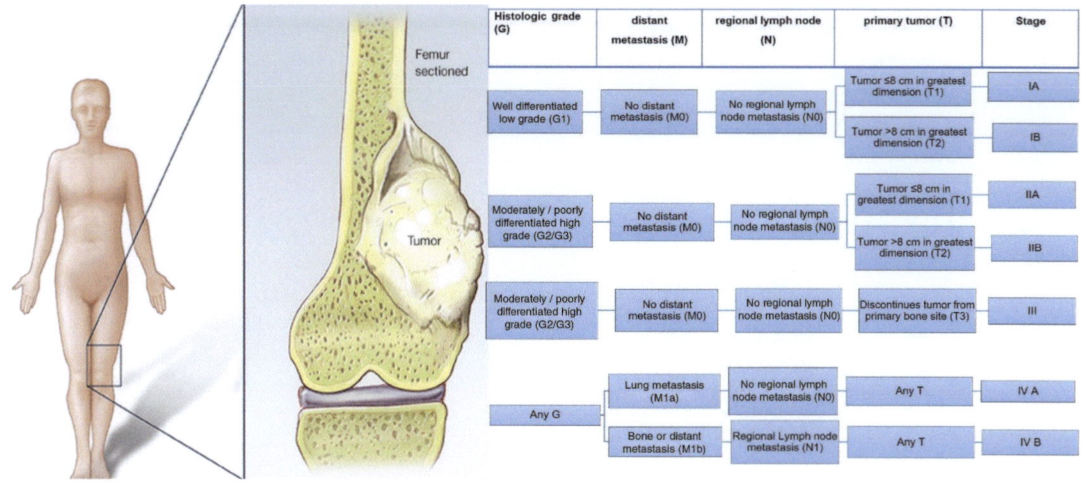

Fig. 56.3 AJCC stage for bone sarcoma in the appendicular skeleton

Now, in Order to Recall, Let Us Do Some Practical Problems on the Subject

Case Example

Case 1: An 18-year-old male presented with pain over the right knee and swelling over the right knee for 12 months. On examination, there was a diffuse swelling on medial aspect of distal thigh and knee of 8 × 6 cm, soft to firm consistency with ill-defined border, tender, fixed to the bone, and free from the skin. No regional lymph node was palpable. A plain radiograph revealed an eccentric expansile lytic lesion on metaphysio-epiphyseal region of distal femur over medial condyle, with intact cortex. Magnetic resonance imaging (MRI) revealed solid tumor of medial condyle of distal femur with intact cortex and without joint extension. Histopathology was suggestive of giant cell tumor.

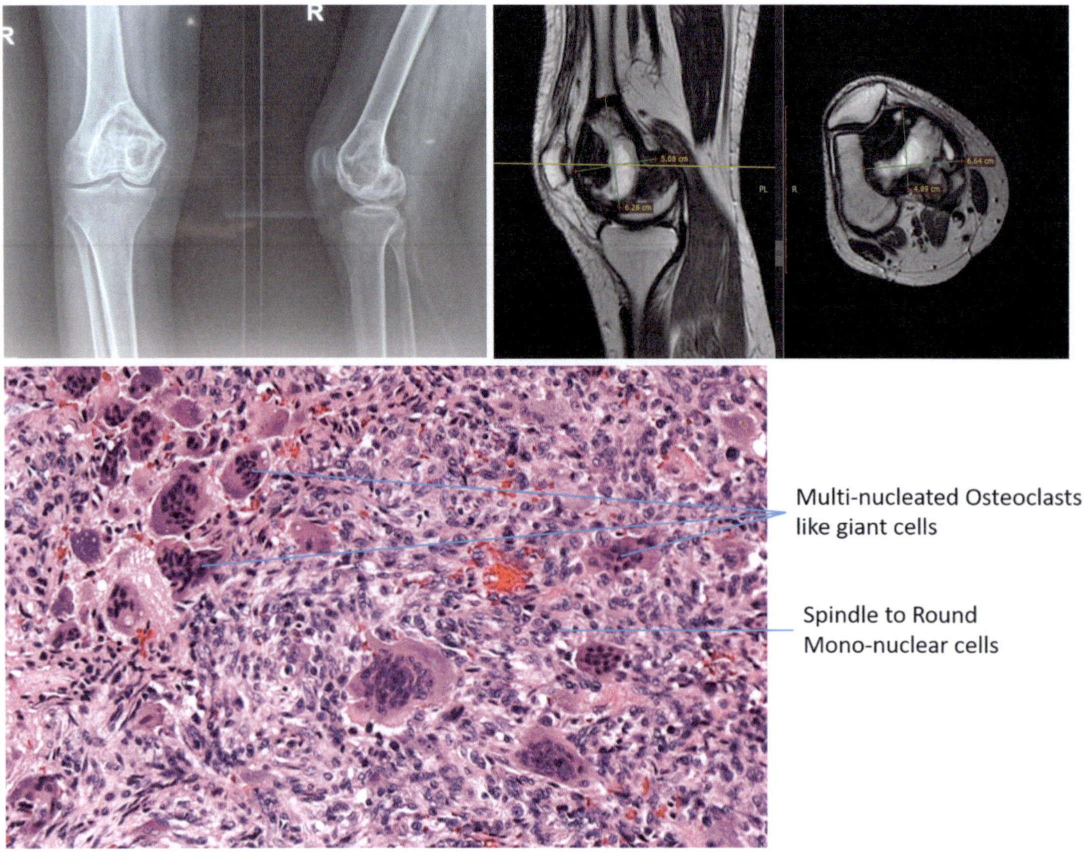

How to classify and stage tumor?

WHO Classification:

- Histology-based
- Osteoclastic giant-cell-rich tumors–intermediate (locally aggressive)–giant cell tumor of bone

Enneking:

- Histology, local morphology, and distant metastatic imaging-based
- Stage: benign; aggressive
  - Indistinct borders

AJCC:

Not applicable as it is the classification of malignant tumors.

Case 2: An 18-year-old male presented with pain and swelling over the left proximal leg for 6 months. On examination, swelling of size 3 × 3 cm can be appreciated over the anteromedial aspect of the proximal leg, which is bony hard, tender, non-fluctuant, attached to the underlying bone, and free from the overlying skin. No regional lymph node was palpable. A plain radiograph revealed lytic and sclerotic-type mixed destructive lesions with extensive periosteal reaction on the medial aspect of the proximal tibia. MRI revealed a solid tumor of the proximal tibia without the involvement of soft tissue and neurovascular structures. Contrast-enhanced computed tomography (CECT) of thorax and abdomen and bone scan for metastatic workup are negative for metastasis. Histopathology was suggestive of conventional osteosarcoma.

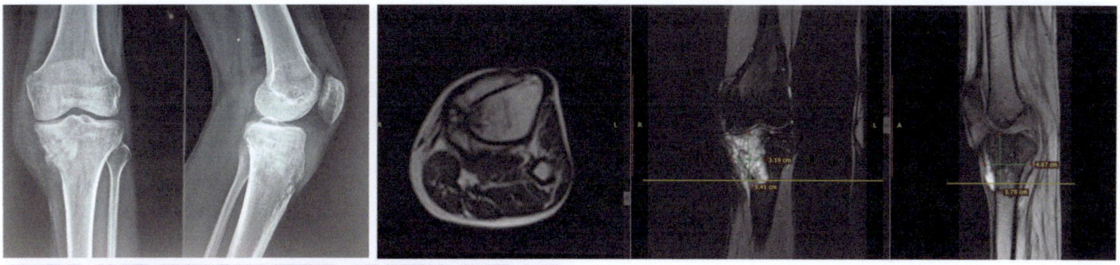

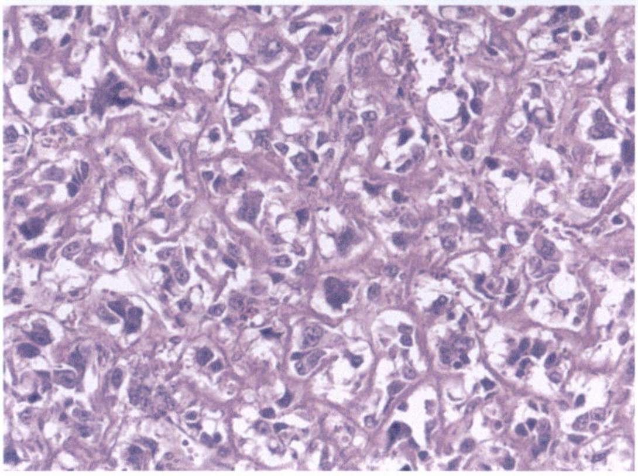

How to classify and stage tumor?

WHO Classification:

- Histology-based
- Osteogenic tumor–malignant–conventional osteosarcoma

Enneking:

- Histology, local morphology, and distant metastatic imaging-based
- Stage: malignant stage II
  - High grade (G2)
  - Intra-compartmental (T1)
  - No metastasis (M0)

AJCC:

- Morphology, lymph node status, distant metastatic imaging, and histology-based
- Stage: II A
  - T1 tumor <8 cm in greatest dimension
  - N0 no regional lymph node metastasis
  - M0 no distant metastasis
  - G2 moderately differentiated, high grade

Case 3: A 12-year-old female presented with pain over the right knee and progressive swelling over the right knee for 6 months. On examination, large swelling present over the right mid-thigh extending up to mid-leg of 30 × 25 × 20 cm size, with tense skin with venous engorgement. Swelling is firm to hard, nonmobile, tender, fixed to the bone, and free from the skin. No regional lymph node was palpable. A plain radiograph revealed a lytic and sclerotic type mixed destructive lesion with extensive periosteal lifting and sun-burst appearance on the proximal tibia, involving the proximal fibula also. MRI revealed a solid tumor of the proximal tibia with extensive involvement of soft tissue and neurovascular involvement. CECT of thorax and abdomen revealed pulmonary done on left lower zone, and bone scan shows a lesion on the left proximal tibia and left lower zone of lung suggestive of metastasis. Histopathology was suggestive of conventional osteosarcoma.

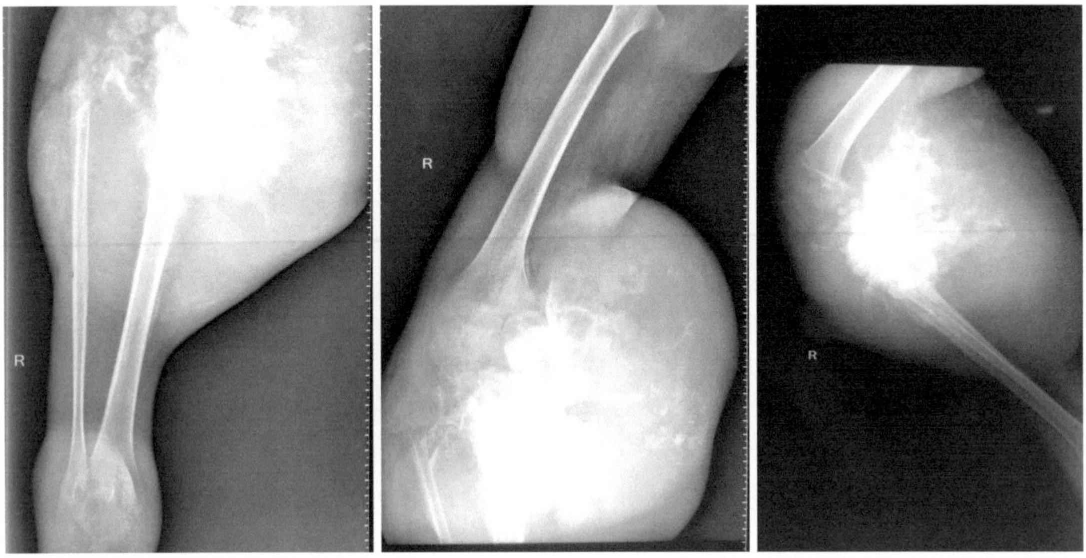
R
R
R

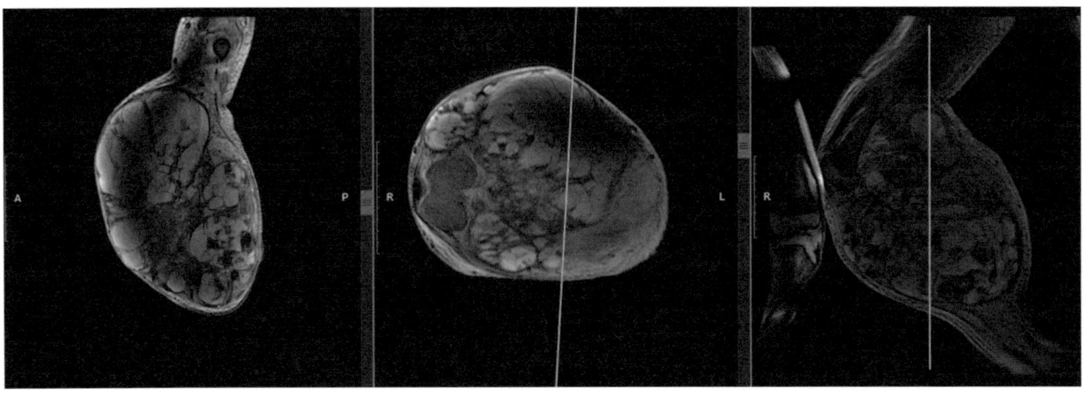
A
P
R
L
R

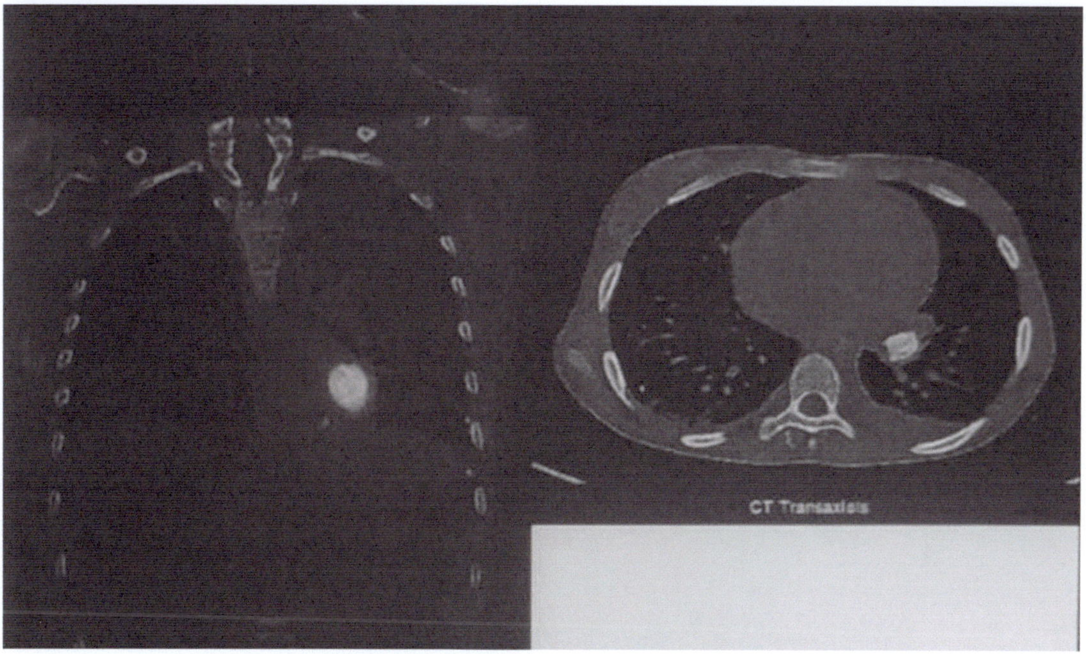

CT thorax showing a large node in the left hemithorax

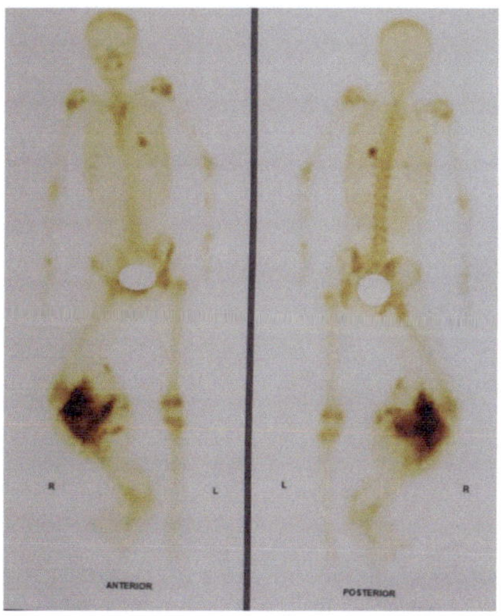

Bone scan showing primary tumour in the leg with a single metastasis in the left lung

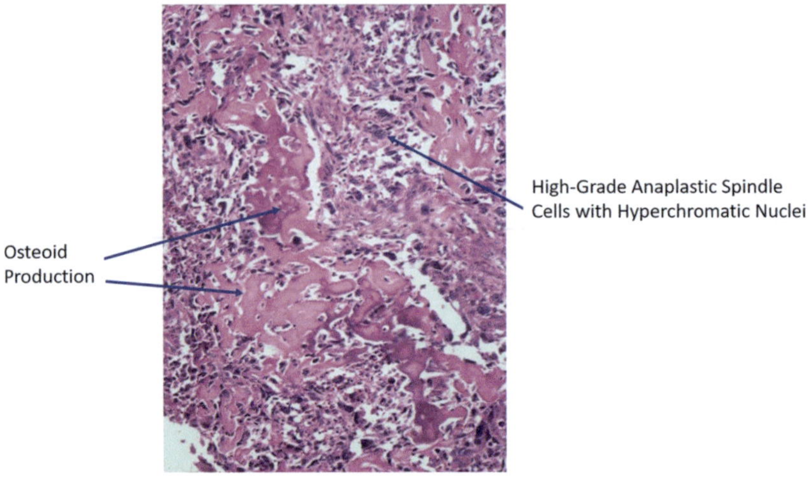

How to classify and stage tumor?

WHO Classification:

- Histology-based
- Osteogenic tumor–malignant–conventional osteosarcoma

Enneking:

- Histology, local morphology, and distant metastatic imaging-based
- Stage: malignant stage III
  - High grade (G2)
  - Extra-compartmental (T2)
  - Regional or distant metastasis (M1)

AJCC:

- Morphology, lymph node status, distant metastatic imaging, and histology-based
- Stage: IV A
  - T2 Tumor >8 cm in greatest dimension
  - N0 No regional lymph node metastasis
  - M1a Lung
  - G3 Poorly differentiated, high grade

Multiple Choice Questions

1. Surgical staging of bone tumors is by:
   (a) Edmonton
   (b) Manchester
   (c) Enneking
   (d) TNM
2. Commonest benign bone tumor is:
   (a) Bone cyst
   (b) Blastoma
   (c) Chordoma
   (d) Osteoma
3. MC malignant bone tumor:
   (a) Osteosarcoma
   (b) Ewing sarcoma
   (c) Multiple myeloma
   (d) Metastasis
4. MC non-hematogenic primary malignant bone tumor:
   (a) Osteosarcoma
   (b) Ewing sarcoma
   (c) Multiple Myeloma
   (d) Metastasis

Metastases>multiple myeloma>osteosarcoma is order of bone malignancy

5. Match the following:

I. Ewing tumor	(i) Flat bones
II. Chondrosarcoma	(ii) Diaphysis
III. Osteosarcoma	(iv) Epiphysis
IV. Giant cell tumor	(iii) Metaphysis

Options:
   (a) I (i) II (ii) III (iii) IV (iv)
   (b) I (ii) II (i) III (iii) IV (iv)
   (c) I (ii) II (i) III (iv) IV (iii)
   (d) I (ii) II (iii) III (iv) IV (i)

6. Bone tumor arising from epiphysis and recurs till epiphysis fuse:
   (a) Osteoclastoma

   (b) Chondroblastoma
   (c) Osteoid osteoma
   (d) Osteoblastoma
7. The differential diagnosis of lesion, histologically resembling giant cell tumor in the small bones of the hands or feet, includes all of the following except:
   (a) Aneurysmal bone cyst
   (b) Fibrosarcoma
   (c) Osteosarcoma
   (d) Hyperparathyroidism
8. According to a newer hypothesis, Ewing sarcoma arises from:
   (a) Epiphysis
   (b) Diaphysis
   (c) Medullary cavity
   (d) Cortex
9. Giant cell tumor comes on which staging of tumor by Enneking system?
   (a) Benign latent
   (b) Benign active
   (c) Benign aggressive
   (d) Malignant
10. A 15-year-old boy is injured while playing cricket. X-rays of the leg rule out possible fracture. Radiologist reports that the boy has an evidence of aggressive bone tumor with both bone destruction and soft tissue mass. The bone biopsy reveals bone cancer with neural differentiation. What is most likely diagnosis?
   (a) Ewing sarcoma
   (b) Aneurysmal bone cyst
   (c) Osteoblastoma
   (d) Giant cell tumor

Answers: 1. (c), 2. (d), 3. (d), 4. (a), 5. (c), 6. (a), 7. (c), 8. (c), 9. (c), 10. (a)

References

1. Choi JH, Ro JY. The 2020 WHO classification of tumors of bone: an updated review. Adv Anat Pathol. 2021;28(3):119–38.
2. Jawad MU, Scully SP. In brief: classifications in brief: enneking classification: benign and malignant tumors of the musculoskeletal system. Clin Orthop Relat Res. 2010;468:2000–2.
3. Tanaka K, Ozaki T. New TNM classification (AJCC eighth edition) of bone and soft tissue sarcomas: JCOG Bone and Soft Tissue Tumor Study Group. Jpn J Clin Oncol. 2019;49(2):103–7.

57 Approach to a Patient

Mohit Dhingra and Vikas Maheshwari

57.1 Dedicated to 'Naina'Introduction

Any patient with pain, swelling, or fracture without significant trauma coming to the clinic should be suspected to be suffering from tumour pathology. These conditions can be classified as follows:

(a) Primary (developing de novo from the bone) which is further classified as follows:
  - Benign (Fig. 57.1)
  - Malignant (Fig. 57.2)

(b) Secondary (arising from some other organs of the body and migrating to the bone). These are mostly malignant in nature.

The usual presentation of these tumours is as follows:

(a) Swelling preceding pain
  - The patient presents with swelling which is initially small and increases gradually or rapidly.
  - The speed of growth depends on the nature of the tumour (benign or malignant).
  - Pain is noticed due to either insidious trauma to the swelling or a sudden increase in size.

(b) Pain preceding swelling

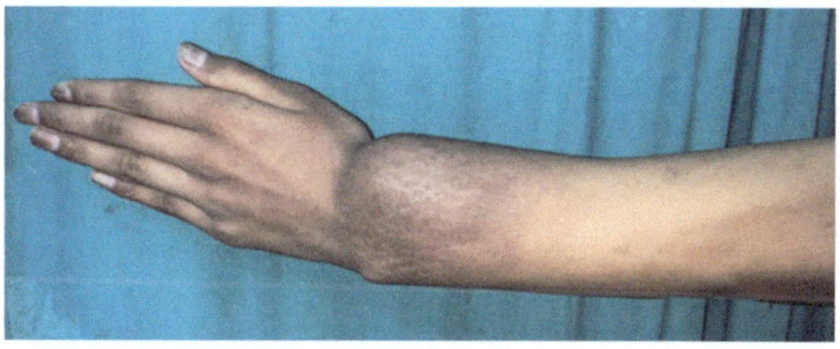

Fig. 57.1 Benign non-aggressive lesion of distal forearm

  - Patient presents with a history of pain which may be dull aching in nature followed by the appearance of swelling in the same area.
  - Pain may be due to the slow weakening of the bone due to primary or metastatic pathology.

(c) Fracture without a history of significant trauma (pathological fracture)
  - Occurs in cases of weakening of bone due to benign cyst in children or due to metastasis in adults where the patient had no symptoms before the insidious trauma and the pathology is only detected once a pathological fracture occurs.

In addition to history, a few determinants are important to reach a diagnosis for bone tumours. Among them, the important ones are as follows:

M. Dhingra (✉) · V. Maheshwari
Department of Orthopedics, All India Institute of Medical Sciences, Rishikesh, Uttarakhand, India

V. Kumar et al. (eds.), *A Quick Guide to Essential Orthopedics*,
https://doi.org/10.1007/978-981-95-2676-5_57

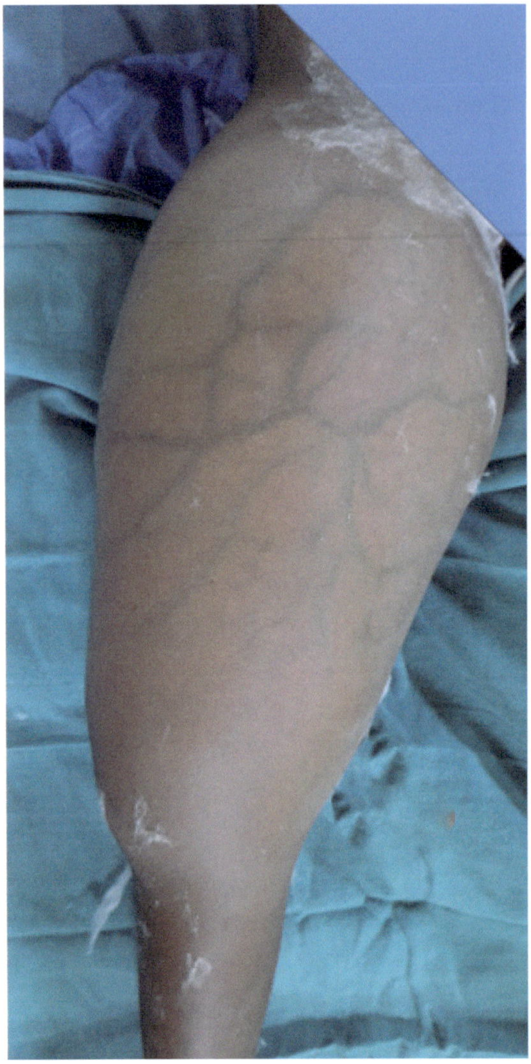

Fig. 57.2 Malignant swelling of thigh with tense shiny skin and dilated veins

(i) *Age of the patient*: Most of the bone tumours follow a particular age pattern with rare exceptions. So, if a child of growing skeleton walks in your out patient department (OPD) with a bony swelling, the most common differential diagnosis which should come is illustrated in Table 57.1.

Table 57.1 Age-wise distribution of tumours

Age	Benign	Malignant
0–10 years	Simple bone cyst Eosinophilic granuloma Aneurysmal bone cyst	Ewing sarcoma Neuroblastoma Langerhans cell histiocytosis (LCH) Haematological malignancy Eosinophilic granuloma
11–20 years	Osteoid osteoma Non-ossifying fibroma Fibrous dysplasia Simple bone cyst Aneurysmal bone cyst Osteochondroma Chondroblastoma Chondromyxoid fibroma	Osteosarcoma Ewing sarcoma
20–40 years	Enchondroma Giant cell tumour Adamantinoma	Chondrosarcoma Parosteal osteosarcoma Fibrosarcoma Pleomorphic sarcoma
>40 years		Metastasis Multiple myeloma Plasmacytoma Chondrosarcoma Osteosarcoma Fibrosarcoma Pleomorphic sarcoma Lymphoma

57.1.1 Clinical Examination

After detailed history, the salient points to be noted in clinical examination are as follows:

1. *Mono-ostotic presentation or polyostotic presentation*: Most of the bone tumours present as mono-ostotic (only in one bone) with the exception of osteochondroma, enchondroma, and fibrous dysplasia in benign tumours and

Table 57.2 Tumour association with particular bones

Bone	Benign	Malignant
Skull	–	Eosinophilic granuloma Myeloma Metastasis
Mandible	Dentogenic cyst	Adamantinoma
Humerus	Simple bone cyst Fibrous dysplasia	Chondrosarcoma Metastasis
Distal radius	Giant cell tumour	Eosinophilic granuloma
Phalanges	Enchondroma	
Ribs	Enchondroma	Metastasis Chondrosarcoma
Spine	Osteoblastoma Aneurysmal bone cyst Haemangioma	Metastasis Myeloma
Pelvis	Simple bone cyst	Chondrosarcoma Ewing sarcoma Lymphoma Multiple myeloma
Proximal femur	Simple bone cyst Fibrous dysplasia	Ewing sarcoma Eosinophilic granuloma
Bones around knee	Giant cell tumour Osteochondroma Aneurysmal bone cyst	Ewing sarcoma Osteosarcoma Synovial sarcoma
Tibia shaft	Osteoid osteoma Fibrous dysplasia Non ossifying fibroma	Adamantinoma
Calcaneum	Simple bone cyst Giant cell tumour	Ewing sarcoma

metastasis in malignant tumours which can present as polyostotic.

2. *Bone involvement*: Most of the bone tumours have a higher tendency to occur in a particular bone. Here is the tabular presentation of the common bones involved in different tumours (Table 57.2 and Fig. 57.3).
3. *Site of bone involvement*: The long bones are divided into three parts namely epiphysis, metaphysis, and diaphysis. Bone tumours have a tendency to involve particular sites of the bone, and the differential diagnosis is based on the site of the bone involved. Fig. 57.4 identifies different sites of the bone involved in cases of various bone tumours.
4. *Clinical examination* of the swelling is then carried out in the following steps:
   (a) Inspection of the swelling depicting its
   - Site—epiphysis, metaphysis, diaphysis, or combination of any two (epiphyseal–metaphyseal)
   - Look
     - Indolent in cases of benign lesion
     - Angry look in cases of malignant lesion
   - Involvement of the nearby joint
   - Involvement of the soft tissues overlying the swelling
   - Presence of any discharge or fungation from the swelling

   (b) Palpation aims at confirming the findings of inspection. In addition to it, the points to be looked are as follows:
   - fixity of the swelling to the underlying bone
   - consistency of the swelling
     - soft
     - firm
     - hard
   - margins of the swelling
   - abnormal mobility in cases of fracture

   (c) Movement of the nearby joint.

   (d) Examination of distal neurovascular status in comparison with opposite limb is important to assess the encasement of neurovascular structures around the swelling.

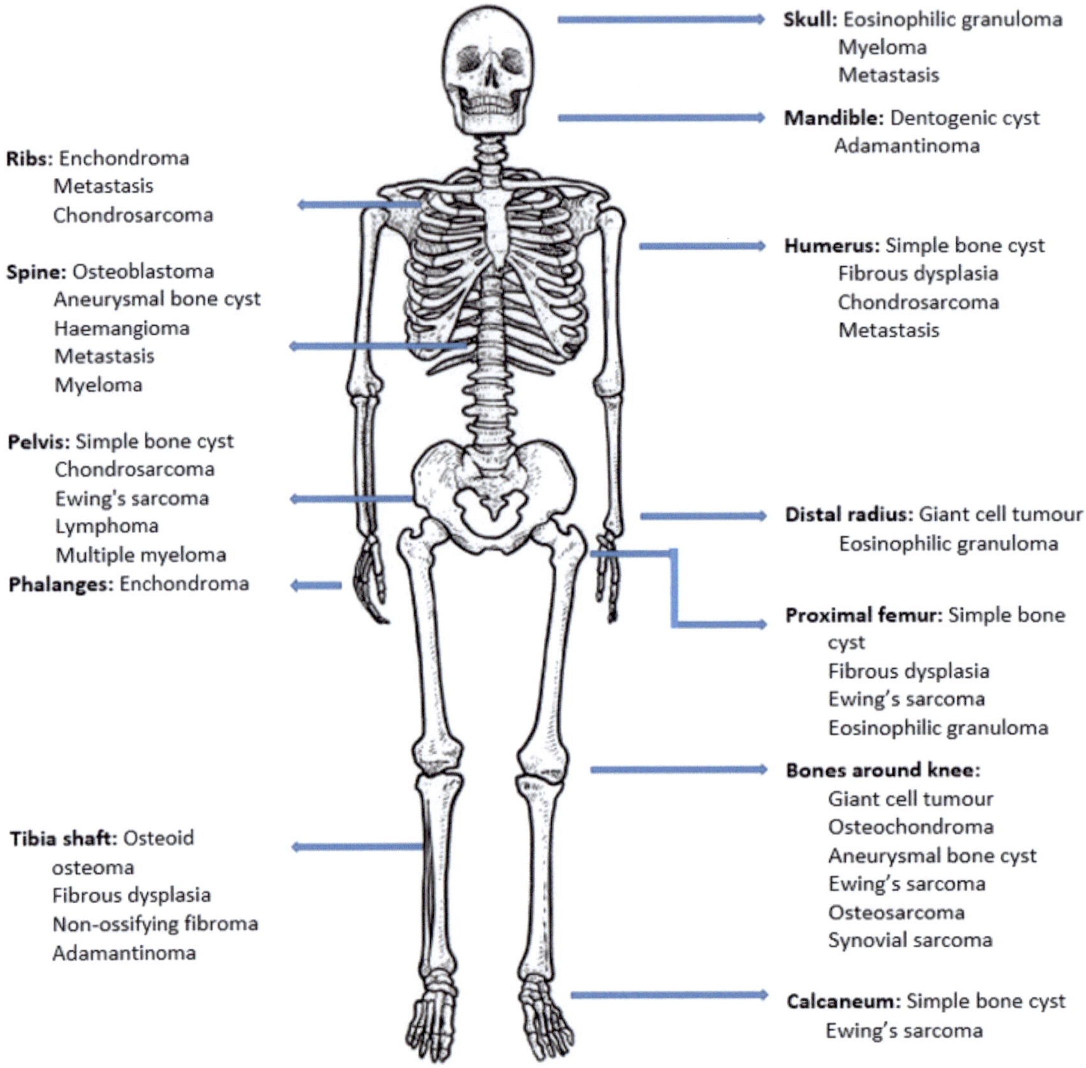

Fig. 57.3 Bone tumours in relation to bone involvement

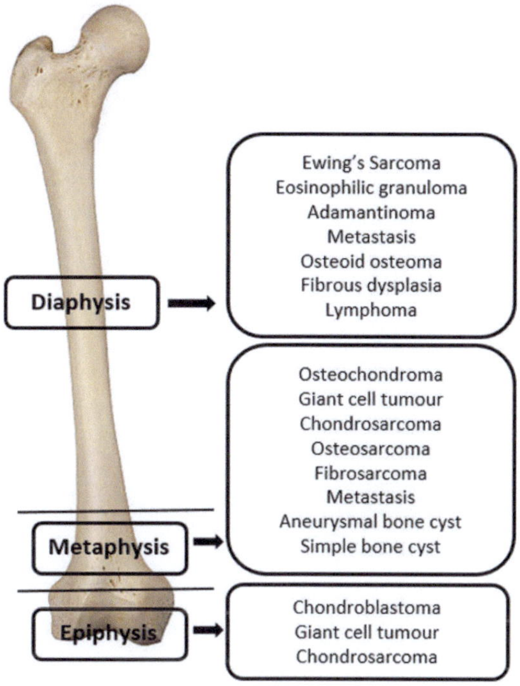

Fig. 57.4 Bone tumours in relation to site of involvement

57.2 Investigations

The history and clinical examination are followed by

(a) *Blood Investigations*

Its role in the diagnosis of bone tumours is of not much importance. Few investigations which may of use are as follows:

- Alkaline phosphatase (ALP) and lactate dehydrogenase (LDH) are the markers of increased bone turnover in primary malignant bone tumours.
- Various other enzymes like prostate-specific antigen (PSA) and alpha-fetoprotein are the markers of solid tumours and raised in metastasis of these solid organs.

(b) *Radiological Examination*

- *Plain radiographs* play an important role in the diagnosis of bone tumours. Ordering a complete orthogonal view is important for reaching a diagnosis. Points to be kept in mind while reading a radiograph which helps to reach an appropriate differential diagnosis consist of the following:
  - The *bone* involved (tubular bones, flat bones, or spine).
  - The *site of bone* involved (epiphysis, metaphysis, or diaphysis) (Fig. 57.5).
  - *Type of bone destruction*: It can be geographic (in cases of benign bone tumours) and moth-eaten or diffuse (in cases of malignant bone tumours) (Fig. 57.6).
  - *Zone of transition* (the intermediate zone between the tumour matrix and the normal bone). In cases of malignant bone disease, there is a wide zone of transition and a narrow zone of transition in cases of benign bone tumours.
  - *Matrix of the tumour*: Discrete calcification is a typical feature of cartilaginous tumours (Fig. 57.7).
  - *Periosteal reaction*: Dense periosteal reaction, which is the response of the body to the tumour in the form of sunray or fusiform appearance in cases of osteosarcoma or Ewing sarcoma, respectively.
- *Magnetic resonance imaging (MRI)*: Role of contrast-enhanced MRI is very crucial to know the actual extent of the tumour. The various additional information gathered from MRI are as follows (Fig. 57.8):
  - Extramedullary extent into the soft tissues around the tumour
  - Intramedullary extent into the diaphysis of the bone
  - Presence of skip lesion (lesion appearing as tumour in the same bone but with normal bone matrix in between)
  - Presence of satellite lesion (presence of tumour tissue in the vicinity of main tumour)

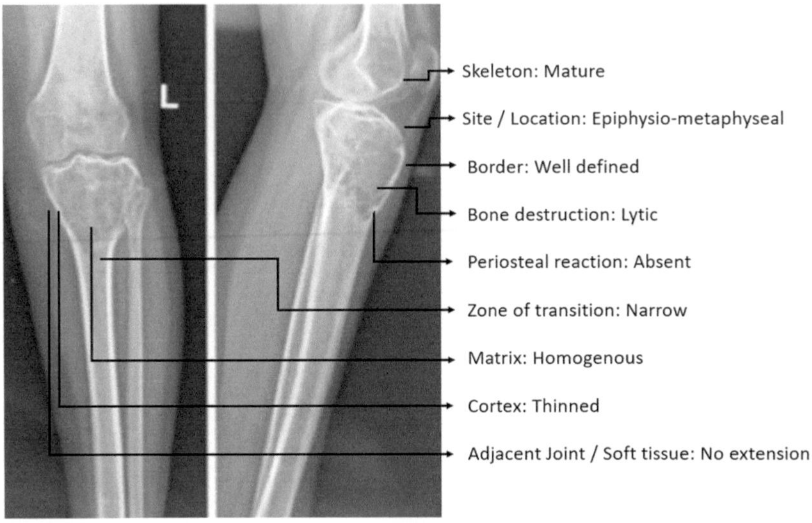

Fig. 57.5 Plain radiograph of benign lytic lesion proximal tibia

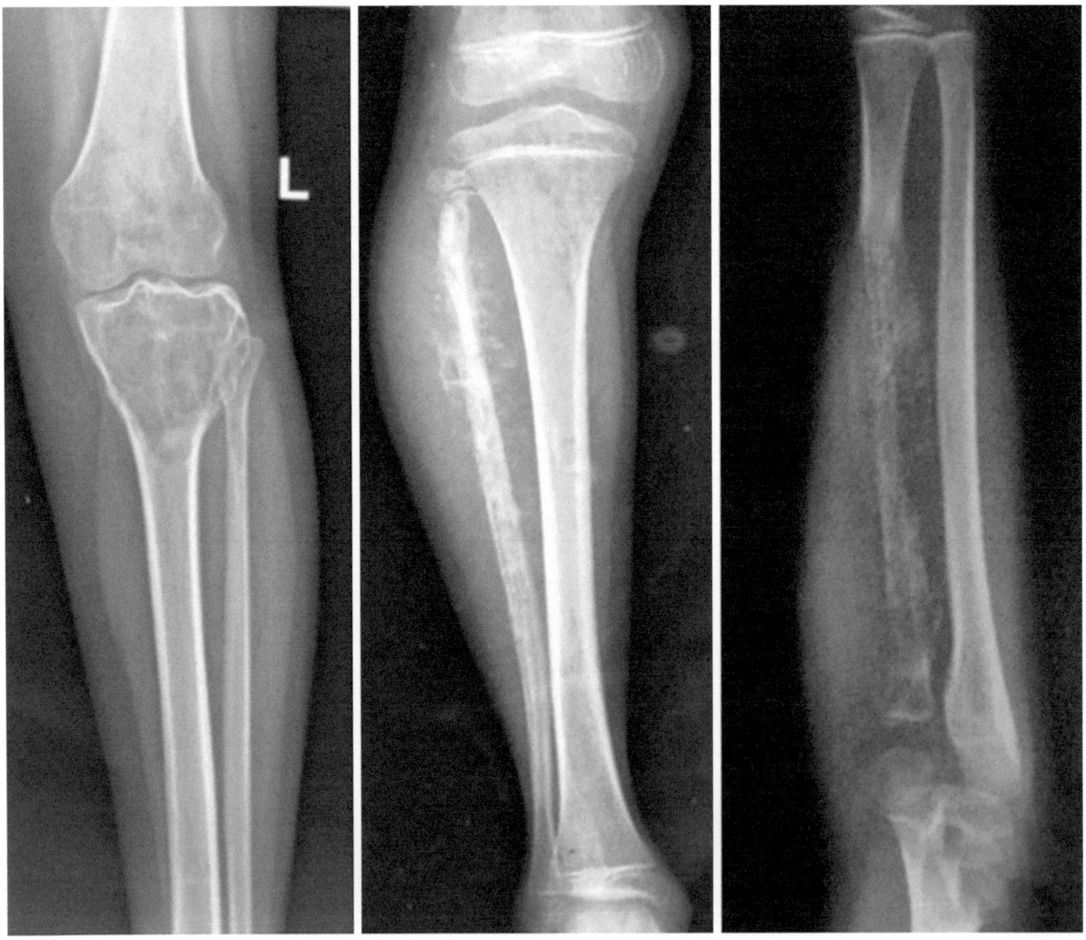

Fig. 57.6 Plain radiograph showing type of bone destruction

   – Involvement of important neurovascular structures in and around tumour
   – Pick up early changes which might not appear in X-ray
- *Computed tomography (CT) scan*: It is an important investigation in cases of (Fig. 57.9)
   – Osteoid osteoma to identify the nidus.
   – Various tumours to identify the true bony margins of the leftover bone after destruction.

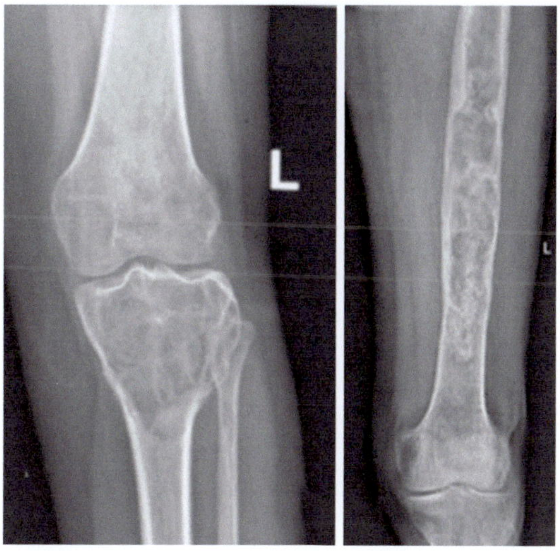

Fig. 57.7 Plain radiograph showing type of matrix

   – Can be added with angiography of vascular structures to help in identifying the true anatomical relationship of the main vessel to the tumour.
   – It is also important to identify the visceral metastasis in chest and abdomen in cases of primary malignant bone tumours.
- *Bone scan*: Functional scan done with the use of radioactive material (technetium 99) to identify the metabolic activity in all the bones of the body in one go. It can pick up very early metastasis of bone of malignant tumours of bone and other visceral organs (Fig. 57.10).

(c) *Histopathological Examination*
- *Fine-needle aspiration cytology (FNAC)*: Needle aspiration has not much role to play in musculoskeletal tumours except in cases of soft tissue sarcoma where it can be of some value.
- *Biopsy*: It is the most essential investigation to reach to final diagnosis and is done after all local investigations particular to the tumour. It is of three types.
   – *Incisional*, where part of the tumour is removed and sent for examination

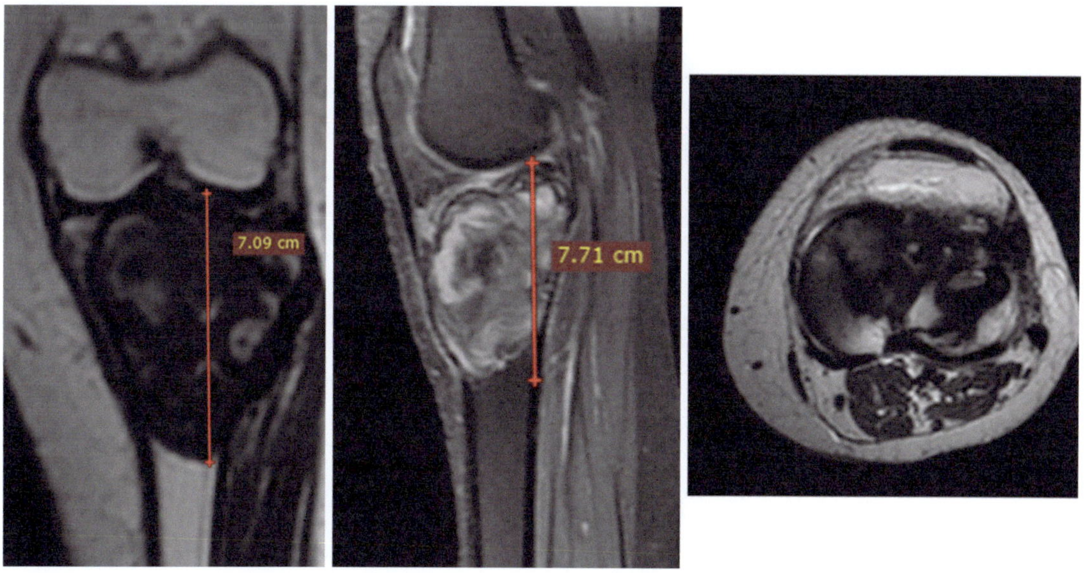

Fig. 57.8 MRI of proximal tibia of the same patient whose plain radiograph is shown in Fig. 57.5, showing the dimension of the lesion, soft tissue extension, and sparing of neurovascular bundle

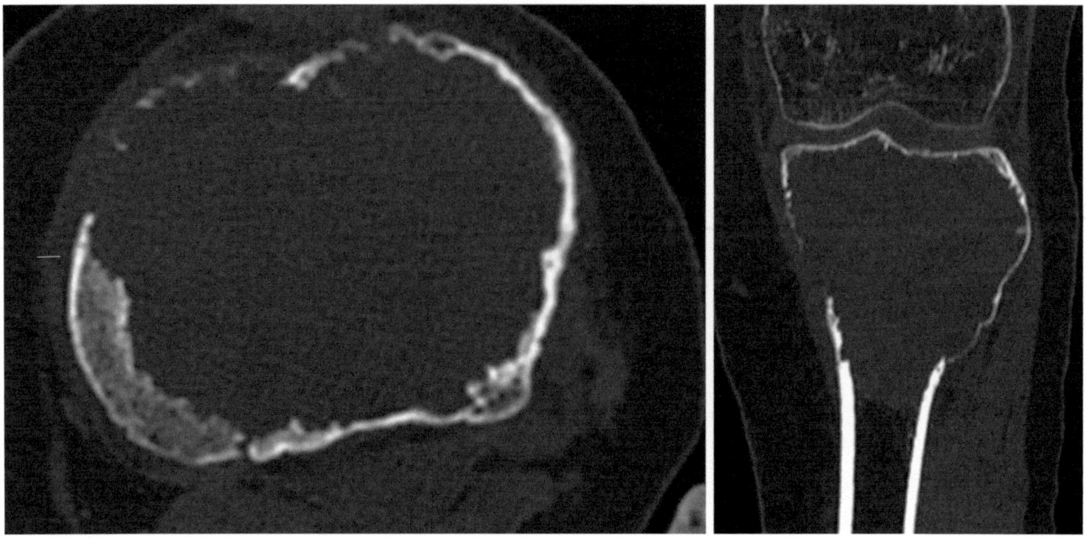

Fig. 57.9 Non contrast computerized tomography (NCCT) of proximal tibia showing the dimension of the lesion and cortical breach of medial border without calcification

- *Excisional*, where the whole tumour along with surrounding reactive zone is removed and sent for diagnosis
- *Core biopsy*: It is the most commonly used method in present times. Three to four good cores are taken with the help of sheathed tubes like Jamshidi needles and sent for histological diagnosis (Fig. 57.11).

Biopsy should be done with certain guidelines:

(a) Biopsy should be done by the surgeon who plans to do final surgery.
(b) The incision should be always in line with the incision of final surgery planned.
(c) Biopsy should be done through one single compartment.
(d) Biopsy should be done through the shortest possible route in order to minimize contamination with the tumour cells.
(e) Hemostasis should be achieved in order to avoid any infection resulting from hematoma formation.

The algorithm shown here will guide to reach a final diagnosis and classify these tumours. The primary aim is to classify them into

- Benign
- Malignant

Then, they are further classified by Enneking classification which will be covered in detail in chapter on classification of bone tumours. The summary of classification is given as follows:

1. *Benign tumours*
   - *Latent*: Tumours with well-defined margins. They grow or may not grow but overall the growth is slow.
   - *Active*: They too have well-defined margins, but the thinning of margins is seen at places. The tumour still remains intracapsular.
   - *Aggressive*: Margins may show breakage of cortex at places with diffuse local spread outside the bone barriers. Sometimes, it may show distant metastasis as well.
2. *Malignant bone tumours*
   - *Grade IA*: low-grade tumours which are intra-compartmental (histologically low grade-sarcoma limited to the bone)
   - *Grade IB*: low-grade sarcoma which has gone extra-compartmental (histologically low-grade sarcoma going outside the bony compartment)

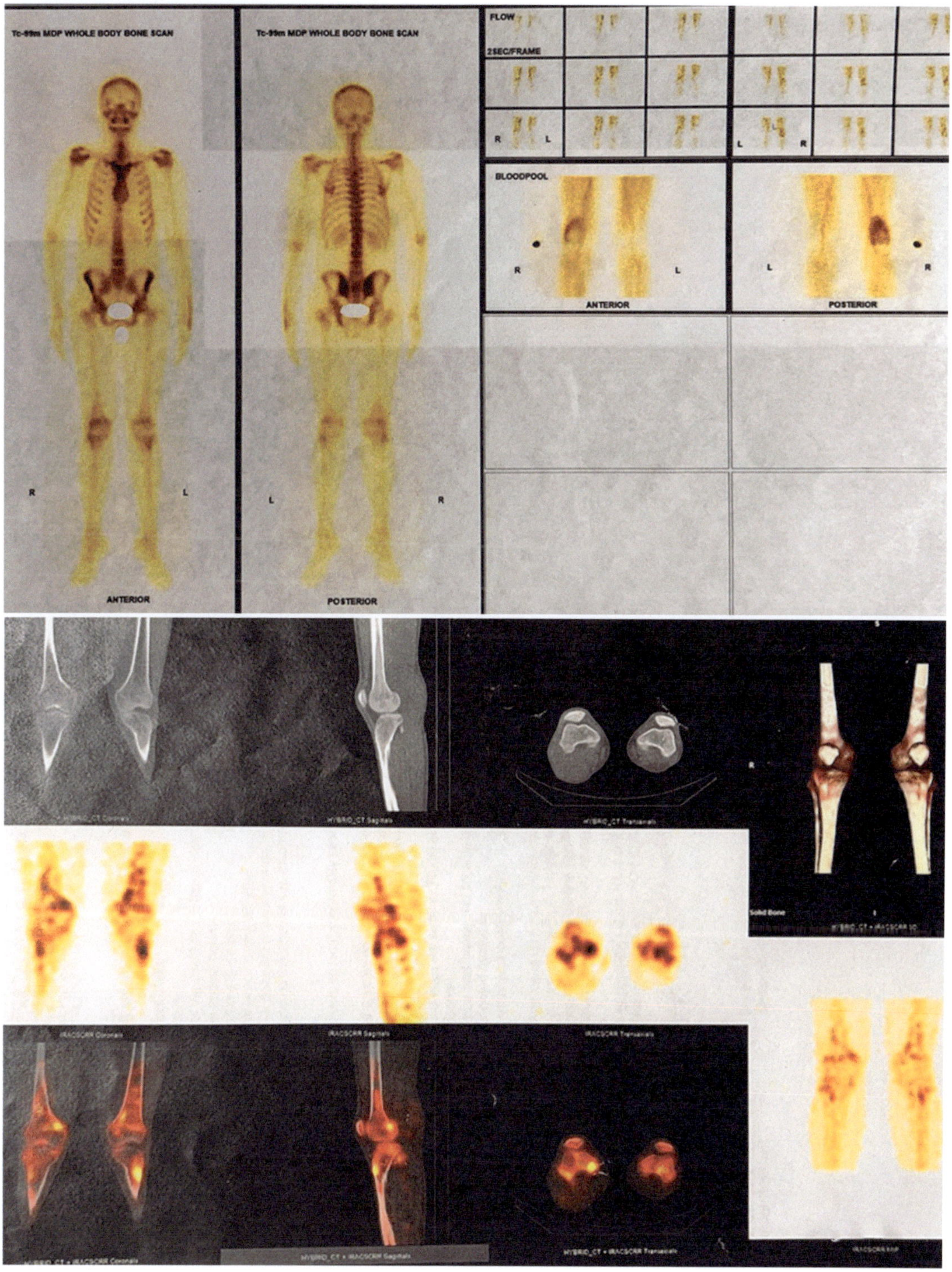

Fig. 57.10 Bone scan with increased uptake around the knee

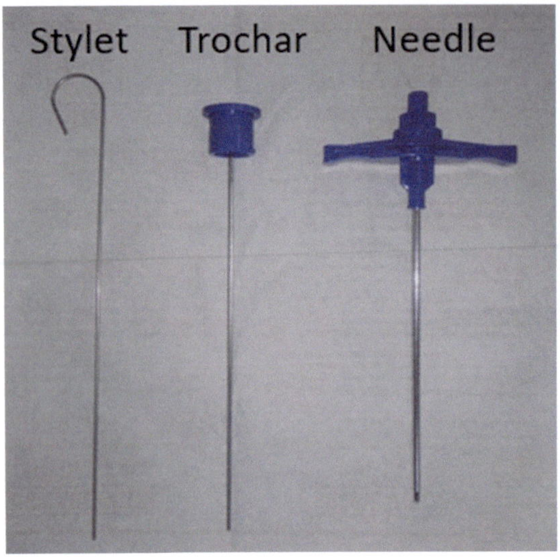

Fig. 57.11 Parts of core biopsy needle

- *Grade IIA*: high-grade sarcoma which are intra-compartmental (histologically high-grade sarcoma limited to the bone)
- *Grade IIB*: high-grade sarcoma which has gone extra-compartmental (histologically high-grade sarcoma going outside the bony compartment)
- *Grade III*: sarcoma of any histological grade and involving one of multiple compartments will be graded as III if visceral or bony metastasis is found in CT or bone scan.

The approach described helps us to reach a final diagnosis of the type of tumour we are dealing with and management is planned accordingly.

Multiple Choice Questions

1. An 11-year-old male with isolated proximal tibia osteosarcoma that extends to soft tissue with high-grade lesion on biopsy without metastasis. What is stage as per musculoskeletal tumour society (MSTS) (Enneking staging)?
   (a) IA
   (b) IIA
   (c) IB
   (d) IIB
2. When performing an open incisional biopsy, which of the following principles do not apply?
   (a) Should be done by the surgeon who plans to do final surgery
   (b) The incision should be always in line with the incision of final surgery planned
   (c) Should be done via intra-compartmental plane
   (d) Should be done through one single compartment
3. In a 15-year-old girl with right groin pain, X-ray shows lytic lesion in proximal femur. What should be the next step in treatment?
   (a) Wait and watch
   (b) Surgery
   (c) MRI of bone
   (d) Biopsy of lesion
4. In a 12-year-old boy with right thigh pain, X-ray shows permeative lesion of shat of femur with onion peel periosteal reaction and MRI shows lesion-involving shaft of femur without any skip lesion and large soft tissue component. What should be the next step in treatment?
   (a) Wait and watch
   (b) Surgery
   (c) Exercise
   (d) Biopsy of lesion

5. In a 25-year-old male with left knee pain with plain radiograph shown below, what is the most likely classification according to Enneking grading?

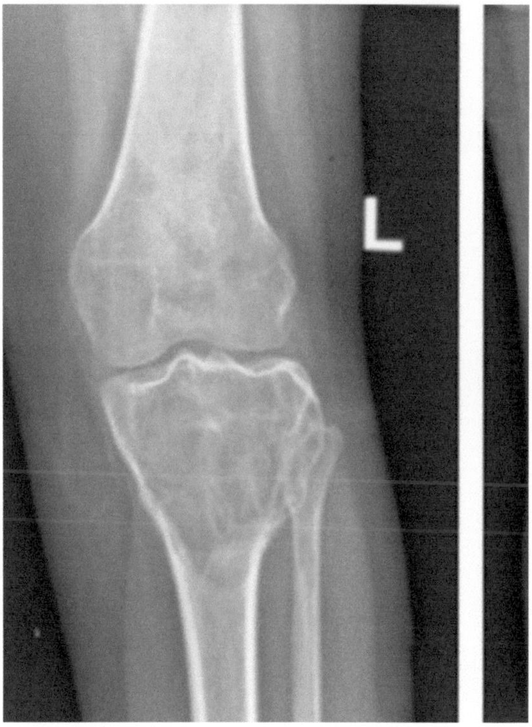

(a) Benign latent
(b) Benign aggressive
(c) Malignant
(d) None of the above

Answers: 1. (d), 2. (c), 3. (c), 4. (d), 5. (b)

Benign Bone Tumors

58

Mohit Dhingra, Vikas Maheshwari,
and Hawaibam Nongdmaba

58.1 Dedicated to 'Naina'Introduction

Bone tumours as already discussed can be benign or malignant in nature. The benign nature is defined by the indolent nature in terms of aggressiveness and typical features radiologically where they are differentiated on the basis of

- Well-circumscribed lesion
- No or minimal periosteal reaction
- Narrow zone of transition
- No or minimal evidence of aggression in the surrounding soft tissues (Fig. 58.1)

Benign bone tumours can be further differentiated into

- Benign bone tumours
  - Osteoma
  - Osteoid osteoma
  - Giant cell tumour (GCT)
  - Other uncommon tumours like
    - Osteoblastoma
    - Chondroblastoma
    - Haemangioma
- Tumour-like conditions

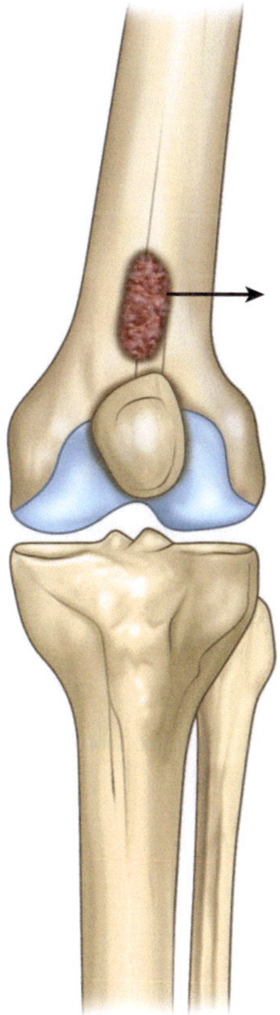

Fig. 58.1 A diagrammatic representation of well-circumscribed lesion with narrow zone of transition

M. Dhingra (✉) · V. Maheshwari · H. Nongdmaba
Department of Orthopedics, All India Institute of Medical Sciences, Rishikesh, Uttarakhand, India

V. Kumar et al. (eds.), *A Quick Guide to Essential Orthopedics*,
https://doi.org/10.1007/978-981-95-2676-5_58

- Osteochondroma
- Enchondroma
- Simple bone cyst
- Aneurysmal bone cyst (ABC)
- Fibrous dysplasia (FD)

58.2 Osteoma

58.2.1 Introduction

It presents as a swelling of flat bones of the skull or face and is composed of well-defined bone. The swelling is sclerotic in morphology and protrudes outside the boundaries of the bones. Normally, it does not need any treatment unless it grows into the sinus cavities of skull producing obstructive symptoms.

58.2.2 Treatment

Generally, no treatment is required unless done for cosmetic purposes or obstruction of sinuses. Simple excision is done in most of cases.

58.3 Osteoid Osteoma

58.3.1 Introduction

It is the most common true benign bone tumour. It most commonly affects in the age group of 5–25 years and involves the diaphysis of the long bones. The size is not more than 1.5 cm and consists of central nidus, an aggregate of mineralized osteoblasts surrounded by dense sclerotic bone.

58.3.2 Clinical Presentation

- Affects diaphysis of long bones
- Nagging dull aching pain worst at night and relieved by salicylates.
- Minimal or no clinical signs except tenderness at the site or swelling if the lesion is superficial.

58.3.3 Diagnosis

It is generally confirmed on X-ray. The lesion appears to be less than 1.5 cm with dense sclerotic margins. Computed tomography (CT) scan is also helpful for delineating the pathology effectively (Fig. 58.2).

58.3.4 Histology

Histologically, it consists of small yellowish-to-red nidus of osteoid and woven bone with interconnected trabeculae and a background of highly vascularized fibrous connective tissue. Various degree of sclerosis may be present around the tissue (Fig. 58.3).

58.3.5 Treatment

Radiofrequency ablation (RFA) is the treatment of choice nowadays wherever feasible (Fig. 58.4). It is a less invasive procedure where the probe is introduced into the tumour through the cannulated system and the tumour is burnt with the

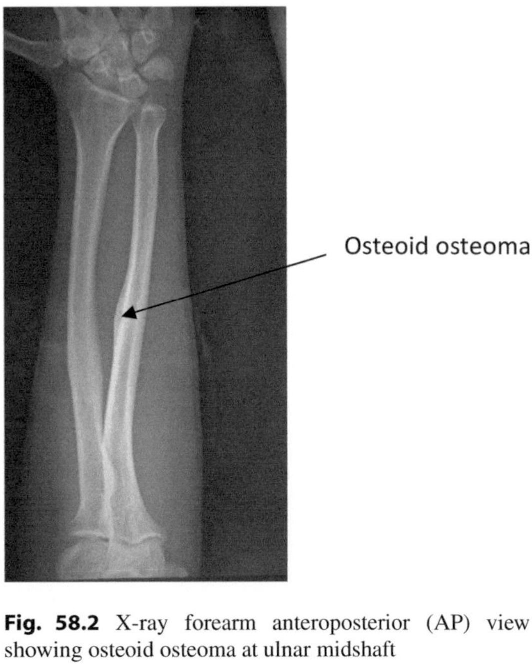

Fig. 58.2 X-ray forearm anteroposterior (AP) view showing osteoid osteoma at ulnar midshaft

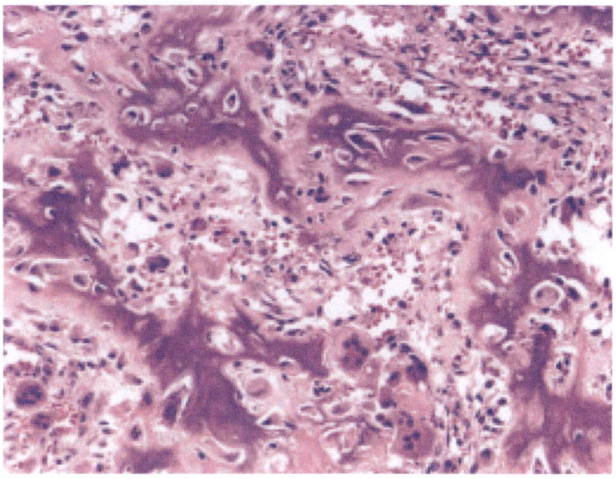

Fig. 58.3 Histological picture of osteoid osteoma showing mature osteoblast in the centre surrounded by fibrous tissue

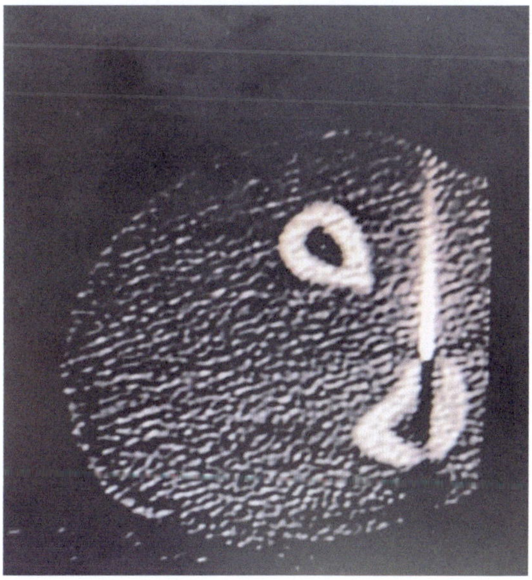

Fig. 58.4 Introduction of RFA probe in the ulna of the same patient as shown in Fig. 58.2

application of heat. Other treatment includes nonsteroidal anti-inflammatory drugs (NSAIDs) if conservative treatment is chosen. Local curettage/resection of the nidus is also carried out in cases of failed RFA or unavailability of the modality.

58.4 Giant Cell Tumour

58.4.1 Introduction

Giant cell tumour also known as osteoclastoma (as it has abundant osteoclastic cells) is one of the most common benign bone tumours that exhibit local aggressiveness and high rate of recurrence. It accounts for 4–5% of all primary bone neoplasm and around 20% of all benign bone tumours. Metastasis is rare (1–5%) and is seen mostly in the lungs.

58.4.2 Anatomic Location

Giant cell tumours (GCTs) are usually found in an eccentric position at the end of long bones. Epiphysis is primarily affected but may involve metaphysis as well. The most commonly affected bones include the following:

- Distal femur and proximal tibia: 50–65%
- Distal radius: 10–12%
- Proximal humerus: 4–8%
- Sacrum: 4–9%
- Vertebral bodies: 3–6% (most commonly thoracic spine, followed by cervical and lumbar spines)

Less frequently, GCTs may occur in other locations such as hands and feet, as well as the innominate bones of the pelvis.

58.4.3 Pathophysiology

The destruction of bone in giant cell tumour is due to the activation of osteoclastic cells via cathepsin K and matrix metalloproteinase pathway as shown in Fig. 58.5.

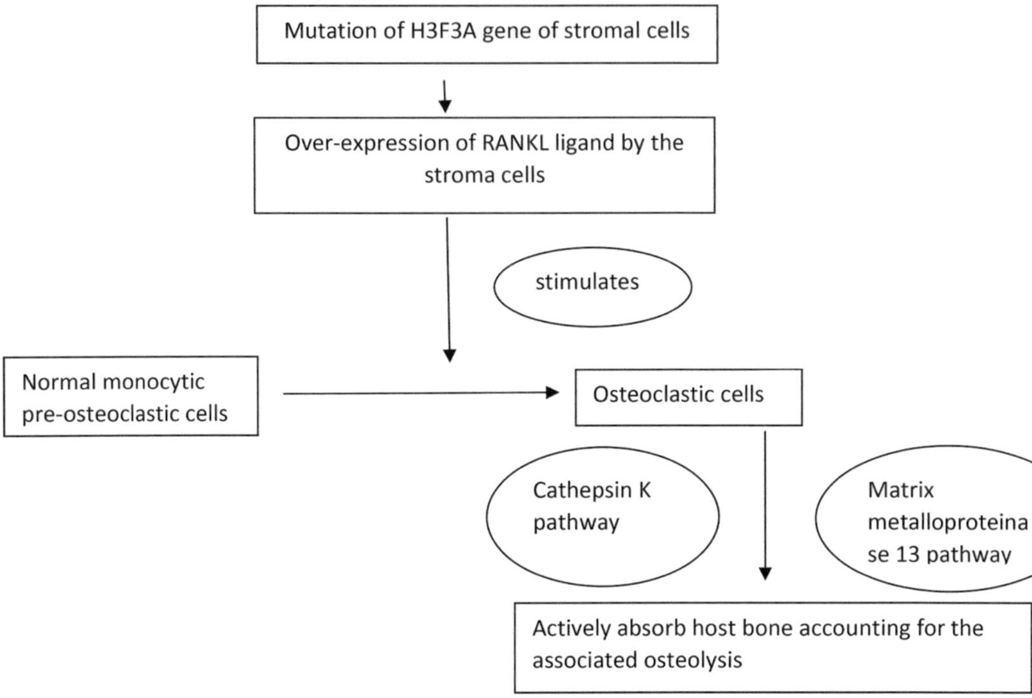

Fig. 58.5 The pathogenesis of destruction of bone in giant cell tumour

58.4.4 Clinical Features

- Pain: Pain is the most common presenting symptom which is caused by mechanical insufficiency due to the destruction of bone. It is insidious in onset, mostly dull aching in nature, and aggravates with activity.
- Swelling: Swelling is firm to hard in consistency, fixed to the underlying bone, and tender to touch.
- Decrease range of movement of the joint: Due to the involvement of the juxta-articular area, joint movement may be affected remarkably.
- Pathological fracture: Pathological fractures are present in approximately 12% of patients at the time of diagnosis and signify aggressive disease.

58.4.5 Evaluation

- *X-ray:* The common features in the X-ray includes the following (Fig. 58.6):
  - Eccentric expansile lytic lesion (soap bubble appearance)
  - Involvement of epiphysis
  - Cortical thinning or cortical breakthrough
  - Narrow zone of transition (benign in nature)
  - No surrounding sclerosis (unless treated by drugs such as denosumab)
  - No mineralization of matrix
  - Pathological fracture may be present
  - Minimal periosteal reaction
- *CT scan:* Although magnetic resonance imaging (MRI) is a better modality for further characterizing the tumour, CT scan may be helpful in few cases to characterize the cortical margins or indolent pathological fractures. Matrix mineralization may also be seen better in CT scan.
- *MRI:* Useful tool in evaluating the following(Fig. 58.7):

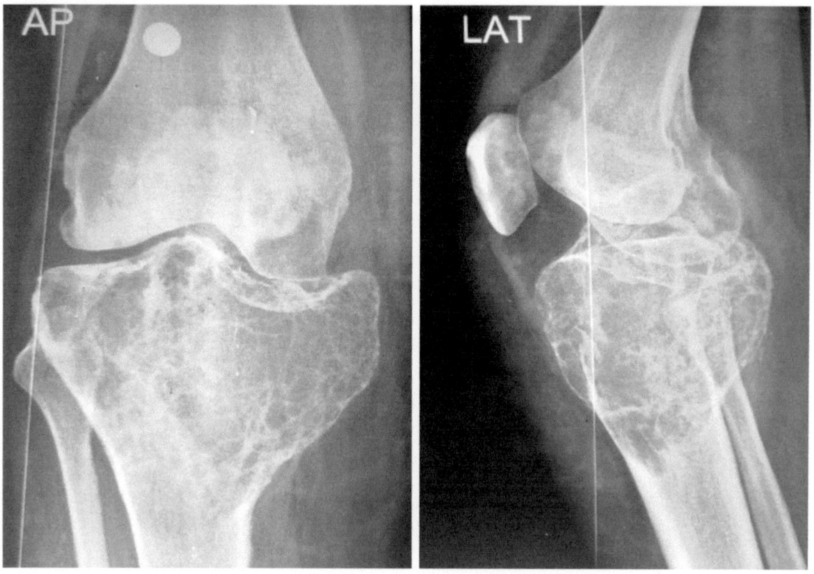

Fig. 58.6 X-ray knee AP and lateral view showing eccentric, lytic lesion in the epiphyseo-metaphyseal region, with thinning of cortex with narrow zone of transition s/o GCT proximal tibia

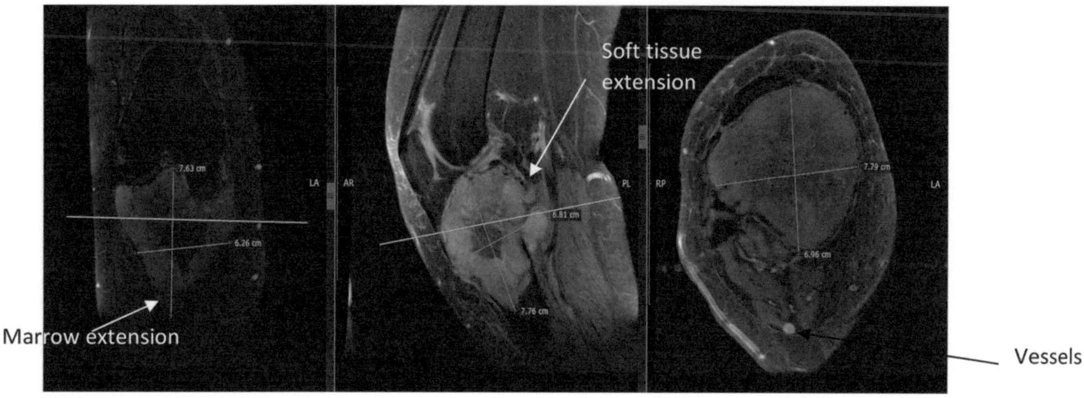

Fig. 58.7 T2 weighted MRI of the X-ray as shown in Fig. 58.6 showing heterogenous intensity lesion with soft tissue extension

- Soft tissue extension
- Subchondral extension into adjacent joints
- Neurovascular structure involvement
- Intramedullary extensions of the tumour

58.4.6 Histopathology

Gross Features

- Yellow to chocolate brown in colour due to presence of hemosiderin
- Soft, spongy, and fragile
- Cystic blood-filled cavity can be seen
- Cortical expansion/breech with intact periosteum (Fig. 58.8)

Microscopic Features

Reveals numerous osteoclastic giant cells, as well as a smaller number of neoplastic mononuclear cells without atypia (Fig. 58.9)

There are three types of cells present histologically

- Type I: These are stromal cells that are spindle in shape and resemble interstitial fibroblast. It has features of mesenchymal stem cells.
- Type II: These are precursors of giant cells. These cells are from the monocyte/ macrophage family recruited from peripheral blood.
- Type III: These are hallmark of this lesion constitute giant cells with multiple nuclei.

58.4.7 Differential Diagnosis

- Brown tumour
- Aneurysmal bone cyst
- Telangiectatic osteosarcoma
- Giant cell-rich osteosarcoma
- Chondromyxoid fibroma
- Chondroblastoma

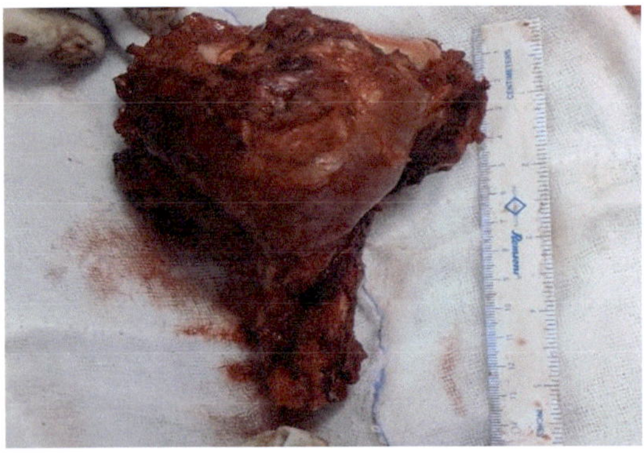

Fig. 58.8 Gross specimen of GCT proximal tibia showing cystic blood-filled cavity with soft, spongy, and fragile capsule

58.4.8 Treatment

58.4.8.1 Non-operative

Medical management: It consists of

- Denosumab, monoclonal antibody, acts by binding to receptor activator of nuclear factor kappa ligand (RANKL) and preventing osteoclastic effect.
- Bisphosphonates induce apoptosis of osteoclast-like giant cell.
- Interferons inhibit vascular endothelial factor and thus decrease the vascularity and size of the tumour.

Overall, these drugs when given before the surgery as neoadjuvant act to limit tumour progression, lower recurrence rate, and decrease micro-metastasis.

58.4.8.2 Operative (Figs. 58.10 and 58.11)

There are various surgical procedures done:

- Extended curettage and bone grafting/ cementing
- Wide resection of tumour and reconstruction with megaprosthesis/allograft

58.4.9 Radiotherapy

Radiation therapy is recommended for inoperable (sacral tumours) or multiple recurrent GCTs.

Fig. 58.9 Image showing histopathology slide of GCT

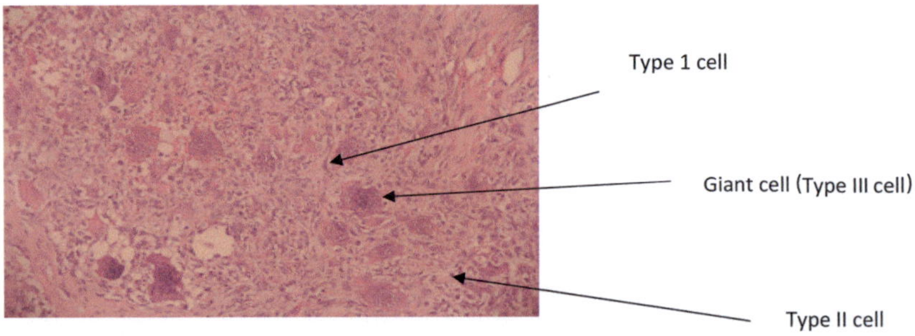

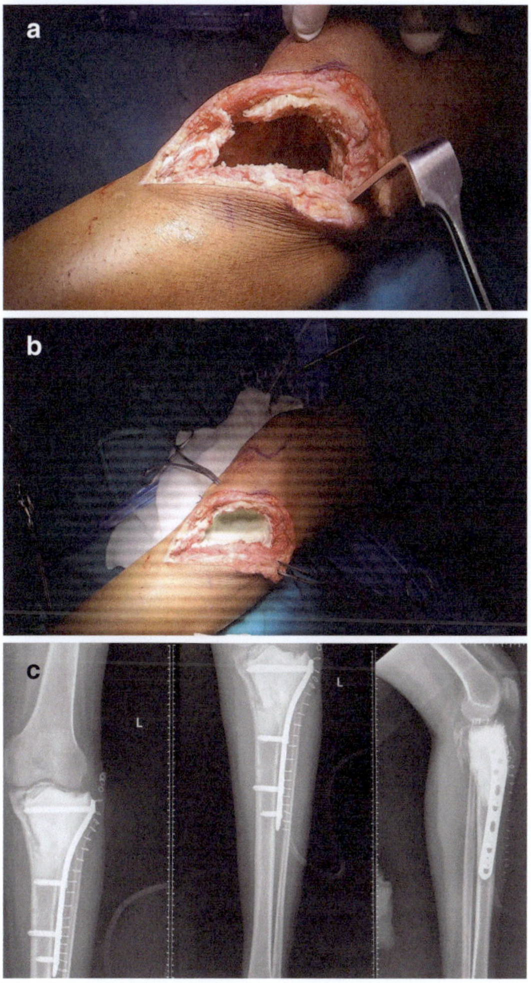

Fig. 58.10 (a–c) Extended curettage of the proximal tibia and filling of defect with bone cement and post-operative radiograph

It results in relief of pain and tumour shrinkage and local control of tumour. It is also associated with malignant transformation in 15% of the cases.

58.4.10 Complications of GCT

- Recurrence
- Secondary ABC
- Pathological fractures
- Malignant transformation to high-grade sarcoma

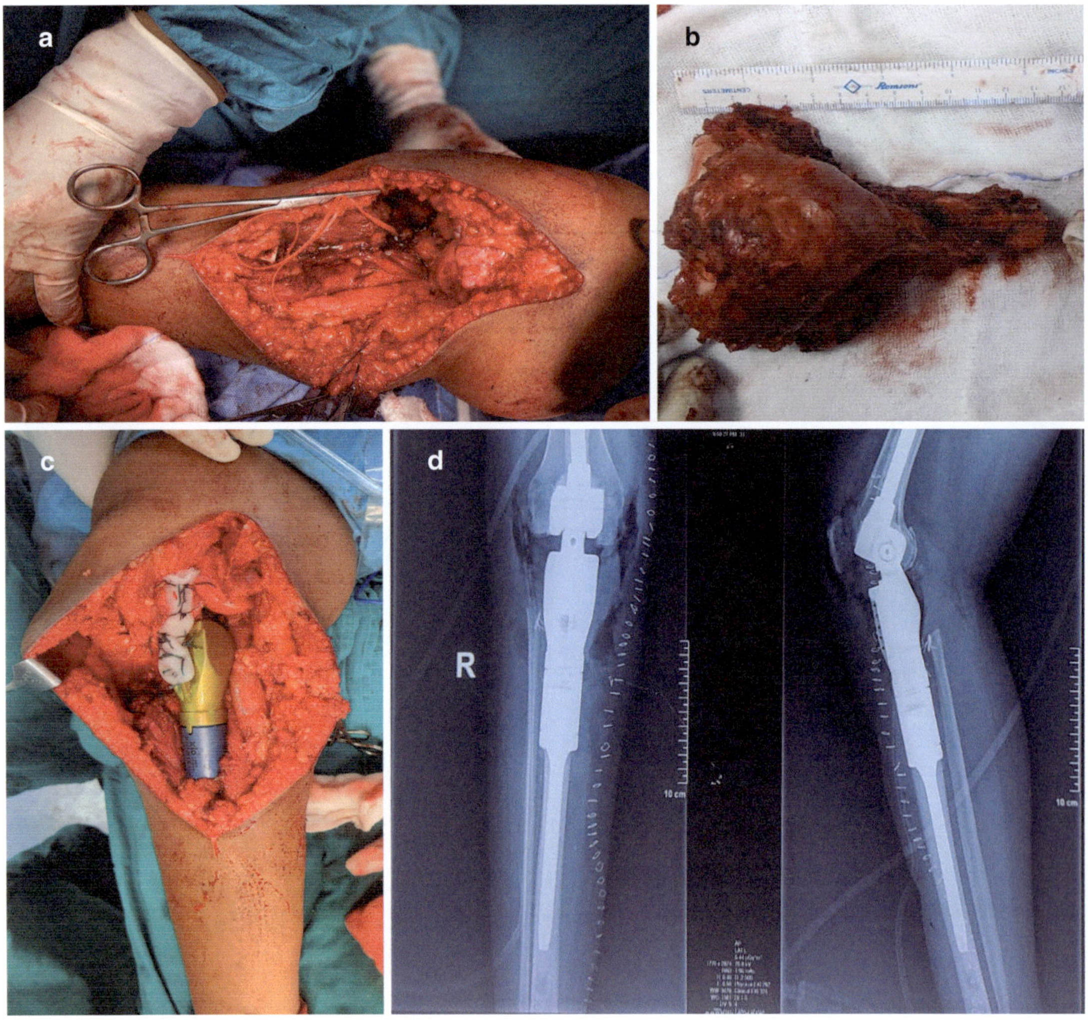

Fig. 58.11 (**a–d**) Resection of proximal tibia and reconstruction with megaprosthesis

58.5 Simple Bone Cyst (Unicameral Bone Cyst)

58.5.1 Introduction

Unicameral bone cysts (UBCs) are true cysts with unknown origins. Unicameral bone cysts (UBCs), also known as simple or solitary bone cysts, were first described by Virchow in 1891 as 'cystic structures' believed to be caused by abnormalities in local circulation. These cysts can occasionally have multiple compartments. They are characterized by benign cavities filled with fluid that gradually enlarge, leading to bone thinning. Typically, UBCs are found in the metaphyseal regions of long bones with open growth plates.

58.5.2 Epidemiology

Approximately 85% of UBCs are observed in children and adolescents. The peak incidence occurs between the ages of 3 and 14 years. The mean age at diagnosis is approximately 9 years and is more common in boys.

58.5.3 Site

Unicameral bone cysts (UBCs) can be found in various bones throughout the body, but the majority (over 95%) occur in long bones. Among these cases, the proximal humerus and femur are the most commonly affected, accounting for nearly 90% of UBCs. In the proximal humerus, where most of the bone's growth takes place, UBCs tend to be more prevalent and often resolve after puberty.

58.5.4 Clinical feature

Pathologic fractures and incidental findings are the most common ways they are presented. The majority (80%) of UBC patients do not experience any symptoms unless a pathologic gross fracture or undisplaced stress fracture occurs. In cases without a history of trauma, symptoms may include mild pain, local tenderness, and occasional swelling.

58.5.5 Evaluation

- *Radiographs* of UBCs show radiolucent central metaphyseal lesions with mild expansion and a narrow zone of transition. UBCs tend to abut growth plates and move away with skeletal growth. Approximately 5% of lesions show a 'fallen leaf' sign where a fracture fragment falls to the dependent portion of the lesion.
- *CT scans* are useful for identifying loculations and pathologic fractures, while *MRI* shows low T1 and high T2 signal with rim enhancement typical of a cyst (Fig. 58.12).

58.5.6 Histology

UBCs consist of a single layer of mesothelial cells comprising the cyst wall and pressurized serous fluid. Osteoid may be observed in cases of pathologic fracture.

58.5.7 Treatment

They tend to elongate with skeletal growth and spontaneously fill in at maturity, making conservative observation an option for most cases with pathologic fractures.

Treatment in the form of intervention may be considered for patients with large lesions at a young age or multiple fractures. Aspiration of the brown fluid for cytologic diagnosis followed by injection of various substances (e.g. steroids, bone marrow aspirate, demineralized bone matrix, and polidocanol) can be attempted to stimulate healing and spontaneous filling. Multiple injections are often required.

Curettage and grafting with or without internal fixation are performed in older children and adolescents.

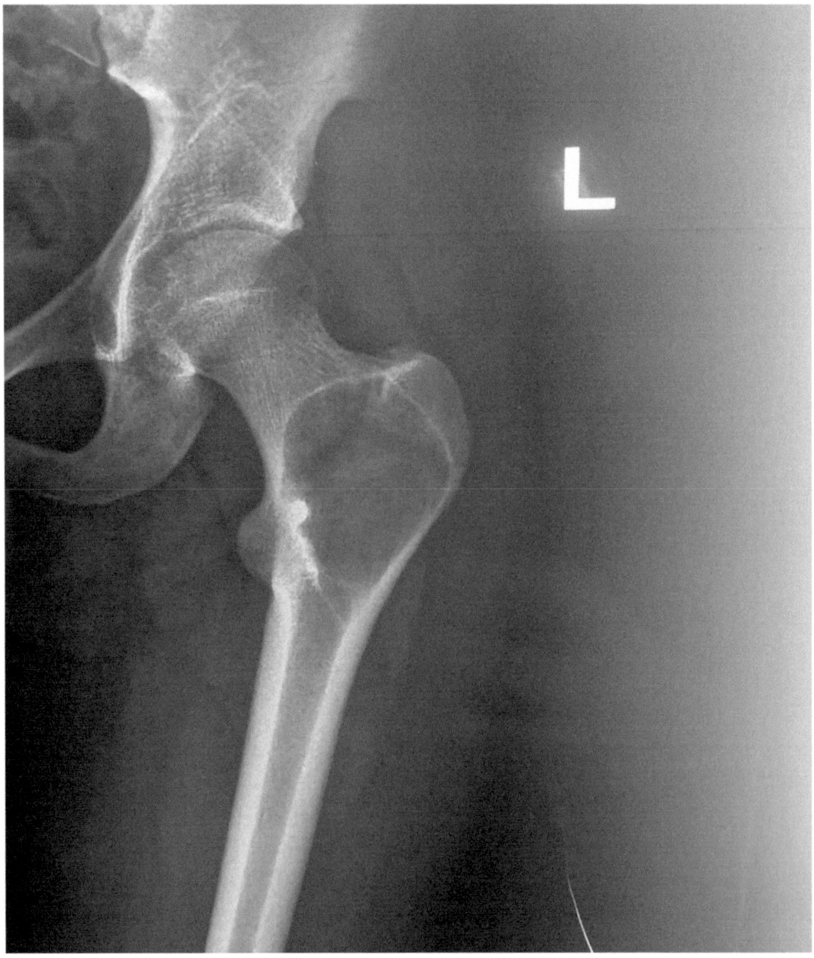

Fig. 58.12 A well-circumscribed lesion in the metaphysis of proximal femur s/o simple bone cyst

58.6 Osteochondroma

58.6.1 Introduction

Osteochondroma is the most common benign bony tumour, accounting for approximately 20–50% of all benign bony tumours and 10–15% of all bony tumours. They are surface bone lesions composed of both cortical and medullary bone with hyaline cartilage caps. They can occur as solitary or in multiple forms (Fig. 58.13).

58.6.2 Epidemiology

- Osteochondromas are commonly discovered in childhood, with 75–80% of cases diagnosed before the age of 20.
- The hereditary form of osteochondroma follows an autosomal dominant inheritance pattern with incomplete penetrance in females.
- Hereditary multiple exostoses (HME) patients are more likely to experience symptoms and

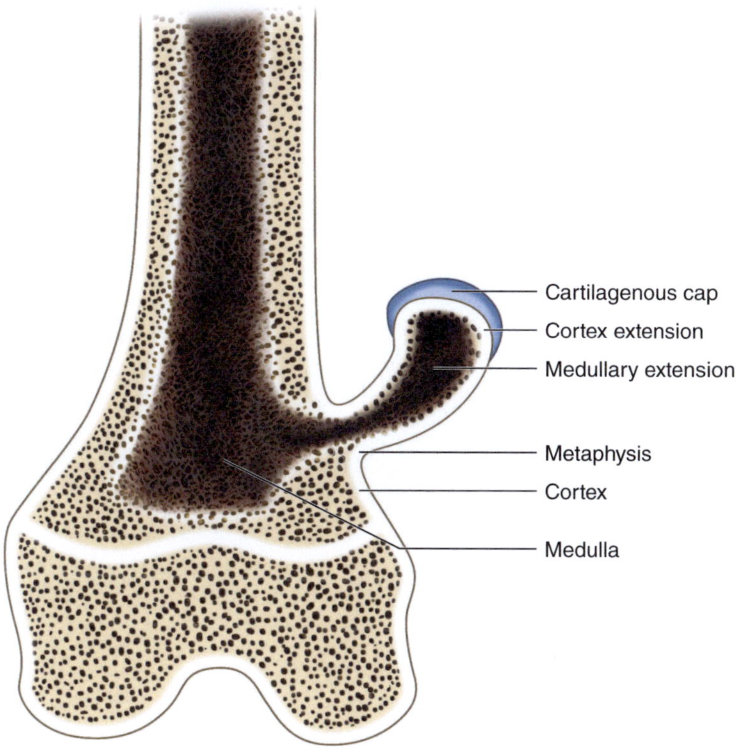

Fig. 58.13 Parts of pedunculated osteochondroma of distal femur

have a more severe presentation, often at a younger age.

- Osteochondromas can develop in any bone that undergoes enchondral ossification.
- Site: Majority of cases (50%) involve long bones, with a higher prevalence in the lower extremities compared to the upper, most commonly around the knee.

58.6.3 Aetiology

Solitary Osteochondroma The proposed hypothesis is that when a fragment of the growth plate separates and protrudes through the periosteum and continues to grow, result in the formation of an osteochondroma either spontaneously, known as primary osteochondroma, or as a secondary osteochondroma due to factors like irradiation, surgery, or fractures.

Hereditary Multiple Exostoses This condition is inherited in an autosomal dominant manner, with a penetrance of 96% in females and 100% in males. Mutations in the EXT1, EXT2, and EXT3 genes, which are tumour suppressor genes, result in decreased heparin sulphate production by chondrocytes at the physis. Individuals with the EXT1 mutation tend to have a more severe presentation compared to those with the EXT2 mutation.

58.6.4 Clinical Features

- Osteochondroma is a bone lesion with a lobulated, cauliflower-like appearance.
- It can be sessile or pedunculated, arising from the bone surface. In children, a cartilage cap thickness of 1–3 cm is normal due to ongoing

growth, while in adults, a cap thickness exceeding 2 cm may indicate malignancy.
- Solitary osteochondromas are typically asymptomatic and are often incidentally discovered on radiographs taken for unrelated reasons.
- However, if symptoms are present, they may be due to various complications such as fracture, malignant transformation, compression of nearby neurovascular structures, bursitis, or the presence of a palpable mass.
- In individuals with hereditary multiple exostoses (HME), the condition is generally more severe, and patients tend to present at a younger age with multiple skeletal abnormalities, including limb bowing, short stature, leg length discrepancy, and deviations such as coxa valgus or genu valgus.

58.6.5 Evaluation

- *X-ray:* Osteochondromas can be sessile or pedunculated lesions found on the bone surface with merged cortex and medulla of parent bone, pointing away from the joint.
- *MRI*: Most effective imaging method for detecting bone or adjacent soft tissue oedema and visualizing nearby neurovascular structures, for evaluating cartilage thickness, and to assess potential malignant transformation (thickness exceeding 2 cm after skeletal maturity raises suspicion for malignancy) (Figs. 58.14 and 58.15).

58.6.6 Treatment

Approach for osteochondromas varies depending on the patient's condition.

- In the case of solitary osteochondromas that are small, asymptomatic, and lack suspicious imaging features, regular follow-up is typically sufficient.
- If a solitary osteochondroma becomes symptomatic or exhibits suspicious imaging features, further assessment with cross-sectional imaging is necessary.
- Surgical excision is generally easier for pedunculated lesions compared to sessile

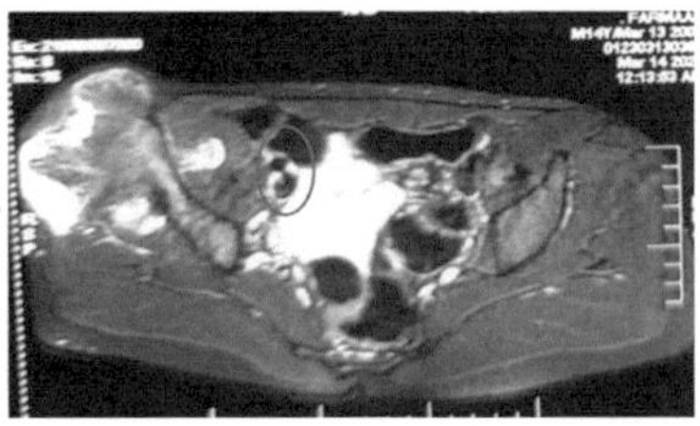

Fig. 58.15 MRI pelvis axial section with osteochondroma of pelvic with cartilagenous cap

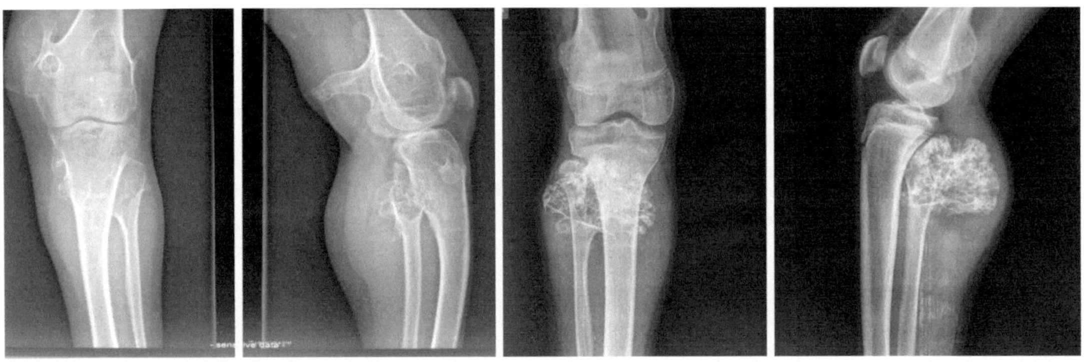

Fig. 58.14 Plain radiograph with multiple exostoses around knee

lesions. Following surgical resection, the reported recurrence rate in the literature is around 2%.
- Patients with hereditary multiple exostoses (HME) have a higher risk of malignant transformation and more severe osseous deformities; thus, surgical intervention is more common in these cases. Surgical intervention in HME patients may aim to correct or improve associated osseous deformities.

58.7 Enchondroma

58.7.1 Introduction

Enchondromas are benign tumours that develop in the hyaline cartilage of bones formed through endochondral ossification.

58.7.2 Epidemiology

They account for approximately 3 percentage of bone tumours and up to 13 percentage of benign bone tumours. They typically appear as solitary lesions located centrally in the metaphysis of tubular bones. The small bones of the hands and feet are the most commonly affected, followed by the femur and humerus.

Enchondromas usually arise during childhood from remnants of growth plate cartilage or chondrocytes. They undergo growth and enlargement during this period but eventually cease growing. However, they persist into adulthood without further growth. Enchondromas are the second most common benign cartilage lesions, following osteochondromas. They affect both males and females equally, with a male-to-female ratio of 1:1. Enchondromas are most frequently observed in individuals within the age range of 20–50 years old.

58.7.3 Types

- *Solitary Enchondroma*: This refers to a single enchondroma present in an individual.
- *Two syndromes* associated with enchondroma are as follows:
  1. *Ollier disease (multiple enchondromatosis):* Ollier disease is characterized by the presence of multiple enchondromas. It occurs sporadically. Enchondromas are found throughout the metaphyses and diaphyses of long bones. The affected bones may exhibit dysplasia, resulting in shortening and bowing. The risk of malignant transformation in Ollier disease is less than 30%.
  2. *Maffucci syndrome:* Maffucci syndrome is a sporadic condition consisting of multiple enchondromas and soft tissue angiomas. Individuals with Maffucci syndrome have an increased risk of developing visceral malignancies such as astrocytoma and gastrointestinal malignancies. In Maffucci syndrome, the risk of developing any malignancy can be as high as 100%.

58.7.4 Clinical Feature

Enchondromas are typically discovered incidentally and should not be mistaken for more aggressive lesions. They are usually asymptomatic; however, enchondromas in the hands or feet can cause pain due to pathological fractures or the risk of impending fractures.

Malignant transformation into low-grade chondrosarcoma is uncommon but can occur in rare cases. The presence of pain may be indicative of malignant transformation. It is important to maintain a high level of clinical suspicion and consider further evaluation if there are concerning symptoms or signs suggestive of malignancy.

58.7.5 Evaluation

- *Radiographs:* Enchondromas appear as well-defined, lucent, central medullary lesions that calcify over time, with characteristic features such as 'popcorn' stippling and minimal endosteal erosion. In Ollier disease and Maffucci syndrome, enchondromas markedly expand the bone and may lead to dysplastic changes, shortening, and bowing.
- *Bone scan:* Bone scans can help differentiate chondrosarcoma from enchondroma and identify polyostotic disease, although they rarely provide additional useful information as most enchondromas show lower uptake compared to chondrosarcomas.
- *MRI:* While usually not necessary for diagnosis, MRI can be helpful in assessing the size, intramedullary extent, and soft tissue extension of enchondromas, showing lobular and bright signals on T2-weighted images without bone marrow oedema or periosteal reaction. A medullary fill of over 90% suggests the possibility of chondrosarcoma rather than enchondroma (Fig. 58.16).

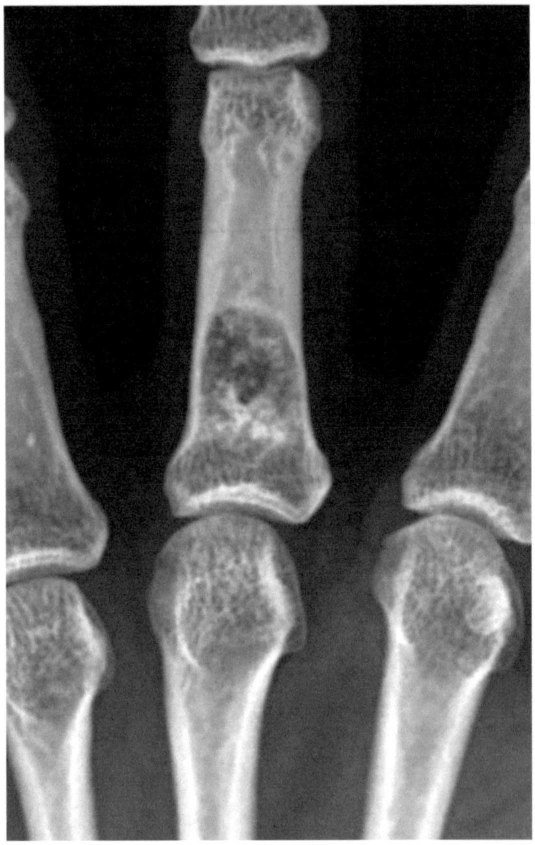

Fig. 58.16 Plain radiograph of finger with enchondroma with popcorn stippled calcification

58.7.6 Histology

Enchondromas exhibit a gross appearance of blue-grey, lobulated hyaline cartilage with scattered calcifications. This characteristic histological feature reflects the cartilaginous nature of the tumour and the presence of calcified areas within the tissue.

58.7.7 Management

Nonoperative management through observation is the recommended approach for asymptomatic enchondromas, with regular follow-up and radiographic monitoring. For symptomatic cases or those showing changes on X-rays, as well as pathologic fractures, operative intervention with intralesional curettage and bone grafting may be necessary. Immediate surgical treatment is preferred for pathologic fractures. Long-term follow-up is essential, especially for patients with multiple enchondroma syndromes. Surgical management is associated with low rates of local recurrence, and there is no significant difference in outcomes between delayed and immediate intervention. In cases of large lesions or when low-grade chondrosarcoma is suspected based on radiographic findings, surgical treatment may be considered.

58.8 Aneursymal Bone Cyst

58.8.1 Introduction

Benign bone lesion characterized by blood-filled cystic spaces and is most commonly found in the meta-diaphysis of the long bones and posterior elements of the vertebrae. Femur and tibia are the most common sites involved.

58.8.2 Epidemiology

- Its annual prevalence is 0.32 per 100,000 young population and 0.14 per 100,000 general population.
- It comprises about 2.5% of all bone tumours.
- ABC has an equal distribution among male and female patients.
- It most commonly occurs in skeletally immature patients, especially in the first two decades of life.

58.8.3 Anatomic Locations

- The lesions are usually found in the metaphysio-diaphyseal region of bones.
- More than 60% of aneurysmal bone cysts occur in long bones, with the femur and tibia being the most common sites.
- A total of 51% of aneurysmal bone cysts occur in the lower extremities, while 22.5% occur in the upper extremities.
- 15% of aneurysmal bone cysts occur in the spine.
- The most common locations in the foot are the metatarsal and calcaneus bones.

58.8.4 Aetiology

- Historically, ABC was believed to develop due to vascular events, increased venous blood flow, or prior trauma.
- Recent molecular findings have identified a recurrent rearrangement involving the USP6 gene (chr.17p13.2 locus) in primary ABC.
- The most commonly described translocation leading to primary ABC is t(16;17)(q22;p13), which results in the juxtaposition of the CDH11 promoter region on 16q22.6
- Due to this discovery, ABC is now considered a neoplasm rather than a reactive lesion.
- Secondary ABC is not considered a neoplasm because no known translocation has been identified.
- ABC is sometimes associated with other bone tumours such as
  1. Giant cell tumour
  2. Chondroblastoma
  3. Fibrous dysplasia
  4. Chondromyxoid fibroma
  5. Non-ossifying fibroma (NOF)

58.8.5 Clinical Presentation

- Pain and swelling are the most common symptoms.
- Can present with pathological fracture especially in tubular long bones of extremities.
- The initial presentation of vertebral lesions may include symptoms of compression of the spinal cord or nerve roots. These symptoms can vary depending on the location and extent of the lesion.

58.8.6 Evaluation

- *X-ray:* Eccentric, expansile lytic lesion with multiple septation at metaphysis impart a characteristics multilocular or 'soap bubble appearance'. Thin surrounding rim of periosteal new bone formation is usually present. There is no matrix mineralization. 'Finger in the balloon' sign seen in tubular bones of hands and feet. 'Blow out' lesion seen in ABC of vertebral body.
- *CT scan:* Well-delineated lytic lesion with mean density higher than fat. Surrounding thin rim of reactive bone can be seen. Soft tissue extension and cortical breech can be appreciated. Fluid–fluid level can also be seen.
- *MRI:* Best imaging modality to identity fluid–fluid level.
  - MRI can show characteristic fluid–fluid levels and identify solid components or

concerning features of other tumour entities.

- Fluid–fluid levels are not pathognomic of aneurysmal bone cysts, which can also be seen in other benign and malignant bone tumours.
- Signal characteristics of cysts on MRI include variable T1 and T2 signals, with a low signal rim and high signal areas representing blood of varying ages.
- Septations in aneurysmal bone cysts may enhance on T1 images (Figs. 58.17, 58.18, and 58.19).

58.8.7 Histopathology

Gross Specimen shows

- Well-demarcated, spongy, haemorrhagic lesion.
- Variably sized multiloculations with cystic spaces ranging from less than one millimetre to several centimetres in size.
- Irregular and sharply demarcated borders with a thin shell of reactive bone surrounding it.
- A variable amount of solid component may be present, especially in the digits (Fig. 58.20).

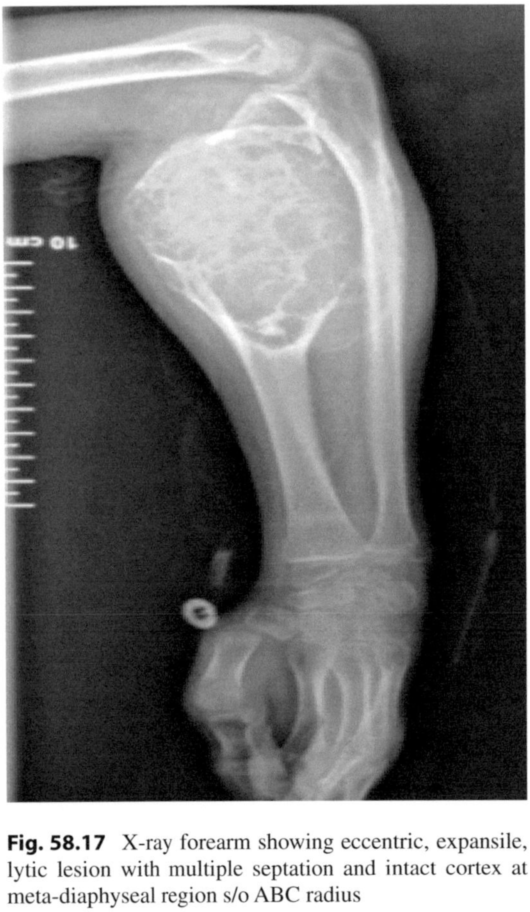

Fig. 58.17 X-ray forearm showing eccentric, expansile, lytic lesion with multiple septation and intact cortex at meta-diaphyseal region s/o ABC radius

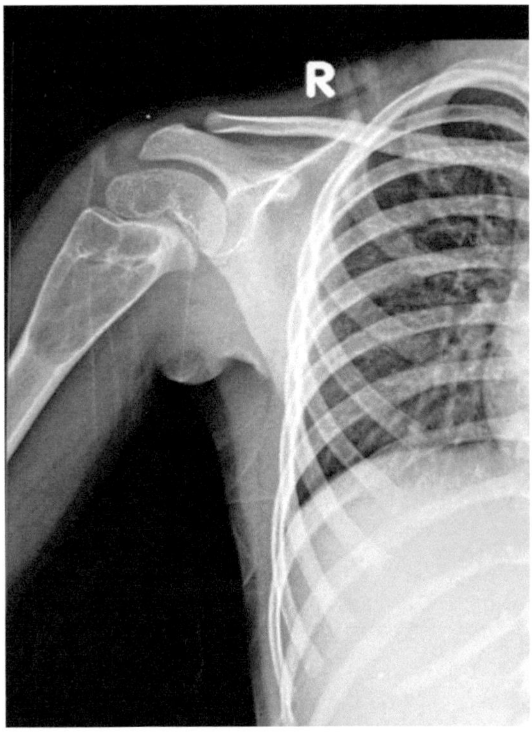

Fig. 58.18 X-ray right shoulder AP view showing expansile lytic lesion (soap bubble appearance) at meta-diaphyseal region most likely ABC

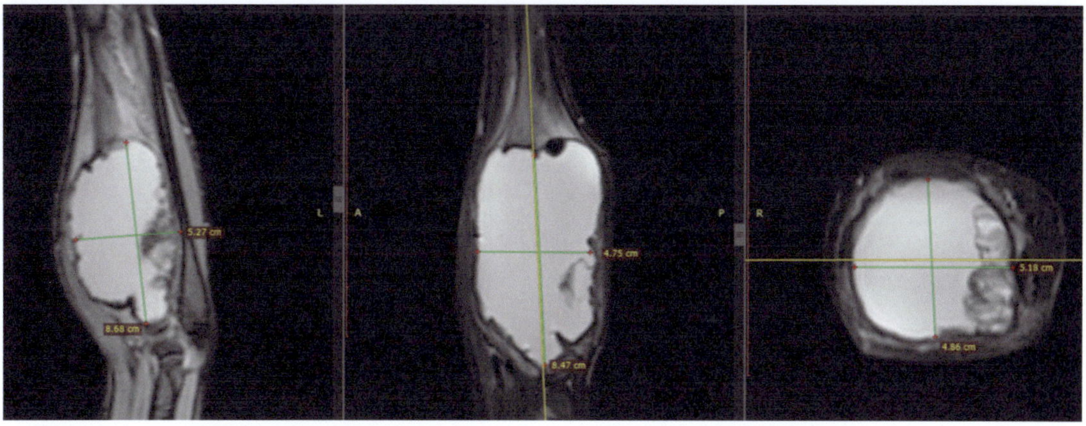

Fig. 58.19 T2-weighted MRI image showing hyperintense lesion with fluid–fluid levels

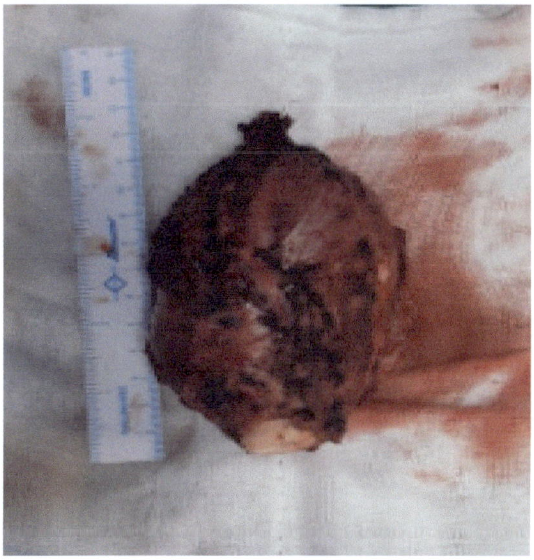

Fig. 58.20 Gross specimen of ABC tumour

Microscopy shows

- Multiloculated blood-filled spaces without endothelial lining separated by septa.
- The fibrous—a mixture of inflammatory cells, reactive fibroblasts, woven bone, and some areas of blood vessel formation.
- The lesion is surrounded by a thin reactive bone formation that is rich in multinucleated osteoclast-like giant cells (Fig. 58.21).

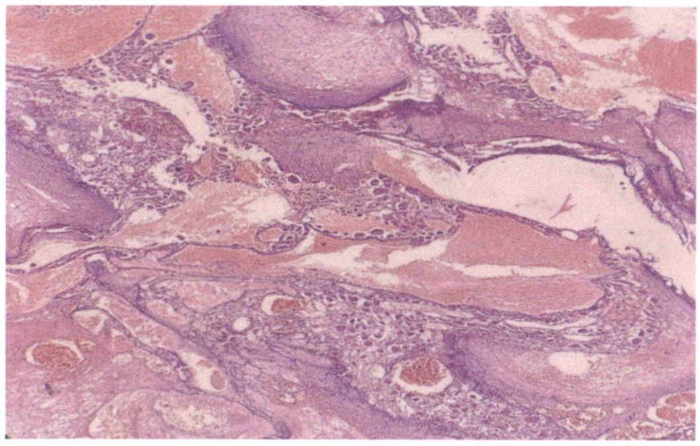

Fig. 58.21 Microscopy: blood-filled spaces lined by fibrohistiocytic cells with osteoclastic giant cells and variable bony tissue with calcification

58.8.8 Treatment

58.8.8.1 Non-operative

1. Intralesional steroid injection.
2. Percutaneous injection of doxycycline.
3. Sclerotherapy: intralesional injection with polidocanol.
4. Bisphosphonates and denosumab also can be given.
5. Arterial embolization (Fig. 58.22).

58.8.8.2 Operative

1. Extended curettage and bone grafting
2. Wide excision and reconstruction
3. Curopsy: curettage + biopsy

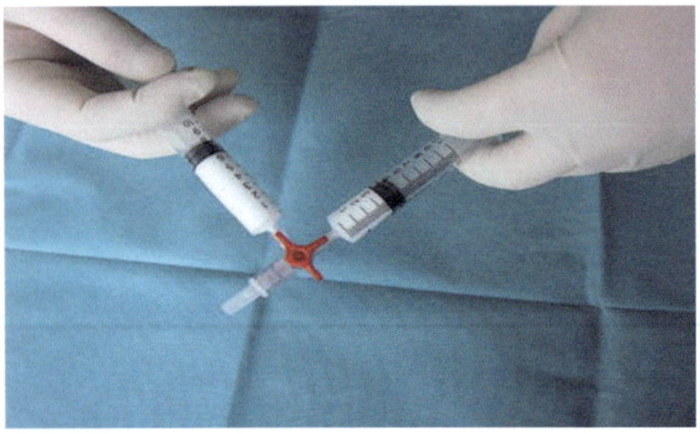

Fig. 58.22 Preparation of sclerotherapy (polidocanol) for intralesional injection

58.8.9 Differential Diagnosis

1. Giant cell tumour
2. Chondroblastoma
3. Fibrous dysplasia
4. Chondromyxoid fibroma
5. NOF

58.9 Fibrous Dysplasia

58.9.1 Introduction

Fibrous dysplasia is a benign intramedullary fibro-osseous lesion, which represents approximately 5% to 7% of benign bone tumours and can occur in one bone (monostotic) or multiple bones (polyostotic). Lesions develop during skeletal formation and growth. Clinical presentation can occur at any age, but most commonly detected by the age of thirty with no gender predilection. Common sites of skeletal involvement include long bones, ribs, craniofacial bones, and the pelvis.

58.9.2 Aetiology

Fibrous dysplasia results from a failure in the normal bone remodelling process and a lack of response to mechanical stress during skeletal development. The affected bone contains a mass of immature trabeculae and dysplastic fibrous tissue that never fully completes the remodelling process.

58.9.3 Anatomic Locations

- *Monostotic form:* Ribs are the most common location (28%); proximal femur (23%), tibia, craniofacial bones (10–25%), and humerus can also be affected.
- *Polyostotic form:* Often affects one limb, monomelic (unilateral). Femur is the most commonly affected bone.

58.9.4 Clinical Presentation

- Asymptomatic: Monostotic lesions are often asymptomatic and discovered incidentally on radiographs taken for other reasons.
- Pain: Localized pain is a common presenting symptom in dysplastic bone with fatigue fractures, particularly in the femoral neck.
- Deformity: Deformity depends on the extent and site of the lesion, age of the patient, and whether the disease is monostotic or polyostotic. Polyostotic fibrous dysplasia can lead to bowing deformities, with the classic shepherd's crook deformity of the proximal femur being a common example.

58.9.5 Evaluation

- *X-ray:* centric, lytic lesion involving medullary canal of metaphysio-diaphyseal region of bone. Typically, normal bone is replaced by tissue that is more radiolucent with a homogeneous, 'ground-glass' pattern. Shepherd's crook deformity of femoral neck.
- *Computed tomography scanning:* CT scan is the best technique for demonstrating the radiographic characteristics of fibrous dysplasia, with the extent of the lesion clearly visible and the cortical boundary depicted with more detail than on radiographs or magnetic resonance images.
- *Magnetic resonance imaging:* MRI is a sensitive means of establishing the lesion's shape and content and the size of the affected region. On T1-weighted MRI, fibrous dysplasia typically appears as an intermediate-to-low signal intensity with a heterogeneous pattern. On

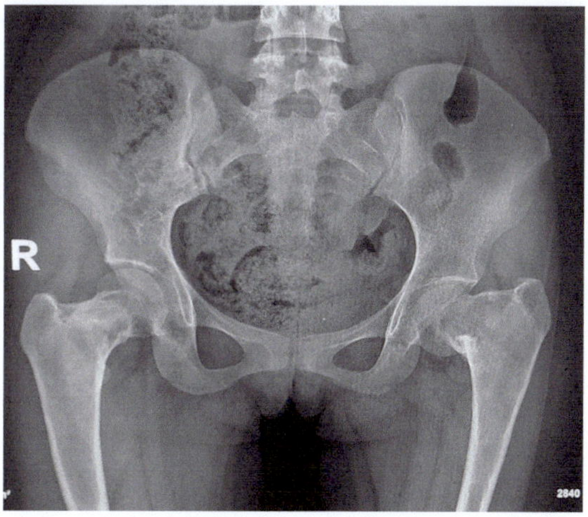

Fig. 58.23 X-ray pelvis with bilateral hip showing ground grass appearance lesion on B/L proximal femur with varus deformity (shepherd's crook deformity)

T2-weighted MRI, the signal intensity can vary (Fig. 58.23).

58.9.6 Histopathology

Gross Features Lesions are intramedullary, well-circumscribed, and expansile and have an abnormal whitish or tannish-grey colour and gritty consistency.

Microscopic Features Fibrous dysplasia exhibits a characteristic appearance of 'alphabet soup' or 'Chinese letters' due to the presence of delicate trabeculae of immature bone enmeshed within a bland fibrous stroma of dysplastic spindle-shaped cells (Fig. 58.24).

58.9.7 Differential Diagnosis

1. Eosinophilic granuloma
2. Lymphoma
3. Leukaemia
4. Enchondroma/Ollier disease/Maffucci syndrome

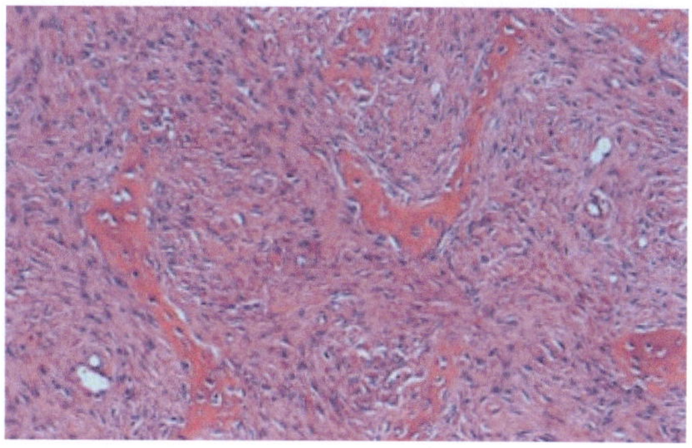

Fig. 58.24 Image showing slide of fibrous dysplasia with characteristics dysplastic trabeculae that are disconnected and have bizarre contours.

5. Osteochondroma/hereditary multiple exostoses (HME)
6. Non-ossifying fibroma/Jaffe-Campanacci syndrome
7. Hemangioendothelioma

58.9.8 Management

58.9.8.1 Observation

- For asymptomatic patients in which FD are incidentally discovered on radiographs.
- Clinical observation is warranted for these lesions.
- Follow-up radiographs should be made every six months.
- Bone scan is needed to exclude a diagnosis of polyostotic disease in newly identified cases.
- Referral to an endocrinologist for endocrine and metabolic testing is paramount if polyostotic disease is found.

58.9.8.2 Bisphoshonate

- Used for patients with symptomatic polyostotic disease.
- Decreases bone pain and has a lasting effect on bone turnover.
- Radiographic changes are seen in some patients.

- Side effects include transient fever, symptomatic hypocalcaemia, and transient diffuse bone pain.
- Osteonecrosis of the jaw is a potentially serious reaction to bisphosphonate therapy, mainly in patients with cancer, related to intravenous zoledronic acid.
- Oral alendronate and intravenous pamidronate are commonly used at dose of 70 mg weekly and 180 mg 6 monthly, respectively.

58.9.8.3 Operative

Indications:

- Eradication of symptomatic lesions
- Correction of deformity
- Prevention of pathologic fracture
- Neurologic compromise in spine

Surgical procedures are as follows:

1. Curettage and bone grafting with internal fixation
   - Intermedullary nailing preferred over plate in lower extremities
   - Cortical graft preferred over cancellous graft.
2. Osteotomies
   - Intertrochanteric osteotomies to correct coxa-vara deformity (Fig. 58.25).

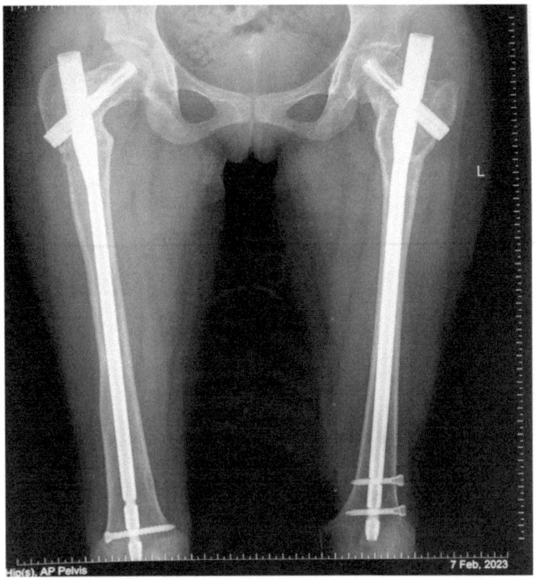

Fig. 58.25 Postoperative X-ray pelvis with hip and thigh showing varus deformity correction done with osteotomies and intramedullary nail fixation

Multiple Choice Questions

1. A 16-year-old male with constant pain over mid diaphysis of left tibia. Pain is worse at night and relieved on anti-inflammatory; radiograph shows thickened reactive cortex around a small radiolucent nidus. What is the likely diagnosis?
   (a) Osteosarcoma
   (b) Ewing sarcoma
   (c) Osteoid osteoma
   (d) Metastasis
2. A 25-year-old male with right knee pain, Radiograph of knee as shown in figure. MRI shows T1 hypointense and T2 hyperintense lesion without soft tissue involvement. What should be the next step in treatment?

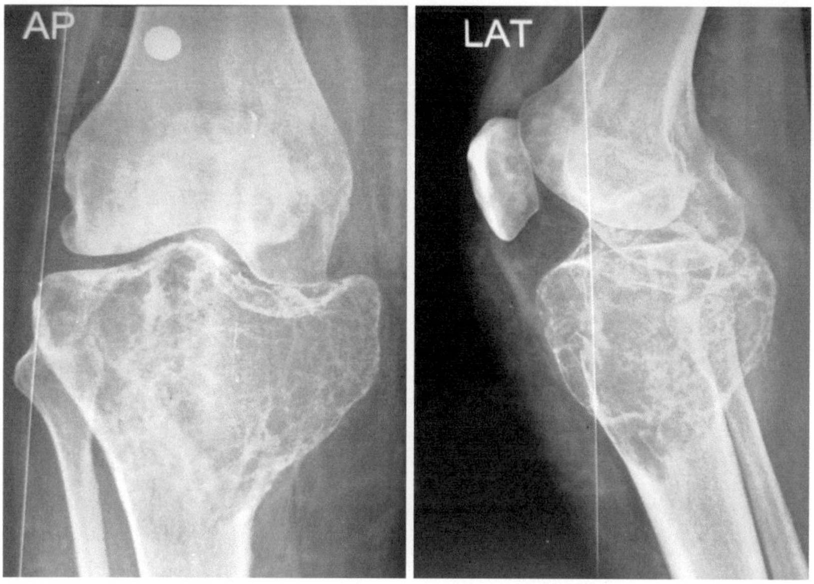

(a) Wait and watch
(b) Surgery
(c) Exercise
(d) Biopsy of lesion

3. A 13-year-old female with right shoulder pain and plain radiograph shown below. MRI shows multiple fluid–fluid levels with septations. And biopsy shows blood-filled spaces without endothelial lining with numerous giant cells. What is the likely diagnosis?

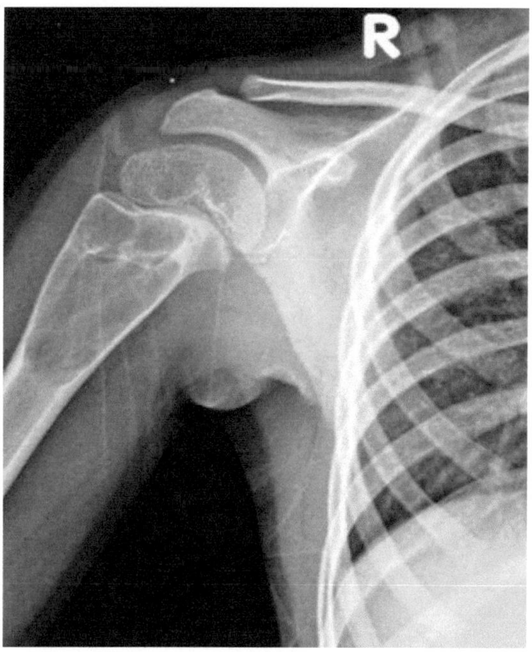

(a) Osteosarcoma
(b) Giant cell tumour
(c) Aneurysmal bone cyst
(d) Simple bone cyst

4. Multiple enchondroma associated with soft tissue angioma seen in which condition?
(a) Ollier disease
(b) Hereditary multiple exostoses
(c) Mazabraud syndrome
(d) Maffucci syndrome

5. EXT 1 and EXT 2 gene mutation with following radiograph seen in which disease?

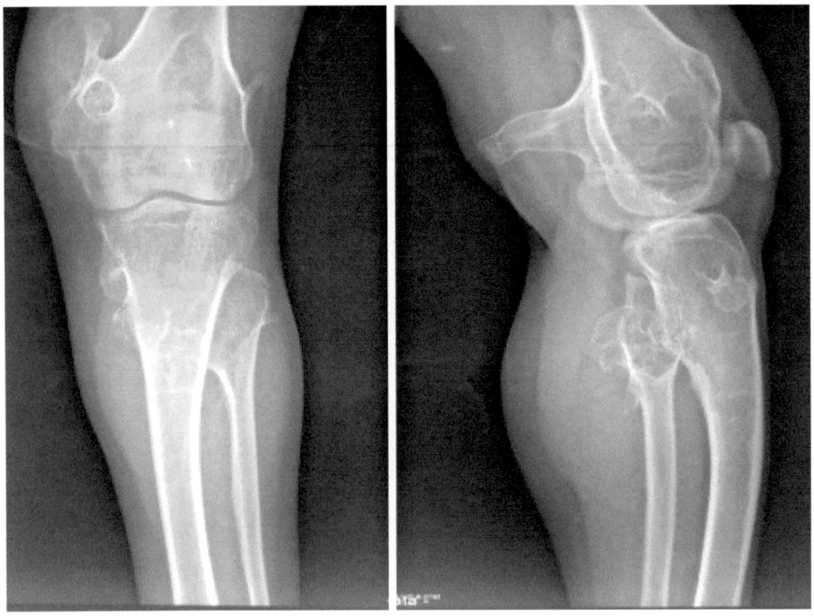

   (a) Ollier disease
   (b) Hereditary multiple exostoses
   (c) Mazabraud syndrome
   (d) Maffucci syndrome

Answers: 1. (c), 2. (d), 3. (c), 4. (d), 5. (b)

Malignant Bone Tumors

59

Mohit Dhingra and Anil Regmi

59.1 Introduction

Malignant bone tumours are rare but serious neoplastic lesions affecting the skeletal system. They can be primary tumours, which originate de novo from the bone, or secondary as a result of metastasis from tumour in other organs of the body.

The most common types of primary malignant bone tumours are as follows:

- Multiple myeloma (MM; most common bone tumour)
- Osteosarcoma (OS; most common non-haematogenous bone tumour)
- Chondrosarcoma
- Ewing sarcoma

These tumours typically occur in children and young adults, although they can also occur in older ones.

Secondary bone tumours, also known as metastatic bone tumours, are more common than primary bone tumours and are usually caused by the spread of tumour from another part of the body, such as the breast, prostate, lung, or kidney.

In this chapter, we will discuss the three most common malignant bone tumours that we commonly encounter in our daily practice. Here, we will discuss osteosarcoma, chondrosarcoma, Ewing sarcoma, and multiple myeloma.

59.2 Osteosarcoma

Osteosarcoma (OS) is the second most common primary malignant tumour of bone, following multiple myeloma, and is considered the most common non-haematologic primary malignancy of bone. It is a highly aggressive cancer that arises from the bone-forming cells, known as osteoblasts.

59.2.1 Epidemiology

OS is relatively rare, accounting for approximately 1% of all cancers and approximately 20% of primary bone cancers. It predominantly affects children and young adults of the second decade. However, it has a bimodal age distribution, with the first peak occurring during adolescence and the second peak in older adults. There is a slight male predominance in the incidence of osteosarcoma.

59.2.2 Aetiology and Risk Factors

The exact cause of OS is unknown. However, several risk factors have been identified, including

M. Dhingra (✉) · A. Regmi
Department of Orthopedics, All India Institute of Medical Sciences, Rishikesh, Uttarakhand, India

V. Kumar et al. (eds.), *A Quick Guide to Essential Orthopedics*,
https://doi.org/10.1007/978-981-95-2676-5_59

genetic predisposition, prior exposure to radiation, certain inherited conditions (such as Li-Fraumeni syndrome and hereditary retinoblastoma), and certain bone diseases (such as Paget's disease and hereditary multiple exostoses).

59.2.3 Classification

Grossly osteosarcoma is classified as primary and secondary osteosarcoma.

- Primary osteosarcomas are subcategorized as follows:
  - Conventional osteosarcoma
  - Low-grade intramedullary osteosarcoma
  - Parosteal osteosarcoma
  - Periosteal osteosarcoma
  - High-grade surface osteosarcoma
  - Telangiectatic osteosarcoma
  - Small cell osteosarcoma
- Secondary OS: OS can be secondary to Paget's disease, or due to radiation at the previous radiation site.

59.2.4 Clinical Presentation

The clinical presentation of OS often includes bony pain, which may initially be attributed to sports injuries or growth spurts. Swelling, tenderness, and limited range of motion in the affected area are also common. In some cases, pathologic fractures may occur.

59.2.5 Diagnostic Methods

The diagnosis of OS involves a combination of imaging studies and histopathological examination. Radiographic techniques such as X-rays, computed tomography (CT) scans, and magnetic resonance imaging (MRI) scans help visualize the bone lesion and evaluate its extent. A biopsy is necessary to confirm the diagnosis and determine the histological subtype.

- X-rays: Typical appearances of conventional high-grade osteosarcoma include medullary and cortical bone destruction with a wide zone of transition, permeative or moth-eaten appearance, aggressive periosteal reaction leading to the formation of sunburst appearance, or Codman triangle or less frequently seen lamellated (onion skin) reaction. In addition to bony changes, it also includes soft tissue mass and tumour matrix ossification/calcification. In addition to the imaging of involved extremities, we should get a routine chest X-ray done to look for lung and nodal metastases which appear to be ossified (Fig. 59.1).
- CT scan: The role of CT scan is predominantly utilized in assisting biopsy and staging. CT adds little to plain radiography and MRI in the direct assessment of the tumour. In the case of contrast imaging by CT angiography, we can appreciate the vascular involvement of the tumour. Also, it helps in identifying the feeding vessels, which helps in planning preoperative embolization for highly vascular (Telangiectatic) OS. Contrast-enhanced computed tomography (CECT) of thorax and abdomen is useful for metastatic workup of patients.
- MRI: MRI is proving an essential tool to determine accurate local staging and assessment for limb-sparing resection, particularly for the evaluation of intraosseous tumour extension and soft tissue involvement. T1 is the best sequence to evaluate intramedullary tumour extension which may be overestimated on T2. Ossified tumour tissue appears low signal intensity with peritumoral oedema appearing intermediate signal intensity and nonmineralized soft tissue as intermediate signal intensity in T1. Ossified tumour tissue appears low signal intensity with peritumoral oedema appearing high signal intensity and nonmineralized soft tissue as high signal intensity in T2 (Fig. 59.2).
- Bone scintigraphy: Bone scintigraphy can show increased activity (hot) at the site of the

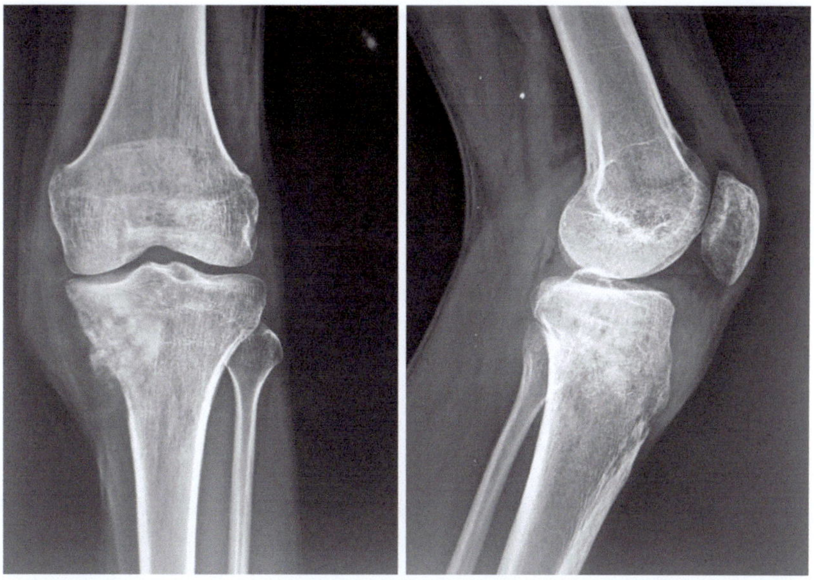

Fig. 59.1 Plain radiograph of left knee anteroposterior (AP) and lateral view of 16-year-old male showing conventional osteosarcoma. It shows soft tissue swelling on the anteromedial aspect of the proximal leg with a wide zone of transition and periosteal reaction

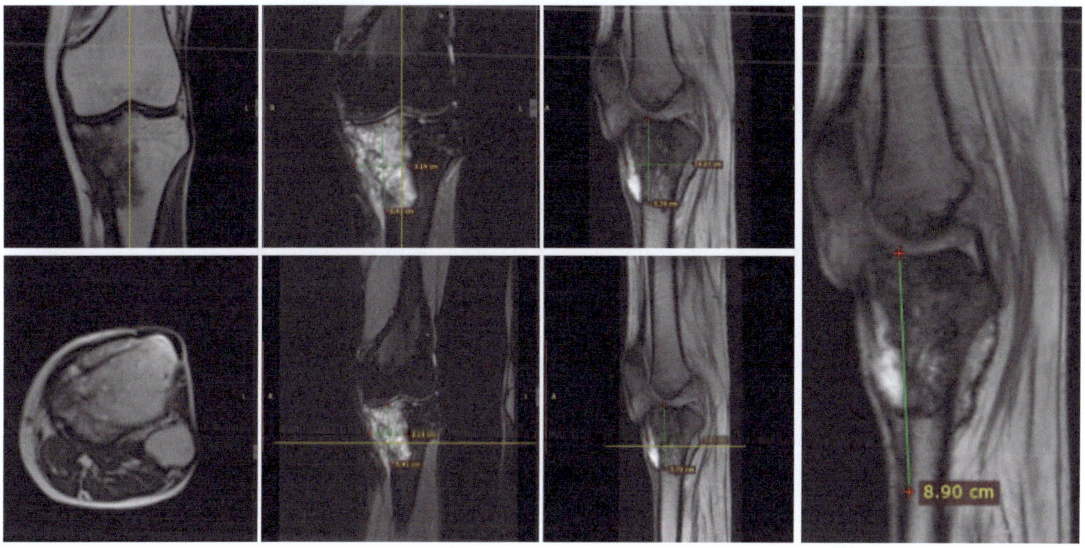

Fig. 59.2 MRI of osteosarcoma of left proximal tibia showing low signal intensity ossified tumour with intermediate signal intensity peritumoral oedema and intermediate signal intensity nonmineralized soft tissue in T1 and low signal intensity ossified tumour tissue with high signal intensity peritumoral edema and high signal intensity nonmineralized soft tissue in T2

primary tumour as well as sites of bone and systemic metastases, for example lung.

- Flouro-deoxy glucose-positron emission tomography (FDG-PET): FDG-PET is better than bone scintigraphy in the detection of bone metastases. It will show increased standardized uptake value (SUV) at sites of distant metastases. As there is no definite cut-off value for SUV level, it can be used in follow-up to evaluate the response to chemotherapy.
- Histology: Histology is obtained after an appropriate bone biopsy sample for final diag-

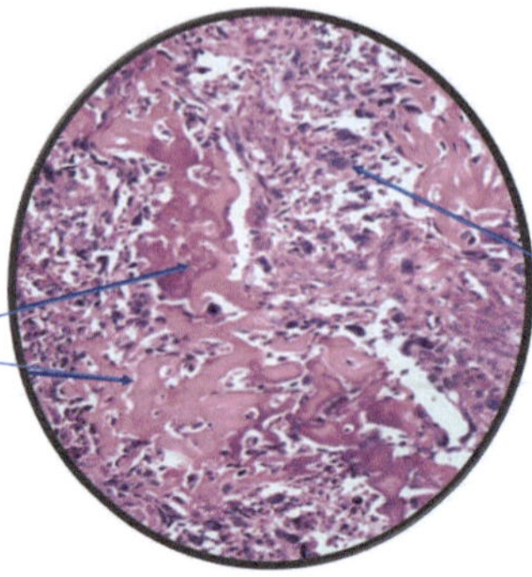

Fig. 59.3 Histology image of osteosarcoma, showing characteristic osteoid formation and high-grade anaplastic spindle cells with hyperchromatic nuclei

nosis. The histological feature varies according to the classification of the tumour. The conventional OS is characterized by the presence of malignant cells producing osteoid, which is the hallmark of this tumour. The osteoid can appear as a lace-like network or irregular trabeculae surrounded by malignant osteoblasts. Other features may include cellular pleomorphism, mitotic activity, and areas of necrosis (Fig. 59.3).

- Immunohistochemistry and molecular markers: Immunohistochemistry can aid in the diagnosis of OS and its subtypes by identifying specific markers associated with osteoblastic differentiation, such as osteocalcin and osteonectin. Additionally, molecular markers, including TP53 mutations, RB1 alterations, and abnormalities in various signalling pathways, can provide valuable prognostic information.

59.2.6 Treatment

The primary treatment for osteosarcoma is neoadjuvant chemotherapy followed by surgical resection of the tumour.

- Chemotherapy: Chemotherapy plays a crucial role in the treatment of osteosarcoma. It is an integral part of the multimodal approach that includes neo-adjuvant (pre-operative) chemotherapy, surgical resection of the tumour, and adjuvant (post-operative) chemotherapy.
  - Neoadjuvant chemotherapy: Neoadjuvant chemotherapy aims to reduce tumour burden, eradicate micrometastases, and improve surgical outcomes. The most commonly used chemotherapy agents in neoadjuvant regimens for osteosarcoma include the following:
    - High-dose methotrexate
    - Doxorubicin (Adriamycin)
    - Cisplatin
    - Ifosfamide

  Various regimens have been employed for osteosarcoma treatment, including the following:

- MAP (methotrexate, doxorubicin, cisplatin)
- MAP+Ifosfamide,
- IE (ifosfamide, etoposide)
- T-ICE (high-dose methotrexate, ifosfamide, cisplatin, etoposide).

These regimens are tailored based on patient characteristics, tumour stage, and institutional protocols. These drugs are administered in combination over several cycles before surgery.

- Adjuvant chemotherapy: After surgical resection of the tumour, adjuvant chemotherapy is given to further eliminate residual tumour cells and reduce the risk of recurrence. The same chemotherapy agents used in neoadjuvant therapy are often continued in the adjuvant setting. The duration and number of cycles may vary depending on the individual patient's response and risk factors.
- Surgery: The goal of surgery is complete resection of the primary tumour while preserving limb function whenever possible. The

primary goal of surgery in osteosarcoma is achieving complete tumour resection with negative margins (margins free of tumour histopathologically). Adequate surgical margins are essential to minimize the risk of local recurrence. The surgical approach may vary depending on the tumour location, size, and extent of involvement. Advancements in surgical techniques, imaging modalities, and preoperative planning have improved surgical precision and outcomes in osteosarcoma treatment. Techniques such as computer-assisted surgery, three-dimensional (3D)-printed models for surgical planning, and intraoperative navigation systems have facilitated accurate tumour resection and reconstruction. The surgical approach can be of two types:

- Limb salvage surgery: Limb salvage surgery, also known as limb-sparing or limb-preserving surgery, is the preferred approach whenever feasible. It involves the removal of the tumour while preserving as much healthy bone and soft tissue as possible. The resected bone is usually reconstructed using various techniques, such as endoprosthetic replacement, allograft transplantation, or biological reconstruction with autografts (Fig. 59.4).
- Amputation: In certain cases, where limb salvage surgery is not possible due to extensive tumour involvement or unsatisfactory oncological margins, amputation may be considered. Amputation involves the complete removal of the affected limb and is performed to ensure complete tumour eradication. Advances in prosthetic technology and rehabilitation have significantly improved the quality of life for individuals undergoing amputation (Fig. 59.5).

59.2.7 Prognosis

The prognosis of osteosarcoma depends on various factors, including the tumour stage at diagnosis, histological response to chemotherapy, and the presence or absence of metastasis. Overall, the survival rates for localized osteosarcoma have improved significantly over the years due to advancements in multimodal treatment approaches.

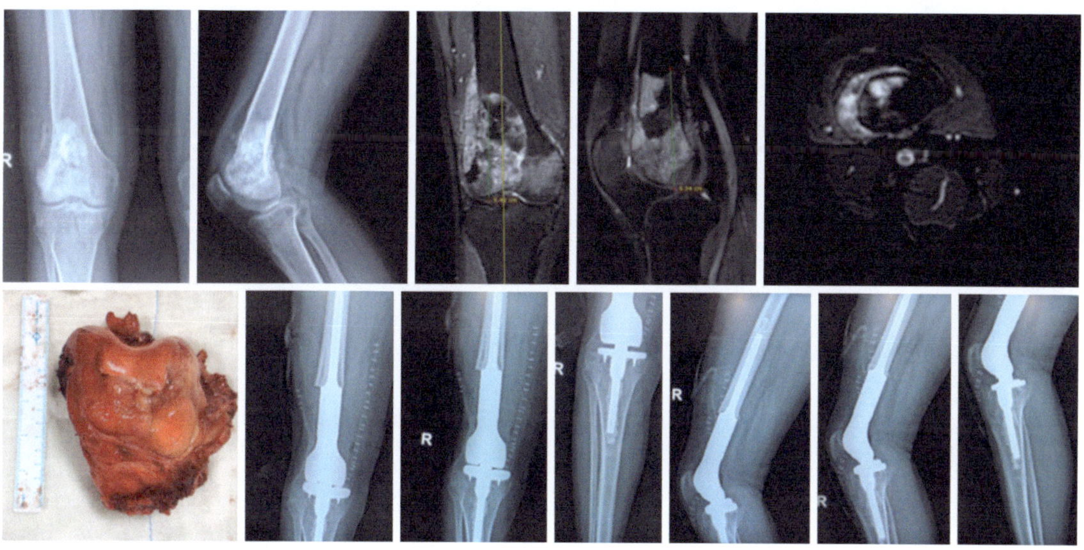

Fig. 59.4 Example of limb salvage surgery: a 26-year-old male with osteosarcoma of right distal femur without neurovascular involvement underwent wide excision and reconstruction by megaprosthesis application

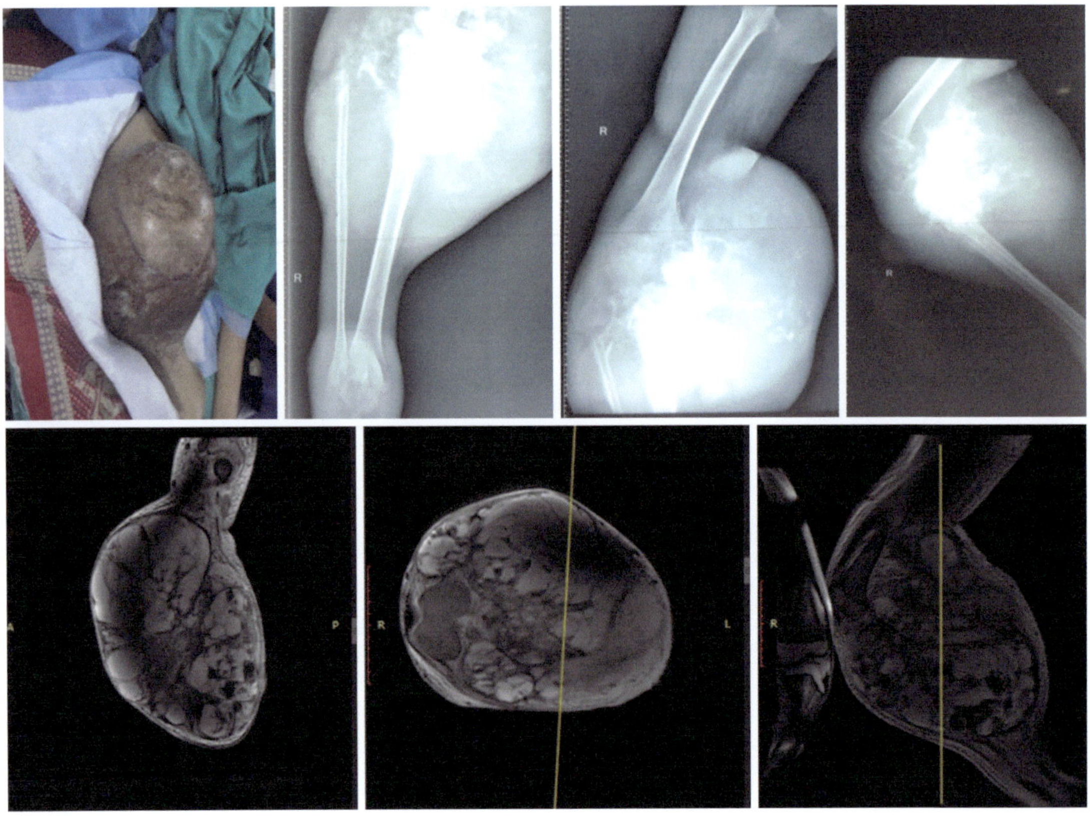

Fig. 59.5 Case example of amputation: a 12-year-old female with large osteosarcoma of right proximal tibia with neurovascular involvement underwent amputation

59.3 Chondrosarcoma

Chondrosarcoma is a malignant bone tumour that arises from cartilage-forming cells. It is the second most common primary bone sarcoma, accounting for approximately 20% of all bone sarcomas.

59.3.1 Epidemiology

Chondrosarcoma primarily affects adults, with a peak incidence in the fifth to seventh decades of life. It is rare in children and adolescents. Chondrosarcomas can occur in any bone but is most commonly found in the pelvis, proximal femur, and shoulder girdle.

59.3.2 Aetiology and Risk Factors

The exact cause of chondrosarcoma is unknown, and most cases occur sporadically. However, certain risk factors have been identified, including previous radiation therapy, certain genetic syndromes (such as Ollier disease and Maffucci syndrome), and hereditary conditions like multiple enchondromatosis and familial chondrosarcoma.

59.3.3 Classification

Chondrosarcomas can be classified into the following subtypes:

- Conventional chondrosarcoma
- Dedifferentiated chondrosarcoma
- Mesenchymal chondrosarcoma
- Periosteal chondrosarcoma
- Clear cell chondrosarcoma
- Extraskeletal chondrosarcoma

59.3.4 Clinical Presentation

The clinical presentation of chondrosarcoma is often insidious, with symptoms developing slowly over time. Common symptoms include localized pain, swelling, and a palpable mass in the affected area. In some cases, pathological fractures may occur. Chondrosarcomas are generally low-grade tumours with a slow growth rate, but high-grade tumours can exhibit more aggressive behaviour.

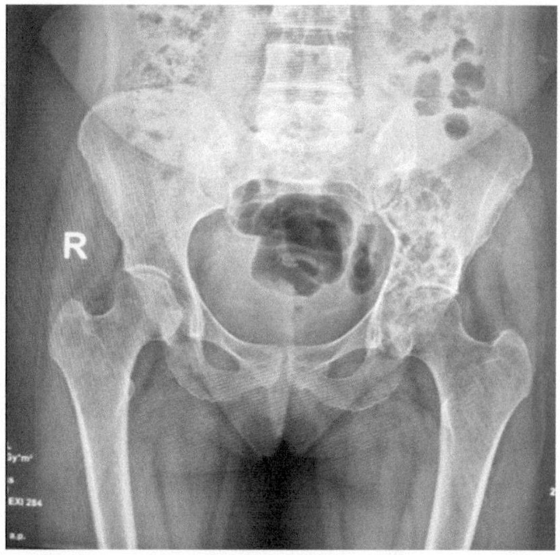

Fig. 59.6 Plain radiograph of pelvis with a bilateral hip of a 62-year-old female with chondrosarcoma in the left pelvis. It shows a lytic lesion with intralesional calcifications (popcorn calcification) on the left pelvis in the ilium and periacetabular region

59.3.5 Diagnostic Methods

Imaging studies play a crucial role in the diagnosis and evaluation of chondrosarcoma. X-rays, CT scans, and MRI scans are used to assess the extent of the tumour, its relationship to surrounding structures, and the presence of any metastases. A definitive diagnosis is made through histopathological examination of a biopsy specimen.

- X-rays: Plain radiographs appears to be the lytic lesion with intralesional calcifications (rings and arcs calcification or popcorn calcification) along with endosteal scalloping, which affects more than two-thirds of the cortical thickness, moth-eaten appearance, or permeative appearance in higher grade tumours. Along with these findings, cortical remodelling, thickening, and periosteal reaction are also useful in distinguishing between an enchondroma and low-grade chondrosarcoma (Fig. 59.6).
- CT scans: The features seen on CT are the same as on plain film but features such as matrix calcification, endosteal scalloping, cortical breach, and soft tissue mass are better seen. CECT (thorax and abdomen) is useful for metastatic workup of patients.
- MRI: MRI demonstrates low-to-intermediate signal in T1 and very high intensity in non-mineralized/calcified portions in T2 as the cartilage is a hydrophilic tissue with high water content. It helps to delineate the soft tissue and marrow extension of the tumour (Fig. 59.7).
- Bone scan: Typically, chondrosarcomas demonstrate increased uptake on bone scan, seen in over 80% of cases, and usually, the uptake is quite intense. This is useful in helping to distinguish low-grade chondrosarcoma from an enchondroma.
- Histology: Histology is obtained after an appropriate bone biopsy sample for final diagnosis. The tumour can exhibit various histological subtypes, including conventional chondrosarcoma, dedifferentiated chondrosarcoma, clear cell chondrosarcoma, mesenchymal chondrosarcoma, and myxoid chondrosarcoma. The most common type, conventional chondrosarcoma, is characterized by the presence of malignant chondrocytes arranged in lacunae within a hyaline cartilage matrix. The tumour cells exhibit

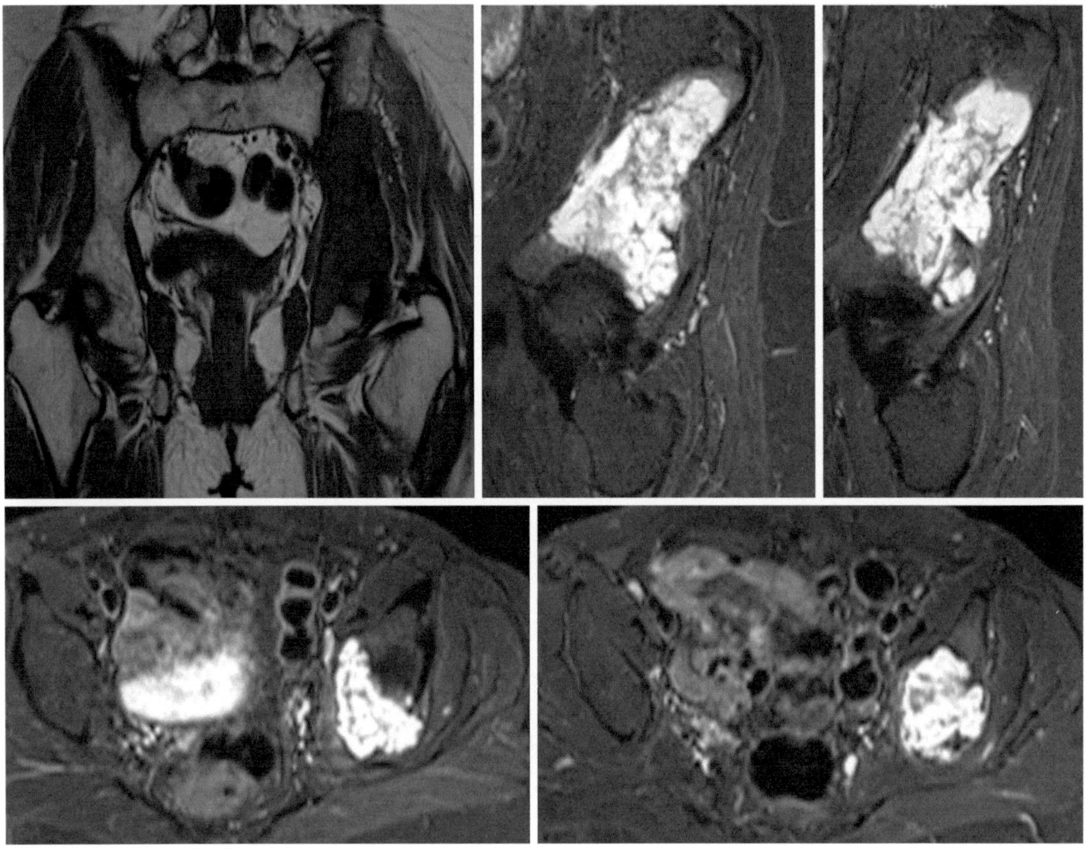

Fig. 59.7 MRI of pelvis showing chondrosarcoma of pelvis, showing multilobulated heterogeneously enhancing lesion involving left ilium, acetabulum extending to hip joint, and soft tissue in pelvis. The tumour tissue abuts left internal iliac vessels with loss of fat planes

varying degrees of cellular atypia, with enlarged and hyperchromatic nuclei. The hyaline cartilage matrix may show areas of calcification and ossification (Fig. 59.8).

59.3.6 Treatment

The treatment of chondrosarcoma involves a multidisciplinary approach, including surgery, radiation therapy, and occasionally chemotherapy.

- Surgical management: Surgery is the mainstay of treatment for chondrosarcoma and aims to achieve complete resection of the tumour with negative margins. The extent of surgical resection depends on tumour location, grade, and patient-specific factors. For low-grade chondrosarcomas, marginal/wide local excision is performed to preserve limb function whenever possible. In high-grade or aggressive chondrosarcomas, more extensive resections, such as amputation, may be necessary. In cases where complete resection is not feasible, surgical debulking may be performed to alleviate symptoms and facilitate adjuvant therapies.
- Radiation therapy: Radiation therapy is used as an adjuvant treatment modality for chondrosarcoma in certain situations. It is particularly considered when the tumour is incompletely resected, there is a high risk of local recurrence, or in cases where surgery is not feasible due to tumour location or patient

Fig. 59.8 Histopathology image of chondrosarcoma showing pleomorphic chondrocytes with adjacent foci showing small tumour cells with round nuclei

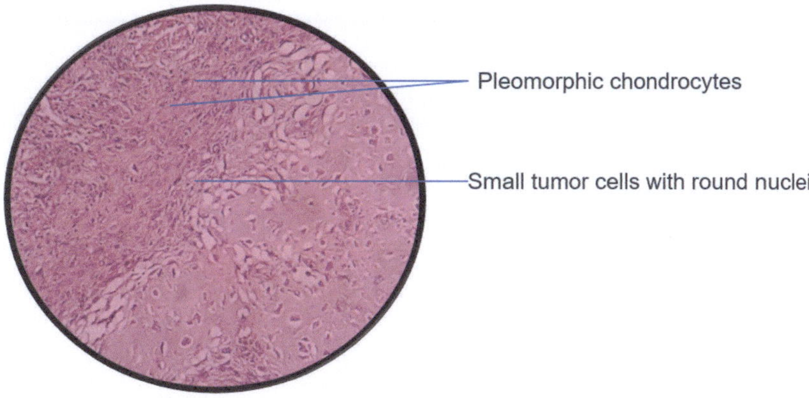

factors. External beam radiation therapy is commonly employed, delivering targeted radiation to the tumour site. Proton therapy may be utilized to minimize radiation exposure to surrounding healthy tissues and critical structures.

- Chemotherapy: The role of chemotherapy in the management of chondrosarcoma is limited, and primarily reserved for unresectable, metastatic, or recurrent cases. Chemotherapy regimens typically consist of agents such as doxorubicin, cisplatin, ifosfamide, and etoposide. The effectiveness of chemotherapy in chondrosarcoma is variable, and individualized treatment plans are tailored based on patient factors, tumour characteristics, and response to treatment.

59.3.7 Prognosis

The prognosis of chondrosarcoma varies depending on factors such as tumour grade, size, location, and the presence of metastasis. Low-grade chondrosarcomas generally have a better prognosis, while high-grade and dedifferentiated chondrosarcomas have a poorer prognosis. Local recurrence and metastasis, most commonly to the lungs, are the main factors affecting overall survival.

59.4 Ewing Sarcoma

Ewing sarcoma is a rare and aggressive malignant bone tumour that primarily affects children and young adults. It accounts for approximately 1–3% of all childhood cancers. Ewing sarcoma is characterized by a translocation between chromosomes 11 and 22, resulting in the formation of an abnormal fusion gene.

59.4.1 Epidemiology

Ewing sarcoma primarily affects children and young adults, with a peak incidence in the second decade of life. It is more common in males than females, and there is a higher incidence in Caucasians compared to other ethnic groups. Ewing sarcoma can arise in any bone, but it most commonly affects the long bones of the extremities, pelvis, and chest wall.

59.4.2 Aetiology and Risk Factors

The exact cause of Ewing sarcoma is unknown. However, it is believed to arise from primitive mesenchymal cells with a neural crest origin. Several genetic predispositions and environmental factors have been implicated, including radiation exposure, certain chromosomal abnormalities, and specific genetic syndromes (e.g. Li-Fraumeni syndrome).

59.4.3 Clinical Presentation

The clinical presentation of Ewing sarcoma can vary depending on the location and size of the tumour. Common symptoms include pain, swelling, and tenderness at the site of the tumour. Patients may also experience fatigue, fever, and weight loss. In some cases, the tumour may cause compression of nearby structures, leading to neurological deficits, respiratory distress, or bowel or bladder dysfunction.

59.4.4 Diagnosis

The diagnosis of Ewing sarcoma is established through a combination of clinical examination, imaging studies, and biopsy. Imaging studies such as X-rays, CT scans, and MRIs are used to visualize the tumour and assess its size and extent.

- X-rays: The appearance of these tumours is very variable, but they usually have an aggressive appearance. Common findings include permeative lesions with lamellated (onion skin) periosteal reaction and sclerosis. They occasionally demonstrate other appearances, including Codman triangles, spiculated (sunburst) or thick periosteal reaction, and even bone expansion or cystic components (Fig. 59.9).
- CT scan: The features seen on CT are the same as on plain film but they are slightly sensitive. CECT (thorax and abdomen) is useful for metastatic workup of patients.
- MRI: In MRI Ewing's sarcoma has low to intermediate signal in T1 and high signal in T2 (Fig. 59.10).
- Bone scans: Ewing sarcomas demonstrate increased uptake on both gallium-67 citrate and all three phases of technetium99m methylene diphosphonate bone scans.
- Histology: A biopsy is performed to confirm the diagnosis and determine the tumour's histological subtype. Ewing sarcoma is characterized by the presence of small round blue cells with a high nuclear-to-cytoplasmic ratio. These cells are uniform in size and shape, typically measuring 10 to 20 μm in diameter. The nuclei are round to ovoid, often exhibiting finely dispersed chromatin and one or more prominent nucleoli. The cytoplasm is scant, pale to eosinophilic, and may show occasional vacuolation (Fig. 59.11).

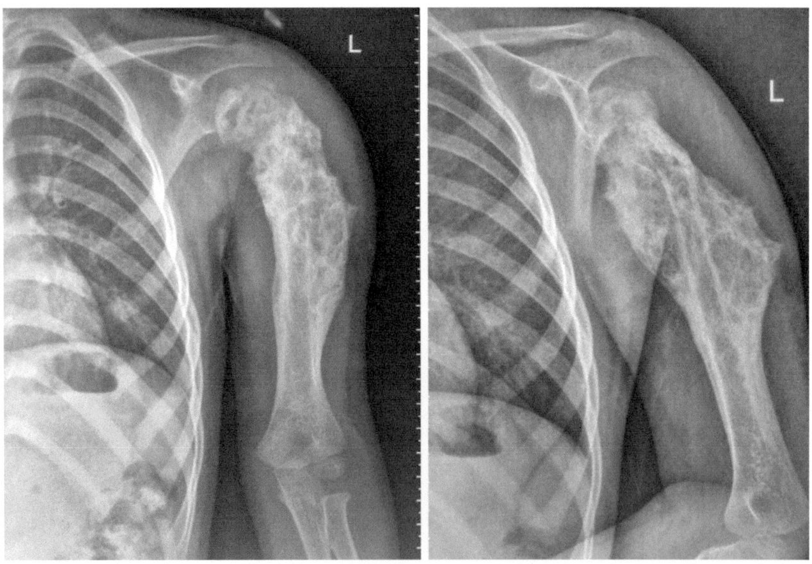

Fig. 59.9 Plain radiograph of left arm AP and lateral view of a 10-year-old male with Ewing sarcoma of left humerus. It shows a permeative lesions with lamellated (onion skin) periosteal reaction appearing Codman triangles due to thick periosteal reaction

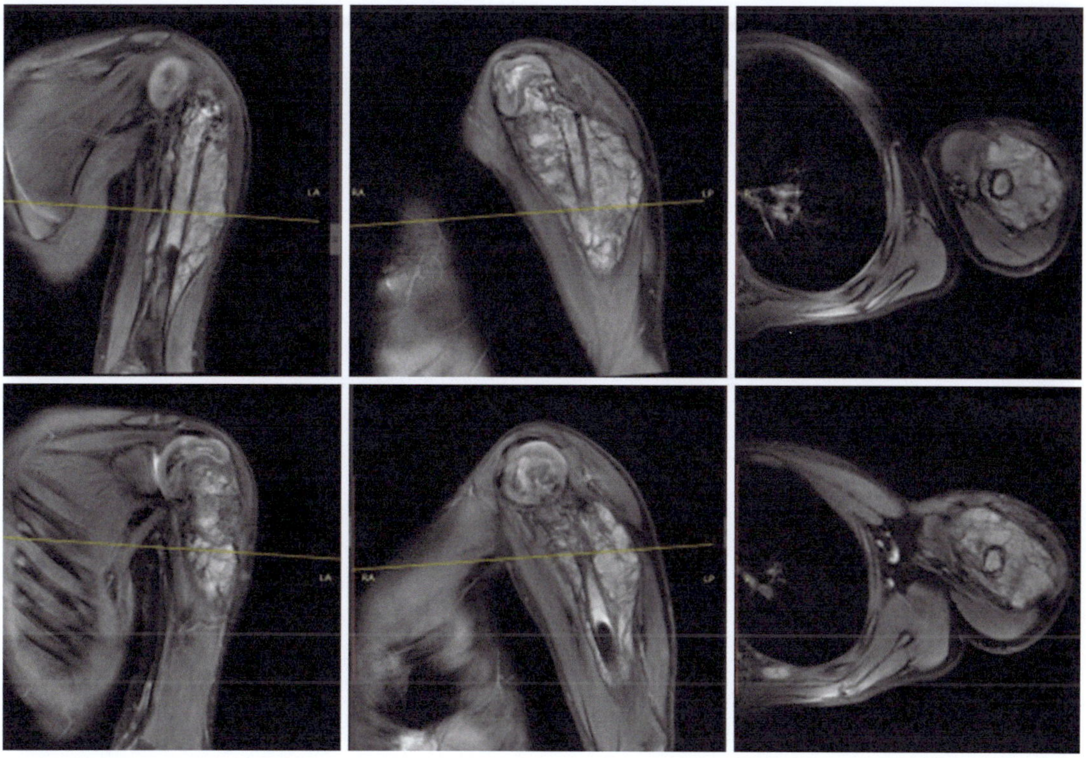

Fig. 59.10 MRI image of Ewing sarcoma of left humerus showing T1 and heterogeneously high signal, and low signal striations in T2

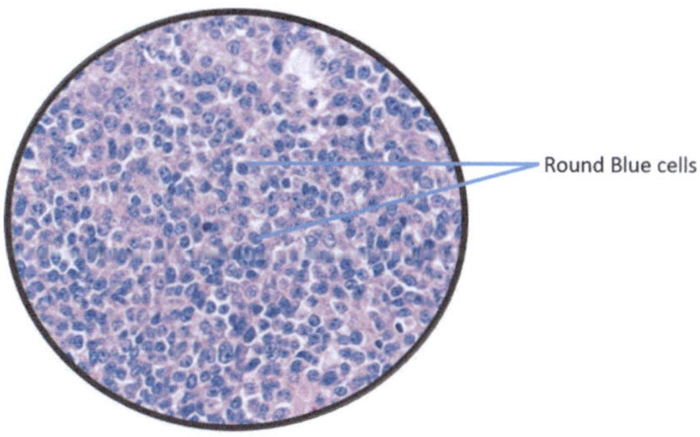

Fig. 59.11 Histopathology image of Ewings sarcoma showing small round blue cells with a high nuclear-to-cytoplasmic ratio

- Immunohistochemical staining: Immunohistochemistry plays a supportive role in the diagnosis of Ewing sarcoma. The tumour cells typically express markers such as CD99 and Friend leukaemia integration-1 transcription factor (FLI1). CD99 is considered the most sensitive and specific marker for Ewing sarcoma and shows membranous and cytoplasmic staining. FLI1, a transcription factor involved in Ewing sarcoma-specific gene fusion, is also commonly positive.

59.4.5 Treatment

The management of Ewing sarcoma requires a multidisciplinary approach involving surgery, radiation therapy, and chemotherapy. Treatment plans are tailored based on various factors, including tumour location, size, grade, and the presence of metastasis.

- Surgical management: Surgery is an essential component of the treatment of Ewing sarcoma and aims to achieve complete resection of the tumour with negative margins. The extent of surgical resection depends on tumour location, size, and patient-specific factors. In some

cases, limb-sparing surgery may be performed to preserve limb function, while in other cases, amputation may be necessary.
- Radiation therapy: Radiation therapy is used as an adjuvant treatment modality for Ewing sarcoma in certain situations. It is particularly considered when the tumour is incompletely resected, there is a high risk of local recurrence, or in cases where surgery is not feasible due to tumour location or patient factors. External beam radiation therapy is commonly employed, delivering targeted radiation to the tumour site.
- Chemotherapy: Chemotherapy is a critical component of the management of Ewing sarcoma and is typically administered before or after surgical resection and radiation therapy. Chemotherapy regimens typically consist of agents such as vincristine, doxorubicin, cyclophosphamide, and ifosfamide. The effectiveness of chemotherapy in Ewing sarcoma is variable, and individualized treatment plans are tailored based on patient factors, tumour characteristics, and response to treatment.

59.4.6 Prognosis

The prognosis of Ewing sarcoma is influenced by various factors, including tumour size, location, grade, and the presence of metastasis. Overall, the survival rates for Ewing sarcoma have improved significantly over the last few decades, with current five-year survival rates approaching 70–80%. Long-term outcomes can be influenced by treatment-related complications.

To summarize, the differences between osteosarcoma, chondrosarcoma, and Ewing sarcoma are tabulated as follows (Table 59.1):

Table 59.1 Summary of malignant bone tumours

Aspect	Osteosarcoma	Chondrosarcoma	Ewing Sarcoma
Age group	Primarily affects teenagers and young adults (10–20 years)	Predominantly affects adults, rare in children (30–40 years)	Primarily affects children and young adults (5–15 years)
Common sites	Distal femur, proximal tibia, humerus	Pelvis, proximal femur, proximal humerus, ribs, shoulder girdle	Femur, pelvis, tibia, humerus, ribs
Location	Metaphysis of long bone	Flat bones	Diaphysis of long bone
Tumour origin	Arises from osteoblasts	Arises from chondrocytes	Arises from primitive mesenchymal cells
Genetic alterations	Variable, including TP53 gene mutations	IDH gene mutations	EWSR1 gene translocation
Histological features	Variable, including production of osteoid	Variable, including chondroid matrix	Small round blue cells
Radiographic findings	Mixed lytic and sclerotic bone lesions	Predominantly lytic or sclerotic bone lesions	Lytic or permeative bone destruction
Metastatic potential	Potential for both local and distant spread	Metastasis is less common	High propensity for distant metastasis
Treatment	Chemotherapy, surgery, and radiation therapy	Surgery (wide/local excision), sometimes radiation or chemotherapy	Chemotherapy, surgery, and radiation therapy
Prognosis	Variable, influenced by tumour grade, extent, and response to treatment	Variable, influenced by tumour grade, size, location, and presence of metastasis	Variable, influenced by factors such as tumour stage, size, and response to treatment

59.5 Multiple Myeloma

Multiple myeloma is a haematological malignancy characterized by the clonal proliferation of plasma cells in the bone marrow. It is the second most common haematological cancer and primarily affects older adults.

59.5.1 Epidemiology

Multiple myeloma accounts for approximately 1% of all cancers and 10% of haematological malignancies. It occurs predominantly in individuals over the age of 60, with a slight male predominance. The incidence of multiple myeloma varies geographically, with higher rates observed in Western countries.

59.5.2 Aetiology and Risk Factors

The exact cause of multiple myeloma is unknown. However, certain risk factors have been identified, including advanced age, male gender, family history of multiple myeloma or monoclonal gammopathy of undetermined significance (MGUS), exposure to radiation or certain chemicals (e.g. benzene), obesity, and certain genetic abnormalities (e.g. chromosomal translocations involving the immunoglobulin heavy chain locus)

59.5.3 Pathophysiology

Multiple myeloma arises from malignant transformation of plasma cells, resulting in the production of monoclonal immunoglobulins (M-proteins). The abnormal plasma cells accumulate in the bone marrow, leading to bone destruction, anaemia, immunodeficiency, and other organ dysfunction. Various genetic and molecular abnormalities, such as mutations in the RAS pathway and dysregulation of cyclin D genes, contribute to the pathogenesis of multiple myeloma.

59.5.4 Clinical Presentation

The clinical presentation of multiple myeloma is diverse and can vary from asymptomatic to symptomatic disease. Common symptoms include bone pain, fatigue, recurrent infections, anaemia, renal dysfunction, hypercalcaemia, and neuropathy. Some patients may present with pathological fractures or spinal cord compression due to bone involvement.

59.5.5 Diagnostic Methods

The diagnosis of multiple myeloma requires a combination of clinical evaluation, laboratory tests, imaging studies, and bone marrow examination.

- Laboratory tests include the following:
  - Serum and urine protein electrophoresis (Fig. 59.12)
  - Serum-free light chain assay,
  - Beta-2 microglobulin
  - Lactate dehydrogenase
- Imaging modalities such as X-rays, CT scans, MRI scans, and PET scans are used to assess bone lesions and evaluate disease extent.
- Definitive diagnosis is made through bone marrow aspiration and biopsy, demonstrating clonal plasma cell infiltration, presence of M-proteins, and specific immune-phenotypic characteristics

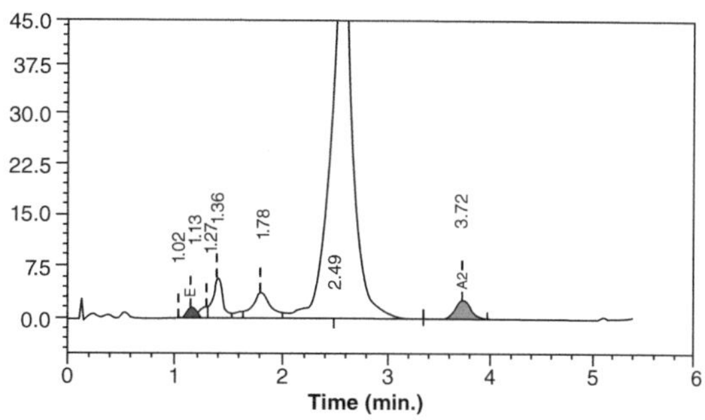

Fig. 59.12 Diagnosis of multiple myeloma by serum protein electrophoresis

59.5.6 Orthopaedic Implications

Flat bones are involved primarily including the spine. The clinical presentation is primarily due to dull pains/fractures. Sometimes, patient may present with neurological deficit due to collapse of vertebra.

X-rays shows multiple 'punched-out' lytic lesions due to osteoclastic bone resorption and lack of osteoblastic activity (Figs. 59.13 and 59.14).

MRI: indicated for pelvis and spine lesions, where the lesion appears to be hypointense on T1 and on T2 (Fig. 59.15).

Bone scans: Bone scans are 'hot' due to radiotracer integration into the inorganic phase of bone caused by osteoblastic activity.

FDG-PET: More sensitive in diagnosing/screening for MM, uptake into cancer cells due to increased glucose metabolism in most types of tumours may uncover additional sites in 'solitary' plasmacytoma.

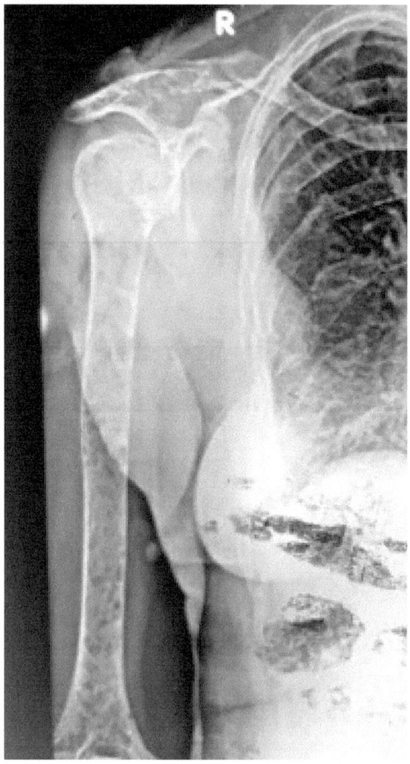

Fig. 59.14 Plain radiograph of left humerus of a multiple myeloma case showing lytic lesion and punched-out lesion

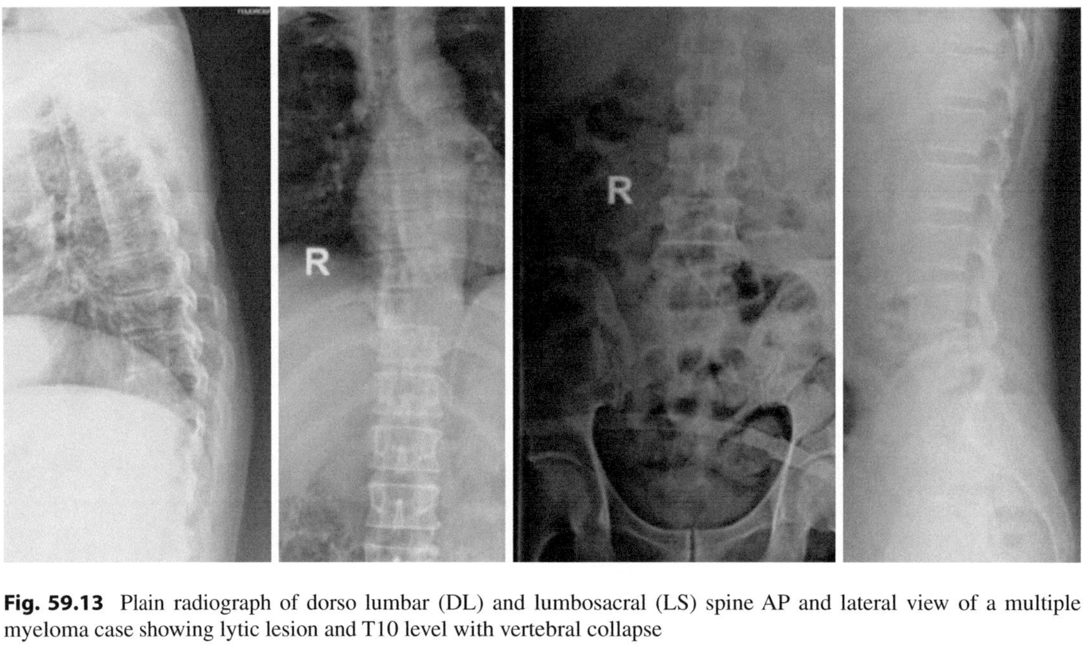

Fig. 59.13 Plain radiograph of dorso lumbar (DL) and lumbosacral (LS) spine AP and lateral view of a multiple myeloma case showing lytic lesion and T10 level with vertebral collapse

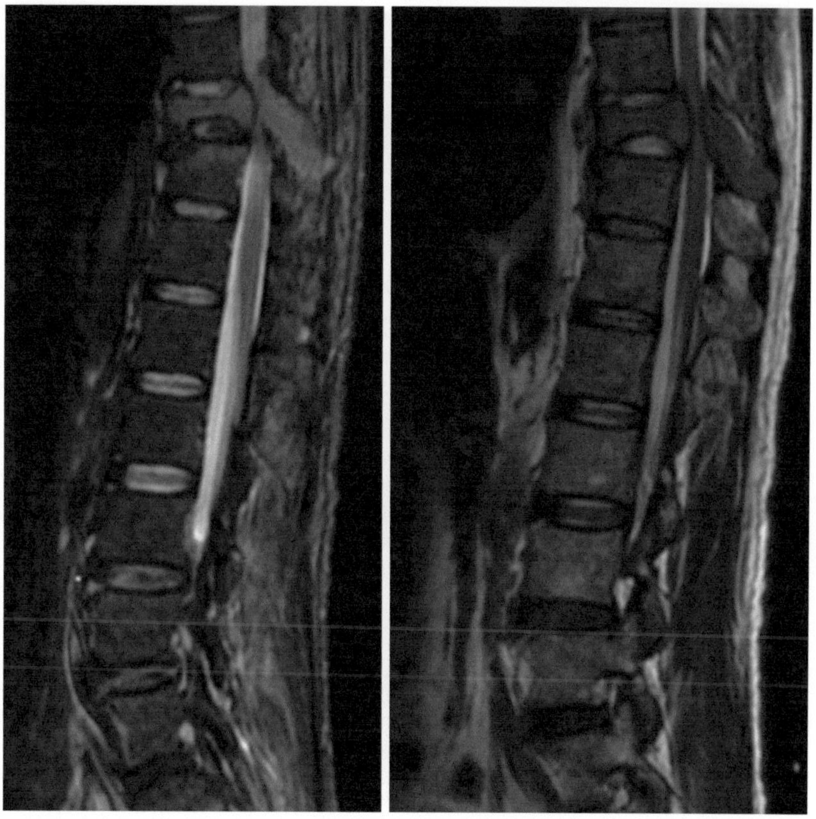

Fig. 59.15 MRI of DL spine of a multiple myeloma vertebral lesion with enhancing paravertebral components with collapse of D10 vertebra with compressive myelopathy

59.5.7 Treatment

The management of multiple myeloma involves a combination of chemotherapy, immunomodulatory drugs, proteasome inhibitors, stem cell transplantation, and supportive care measures.

- Induction therapy aims to achieve deep remission and consists of combination chemotherapy regimens such as bortezomib, lenalidomide, and dexamethasone.
- Autologous stem cell transplantation may be performed in eligible patients.
- Maintenance therapy is often recommended to prolong remission. Supportive care includes bisphosphonates for bone protection, management of infections, and treatment of renal dysfunction.
- Novel therapies and targeted agents: Advancements in the understanding of the molecular basis of multiple myeloma have led to the development of targeted therapies. Monoclonal antibodies, such as daratumumab and elotuzumab, have shown efficacy in the treatment of multiple myeloma. Other promising agents include immunotherapies, such as chimeric antigen receptor (CAR) T-cell therapy and immune checkpoint inhibitors.

Operative: Surgical stabilization and external beam radiation therapy

- Surgical stabilization is indicated if life expectancy >3 months
  - In appendicular skeleton: complete or impending fractures
  - In axial skeleton: vertebral compression fractures with instability or neural compression resistant to radiation

59.5.8 Prognosis

The prognosis of multiple myeloma varies widely depending on factors such as age, stage, cytogenetic abnormalities, and response to treatment. The International Myeloma Working Group (IMWG) has defined response criteria, including stringent complete response, complete response, very good partial response, and partial response. Regular follow-up visits, including laboratory monitoring and imaging studies, are important to assess treatment response, detect relapse, and manage any treatment-related complications.

Multiple Choice Questions

1. A 7-year-old boy with a history of trauma 2 months back now presents with fever and acute pain over thigh. On X-ray, femoral shaft shows lesions with multiple laminated periosteal reaction. Next line of management:
   (a) CRP measurements
   (b) MRI
   (c) Biopsy
   (d) CT scan
2. OGS-12 protocol of treatment of osteosarcoma includes all of the following except
   (a) Methotrexate
   (b) Cisplatin
   (c) Adriamycin
   (d) Ifosfamide
3. Children with germline retinoblastoma are more likely to develop other primary malignancies in their later life. Which of the following can occur in such patients?
   (a) Thyroid carcinoma
   (b) Chondrosarcoma
   (c) Ewings tumour
   (d) Osteosarcoma
4. Which of the following is correct description about bone destruction in Ewing sarcoma
   (a) Non-permeative
   (b) Moth eaten
   (c) Geographic
   (d) Sunburst appearance
5. All of the following investigations are needed for the diagnosis of osteosarcoma except:
   (a) CT chest
   (b) MRI of femur
   (c) Bone marrow biopsy
   (d) Bone scan
6. Which of the following is the most common cause of secondary osteosarcoma?
   (a) Bone infarcts
   (b) Paget's disease
   (c) Osteogenesis imperfecta
   (d) Osteomyelitis
7. A 55-year-old male having bone pains for last two years. On X-ray, skull shows punched-out lytic lesions. What is the most probable diagnosis?
   (a) Osteosarcoma
   (b) Multiple myeloma
   (c) Thalassemia
   (d) Haemangiomas
8. A 15-year-old boy is injured while playing cricket. X-rays of the leg rule out possible fracture. Radiologist reports that boy has an evidence of aggressive bone tumour with both bone destruction and soft tissue mass. The bone biopsy reveals bone cancer with neural differentiation. What is the most likely diagnosis?
   (a) Ewing sarcoma
   (b) Aneurysmal bone cyst
   (c) Osteoblastoma
   (d) Giant cell tumour
9. A patient with pain in back. Laboratory investigation shows elevated erythrocyte sedimentation rate (ESR). X-ray skull shows multiple punched-out lytic lesions. What is the most important investigation to be done?
   (a) Serum acid phosphatase
   (b) Serum electrophoresis
   (c) Whole-body scan
   (d) CT head
10. A 60-year-old male has bone pain, vertebral collapse, and pathological fracture in pelvis. What is the most probable diagnosis?
   (a) Ewing sarcoma
   (b) Chronic osteomyelitis
   (c) Tuberculosis (TB)
   (d) Secondaries

Answers: 1 (b), 2. (a), 3. (d), 4. (b), 5. (c), 6. (b), 7. (b), 8. (a), 9. (b), 10. (d)

Metastasis

60

Mohit Dhingra, Hawaibam Nongdamba, and Gobinder Singh

60.1 Introduction

Metastatic bone tumors are more common than primary bone tumors, with bone metastasis ranking as the third most frequent site of metastasis following the lungs and liver. This condition is most commonly associated with prostate and breast cancer, contributing to up to 70% of skeletal metastases. The incidence of bone metastasis varies by tumor type, with breast and prostate cancers leading the list at 65–75%, followed by thyroid, lung, bladder, renal cell carcinoma, and melanoma. Notably, bone metastases tend to occur more frequently in the spine, followed by the proximal femur and humerus. These metastases can lead to various complications, including pain, fractures, impaired mobility, and other serious health issues.

60.2 Pathogenesis of Bone Metastasis

Metastasis to bone involves a complex process driven by several mechanisms. Factors such as the hematopoietically active red bone marrow and the paravertebral network contribute to bone metastases' prevalence in the axial skeleton. The tumor microenvironment also plays a role in facilitating tumor cell survival within the bone. Successful extravasation of circulating tumor cells involves interactions with endothelium through chemo attractive and adhesion molecules. Essential molecules such as vascular cell adhesion molecule (VCAM), E-selectin, chemokines, integrin, osteopoitin, and collagen type I influence cancer cell retention and colonization. Unique expressions in different cancers, like receptor activator of nuclear

Dedicated to "Naina"

M. Dhingra (✉)
Department of Orthopedics, All India Institute of Medical Sciences, Rishikesh, Uttarakhand, India

H. Nongdamba
Department of Orthopedics, RIMS, IMPHAL, India

G. Singh
Department of Orthopedics, B R Ambedkar institute of medical sciences, Mohali, India

V. Kumar et al. (eds.), *A Quick Guide to Essential Orthopedics*,
https://doi.org/10.1007/978-981-95-2676-5_60

factor - kB ligand (RANK) in breast cancer and sialoprotein in non-small-cell lung cancer, facilitate binding to bone structures. The bone microenvironment further supports metastatic growth through bone formation and reabsorption, releasing growth-promoting factors.

60.3 Epithelial–Mesenchymal Transition

Cancer cells can undergo an epithelial–mesenchymal transition, enabling them to acquire invasive characteristics. Although this process is typical during embryogenesis, in cancer cells, it promotes an invasive phenotype, facilitating migration to new environments.

60.4 Types of Bone Metastasis Lesions

Bone metastases are classified into three main types: osteolytic, osteoblastic, and mixed. Osteolytic metastases involve the destruction of normal bone and are common in multiple myeloma, melanoma, lung cancer, and more. Osteoblastic metastases are characterized by new bone deposition and are prevalent in prostate cancer, carcinoid tumors, and others. Mixed metastases feature both osteolytic and osteoblastic components.

60.5 Clinical Features

Clinical manifestations of bone metastasis can vary based on location, extent, and primary cancer type. Common symptoms include pain (often worse at night or during activity), pathological fractures, decreased mobility, spinal cord compression, nerve compression, and hypercalcemia. A Mirel scoring system aids in predicting fracture risk (Table 60.1).

Prophylactic fixation is indicated for a lesion with overall score ≥ 9.

Table 60.1 Mirel scoring system for pathological fracture prediction

Score	1	2	3
Site	Upper limb	Lower limb	Trochanteric
Pain	Mild	Moderate	Functional
Type of lesion	Blastic	Mixed	Lytic
Size of lesion	< 1/3rd cortex	1/3rd– 2/3rd cortex	>2/3rdcortex

60.6 Evaluation

Evaluating suspected bone metastasis involves medical history, physical examination, blood tests (complete blood count [CBC], liver function tests [LFTs], prostate-specific antigen [PSA], carcinoembryonic antigen [CEA], CA 15-3), imaging (X-rays, computed tomography [CT], magnetic resonance imaging [MRI], bone scans, positron emission tomography [PET]), and biopsy. Blood tests help detect abnormalities, while imaging provides detailed insights into bone lesions. Biopsy confirms the diagnosis.

60.7 Blood Test Evaluation

Blood tests hold a crucial role in the diagnostic process of bone metastasis. Routine blood assessments encompass essential components like complete blood count (CBC), liver function tests (LFTs), serum calcium levels, alkaline phosphatase levels, and specialized tumor markers. In the case of men, prostate-specific antigen (PSA) levels are evaluated, while carcinoembryonic antigen (CEA) and CA 15-3 levels are analyzed for women. Elevated levels of alkaline phosphatase and calcium often serve as indicators of potential bone metastasis. Similarly, elevated PSA, CEA, and CA 15-3 levels provide valuable insights into potential underlying prostate, colorectal, and breast cancers. Additional markers, such as serum lactate dehydrogenase (LDH), C-reactive protein (CRP), erythrocyte sedimentation rate (ESR), and serum/urine immunoelectrophoresis (SPEP, UPEP), can contribute to both confirming the diagnosis and monitoring the progression of the disease.

60.8 Imaging Techniques

The evaluation of bone metastasis relies on a diverse range of imaging techniques:

- Plain radiography: Often constituting the initial step, plain radiography yields preliminary insights into lesion types and any associated fractures (Figs. 60.1 and 60.2).
- Computed tomography (CT) scans: CT scans provide intricate cross-sectional information, offering detailed views of bone structures and adjacent soft tissues. Their efficacy is particularly pronounced in identifying bone degradation and gauging the extent of bone involvement. For individuals above 50 years, CT scans of the thorax, abdomen, and pelvis are recommended to comprehensively assess potential primary lesions that might be linked to bone metastasis (Fig. 60.3).
- Magnetic resonance imaging (MRI): This technique emerges as a sensitive tool for the early detection of bone metastases. MRI yields intricate anatomical data encompassing bones and the encompassing soft tissues, enabling the identification of even the minutest lesions. MRI's capabilities extend to the detection of bone marrow involvement, evaluating the scope of soft tissue impact, and ruling out spinal cord compression, a particularly relevant consideration in cases of suspected spinal bone metastases (Fig. 60.4a, b).
- Bone scintigraphy: Employing a radioactive tracer injected into the bloodstream, bone scintigraphy highlights potential metastatic sites by accumulating within bones. This method's capacity to detect metastases prior to their visibility in plain radiography sets it apart, with the capability to identify lesions as small as 1 centimeter. It is worth noting that while bone scintigraphy offers notable benefits, its results may entail a degree of ambiguity compared to other imaging techniques, occasionally indicating elevated tracer uptake in nonmalignant conditions like arthritis or infection (Fig. 60.5).
- PET imaging: The significance of positron emission tomography (PET) imaging lies in its ability to identify metastases in soft tissues and organs, including bones. Often integrated with CT or MRI scans, PET provides an advanced understanding of metastatic location and extent.

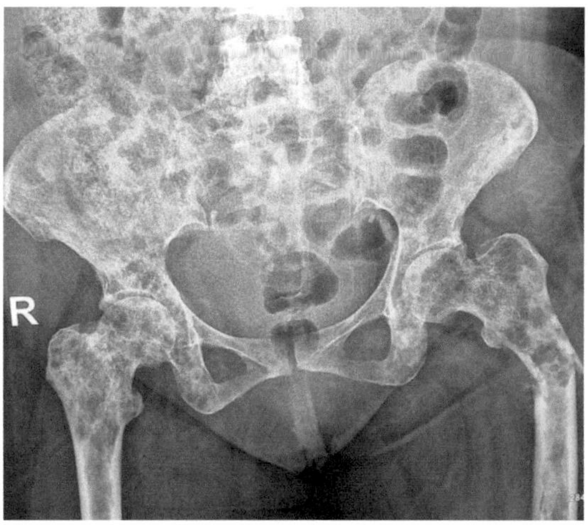

Fig. 60.1 X-ray pelvis with b/l hip showing multiple lytic lesion at b/l proximal femur and pelvic bone with pathological subtrochanteric fracture left side in a case of breast carcinoma s/o metastatic bone lesion

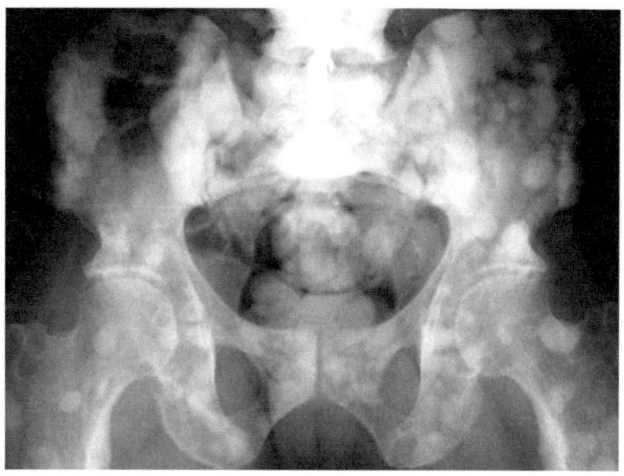

Fig. 60.2 X-ray pelvis with b/l hip showing sclerotic (blastic lesion) at b/l proximal femur and pelvic bone in a case of prostate cancer

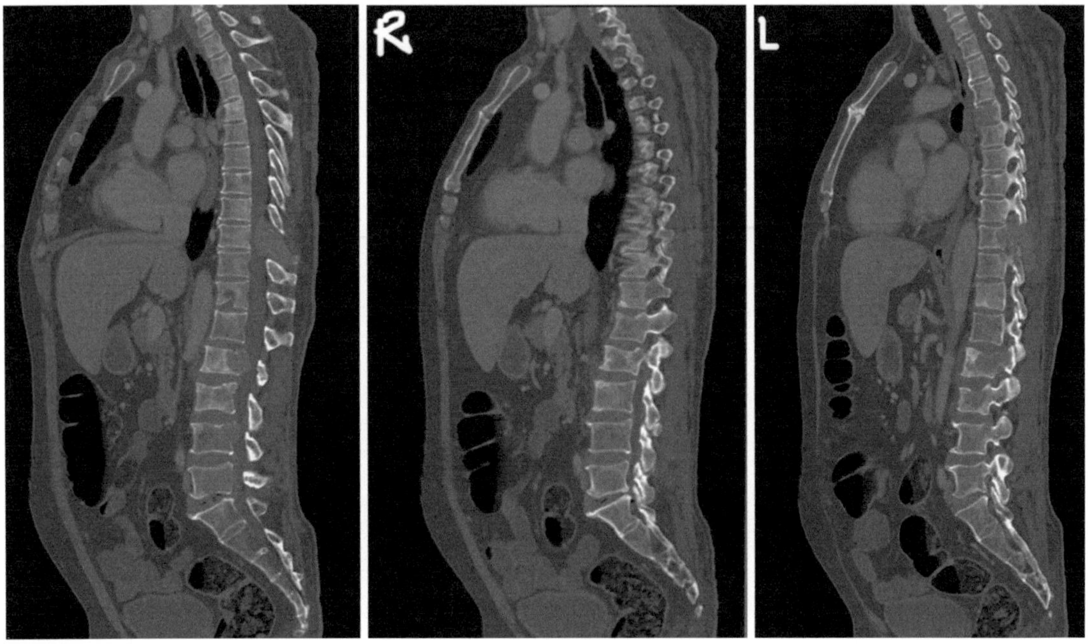

Fig. 60.3 Sagittal CT image of thoracoabdomen showing lytic lesion in multiple vertebrae and compression fracture s/o multiple skeletal metastasis

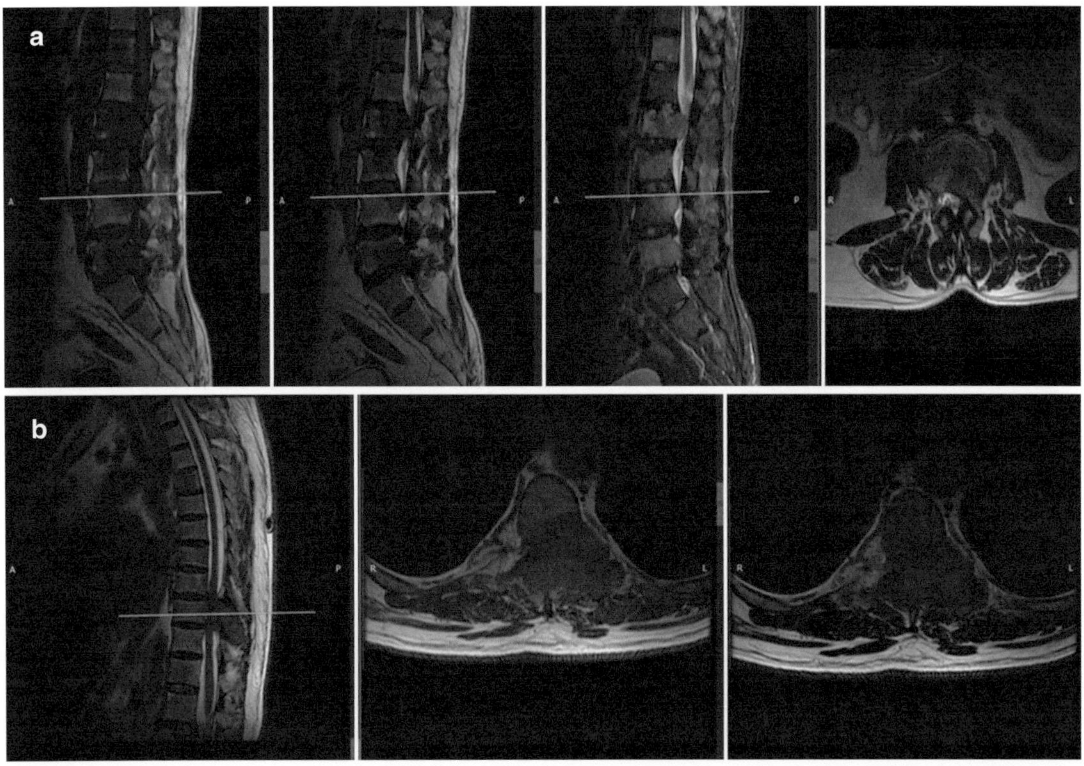

Fig. 60.4 (**a**, **b**) MRI image showing multiple vertebral lesions with enhancing para-osseous components with pathological fracture/collapse of few vertebra and compressive neuropathy multiple lumbar spine level s/o metastatic vertebrae with cord compression

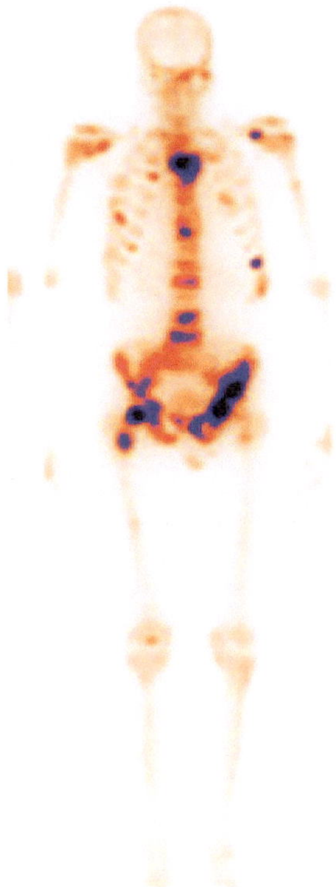

Fig. 60.5 Bone scintigraphy showing metastasis involving pelvic bone, multiple vertebrae in prostate cancer

60.9 Biopsy

Biopsy stands as a pivotal element in definitively confirming the presence of bone metastasis. During a biopsy, a minute tissue sample is extracted from the affected bone and meticulously examined under a microscope by a specialized pathologist. This comprehensive assessment serves the purpose of distinguishing between primary bone tumors and metastatic growths. Beyond establishing the diagnosis, biopsy outcomes provide a wealth of information pertaining to the specific cancer type, its aggressiveness, its responsiveness to treatment, and the overall prognosis.

60.10 Treatment

Nonoperative and operative approaches are used for treatment. Nonoperative options include bisphosphonates, denosumab, radiation therapy, chemotherapy, and hormone therapy. Bisphosphonates and denosumab prevent skeletal events and hypercalcemia. Radiation therapy provides pain relief and local control. Operative treatment includes fracture stabilization (Fig. 60.6), followed by radiation. Prophylactic stabilization may be used for impending fractures. Stereotactic radiosurgery is emerging as an effective option. Bone metastasis in spine with neurological symptoms is managed by neurologic decompression and stabilization of spine followed by postoperative radiotherapy (Fig. 60.7).

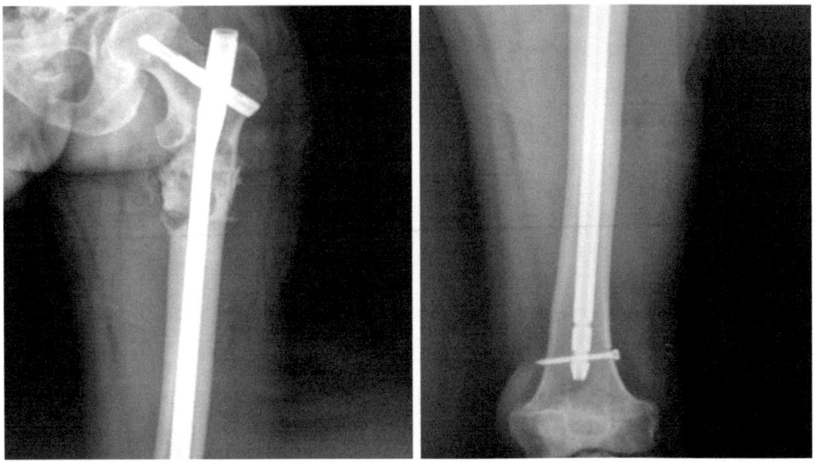

Fig. 60.6 X-ray of left hip with thigh anteroposterior (AP) view showing pathological subtrochanteric fracture in a case of laryngeal cancer managed by cephalomedullary nail

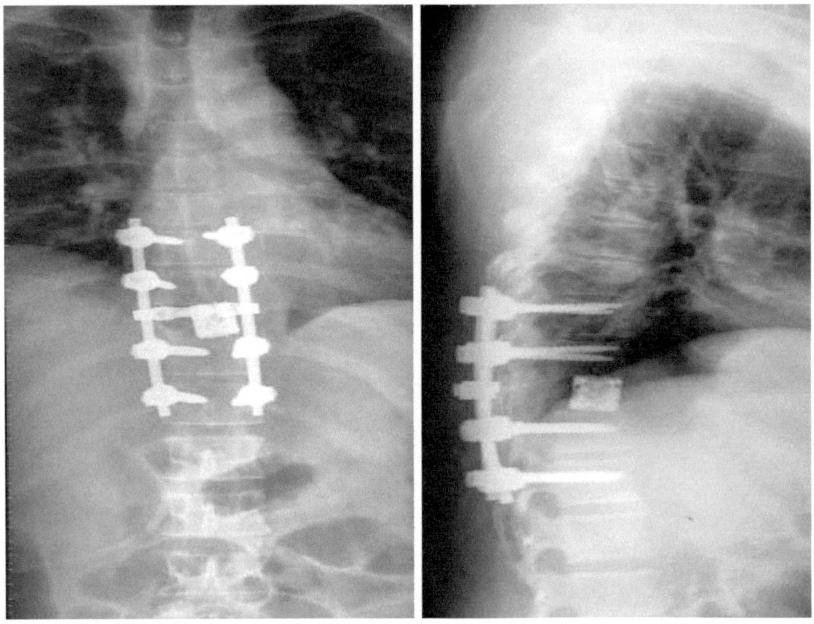

Fig. 60.7 X-ray of dorsal lumbar (DL) spine AP and lateral view showing instrumentation D8-D12 with anteior column re-alignment (ACR) with expandable cage D10 for metastatic D10 vertebrae

60.11 Prognosis

Survival varies by primary cancer site, ranging from 6 months in lung cancer to 48 months in thyroid cancer. Early diagnosis and appropriate treatment can significantly impact survival.

Multiple Choice Questions

1. A 63-year-old male presented with difficulty in lifting objects from right hand with moderate pain with difficulty in breathing and loss of weight of 12 kg in previous

2 months. He was referred to orthopedist for thigh pain for which the doctor advised an X-ray of thigh region. On X-ray, there is lytic lesion involving one-third diameter of femur.
Which classification is used and what is your management plan?
(a) Harington and you will manage him conservatively only
(b) Mirel and you will manage him conservatively only
(c) Harington and you will do prophylactic fixation
(d) Mirel and you will do prophylactic fixation
2. The common sites of bone metastatic lesions
(a) Spine > distal femur > humerus
(b) Spine > proximal femur > proximal tibia
(c) Spine > proximal femur > humerus
(d) Spine > distal femur > proximal tibia
3. Preoperative embolization is used in the treatment of pathological fractures secondary to which cancer?
(a) Renal cell carcinoma
(b) Thyroid
(c) Both
(d) None of the above
4. What type of bone lesion would you expect in Langerhans cell histiocytosis?
(a) Osteolytic
(b) Osteoblastic
(c) Both
(d) No bone lesion
5. Non-small cell lung cancer expresses what protein that facilitates them to bind with type 1 collagen?
(a) Metalloproteinase
(b) Sialoprotein
(c) Integrin
(d) Selectin
6. A 58-Year-old female was recently found to have malignant bone tumor which was found to be metastatic in origin. Which of the following be the most common source of metastasis?
(a) Lung
(b) Ovaries
(c) Kidney
(d) Breast
7. Which is the most common malignant lesion of the bone?
(a) Multiple myeloma
(b) Ewing sarcoma
(c) Osteosarcoma
(d) Metatstasis
8. Which of the following are not false?
(a) 1. Ewing sarcoma is the most common malignant lesion of bone.
(b) 2. In children, neuroblastoma is the most common cause of metastatic bone tumor.
(c) 3. Ewing sarcoma can metastasize from one bone to another.
1. a. Only 1 is correct
2. b. 1 and 3 are correct
3. c. 2 and 3 are correct
4. d. All are correct
9. Which of the following imaging techniques is often used to diagnose bone metastasis and assess its extent?
(a) Electrocardiogram (ECG or EKG)
(b) Magnetic resonance imaging (MRI)
(c) Colonoscopy
(d) Pap smear
10. Which of the following treatments is commonly used to manage bone pain and complications caused by bone metastasis?
(a) Chemotherapy
(b) Radiation therapy
(c) Antibiotic therapy
(d) Psychotherapy

Answers: 1. (d), 2. (c), 3. (a), 4. (a), 5. (c), 6. (d), 7. (d), 8. (c), 9. (b), 10. (b)

Further Reading

1. Chambers A, Naumov G, Varghese H, et al. Critical steps in hematogenous metastasis: an overview. Surg Oncol Clin N Am. 2001;10:243–55.
2. Luzzi KJ, MacDonald IC, Schmidt EE, et al. Multistep nature of metastatic inefficiency: dormancy of solitary cells after successful extravasation and limited survival of early micrometastases. Am J Pathol. 1998;153:865–73.
3. Coleman R. Metastatic bone disease: clinical features, pathophysiology and treatment strategies. Cancer Treat Rev. 2001;27:165–76.
4. Selvaggi G, Scagliotti G. Management of bone metastases in cancer: a review. Clin Rev Oncol Hematol. 2005;56:365–78.

Part VII

Spine Disorders

61 Approach to a Patient with Low Back Pain

Aakash Jain and Vishal Kumar

61.1 Introduction

Low back pain (LBP) is an extremely common problem for patients to seek medical care in both primary care and emergency settings. The etiologies differ depending on the patient population, but most commonly, it is mechanical or nonspecific. Inflammatory disorders, malignancy, trauma, osteoporosis, radiculopathy, degenerative disc disease, sacroiliac joint dysfunction, spine deformity, or infection are all parts of the differential. Distinguishing mechanical back pain from radiculopathy is an essential first step in the diagnosis of back pain. Also, certain conditions such as cauda equina syndrome, tumors, and chronic tubercular infection can present with back pain as the chief complaint. Knowing the typical red flag signs (discussed here) aids in diagnosis. The current chapter will help readers understand the etiology of back pain, how to evaluate and reach a diagnosis based on history and clinical examination alone, and how to treat back pain via pharmacological, interventional, surgical, non-pharmacological, and/or alternative treatment modalities.

A. Jain (✉)
Department of Orthopedics, All India Institute of Medical Sciences, Rishikesh, Uttarakhand, India

V. Kumar
Department of Orthopaedics, PGIMER, Chandigarh, Chandigarh, India

61.2 Etiology

Causes of LBP are broken mainly into five primary categories:

(a) *Mechanical*: Most commonly, this is due to injury to the spine, intervertebral discs, or soft tissues. Disc herniation is a common type of traumatic back pain. Pregnancy is also a mechanical cause of back pain.
(b) *Degenerative:* Osteoarthritis of the spine includes facet joint osteoarthritis, sacroiliac joint osteoarthritis, spinal stenosis, osteoporotic compressive fractures, and degenerative disc disease.
(c) *Inflammatory:* This is caused primarily due to inflammatory (seronegative) spondyloarthropathies such as ankylosing spondylitis. Sacroiliitis is most commonly seen.
(d) *Oncologic:* This is caused by lytic lesions of the spine, cancers of the marrow, or compressive nerve phenomena from adjacent space-occupying lesions, often presenting as a pathological fracture.
(e) *Infections:* Infections of the spine, discs, epidural spaces, or muscular/soft tissue abscesses.

V. Kumar et al. (eds.), *A Quick Guide to Essential Orthopedics*,
https://doi.org/10.1007/978-981-95-2676-5_61

61.3 History and Physical Examination

A thorough history and physical examination are essential in the evaluation of LBP patients in both adult and pediatric populations.

The mechanism of injury, the intensity, and the quality and nature of pain help narrow the differentials. The alleviating and provoking factors of back pain can illuminate. Furthermore, past medical and family history and social history can also change the most likely working diagnosis. The character of the pain can help differentiate neuropathic pain from nociceptive pain, while the duration of pain helps establish the acute or chronic nature of the pain. Radiation of pain is a useful tool to assess radicular symptoms. The severity of pain also gives an insight to the clinician about the impact of the illness or injury on the patient's quality of life. Associated constitutional symptoms such as fever, weight loss, loss of appetite, night bowel, and bladder changes direct toward severe pathology. The history of neurogenic claudication is usually suggestive of lumbar canal stenosis.

Physical examination is done in sitting, standing, and lying positions. It includes inspection, palpation, range of motion, strength testing, provocative maneuvers, and neurological assessment. A straight leg raise test (SLRT) can be completed by raising the patient's leg to 30–70 degrees. Ipsilateral leg pain at less than 60 degrees is a positive test for lumbar disc herniation. Pain with the hyperextension of the back is suggestive of a pars interarticularis defect.

61.4 Further Evaluation

After proper history and physical examination, a provisional diagnosis with few differentials is made. To confirm, the diagnosis patient is subjected to radiological investigations. Anteroposterior and lateral plain radiographs are obtained to evaluate for bony pathology. Magnetic resonance imaging (MRI) aids in the evaluation of soft tissue lesions, disc desiccation, nerve root/cord compression secondary to bulging disc, and infective or malignant lesion. In addition to imaging, laboratory evaluation may be considered in the presence of red flag signs. Complete blood count, erythrocyte sedimentation rate (ESR), and quantitative C-reactive protein (CRPH) are done. Rheumatological assays such as HLA-B27, antinuclear antibody (ANA), rheumatoid factor (RF), and anti-cyclic citrullinated peptide (CCP) are considered in the presence of signs and symptoms suggestive of inflammatory pathology.

61.5 Differential Diagnosis

Below is the list of the conditions which are most likely and most disquieting that make up the differentials:

(a) Lumbosacral muscle strains/sprains: traumatic incident or repetitive overuse, pain worse with movement, better with rest, restricted range of motion, tenderness to palpation of muscles.
(b) Lumbar degenerative disc disease: patient typically is greater than 40 years old; pain may be present or radiate from hips; pain with extension or rotation.
(c) Disk herniation: usually involves the L4 to S1 segments and may include paresthesia, sensory change, loss of strength, or reflexes depending on the severity and nerve root involved.
(d) Infection: tubercular or pyogenic discitis, septic sacroiliitis, epidural abscess, and paraspinal muscle abscess.
(e) Spondylolysis, spondylolisthesis: spondylolisthesis may present back pain with radiation to the buttock and posterior thighs.
(f) Vertebral compression fracture: localized back pain worse with flexion; point tenderness on palpation; may be acute or occur insidiously over time; and age, chronic steroid use, and osteoporosis are risk factors.
(g) Tumor: history of metastatic cancer, unexplained weight loss, and focal tenderness to palpation in the setting of risk factors.

Table 61.1 Red flags

Indications that LBP may involve underlying conditions
(a) Patient demographics
(b) Age > 70 years
(c) History of malignancy
(d) Glucocorticoid or immunosuppressive drug therapy
(e) Alcohol or IV drug abuse
Historical features
(a) Weight loss
(b) Fever
(c) The pain increased with rest
Neurological symptoms
(a) Saddle anesthesia
(b) Bladder or bowel dysfunction
(c) Progressive motor weakness

61.6 Principles of Management of LBP

1. History and physical examination to identify risk factors (Table 61.1). Further evaluation is usually unnecessary in patients without red flags because acute LBP improves in 1 month in the majority of cases.
2. Reassess if pain persists after 4–6 weeks of conservative management. Obtain plain radiographs and basic laboratory studies such as CBC and inflammatory markers to screen for any systemic illness.
3. MRI to confirm for any herniated disc or to evaluate lumbar canal stenosis, neoplasm, infection, and other lesions.
4. Electromyography in selected patients is useful in differentiating lumbar radiculopathy from other causes of radicular leg pain.

61.7 Drug Therapy

Usually, patients start initially with acetaminophen or nonsteroidal anti-inflammatory drugs (NSAIDs) for mild-to-moderate pain. Opioids, muscle relaxants, and tricyclic antidepressants, and gabapentin analogs are used along with NSAIDs.

61.8 Therapeutic Injections for LBP

A couple of injection therapies used most commonly in pain management such as trigger point injections, selective joint injections, and epidural injections with steroids have shown to be effective for pain with a significant inflammatory component.

61.8.1 Physical Modalities of LBP

Therapeutic heat (40–45 degree Celsius): Superficial heat (hot packs) for 20–30 minutes, or deep heat (ultrasound for 5–10 minutes). Cryotherapy, electrotherapy like transcutaneous nerve stimulators (TENS), is mainly used for chronic LBP.

61.8.2 Exercise Rehabilitation for LBP

Active exercises are proven to be more effective than rest since it decreases the amount of adhesion and muscle atrophy and increases tissue circulation and oxygenation. Back and core muscle strengthening exercises are recommended for strength training.

Operative interventions for LBP require a multidisciplinary approach. Microdiscectomy is a standard operation for the prolapsed lumbar disc. More extensive operations like laminectomy or addition of instrumentation or less invasive procedures have to be tailored to specific cases.

Multiple-Choice Questions

1. A 35-year-old female came to OPD with the chief complaint of new-onset LBP. Which of the following is indicative of an organic cause of LBP symptoms?
   (a) Positive straight leg raise test
   (b) Pain with axial loading of the spine

   (c) Lower extremity numbness in a non-dermatomal pattern
   (d) Diffuse tenderness over the paraspinal area
2. Which of the following is the best initial study for the diagnostic evaluation of diskogenic LBP?
   (a) MRI
   (b) Diskography
   (c) CT
   (d) Radiography
3. The structure responsible for maintaining the water content of IVD is
   (a) Aggrecan
   (b) Type 1 collagen
   (c) Type 2 collagen
   (d) Versican
4. Which of the following is not true regarding lumbar canal stenosis?
   (a) Associated with chronic low back pain
   (b) Associated with neurogenic claudication
   (c) Pain relief with spine extension
   (d) Pain relief with spine flexion
5. During a spine examination, the passive elevation of the lower extremity between 30 and 70 degrees causes radiating pain from the patient's low back to distal to the knee. The physical maneuver is known as:
   (a) Femoral nerve stretch test
   (b) Hoffman's test
   (c) Straight leg raise test
   (d) Spurling's test

Answer: 1. (a), 2. (d), 3. (a), 4. (c), 5. (c)

Further Reading

1. Urits I, Burshtein A, Sharma M, Testa L, Gold PA, Orhurhu V, Viswanath O, Jones MR, Sidransky MA, Spektor B, Kaye AD. Low back pain, a comprehensive review: pathophysiology, diagnosis, and treatment. Curr Pain Headache Rep. 2019;23(3):23. https://doi.org/10.1007/s11916-019-0757-1. PMID: 30854609.
2. Duffy RL. Low back pain: an approach to diagnosis and management. Prim Care. 2010;37(4):729–741, vi. https://doi.org/10.1016/j.pop.2010.07.003. PMID: 21050954.
3. Knezevic NN, Candido KD, Vlaeyen JWS, Van Zundert J, Cohen SP. Low back pain. Lancet. 2021;398(10294):78–92. https://doi.org/10.1016/S0140-6736(21)00733-9. Epub 2021 Jun 8. PMID: 34115979.
4. Casiano VE, Sarwan G, Dydyk AM, Varacallo M. Back Pain. 2023. In: StatPearls [Internet]. Treasure Island: StatPearls Publishing; 2023. PMID: 30844200.

Intervertebral Disc Anatomy and Degeneration

62

Aakash Jain

62.1 Introduction

The intervertebral disc (IVD) is a fibrocartilaginous structure with the primary function of shock absorption, transmitting compressive loads between vertebral bodies. IVD is composed of three main components: the cartilaginous endplates, the central nucleus pulposus, and the peripherally located annulus fibrosus.

Cartilaginous endplates are a bilayer of cartilage and bone that separates the IVD from the vertebral body. It typically serves as a growth plate for the vertebral bodies. In infancy, the end plates are thick and thin as the growth progresses and eventually consist of only a 1-mm-thick, avascular layer of hyaline cartilage in adults.

The nucleus pulposus lies between adjacent endplates and forms the gel-like core of the disc. It is a highly hydrated structure predominantly composed of proteoglycans (PGs) interspersed within an irregular mesh of type 2 collagen and elastin fibres. Proteoglycans have numerous highly anionic glycosaminoglycan (GAG) side chains (chondroitin sulfate and keratan sulfate), which allows the nucleus to imbibe water. The primary proteoglycan is aggrecan, a highly hydrophilic molecule that provides the osmotic properties necessary to resist compression. Cells are chondrocyte-like, and they synthesize mostly proteoglycans and type 2 collagen in response to changes in hydrostatic pressure. The nucleus acts as a pressurized deformable sphere that dissipates compressive forces to the annulus and the adjacent vertebral bodies.

The annulus fibrosus surrounds the nucleus and is composed of concentrically arranged primarily type 1 collagen fibres. Fibres of the outer annulus attach to the periphery of the vertebral bodies, whereas inner fibres pass from one endplate to another. Arranged between lamellae are the cells ranging from fibroblasts to chondrocytes. The annulus controls the nucleus pulposus and maintains its pressurization under compressive loads. The tensile properties of the annulus allow the nucleus to regain its original shape once the compressive load is reduced (Fig. 62.1).

A. Jain (✉)
Department of Orthopedics, All India Institute of Medical Sciences, Rishikesh, Uttarakhand, India

V. Kumar et al. (eds.), *A Quick Guide to Essential Orthopedics*,
https://doi.org/10.1007/978-981-95-2676-5_62

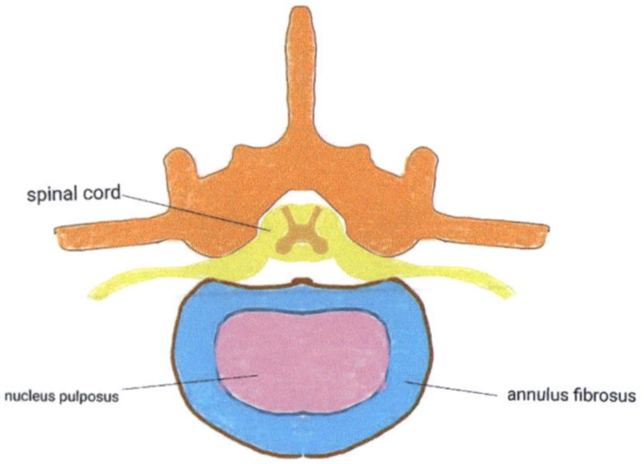

Fig. 62.1 Anatomy of IVD. (Source: Orthobullets)

62.2 Blood Supply and Nutrition

In early foetal life, vascular channels traverse the endplates, but they decrease in size starting at birth until complete disappearance by 5 years of age. In adulthood, IVD derives blood supply from capillary plexuses. As one of the largest avascular structures in the body, intervertebral discs rely almost entirely on diffusion for their nutrition. Small molecules (i.e. glucose and oxygen) readily leave vertebral capillaries and diffuse across the thin vertebral endplates and outer annulus. The oxygen tension in the disc is low, which leads to anaerobic metabolism (i.e. glycolysis) and consequently higher concentrations of lactic acid. Metabolic by-products are also excreted from the disc by diffusion in the opposite direction of nutrient entry.

62.3 Innervation

In a normal disc, only the outer 1–2 mm of atrial fibrillation (AF) is innervated and the rest of the annulus and nucleus are avascular and devoid of any innervation. Endplates are innervated by the basivertebral nerve.

62.4 The Molecular Composition of the IVD

The three major constituents of the disc are water, fibrillar collagens, and aggrecan. The function of the disc depends primarily on the properties of the extracellular matrix (ECM). The ECM provides biomechanical properties and acts as a filter to regulate extracellular fluid composition. The major component of the IVD is water, and its concentration is regulated by the GAG side chains of PGs. The concentrations of the water vary with age, location within the disc, and body position. The nucleus pulposus is most highly hydrated, which decreases as age advances.

62.5 Intervertebral Disc: Ageing and Degeneration

IVD degeneration mimics age-related changes in the discs, but the process occurs prematurely or at an accelerated rate and may result in symptoms. The most physiologically important changes of disc degeneration start in the nucleus. Early changes include increased degradation of aggrecan and other aggregating PGs. This impairs the diffusion of nutrients and oxygen throughout the disc. This diminishes the diffusion capacity of the disc. Loss of proteoglycans and GAGs leads to decreased ability to imbibe water, resulting in reduced swelling pressure, loss of hydration, and loss of disc height. The changes result in altered responses to applied biomechanical loads, ultimately leading to the structural features of degeneration.

IVD degeneration also results in disorganization and destruction of the collagen network. As the overall proteoglycan and water content decreases, there is a corresponding increase in collagen content. The highly organized collagen fibre arrangements of the annulus are also disrupted, and collagen and elastin networks become more haphazard. Kirkaldy-Willis and Farfan hypothesized that the course of disc degeneration is characterized by three stages: temporary dysfunction, instability, and stabilization.

The spectrum of disc degeneration

1. Internal disc disruption
2. Disc herniation
3. Degenerative spondylolisthesis
4. Spinal stenosis
5. Adult spinal deformities

62.5.1 Causes of Disc Degeneration

Disc degeneration was earlier linked to constitutional and environmental causes such as age, sex, occupation, smoking, and vibration. However, genetic factors such as vitamin D receptor polymorphism have also been implemented in the pathogenesis of disc degeneration.

Degeneration of the disc also affects the facets as well as the ligaments and vertebral bodies. Due to loss of disc height, instability, and altered biomechanics, there is an increase in the loads borne by the facets, generating cartilage damage and subluxation of the facet joint. Nociceptive nerve endings have been found around the facet joints, implicating them as a source of pain generator.

62.5.2 Grading of Disc Degeneration

Disc degeneration is primarily graded based on MRI findings (Table 62.1). However, the association between MRI findings and disc-related pain is not direct. Grading can also be done on discography; however, it is not done commonly due to the wider availability of MRI.

Pfirrmann grading of disc degeneration is done on MRI.

Table 62.1 Pfirrmann grading of disc degeneration

Grade	Structure	Annular–nuclear distinction	Signal intensity	IVD height
1	Homogenous bright white	Clear	Hyperintense, isointense to CSF	Normal
2	Inhomogenous with or without horizontal bands	Clear	Hyperintense, isointense to CSF	Normal
3	Inhomogenous grey	Unclear	Intermediate	Slightly reduced
4	Inhomogenous grey to black	Lost	Intermediate to hypointense	Moderate loss
5	Inhomogenous black	Lost	Hypointense	Collapsed disc space

Multiple Choice Questions

1. A 28-year-old male feels a 'pop' in his low back while lifting a heavy object. Four weeks later, he continues to have significant low back pain, with no complaints of symptoms in his leg. A T2-weighted MRI is shown in Figure A with a red arrow identifying abnormal signal intensity in an anatomic structure. What type of collagen is primarily responsible for the biological properties of this anatomic structure?

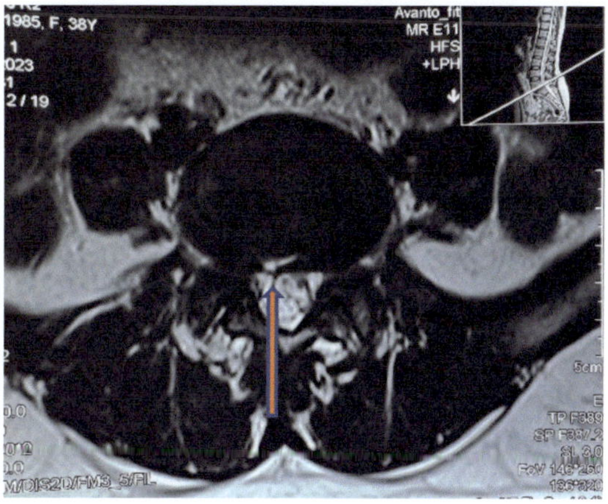

(a) Type I
(b) Type II
(c) Type V
(d) Type IX

2. Which of the following statements is true regarding the nucleus pulposus?
   (a) The nucleus is derived from myotome
   (b) It is primarily composed of type 1 collagen
   (c) It is composed of fibroblast-like cells
   (d) It has a high proteoglycan-to-collagen ratio
3. The structure responsible for maintaining the water content of IVD is
   (a) Aggrecan
   (b) Type 1 collagen
   (c) Type 2 collagen
   (d) Versican
4. Which of the following processes is involved in age-related IVD degeneration?
   (a) Increased proteoglycan content
   (b) Increased disc height
   (c) Increased degradative enzyme activity
   (d) Increased chondroitin sulfate
5. Which of the following is the pathognomonic of IVD degeneration?
   (a) Increased water content in nucleus pulposus
   (b) Decreased thickness of the annulus fibrosis
   (c) Degradation of large proteoglycan molecules in the nucleus pulposus
   (d) Loss of Type X collagen in the nucleus pulposus

Answer: 1. (a), 2. (d), 3. (a), 4. (c), 5. (c)

Further Reading

1. Raj PP. Intervertebral disc: anatomy-physiology-pathophysiology-treatment. Pain Pract. 2008;8(1):18–44. https://doi.org/10.1111/j.1533--2500.2007.00171.x. PMID: 18211591.
2. Theodorou DJ, Theodorou SJ, Gelalis ID, Kakitsubata Y. Lumbar intervertebral disc and discovertebral segment, part 1: an imaging review of normal anatomy. Cureus. 2022;14(6):e25558. https://doi.org/10.7759/cureus.25558. PMID: 35784982; PMCID: PMC9249043.
3. Oichi T, Taniguchi Y, Oshima Y, Tanaka S, Saito T. Pathomechanism of intervertebral disc degeneration. JOR Spine. 2020;3(1):e1076. https://doi.org/10.1002/jsp2.1076. PMID: 32211588; PMCID: PMC7084053.
4. Dowdell J, Erwin M, Choma T, Vaccaro A, Iatridis J, Cho SK. Intervertebral disk degeneration and repair. Neurosurgery. 2017;80(3S):S46–S54. https://doi.org/10.1093/neuros/nyw078. Erratum in: Neurosurgery 2018 Nov 1;83(5):1084. PMID: 28350945; PMCID: PMC5585783.

63 Scoliosis and Kyphosis

Sunny Chaudhary and Pankaj Kandwal

63.1 Introduction

Definition: Scoliosis is a deformity of spine in which the spine is bend sideways and has one or more lateral curves measuring more than 10 degrees. Although the coronal plane deformity is the major component, it also has sagittal and transverse plane deformity. So, the deformity in scoliosis is complex three-dimensional (3D) in nature (Fig. 63.1).

The cause of lateral bending is usually idiopathic, but it may be due to underlying bony or neurological abnormality.

S. Chaudhary (✉)
Department of Spine Surgery, Alberta Children's Hospital, Calgary, AB, Canada
e-mail: sunny.chaudhary@albertahealthservices.ca

P. Kandwal
Department of Orthopedics, All India Institute of Medical Sciences, Rishikesh, India

V. Kumar et al. (eds.), *A Quick Guide to Essential Orthopedics*,
https://doi.org/10.1007/978-981-95-2676-5_63

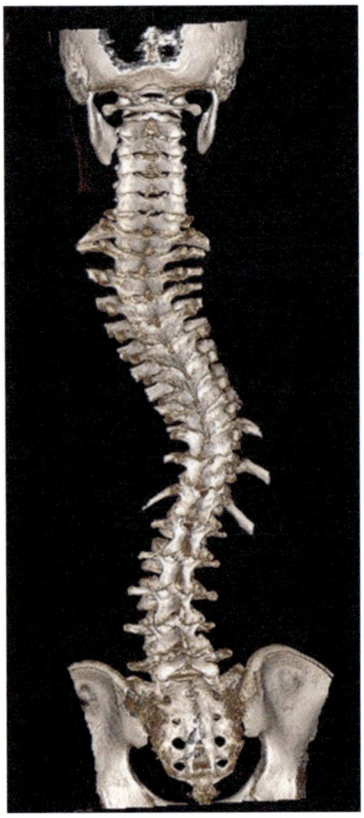

Fig. 63.1 A three-dimensional computed tomography (CT) reconstruction of scoliosis deformity

63.2 Biomechanics

According to Hueter-Volkmann law, bone growth is affected by the forces acting on growing skeleton. There is retardation of growth due to compressive forces, and it accelerates by tensile forces. Initially, the vertebra rotates in axial plane and so uneven loading takes place on it along ventral axis and dorsal axis. Compressive forces are more near ventral axis in thoracic region so there is growth retardation, whereas the part along dorsal axis grows more rapidly due to tensile forces. The difference in height on two sides of vertebrae increases with time, and ventral part forms the concave side, whereas the dorsal part forms the convex side of the curve. This uneven growth further leads to uneven forces, and curve progresses to larger magnitude. Curve progression is usually maximum during growth spurt.

63.3 Clinical Examination

The clinical evaluation of scoliosis is crucial to determine the severity of the condition and develop an appropriate treatment plan. The clinical findings that may be observed in individuals with scoliosis include the following (Fig. 63.2):

1. Spinal curvature: A visible curvature of the spine is typically the most prominent finding in scoliosis. The spine may appear as an "S" or "C" shape when viewed from behind. The degree of curvature may be more noticeable when the individual is standing upright.
2. Asymmetrical shoulders and hips: As scoliosis progresses, the curvature of the spine can lead to unevenness in the shoulders and hips. Limb length discrepancy may be associated, and it can lead to unequal levels of hips and shoulders.
3. Rib prominence: The curvature of the spine in scoliosis can cause the ribs to become more prominent on one side of the body. This may manifest as a bulge or hump on one side of the back.
4. Waistline asymmetry: As the curvature of the spine increases, the waistline may become asymmetrical. The individual may have a more pronounced curve on one side of the waist than the other.
5. Height and arm span should be recorded. Sitting and standing heights should be measured separately. This helps to diagnose Marfan syndrome. The upper-segment-to-lower-segment ratio is decreased and arm-span-to-height ratio is increased in this disease.
6. Clinical signs of hyperlaxity should be evaluated. They help to rule out Marfan syndrome and other collagen tissue disorder.
7. Forward bending test: The forward bend test is a standard technique used to evaluate the curvature of the spine in scoliosis. During the test, the individual is asked to bend forward at the waist with arms hanging freely. The examiner assesses for any asymmetry in the

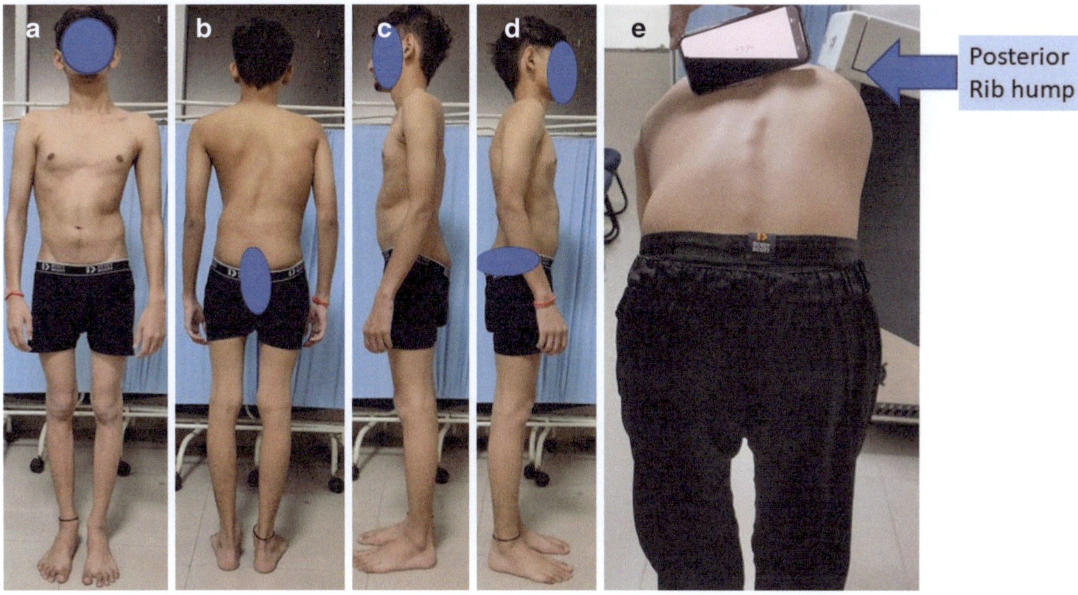

Fig. 63.2 (**a**–**d**) Clinical images of a patient with scoliosis and (**e**) Adam's forward bending test and prominent posterior rib hump

curvature of the spine, rib prominence, or lumbar hump.

8. Neurocutaneous stigmata: Signs of spinal dysraphism such as skin lesions, absence of abdominal reflexes, and tuft of hairs must be ruled out.
9. Neurological examination: Some individuals with scoliosis may experience neurological symptoms such as weakness or numbness in their extremities. Detailed neurological examination should be carried out, and any asymmetry of jerks should be recorded.
10. Flexibility of curves on sideward bending should also be examined.
11. Syndromic evaluation should be done.
12. Remaining growth: It should be calculated as progression of curve is affected by the remaining growth, and it guides us about time of surgical intervention. It is measured by five indices—Risser sign, hand and wrist radiographs, peak height velocity, olecranon apophysis maturity, and menarchal stage in female.

63.4 Radiological Examination

The diagnosis of scoliosis is mainly clinical, but age of onset and radiological studies help to classify it further. Radiological imaging in form of radiographs is often the first investigation. The standing full-length anteroposterior and lateral radiographs are done. Additional radiographs include bending images to assess the flexibility of curves. The number of vertebrae involved in deformity helps to distinguish different types of curves.

1. Short sharp curves (less than four vertebrae in the curve): congenital/NF
2. Four–six vertebrae: idiopathic curves
3. Long C curves (more than six vertebrae): neuromuscular

Computed tomography (CT) scan and magnetic resonance imaging (MRI) are indicated to assess the 3D deformity, bony changes or malformation, and neurological involvement.

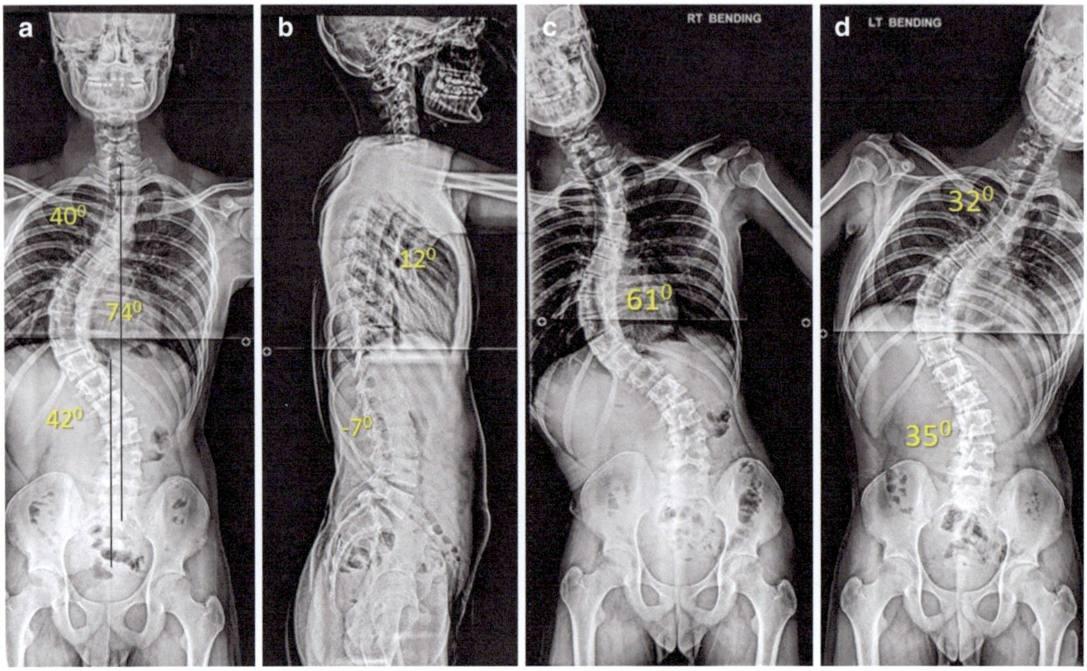

Fig. 63.3 (**a**, **b**) Full-length radiographs of spine and (**c**, **d**) side bending images of spine

Most of the scoliotic curves are idiopathic, but CT scan and MRI help to differentiate them from congenital curves. Congenital curves have neurological or osseous abnormalities (Fig. 63.3).

63.5 Nomenclature and Measurement

The vertebra or disc which is at maximum distance from midline is called the apex. It is that part which has maximum rotation.

A primary curve or major curve is the first curve to develop and is the largest curve. Secondary curves are of smaller magnitude and develop to compensate the primary curve.

A structural curve is a curve which has bony changes, and it cannot be fully corrected with bending.

A nonstructural curve is usually the compensatory curve which can be corrected on bending. A long-standing nonstructural curve may change into a structural curve.

Based on the location of apex of the curve, it is anatomically classified. If the apex lies between T2 and T11/T12 disc, the curve is called a thoracic curve. A thoracolumbar curve has its apex on either T12 or L1 vertebrae. If the apex lies between L1/L2 disc and L4 vertebra, the curve is a lumbar curve (Fig. 63.4).

The vertebrae which are most tilted toward the apex are called the end vertebrae. There are one proximal end vertebra and one distal end vertebra. The end plates of these two vertebrae help us to calculate the Cobb angle. Cobb angle is the angle formed between the superior end plate of superior end vertebra and inferior end plate of inferior end vertebrae. Cobb angle is a measure of magnitude of the scoliotic curve (Fig. 63.5).

Rotation of the vertebra is measured by a method given by Nash and Moe. The rotation is indicated by the position of the pedicle at convex side of curve on frontal radiograph (Fig. 63.6).

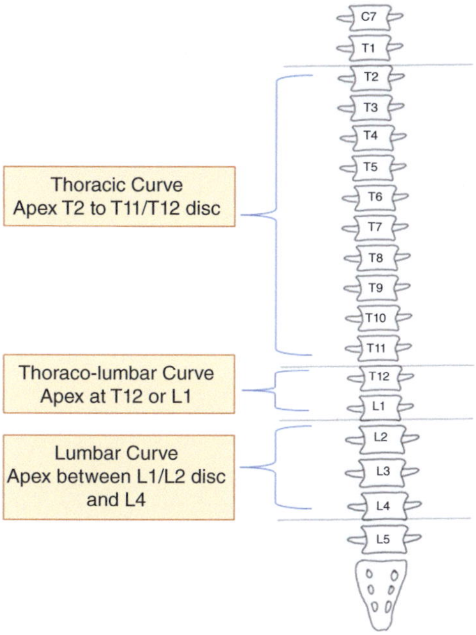

Fig. 63.4 Diagrammatic representation of curve nomenclature based on location of apex of curve

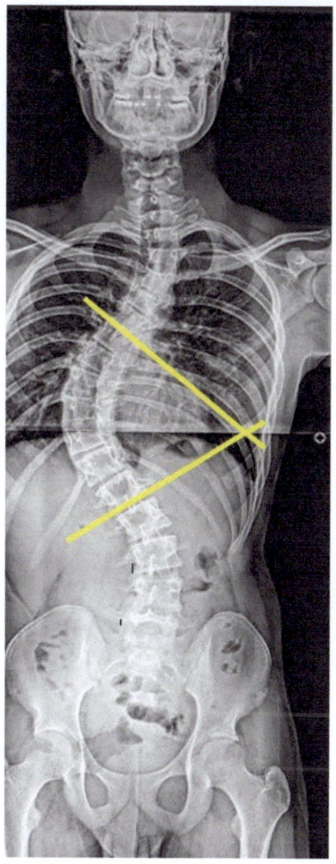

Fig. 63.5 Measurement of Cobb's angle—the angle formed between superior end plate of superior end vertebra and inferior end plate of inferior end vertebra

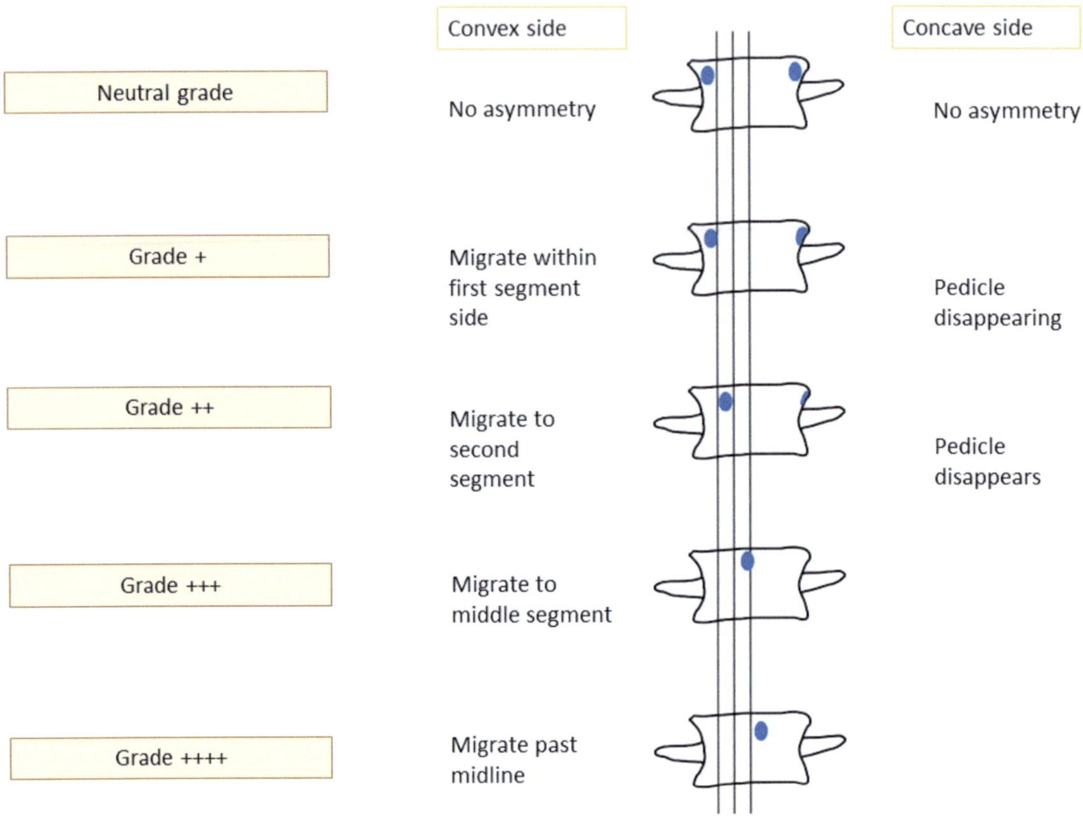

Fig. 63.6 Diagrammatic representation of grading of rotation of vertebrae based on method described by Nash and Moe

63.6 Etiological Classification

Scoliosis curves can be structural or nonstructural.

Nonstructural curves are temporary curves that do not have bony changes in spine. They can be postural, compensatory, or sciatic in nature.

Structural scoliosis is a permanent deformity which may be partially correctible due to flexibility of the curve. It has bony changes and rotation along with coronal plane deformity. It can be either primary or secondary. Primary scoliosis is idiopathic in nature, and it is classified according to the patient's age. Secondary scoliosis is classified based on the cause (Table 63.1).

Table 63.1 Etiological classification of scoliosis

Etiological classification of scoliosis (Scoliosis Research Society) (1969, 1970, and1973)
Idiopathic (80%)
Infantile (age of onset <3 years)
Juvenile (age of onset is in between 3 and 10 years)
Adolescent (age of onset is in between 10 and 18 years)
Congenital (10%)
Osteogenic
Neuropathic
Developmental
Skeletal dysplasia
Skeletal dysostosis
Neuromuscular
Neuropathic (acquired)
Myopathic
Tumor-associated
Osseous
Extraosseous

63.7 Principles of Treatment

The treatment of scoliosis varies with different patient. The magnitude of curve, its progression or tendency to progress in the future, the age of the patient, clinical symptoms, and cosmesis play a major role in guiding about the method and timing of treatment. Various treatment options are observation, bracing, or surgery.

63.7.1 Observation

A patient is followed up at regular intervals to monitor progression of curve. It is mainstay of treatment in adolescent scoliosis patient with

1. < 20 degrees curve in a skeletally immature patient
2. < 30 degrees curve in a skeletally mature patient

63.7.2 Bracing

Bracing has no role in skeletally mature patients. It is advised in a skeletally immature patient of adolescent idiopathic with cobb angle of 20 to 45 degrees. An underarm brace is usually given to patients with apex of the curve below T7. A Milwaukee brace is used when apex of curve is above T7. These braces are prescribed for 18 to 23 hours per day (Fig. 63.7).

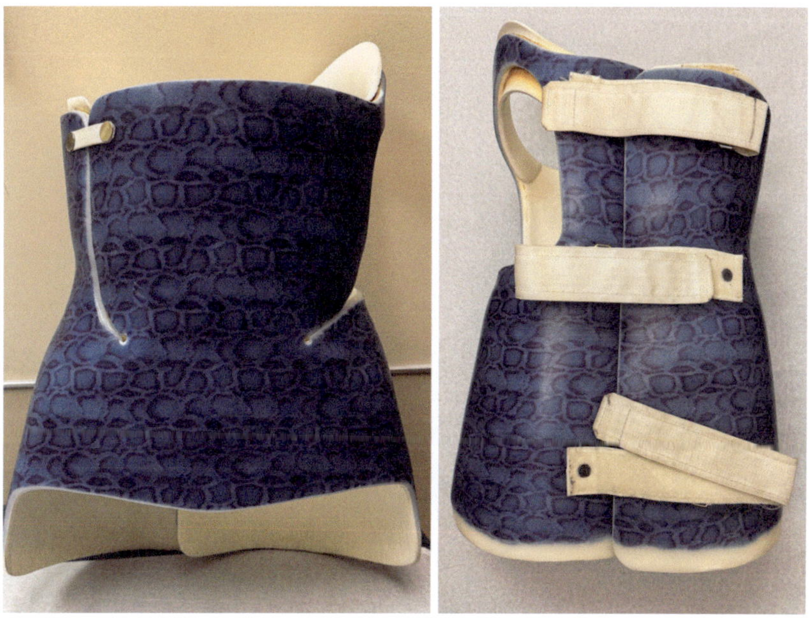

Fig. 63.7 Thoracic lumbar sacral orthosis (TLSO)—front and back

63.8 Surgery

Surgery is mainly needed to stop progression of the curve. It is also used to improve balance of the trunk and to correct the curve. The principle of surgery is to achieve solid fusion and stop progression. The fusion can be achieved from either anterior or posterior approach. Staged procedure for severe curves has been advocated. In severe curves, anterior release is done in first stage and posterior instrumentation and fusion are done later (Figs. 63.8 and 63.9).

It is indicated in following circumstances:

1. If *curve is more than 45 degrees* in a skeletally immature patient with adolescent idiopathic scoliosis.
2. If *curve progresses* even after the use of brace in a skeletally immature patient with adolescent idiopathic scoliosis.
3. If a skeletally immature patient with adolescent idiopathic scoliosis is *not tolerating a brace*
4. For *curve correction* in neuromuscular scoliosis for improvement of seating balance, alleviating pain, or improving respiratory function.
5. In patients with progressive congenital scoliosis and having a short sharp curve.
6. An adult patient with Cobb angle greater than 45 degree, and patient has pain when the curve progresses.

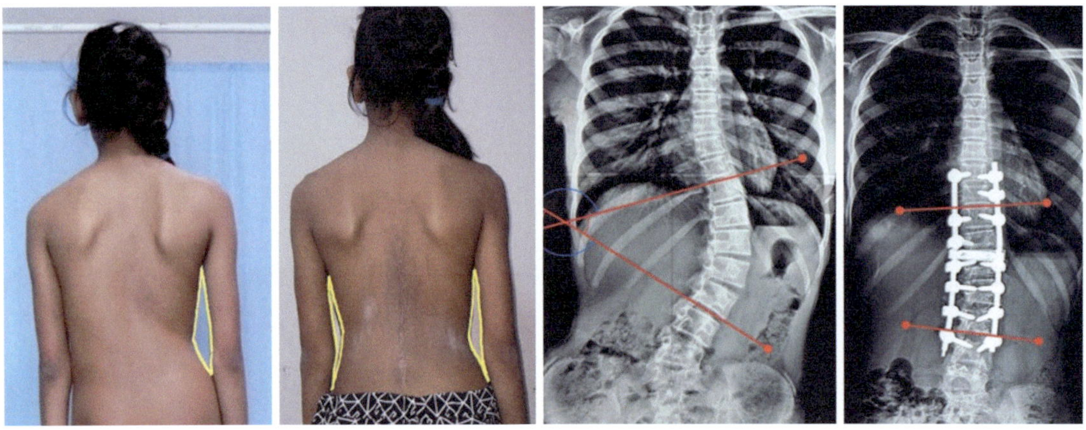

Fig. 63.8 Preoperative and postoperative clinical and radiological images of a patient with scoliosis treated with posterior instrumentation and fusion. Note the improvement in spinal deformity and arm waist triangles

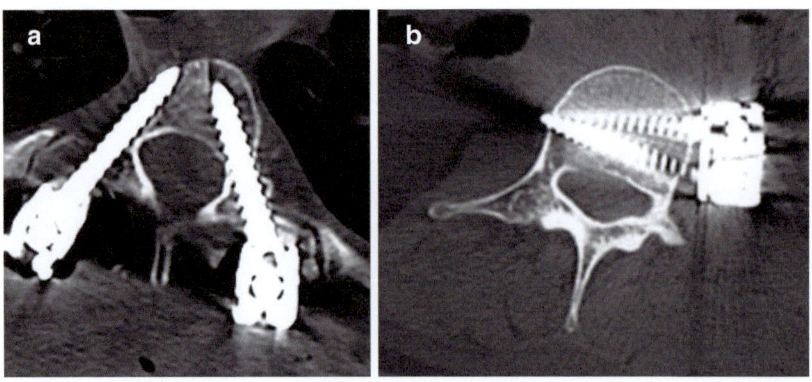

Fig. 63.9 Axial CT images of postoperated cases of scoliosis showing different methods of instrumentation: (**a**) posterior instrumentation (**b**) anterior instrumentation

63.9 Idiopathic Scoliosis

It is diagnosed after the congenital and other causes of scoliosis have been excluded. It has been classified based on the age of onset of scoliosis. The infantile form is between 0 and 3 years, the juvenile form is between 4 and 10 years, and adolescent scoliosis is between 11 and 18 years of age.

63.9.1 Infantile Idiopathic Scoliosis

It is more commonly seen in boys and is left-sided thoracic curve. It is mostly a positional deformity and resolves with age, but in some cases, the deformity progresses. The progression of the curve can be anticipated by measuring the rib vertebral angle difference (RVAD) as described by Mehta. If the difference in between concave and convex side is more than 20 degrees, the curve has a potential to progress. It may also progress if the head of the rib overlaps the vertebral body. The aim of treatment is to decrease the deformity (Flowchart 63.1).

63.9.2 Juvenile Idiopathic Scoliosis

A curve is said to be juvenile when the age of onset is between 4 and 10 years. Boys and girls are equally affected, but the ratio of girls affected increases with age. The curve usually progresses during this period and requires surgery early to prevent development of gross deformity. The fusion surgery which is usually done in adolescent population cannot be done as this will prevent the normal growth of the spine and gain in height. Instrumentation without fusion is performed, and a curve of less than 40 degree is targeted. If the curve cannot be reduced or deformity is gross, then early fusion is also advocated in such cases. Various other procedures such as vertebral expanding prosthetic rib (VEPTR) and Shilla procedure are growth-preserving options in this age-group. The aim of the treatment is to prevent the exaggeration of deformity until the age at which fusion of spinal segments can be done (Flowchart 63.2).

63.9.3 Adolescent Idiopathic Scoliosis

This type of scoliosis is more common in girls. For the curves greater than 20 degrees, the ratio is as high as 5.4:1. Curve progression is more in females and in patients with more growth remaining and initial large curve magnitude. Most of the patients do not require surgery and are observed. Patients with remaining growth and curve between 20 and 40 degrees require bracing. The curves of adolescent idiopathic scoliosis are classified according to Lenke classification into six curve types. Lumbar spine modifiers and thoracic sagittal modifiers further guide about the type of surgical treatment. The aim of treatment is to prevent progression of deformity and to improve the balance of spine. Cosmesis and reduction of pain are also the main factors that guide the treatment (Flowchart 63.3).

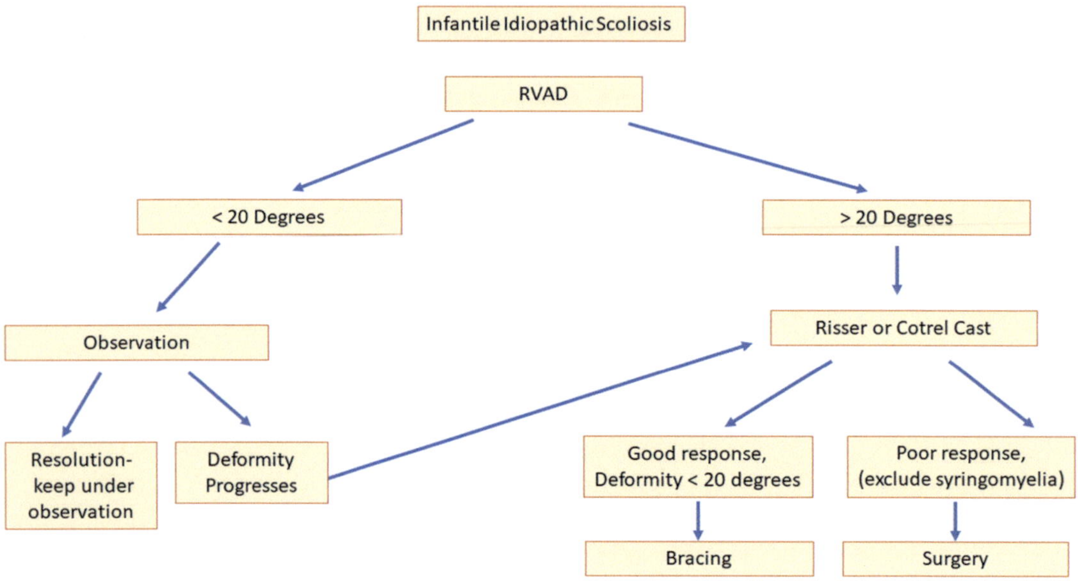

Flowchart 63.1 Treatment of infantile idiopathic scoliosis

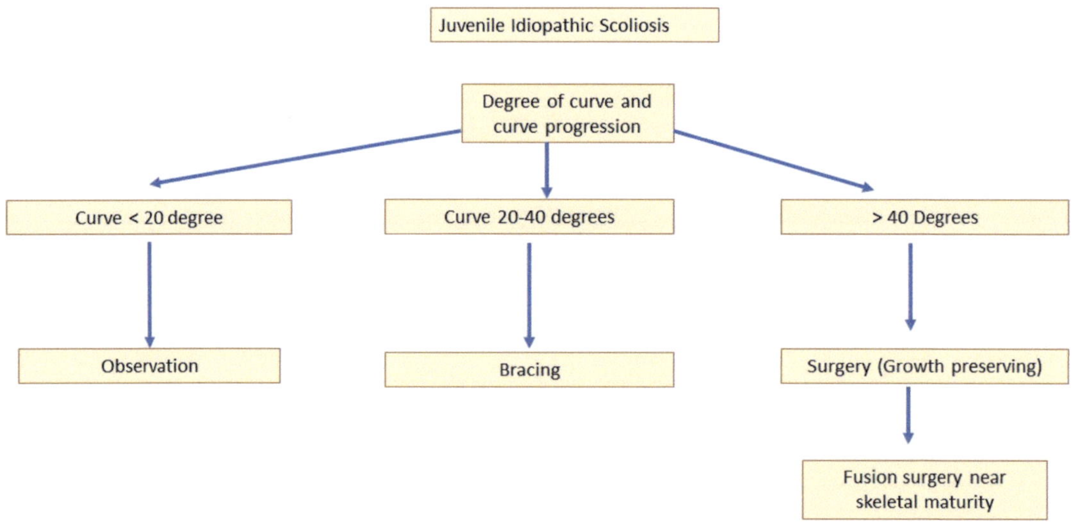

Flowchart 63.2 Treatment of juvenile idiopathic scoliosis

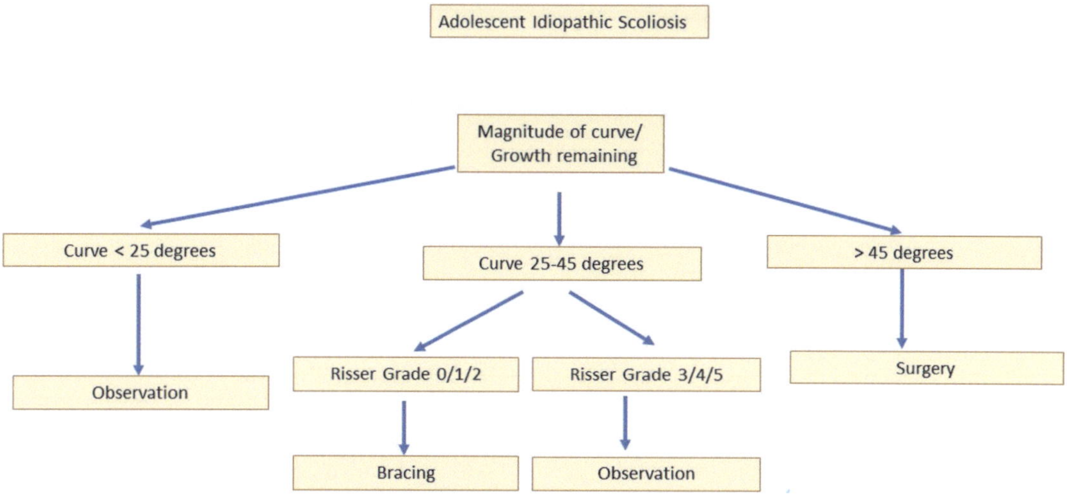

Flowchart 63.3 Treatment of adolescent idiopathic scoliosis

63.10 Congenital Scoliosis

The deformity of congenital may not be present at birth and reveals as the child grows. Abnormal fetal somite formation leads to abnormal spinal and rib development, and this causes deformity. The cause can be either the failure of segmentation or failure of formation or due to both. Abdominal organs are evaluated to rule out any anomaly.

The aim of the treatment is to improve the balance, prevent further progression of deformity, prevent compression of neurological elements, and improve the thoracic cage volume. Bracing is not an effective method of treatment in the presence of vertebral anomalies. Various treatment methods are hemivertebra resection and fusion, distraction by VEPTR or dual rods, vertebral column resection, and instrumentation if deformity is gross.

Multiple Choice Questions

1. According to Hueter-Volkmann law, how does bone growth respond to different forces on the growing skeleton?
   (a) Growth is accelerated by compressive forces
   (b) Growth is accelerated by tensile forces
   (c) Growth is retarded by compressive forces and accelerated by tensile forces
   (d) Growth is retarded by tensile forces and accelerated by compressive forces
2. When is curve progression typically most significant in scoliosis?
   (a) During old age
   (b) At the time of diagnosis
   (c) During growth spurts
   (d) In the early stages of the condition
3. Why is assessing remaining growth important in scoliosis?
   (a) It helps diagnose Marfan syndrome
   (b) It guides the timing of surgical intervention
   (c) It measures arm-span-to-height ratio
   (d) It evaluates flexibility of spinal curves
4. Which additional radiographs are often taken to assess the flexibility of scoliotic curves?
   (a) Lateral radiographs only
   (b) Anteroposterior radiographs only
   (c) Side bending images
   (d) MRI images

5. What is the term for the vertebra or disc at the maximum distance from the midline, which also has the maximum rotation?
   (a) Pivot vertebra
   (b) Apex vertebra
   (c) Central vertebra
   (d) Principal vertebra
6. How is the Cobb angle measured?
   (a) Between the upper end plates of adjacent vertebrae
   (b) Between the lower end plates of adjacent vertebrae
   (c) Between the upper end plate of the superior end vertebra and lower end plate of inferior end vertebra
   (d) Between the lower end plate of the superior end vertebra and upper end plate of inferior end vertebra
7. How is the rotation of the vertebrae measured according to Nash and Moe?
   (a) By assessing the angle of curvature
   (b) By measuring the distance from the midline
   (c) By evaluating the Cobb angle
   (d) By the position of the pedicle at the convex side of the curve on a frontal radiograph
8. Which method is used to assess the rotation of vertebrae in scoliosis?
   (a) Nash and Moe method
   (b) Cobb angle method
   (c) Bend and twist method
   (d) Axial rotation method

Answer: 1. (c), 2. (c), 3. (b), 4. (c), 5. (b), 6. (c), 7. (d), 8. (a)

64 Thoracic Outlet Syndrome

Vishnu R. Unnithan and Sitanshu Barik

64.1 Definition

- Thoracic outlet syndrome is a clinical condition characterized by a group of disorders that ultimately result in compression of the brachial plexus and subclavian vessels exiting the thoracic outlet [1].

64.2 Epidemiology

- Affects 1–2% population [2]
- Female to male ratio is 3:1 [3]

64.2.1 Anatomy

Thoracic outlet—comprised of three distinct spaces.

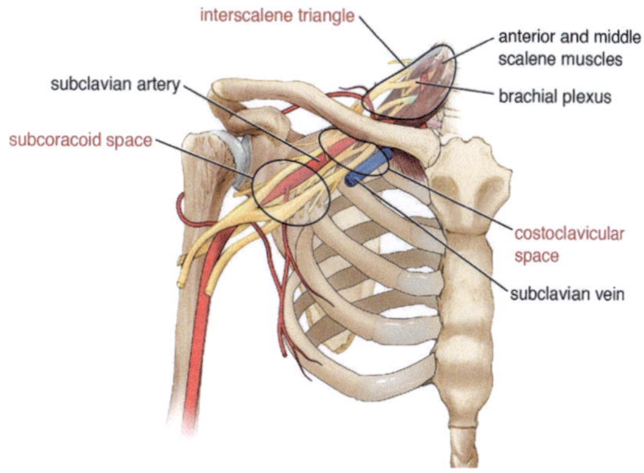

V. R. Unnithan (✉)
PRS Hospital, Karamana, Trivandrum, India

S. Barik
Department of Orthopaedics, AIIMS Nagpur,
Nagpur, Maharashtra, India

V. Kumar et al. (eds.), *A Quick Guide to Essential Orthopedics*,
https://doi.org/10.1007/978-981-95-2676-5_64

Name of space		1. Scalene triangle	2. Costoclavicular space	3. Subcoracoid space
Location		Proximal space	Middle space	Distal space
Borders	Superior			Coracoid
	Anterior	Anterior scalene muscle	Clavicle and subclavius muscle	Pectoralis minor muscle
	Post	Middle scalene muscle	First rib and scalene muscles	Second to fourth ribs
	Inferior	First rib		
	Medial		Costoclavicular ligament	
	Lateral		Upper scapular border	
Contents	Brachial plexus	Trunks	Divisions	Cords
	Vessels	Subclavian artery	Subclavian artery and vein	Axillary artery and vein

64.3 Types:

A. Neurogenic
  - Most common (95%)
  - Due to compression of brachial plexus

B. Vascular—due to constriction of vascular structures
  (a) Arterial
  (b) Venous

64.4 Etiology

- Congenital, acquired, or traumatic
  1. Bony causes:
     (a) Cervical rib
     (b) Prominent C7 transverse process
     (c) Clavicle or first rib—fracture, malunion, tumors
     (d) Acromioclavicular and sternoclavicular joint injuries
  2. Soft tissue causes:
     (a) Abnormalities related to neck muscles—scalene, pectoralis minor
     (b) Tumors—benign and malignant
     (c) Abnormal ligaments and bands
     (d) Chronic repetitive injury—overhead athletes

64.5 Clinical Features

64.5.1 Symptoms

- Usually episodic
- Symptoms usually precipitated by activities involving upper limb and at night (night pains)

A. Neurogenic
  - Non-radicular pain in neck, chest, and arm
  - Pain mainly around trapezius muscle
  - Paresthesia, numbness, and weakness of the upper limb

B. Vascular
  - Venous
    – Swelling and heaviness of the limb along with pain
    – Bluish discoloration of the limb
    – Dilated veins
  - Arterial
    – Pain, numbness
    – Claudication
    – Raynaud's disease like symptoms

C. Associated symptoms
  - Usually seen along with neurogenic thoracic outlet syndrome
  - Facial pain, visual or hearing disturbances, vertigo, tachycardia, sleep disturbances, and occipital headaches

64.5.2 Examination Findings

- Inspection:
  - Anatomical abnormalities of spine or shoulder
  - Skin: pallor, cyanosis, swelling, features of ischemia
  - Atrophy of intrinsic hand muscles
- Palpation
  - Skin—temperature
  - Tenderness over the supraclavicular region
  - Radial and ulnar pulse and symmetry with contralateral limb
  - Loss of peripheral nerve sensations
- Provocation tests
  - Elevated arm stress test
  - Upper limb tension test
  - Adson's test [4]
  - Wright's test
  - Roos test
  - Cyriax test
  - Supraclavicular squeeze test
  - Costoclavicular maneuver

64.5.3 Investigations

1. X-ray chest and cervical spine—cervical rib, elongated C7 transverse process, any fractures, tumors
2. Ultrasound—to assess any mass lesions
3. Nerve conduction studies—nerve conduction velocity (NCV) and electromyography (EMG) to assess nerve damage
4. Computed tomography (CT) scan—for osseous lesions
5. Magnetic resonance imaging (MRI)—for soft tissue lesions
6. Vascular imaging—venous and arterial Doppler, CT angiography, and MR angiography

64.6 Diagnosis

- Clinical diagnosis of the syndrome
- Investigations to identify the cause

64.7 Differential Diagnosis

- Cervical disc disease—more radicular type of pain
- Compression neuropathy of peripheral nerves
- Raynaud's disease
- Venous thrombosis of upper limb
- Dissecting aortic aneurysm

64.8 Treatment

A. Conservative
  - First-line management for all patients
  - Analgesics, anticoagulation
  - Avoiding overhead activities and lifestyle modifications
  - Physiotherapy—muscle strengthening of the cervical spine, core, and shoulder and posture correction

B. Injection Therapy
  - Steroids, anesthetic agents
  - Ultrasound-guided botulinum toxin A injection into scalene muscles

C. Vascular Procedures
  - In combination with conservative/surgical management or as a standalone procedure
  - Anticoagulation, thombectomy, embolectomy, stenting, vascular grafting, vascular bypass procedures

D. Surgery
  - After failure with conservative management
  - Depends on the etiology:
    1. First rib resection with anterior and middle scalenectomy with neurolysis—most common surgical procedure
    2. Cervical rib excision
    3. Elongated C7 transverse process excision
    4. Isolated scalenectomy
    5. Pectoralis minor tenotomy
    6. Release of abnormal ligaments and bands
    7. Correction of bony malunion of clavicle

64.9 Complications

1. Thromboembolic events
2. Aneurysm of the vessel
3. Pneumothorax

Multiple Choice Questions

1. Thoracic outlet consists of all of the following except
   (a) Axillary vein
   (b) Subclavian vein
   (c) Axillary nerve
   (d) Axillary artery
2. Not a content in thoracic outlet
   (a) Brachial plexus roots
   (b) Brachial plexus trunks
   (c) Brachial plexus divisions
   (d) Brachial plexus cords
3. Provocative test for thoracic outlet syndrome
   (a) Phalen's test
   (b) Elevated arm stress test
   (c) Durkan's test
   (d) Mill's test
4. Not a cause of thoracic outlet syndrome
   (a) Cervical rib
   (b) Prominent C7 transverse process
   (c) Abnormalities related to the pectoralis major muscle
   (d) Chronic repetitive Injury
5. Most common Surgical Procedure performed for treating Thoracic Outlet Syndrome
   (a) Cervical rib excision
   (b) Elongated C7 transverse process excision
   (c) First rib resection with anterior and middle scalenectomy with neurolysis
   (d) Pectoralis minor tenotomy

Answer: 1. (c), 2. (a), 3. (b), 4. (c), 5. (c)

References

1. Jones MR, Prabhakar A, Viswanath O, Urits I, Green JB, Kendrick JB, Brunk AJ, Eng MR, Orhurhu V, Cornett EM, Kaye AD. Thoracic outlet syndrome: a comprehensive review of pathophysiology, diagnosis, and treatment. Pain Ther. 2019;8(1):5–18. https://doi.org/10.1007/s40122-019-0124-2. Epub 2019 Apr 29. PMID: 31037504; PMCID: PMC6514035.
2. Moore WS. Vascular and endovascular surgery: a comprehensive review. 8th ed. Elsevier Health Sciences; 2012. p. 524. ISBN 978-1-4557-5386-4.
3. George E, Lee JT. Thoracic outlet syndrome, do women present differently than men? Elsevier eBooks; 2021. https://doi.org/10.1016/b978-0-12-822959-0.00004-3.
4. Huang JH, Zager EL. Thoracic outlet syndrome. Neurosurgery. 2004;55:897–903.

Part VIII

Inflammatory Disorders

65 Approach to a Patient with Polyarthralgia

Arghya Kundu Choudhury and Sitanshu Barik

65.1 Introduction

Polyarthralgia refers to joint pain involving multiple sites. The prefix "poly" indicates multiplicity, while "arthralgia" describes joint pain without necessarily implying inflammation. This distinguishes it from polyarthritis, which involves inflammatory processes affecting several joints, often accompanied by structural joint changes and systemic features.

65.2 Definition

Polyarthralgia: It is characterized by pain involving multiple joints, either symmetric or asymmetric, affecting both large and small joints. The pain may be intrinsic to the joint or arise from periarticular or extra-articular structures, occasionally radiating to the joint area.

Polyarthritis: It involves inflammation in multiple joints with or without accompanying joint destruction. It is commonly associated with systemic inflammatory diseases and autoimmune conditions.

A. Kundu Choudhury (✉)
Department of Hip, Knee and Robotic Joint Replacement, Sarvodaya Hospital and Research Centre, Faridabad, Haryana, India

S. Barik
Department of Orthopaedics, AIIMS Nagpur, Nagpur, Maharashtra, India

65.3 Clinical Evaluation

The assessment of polyarthralgia requires differentiating between articular and nonarticular origins of pain. Joint pain may stem from structures adjacent to the joint, which can mimic intra-articular pathology. Determining whether the etiology is inflammatory or mechanical is essential.

Noninflammatory causes, like osteoarthritis, generally manifest as chronic, activity-related pain without significant warmth, redness, or swelling.

Inflammatory arthritis is suggested by joint swelling, warmth, erythema, stiffness lasting more than 30 minutes in the morning, and systemic features. Confirmatory investigations should be tailored based on the clinical pattern—considering the chronicity, distribution, and number of involved joints.

65.4 Etiologies and Differential Diagnoses

A broad range of conditions can manifest as polyarthralgia:

Nonarticular causes: Hypothyroidism, somatoform disorders, neuropathic pain, and depression.

Periarticular conditions: Tendinitis, bursitis, soft tissue injuries, and fibromyalgia.

V. Kumar et al. (eds.), *A Quick Guide to Essential Orthopedics*,
https://doi.org/10.1007/978-981-95-2676-5_65

Noninflammatory arthritis: Degenerative joint diseases such as osteoarthritis.

Inflammatory arthritis:

Infective: Bacterial (e.g., septic arthritis and Lyme disease), viral (e.g., parvovirus and hepatitis B/C), and postinfectious arthritis.

Autoimmune and connective tissue diseases: Rheumatoid arthritis (RA), systemic lupus erythematosus, vasculitides, and spondyloarthropathies.

Crystal arthropathies: Gout (monosodium urate) and pseudogout (calcium pyrophosphate).

Inherited disorders: Familial Mediterranean fever.

65.5 Pathophysiology

Noninflammatory arthritis primarily involves mechanical wear and abnormal cartilage repair, leading to progressive joint degeneration, osteophyte formation, and eventual functional impairment.

Inflammatory arthritis results from immune-mediated processes or direct infection. In autoimmune conditions, cytokines and autoantibodies initiate synovial inflammation, pannus formation, and joint destruction if left untreated.

65.6 Approach to History Taking

A detailed clinical history is paramount. Key elements include the following:

Duration: Acute (<2 weeks) versus chronic (>2 weeks).

Number of joints: Monoarticular, oligoarticular (2–4), or polyarticular (>5).

Symmetry: Symmetric (common in RA) versus asymmetric (typical of spondyloarthropathies).

Pain characteristics: Inflammatory pain worsens with rest, whereas mechanical pain aggravates with activity.

Pattern: Migratory, additive, or intermittent involvement.

Systemic symptoms: Rashes, oral ulcers, uveitis, and constitutional symptoms.

65.7 Joint Involvement Patterns

Certain conditions have predilection for specific joints:

Disease	Commonly affected Joint
Septic arthritis	Knee
Gonococcal arthritis	Knee
Gout	First metatarsophalangeal joint
Pseudogout	Knee
Rheumatoid arthritis	metacarpophalangeal (MCP) and proximal interphalangeal (PIP) joints
Ankylosing spondylitis	Sacroiliac joints
Hemophilic arthropathy	Knee (especially in children)

65.8 Physical Examination

Inspection: Swelling, redness, deformity.

Palpation: Localized tenderness, warmth, synovial thickening.

Range of motion (ROM): Both passive and active ROM should be assessed.

Signs of inflammation: Erythema, effusion, warmth, and tenderness.

Extra-articular findings: Skin lesions, lymphadenopathy, ocular inflammation, or nail changes may hint at systemic diseases.

65.9 Diagnostic Investigations

65.9.1 Imaging

X-rays: Detect advanced osteoarthritis, joint space narrowing, erosions, and calcifications.

Ultrasound: Effective for detecting joint effusions and guiding arthrocentesis.

Magnetic resonance imaging (MRI): Useful for early detection of inflammatory changes and soft tissue involvement.

Bone scans: Occasionally employed in suspected osteomyelitis or metastatic disease.

65.10 Laboratory Tests

Complete blood count (CBC), erythrocyte sedimentation rate (ESR), and C-reactive protein (CRP): Nonspecific markers of inflammation.

65.10.1 Rheumatologic Workup

Rheumatoid factor (RF), anti-cyclic citrullinated peptide (CCP): RA.

Antinuclear antibody (ANA), anti-dsDNA, anti-Smith: Lupus.

Anti-neutrophil cytoplasmic antibody (ANCA): Vasculitides.

Human leukocyte antigen (HLA)-B27: Seronegative spondyloarthropathies.

65.11 Synovial Fluid Analysis

Normal fluid: Clear, viscous, <200 WBC/μL.

Noninflammatory arthritis: Clear, slightly elevated white blood cell (WBC; 200–2000/μL).

Inflammatory arthritis: Turbid, WBC 2000–50,000/μL, polymorphonuclear neutrophil (PMN) predominance.

Septic arthritis: Purulent, >50,000 WBC/μL.

65.11.1 Crystals

Needle-shaped, negatively birefringent: Gout.

Rhomboid-shaped, positively birefringent: Pseudogout.

65.12 Biopsy

Though rarely required, synovial or soft tissue biopsy may be necessary for diagnosing vasculitis, granulomatous diseases, or persistent undiagnosed arthritis.

65.13 Management

Acute inflammatory arthritis: Prompt nonsteroidal anti-inflammatory drugs (NSAIDs) and corticosteroids as appropriate.

Septic arthritis: Immediate joint aspiration, broad-spectrum intravenous (IV) antibiotics, adjusted based on culture results.

Gout/pseudogout: NSAIDs, colchicine, corticosteroids; consider urate-lowering therapy for recurrent gout.

Autoimmune arthritis: Initiation of disease-modifying antirheumatic drugs (DMARDs) (e.g., methotrexate), escalation to biologics as required. Early treatment is key to preventing joint damage.

A multidisciplinary approach involving rheumatologists, physiotherapists, and patient education is vital for optimal long-term outcomes.

Multiple Choice Questions

1. Which condition is not typically a cause of polyarthralgia?
   (a) Rheumatoid arthritis
   (b) Ankylosing spondylitis
   (c) Osteoarthritis
   (d) Reactive arthritis
2. Needle-shaped, negatively birefringent crystals on synovial fluid microscopy indicate:
   (a) Pseudogout
   (b) Gout
   (c) Tuberculosis
   (d) Rheumatoid arthritis
3. A middle-aged woman with monoarthritis and lymphocytic-predominant synovial fluid suggests:
   (a) RA
   (b) Septic arthritis
   (c) Tubercular arthritis
   (d) Spondyloarthropathy
4. Gold-standard investigation for suspected tuberculosis (TB) arthritis:
   (a) MRI
   (b) X-ray

   (c) Biopsy
   (d) Synovial fluid analysis
5. Most commonly affected joint in a 20-year-old male with hemophilia A:
   (a) Hip
   (b) Shoulder
   (c) Interphalangeal
   (d) Knee

Answer: 1. (c). 2. (b), 3. (c), 4. (c), 5. (d)

References for Further Reading

1. https://pubmed.ncbi.nlm.nih.gov/12702621/
2. https://www.ncbi.nlm.nih.gov/pmc/articles/PMC6812894/
3. https://www.ncbi.nlm.nih.gov/books/NBK537170/
4. https://emedicine.medscape.com/article/336054-overview
5. https://pubmed.ncbi.nlm.nih.gov/18189016/

Rheumatoid Arthritis

66

Arghya Kundu Choudhury and Souvik Paul

66.1 Introduction

Rheumatoid arthritis (RA) is a chronic autoimmune condition characterized by persistent inflammation of the synovial joints, leading to progressive joint damage, deformities, and restricted mobility. It predominantly affects smaller joints like those in the hands and feet but can involve larger joints including knees, hips, and ankles.

Inflammatory arthritis encompasses a group of conditions presenting with painful, swollen joints. This category includes RA, psoriatic arthritis, systemic lupus erythematosus, adult-onset Still's disease, juvenile idiopathic arthritis, scleroderma, and those linked with inflammatory bowel disease.

RA is an autoimmune inflammatory disorder largely influenced by genetic and environmental factors such as tobacco use. It primarily targets synovial joints, where prolonged inflammation results in cartilage loss and bone erosions. Based on symptom duration, RA is classified as early (<6 months) or established (≥6 months) disease.

A. Kundu Choudhury (✉)
Department of Hip, Knee and Robotic Joint Replacement, Sarvodaya Hospital and Research Centre, Faridabad, Haryana, India

S. Paul
AMRI Hospitals, Kolkata, India

66.2 Epidemiology

- Females are affected about three times more than males.
- More common in older women, particularly after 60.
- Uncommon in men under 45.
- Typically involves joints symmetrically, especially peripheral joints.
- Associated conditions:
  – Felty's syndrome
  – Osteoporosis
  – B-cell lymphomas

66.2.1 Risk Factors

- Female gender
- Middle age, though it can occur at any age
- Family history of RA
- Tobacco use, particularly in genetically susceptible individuals
- Obesity

Notably, smoking in individuals with a shared epitope (SE) genotype significantly heightens RA risk by promoting anti-citrullinated protein antibody (ACPA) production.

V. Kumar et al. (eds.), *A Quick Guide to Essential Orthopedics*,
https://doi.org/10.1007/978-981-95-2676-5_66

66.3 Felty's Syndrome Overview

This condition involves the classic triad of RA, pancytopenia, and splenomegaly. It typically arises in chronic RA cases and is associated with high rheumatoid factor levels and extra-articular manifestations. Patients may develop chronic ulcers and recurrent infections.

66.4 Classification Criteria (2010 ACR/EULAR)

Diagnostic classification is based on cumulative scoring derived from four domains:

Classification criteria by the American College of Rheumatology (ACR) and the European League Against Rheumatism (EULAR)—2010

Criteria		Score
Joint involvement:	1 large joint (shoulders, elbows, hips, knees, and ankles)	0
	2–10 large joints	1
	1–3 small joints (metacarpophalangeal joints, proximal interphalangeal joints, the interphalangeal joint of the thumb, second through fifth metatarsophalangeal joint, and wrist) with or without the involvement of large joints	2
	4–10 small joints (with or without the involvement of large joints)	3
	>10 joints (with involvement of at least 1 small joint)	5
Serological parameters	Negative rheumatoid factor (RF) *and* negative anti-citrullinated protein antibody (ACPA)	0
	Low-positive RF *or* low-positive ACPA	2
	High-positive RF or high-positive ACPA	3
Acute phase reactants	Normal erythrocyte sedimentation rate (ESR) and C-reactive protein (CRP)	0
	Elevated ESR and CRP	1
Duration of arthritis	< 6 weeks	0
	≥ 6 weeks	1

Total score is 10
A cumulative score of 6 or more is required for a definitive RA diagnosis

66.5 Etiology

- RA has a strong genetic basis.
- Monozygotic twins show a 15% concordance compared to 5% in dizygotic pairs.
- Heritability estimates: 40–65% for seropositive RA and around 20% for seronegative cases.
- HLA-DRB1 alleles (notably *04, *01, *10) containing a "shared epitope" increase susceptibility.
- Other implicated genes:
- PAD14, PTPN22, CTLA4, IL-2RA, STAT4, TRAF1, CCR6, IRF5.
- SNPs in PSORS1C1, PTPN22, and MIR146A predict severe disease.

Epigenetic alterations (DNA methylation, histone modification) also contribute, particularly influencing fibroblast-like synoviocytes (RA-FLS) behavior and invasiveness via dysregulation of the PTPN11 gene.

66.6 Pathogenesis

RA initiation involves an environmental trigger, such as cigarette smoke, in a genetically predisposed individual, leading to autoimmunity. The inflammatory response begins at mucosal sites like the lungs, gingiva, or gastrointestinal tract, where environmental insults induce citrullination of proteins.

In the lungs, for instance, tobacco exposure upregulates peptidyl arginine deiminase (PAD) enzymes, particularly *PADI4*, which converts arginine residues into citrulline. These neoantigens stimulate the production of ACPA, initiating systemic autoimmunity.

Activated antigen-presenting cells (APCs) stimulate T-lymphocytes, leading to differentiation into Th1 and Th17 subsets. Th1 cells secrete TNF-α, promoting macrophage activation, while Th17 cells release IL-17, IL-1, and TNF-α, perpetuating inflammation and recruiting chondrocytes, osteoclasts, and fibroblasts. Synovial fibroblasts transform into aggressive RA-FLS, which produce pro-inflammatory cytokines and matrix metalloproteinases, leading to extracellular matrix degradation and pannus formation.

Autoantibody production by B-cells and plasma cells contributes to immune complex formation, neutrophil and macrophage activation, joint inflammation, and tissue destruction.

66.7 Clinical Features

66.7.1 Articular Manifestations

Acute: Synovitis with warmth, tenderness, and swelling

Chronic: Joint deformities are seen in advanced cases

66.7.2 Classical Deformities

66.7.2.1 Hand

- *Boutonniere deformity*—flexion of proximal interphalangeal (PIP) and extension of distal interphalangeal (DIP) of the hand due to rupture or incompetency of the extensor tendon.
- *Swan neck deformity*—hyperextension at the PIP joint and flexion at the DIP joint.
- *Z-thumb* consists of hyperextension of the interphalangeal joint, fixed flexion, and subluxation of the metacarpophalangeal joint and gives a "Z" appearance to the thumb.
- *Z-deformity of the wrist*—radial deviation of the wrist with ulnar deviation of the digits, with palmer subluxation of the proximal phalanges.

66.7.2.2 Foot

- Hallux valgus
- Hammer toe
- Windswept deformity (valgus deformity in one knee, varus in the other)

66.7.2.3 Nonarticular and Nonskeletal Manifestations

- Rheumatoid nodules, typically over pressure points
- Interstitial lung disease
- Ocular involvement: secondary Sjögren's syndrome, episcleritis, and scleritis
- Rheumatoid vasculitis affecting small and medium vessels
- Felty's syndrome

66.8 Investigations

66.8.1 Imaging

- *Plain radiographs:* reveal periarticular osteopenia, joint space narrowing, erosions, and soft tissue swelling (Figs. 66.1, 66.2, 66.3 and 66.4).
- *Magnetic resonance imaging (MRI):* sensitive for detecting early synovitis and marrow edema.
- *Ultrasound with Doppler:* identifies active synovitis and vascularity.

66.8.2 Laboratory Tests

- Rheumatoid factor and anti-cyclic citrullinated peptide (CCP) antibodies.
- Erythrocyte sedimentation rate (ESR) and C-reactive protein (CRP) for disease activity monitoring.
- Complete blood count (CBC), renal function test (RFT), liver function test (LFT), and antinuclear antibody (ANA) to assess systemic involvement and medication safety.

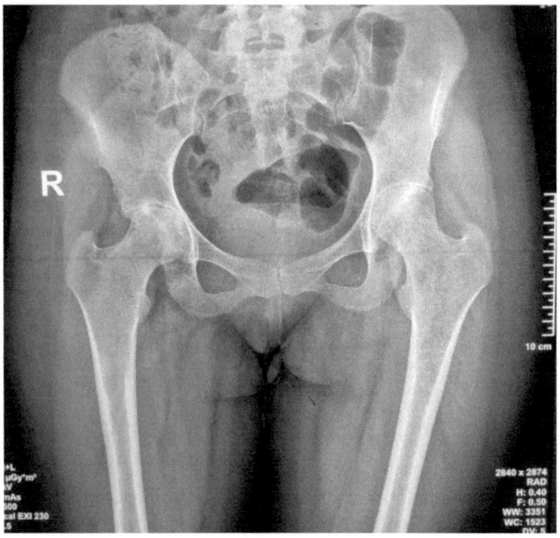

Fig. 66.1 Plain X-ray of pelvis with both hips (anteroperterior (AP) view) showing bilateral symmetrical joint space reduction with sclerosis of the femoral heads suggesting advanced hip arthritis

66.9 Management

66.9.1 Disease Activity Score (DAS28)

A validated tool assessing 28 joints to monitor RA activity and treatment response (Fig. 66.5).

66.9.2 Therapeutic Objectives

- Control synovitis promptly
- Preserve joint function
- Prevent deformities
- Restore mobility
- Alleviate pain
- Optimize quality of life

66.9.3 Pharmacotherapy

- *Nonsteroidal anti-inflammatory drugs (**NSAIDs**):* symptomatic relief
- *Corticosteroids:* for acute flares and severe disease manifestations
- *Conventional **disease-modifying antirheumatic drugs** (DMARDs):* Methotrexate remains first line (7.5–15 mg/week), supplemented with folic acid to mitigate toxicity
- *Biologic DMARDs:* TNF inhibitors (adalimumab, etanercept), IL-6 inhibitors (tocilizumab, sarilumab), T-cell co-stimulation blockers (abatacept), B-cell depleting agents (rituximab)
- *Targeted synthetic DMARDs:* Janus kinase inhibitors (tofacitinib, baricitinib, upadacitinib) for refractory cases

66.9.4 Non-pharmacologic Measures

- Dietary modifications favoring anti-inflammatory nutrients (omega-3 polyunsaturated fatty acids [PUFAs])
- Structured physiotherapy programs

66.9.5 Surgical Management

- Synovectomy for refractory monoarthritis
- Corrective orthopedic procedures for deformities
- Joint replacement in advanced arthropathy

66.9.6 Differential Diagnoses

- Crystal-induced arthritis (gout, pseudogout)
- Osteoarthritis
- SLE-related arthropathy
- Psoriatic arthritis
- Lyme disease
- Reactive arthritis
- Ankylosing spondylitis

66.9.7 Prognosis

- Poor outcomes are linked with:
- High RF and acute-phase reactants
- Subcutaneous nodules
- Early erosive changes
- Persistent high disease activity beyond a year

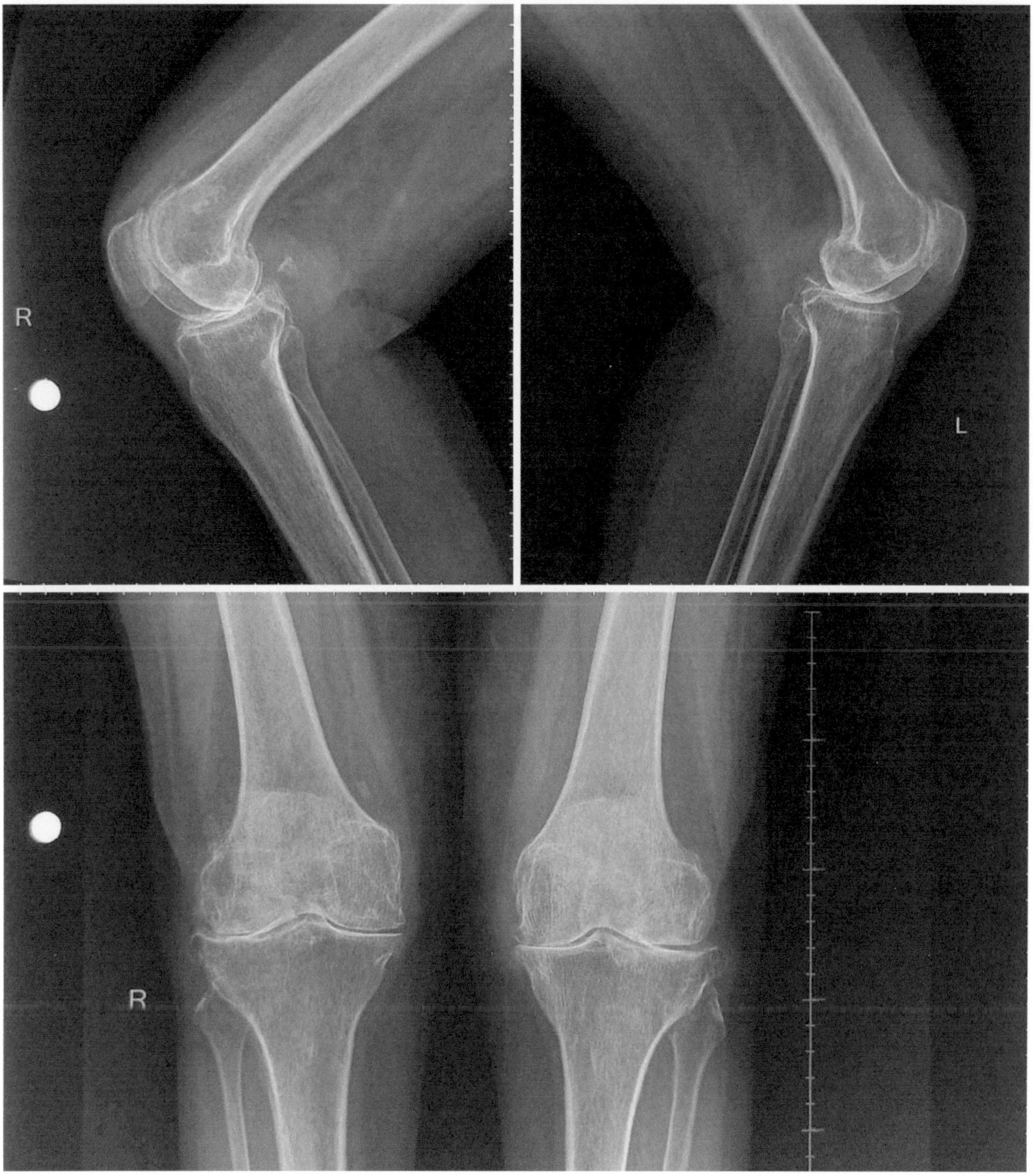

Fig. 66.2 Plain X-ray of bilateral knees (AP and lateral (LAT) views) showing bilateral symmetrical joint space reduction with sclerosis of the distal femur and proximal tibia heads suggesting advanced knee arthritis secondary to RA

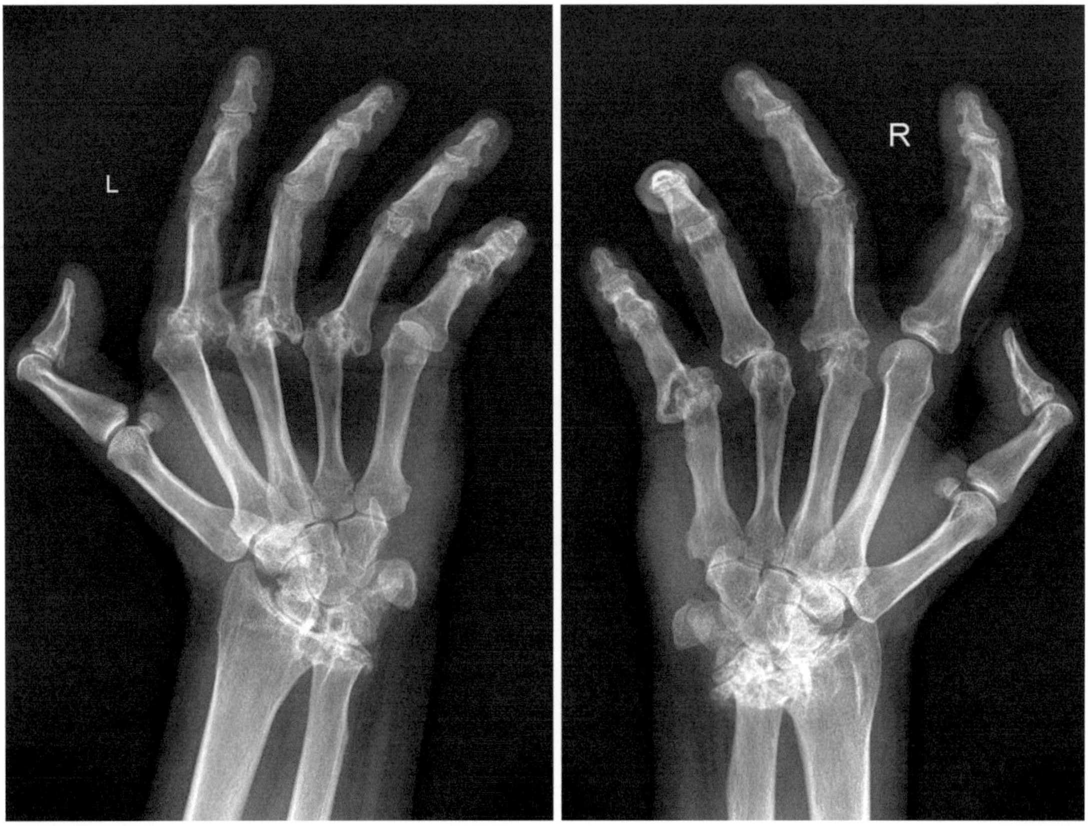

Fig. 66.3 Plain X-ray of bilateral hands with wrists (AP views) showing bilateral symmetrical joint space destruction of the interphalangeal and metacarpal–phalangeal joints with Z-thumbs and advanced arthritis of both wrists

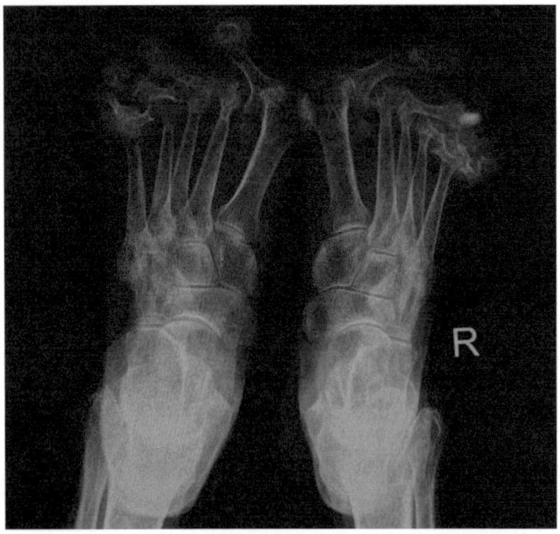

Fig. 66.4 Plain X-ray of bilateral feet (AP views) showing bilateral symmetrical joint space destruction of the interphalangeal and metatarsophalangeal joints with bilateral hallux valgus deformities and advanced arthritis

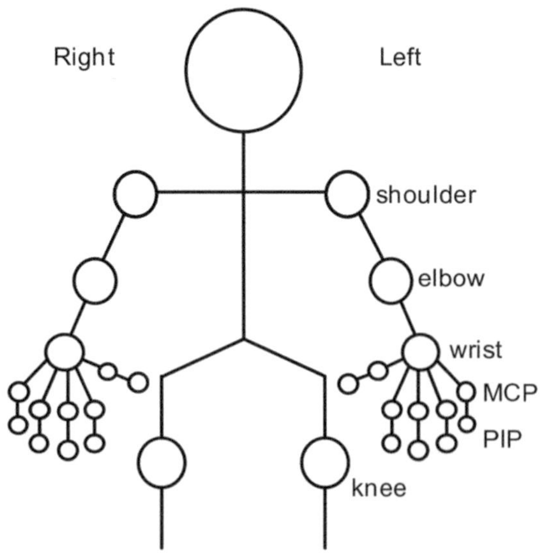

Fig. 66.5 DAS 28 joints scoring system takes into account these 28 joints

Multiple Choice Questions

1. In which of the following deformity, the distal interphalangeal joint is flexed and the proximal interphalangeal joint is extended?
   (a) Boutonniere deformity
   (b) Swan neck deformity
   (c) Z deformity
   (d) Claw hand
2. Rheumatoid arthritis affects which part of the spinal column?
   (a) Cervical
   (b) Thoracic
   (c) Lumbosacral
   (d) Occiputo-cervical
3. Which secondary arthritis causes no periosteal reactions?
   (a) Psoriatic
   (b) Ankylosing spondylitis
   (c) Rheumatoid arthritis
   (d) Reactive arthritis
4. A middle-aged female on treatment for rheumatoid arthritis suddenly developed upper motor neuron symptoms on her bilateral lower limbs, what will be the next investigation of choice?
   (a) Spine lateral view in flexion and extension
   (b) Open mouth view
   (c) Swimmers view
   (d) Broden's view
5. Which of the following is never seen in rheumatoid arthritis?
   (a) Heberden's node
   (b) Swan neck deformity
   (c) Ulnar deviation of the fingers
   (d) Symmetric joint space reduction

Answers: 1. (b), 2. (a), 3. (c), 4. (a), 5. (a)

References for Further Reading

1. https://www.ncbi.nlm.nih.gov/books/NBK441999/#:~:text=Rheumatoid%20arthritis%20(RA)%20is%20a,that%20primarily%20involves%20synovial%20joints.
2. https://my.clevelandclinic.org/health/diseases/4924-rheumatoid-arthritis
3. https://pubmed.ncbi.nlm.nih.gov/34831240/
4. https://pubmed.ncbi.nlm.nih.gov/34831081/
5. https://pubmed.ncbi.nlm.nih.gov/33243118/

67 Ankylosing Spondylitis

Arghya Kundu Choudhury and Vishal Kumar

67.1 Introduction

Ankylosing spondylitis (AS) is also known as *Bekhterev–Strümpell–Marie disease or Bechterew's disease or Pierre–Marie's disease.*

It is a seronegative spondyloarthropathy (SpA) that typically affects the axial skeleton (sacroiliac joint and spine). However, the hips, knees, and shoulder joints can also be affected. Chronic back pain and progressive spinal stiffness are the most common features of this disease. Affected spinal movements, postural abnormalities, hip pain, peripheral arthritis, enthesitis, and dactylitis are all commonly associated with ankylosing spondylitis.

67.1.1 Definition

It is a form of axial spinal arthropathy and chronic inflammation, chiefly affecting young males, that eventually causes ankylosis or fusion of the vertebral and sacroiliac joints.

67.2 Etiology

The cause of ankylosing spondylitis (AS) remains largely idiopathic, but there seems to be a correlation between the prevalence of AS in a given population and the prevalence of human leukocyte antigen (HLA)-B27 in that same population. Among people who are HLA-B27-positive, the prevalence of AS is approximately 5–6%.

67.3 Epidemiology

- Prevalence is 0.1% and 0.8%.
- Onset is typically in young adults (15–25 years).
- Males and females are equally affected, although the disease is picked up by X-ray more commonly in males than in females (3:1).
- HLA-B27 antigen positive in >90% patients of AS.
- High levels of immunoglobulin A (IgA).

A. Kundu Choudhury (✉)
Department of Hip, Knee and Robotic Joint Replacement, Sarvodaya Hospital and Research Centre, Faridabad, Haryana, India

V. Kumar
Department of Orthopaedics, PGIMER, Chandigarh, Chandigarh, India

V. Kumar et al. (eds.), *A Quick Guide to Essential Orthopedics*,
https://doi.org/10.1007/978-981-95-2676-5_67

67.4 Pathogenesis

- Primary involvement of the entheses.
- Enthesitis is associated with edema of adjacent bone marrow and erosive lesion which in time ossify.
- Tumor necrosis factor (TNF) and cytokines like IL-1 are involved in the pathogenesis.
- Ankylosing spondylitis (AS) is a chronic inflammatory disease with an insidious onset. Progressive musculoskeletal, and often extra-skeletal, signs and symptoms are characteristics of the disease. The rate of progression can vary from one patient to the next.
- The primary pathology of spondyloarthropathies is enthesitis with chronic inflammation, including CD4 and CD8 T lymphocytes and macrophages.
- Cytokines, particularly tumor necrosis factor-α (TNF-α) and transforming growth factor-β (TGF-β), are also important in the inflammatory process by leading to inflammation, fibrosis, and ossification at sites of enthesitis (Table 67.1).

Table 67.1 Difference between ankylosing spondylitis and rheumatoid arthritis

	Ankylosing spondylitis	Rheumatoid arthritis
Features of peripheral arthritis	Synovial hyperplasia, lymphoid infiltration, and pannus	Exuberant synovial villi, fibrin deposit, ulcer, and accumulation of plasma cells
Central cartilaginous erosion	Common	Rare

67.5 Prognosis

67.5.1 Poor Prognostic Factors

- Male sex
- Plus 3 of the following in the first 2 years of disease:
  - ESR >30 mm/h
  - Decreased response to nonsteroidal anti-inflammatory drugs (NSAIDs)
  - Limitation of lumbar spine movement
  - Sausage-like fingers or toes
  - Oligoarthritis
  - Early onset (<16 years old)

67.6 Clinical Features

The characteristic type of back pain in AS is "inflammatory" in nature. Inflammatory back pain typically exhibits at least four of the five following characteristics:

age of onset less than 40 years, insidious onset, improvement with exercise, no improvement with rest, and pain at night with an improvement upon arising.

- Chronic dull *low back pain* which can be associated with buttock pain.
  - The pain worsens after a period of rest and improves after activity.
  - The patient complains of pain that is severe enough to awaken them in the second half of night.
  - *Back pain is the first and most common symptom of AS.*
- Limitations in flexibility of the back and neck.

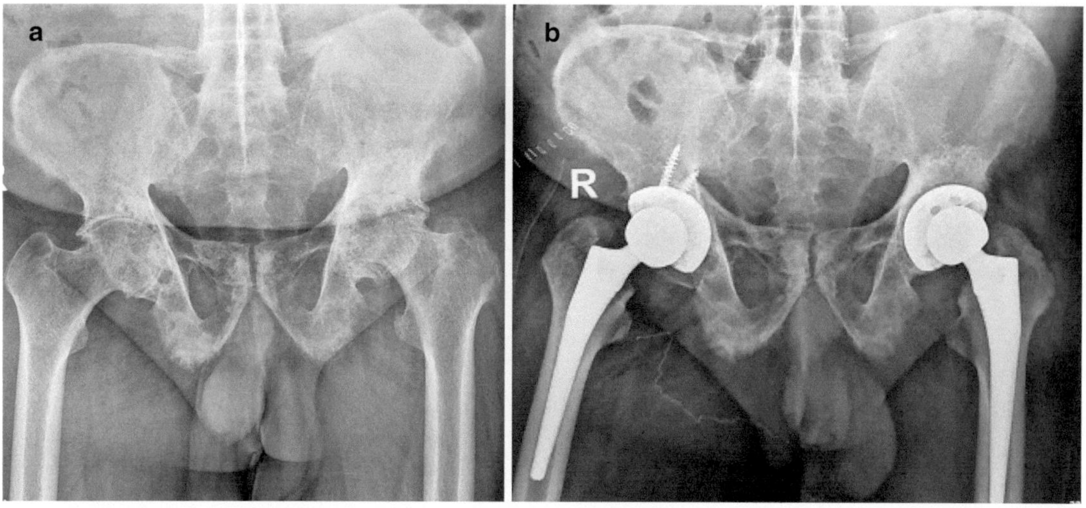

Fig. 67.1 (**a**) Bilateral inflammatory hip arthritis in ankylosing spondylitis, with fused SI joints, and (**b**) bilateral total hip arthroplasty in the same patient

- Irreversible head-forward *"hunchback" (increased thoracic kyphosis)* posture due to involvement of thoracic spine and loss of lumbar lordosis.
- Shoulder pain due to inflammation of the tendon and bone.
- Hip pain due to arthritis of the hip joint.
- Heel pain due to Achilles tendinitis or plantar fasciitis.
- Pain, stiffness, and swelling of other joints like hips, knees, ankles, heels, and feet.
- Fatigue and sleeplessness.
- Spinal fracture with minor trauma can occur in severe disease as the spine and the joints adjoining the pelvis - like hips are often fused, allowing no range of motion (Figs. 67.1 and 67.2).

Juvenile ankylosing spondylitis (JAS) is a rare form of AS which differs from the more common adult form. The following features are seen more in JAS:

- Enthesopathy and arthritis of knee joint are more common than early-morning back pain of adult AS.
- Ankylosing tarsitis of the ankle.
- Seronegative ANA and RF.
- Presence of the HLA B27 allele.

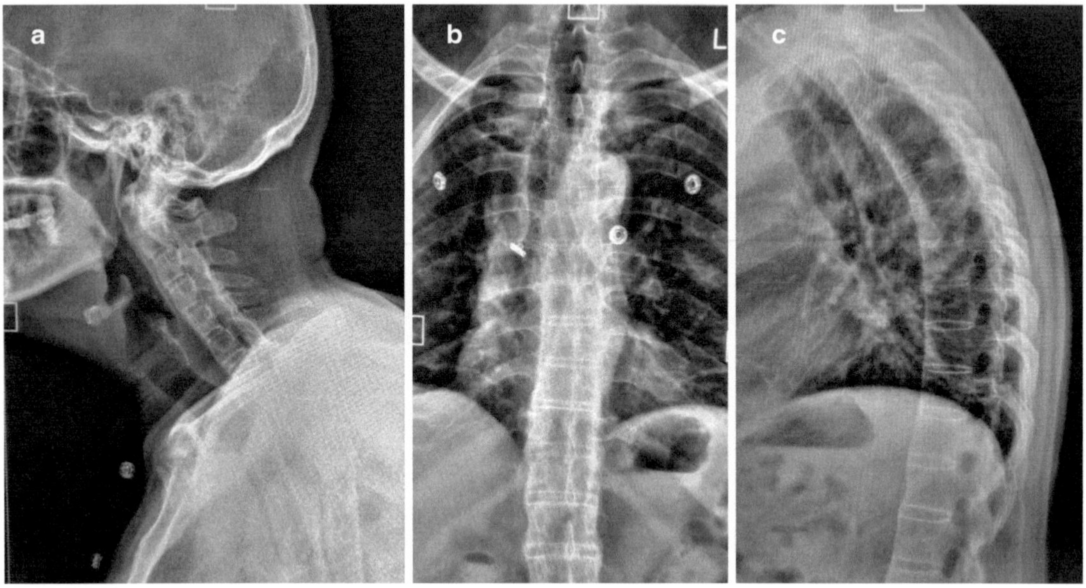

Fig. 67.2 (**a**) Loss of cervical lordosis with marginal syndesmophytes and fusion, (**b**) AP view of thoracic spine—squaring of the vertebra, marginal syndesmophytes—bamboo spine/dagger sign, and (**c**) thoracic hyperkyphosis—with marked fusion

67.6.1 Extra-Skeletal Features of AS

- *Ocular:* Acute anterior uveitis in 30% patients. It is the most common extra-articular manifestation of AS.
- *Cardiovascular:* Inflammation of the aorta, aortic valve insufficiency, or third degree heart block.
- *Pulmonary:* Pulmonary fibrosis.
- *Gastrointestinal:* Inflammatory bowel disease (5–10%).
- *Genito-urinary:* IgA nephropathy, prostatitis.

67.7 Diagnosis

67.7.1 *Assessment of SpondyloArthritis International Society (ASAS)—* 2009—Introduced Axial SpA Criteria

Evidence of sacroiliitis on imaging (radiographic or magnetic resonance imaging [MRI]) is a major inclusion criterion for AS. A standardized plain radiographic grading scale exists for sacroiliitis, which ranges from normal (0) to most severe (IV).

- 0: Normal sacroiliac (SI) joint width, sharp joint margins
- I: Suspicious
- II: Sclerosis, some erosions
- III: Severe erosions, pseudo-dilation of the joint space, partial ankylosis
- IV: Complete ankylosis

67.7.2 Modified New York Criteria

Essential Criteria Grade 2–4 sacroiliitis on both sides or grade 3–4 sacroiliitis on one side on X-rays. The different grades of sacroiliitis on X-ray are as follows:

- Grade 0: normal
- Grade 1: suspicious changes
- Grade 2: minimal definite changes
- Grade 3: distinctive changes
- Grade 4: ankylosis (fusion of the bones)

Supporting Criteria *At least one of the following clinical criteria*

(a) Insidious onset low back pain for at least 3 months, which is improved by exercise and not relieved by rest.
(b) Limitation of the lumbar (low) spine movement in sagittal and frontal plane (Schober test/modified Schober test).
(c) Limitation of chest expansion (<5 cm at fourth inhaled corticosteroid [ICS]).

67.8 Clinical Examination

- Test for sacroiliitis or sacroiliac joint:
  - Gaenslen test
    The patient begins positioned in supine with the painful leg resting on the edge of the treatment table. The examiner sagitally flexes the nonsymptomatic hip, while the knee also flexed (up to 90 degrees). The patient should hold the non-tested (asymptomatic) leg with both arms, while the therapist stabilizes the pelvis and applies passive pressure to the leg being tested (symptomatic) to hold it in a hyperextended position. A downward force is applied to the lower leg (symptomatic side) putting it into hyperextension at the hip, while a flexion-based counterforce is applied to the flexed leg, pushing it in the cephalad direction causing torque to the pelvis. A positive test indicates exacerbation of pain in the affected side of sacroiliac joint (Fig. 67.3).

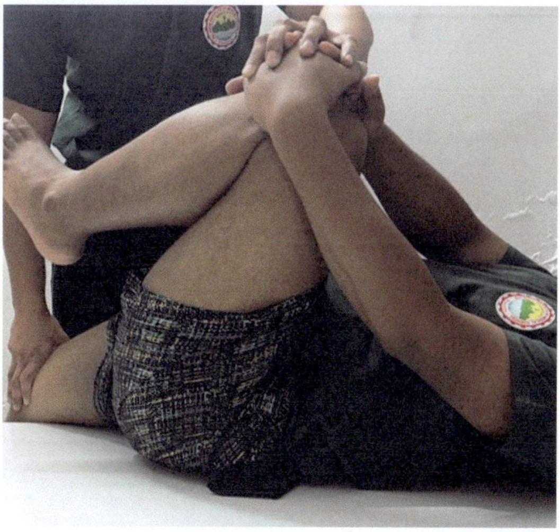

Fig. 67.3 Gaenslen test

  - Patrick/FABER test/figure-of-4 test
    The patient is positioned in supine. The leg is placed in a figure-of-4 position (hip flexed and abducted with the lateral ankle resting on the contralateral thigh proximal to the knee). While stabilizing the opposite side of the pelvis at the anterior superior iliac spine, an external rotation, abduction, and posterior force are then lightly applied to the ipsilateral knee until the end range of motion is achieved. A further few small-amplitude oscillations can be applied to check for pain provocation at the end range of motion. A positive test is one that reproduces the patient's pain or limits their range of movement (Fig. 67.4).

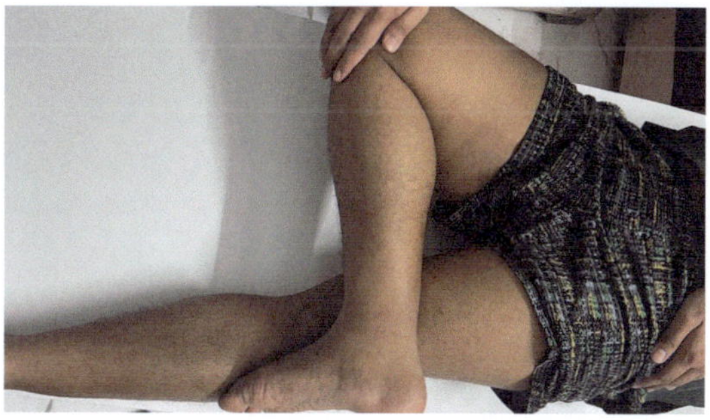

Fig. 67.4 Patrick/FABER test/figure-of-4 test

  - Other provocative tests for SI joint (Table 67.2).
- Test for cervical spine mobility:
  - *Occiput to wall distance or Flesche test*
    Should be normally zero.
  - *Tragus to wall distance*
    With the patient in normal standing position and the head in neutral alignment without allowing any rotations of the neck and the chin drawn in as far as possible, the distance between the tragus and the wall is measured with a rigid ruler.
  - *Cervical spine movements*
    Range of motion of the cervical spine is checked by sideways rotations as well as

Table 67.2 Different clinical tests to detect signs of AS

Tests	Description (positive findings)
Distraction	Pelvic tilt (PT) supine. Examiner applies posterolateral directed pressure to bilateral ASIS. (reproduction of pain)
Compression	Pt lying sideways. Examiner compresses pelvis with pressure applied over the iliac crest directed at the opposite iliac crest. (reproduction of symptoms)
Thigh thrust	Pt supine. Examiner places hip in 90 deg. flexion and adduction. Examiner then applies posteriorly directed force through the femur at varying angles of abduction/adduction. (reproduction of buttock pain)
Sacral thrust	Pt prone. Examiner delivers an anteriorly directed thrust over the sacrum. (reproduction of pain)

forward flexion and extension of the c-spine.

- Test for thoracic spine mobility:
  - *Chest expansion*

    Measured using a graduated measuring tape at the nipple level circumferentially. The difference in maximal inspiration and maximal expiration is calculated.

    Measured at fourth intercostal space, at the nipple level in males and just below the breasts in females.

    Ideally normal is >/= 5 cm

    Abnormal when it is <5 cm.
- Test for lumbar spine mobility:
  - Modified Schober test
    - Patient is standing; examiner marks both posterior superior iliac spine (PSIS) and then draws a horizontal line at the centre of both marks.
    - A second line is marked 5 cm below the first line.
    - A third line is marked 10 cm above the first line.
    - Patient is then instructed to flex forward as if attempting to touch his/her toes; examiner remeasures distance between the top and bottom line.
  - Interpretation

    Less than 5 cm increase in length with forward flexion: Decreased lumbar spine range of motion, in ankylosing spondylitis indicates a positive Schober test.

67.8.1 Radiological Features

67.8.1.1 X-Rays

- Sacroiliac Joint:
  - Erosions causing *pseudo-widening* and juxta-articular sclerosis (earliest change) more on the iliac side of the joint.
  - Later stages show ankylosis (fibrous followed by bony) (Fig. 67.5).
- Spine:
  - Loss of lumbar lordosis
  - Enthesitis and erosion of anterior corners of vertebrae (*squaring* of vertebrae) (Fig. 67.6)
- Bony spur formation (syndesmophyte) which are *vertically* oriented (horizontal orientation is seen in degenerative spine disease) (Fig. 67.7).

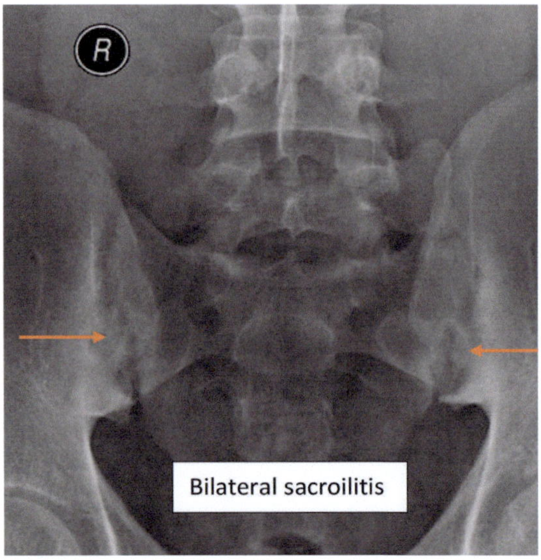

Fig. 67.5 Arrows suggesting bilateral sacroilitis

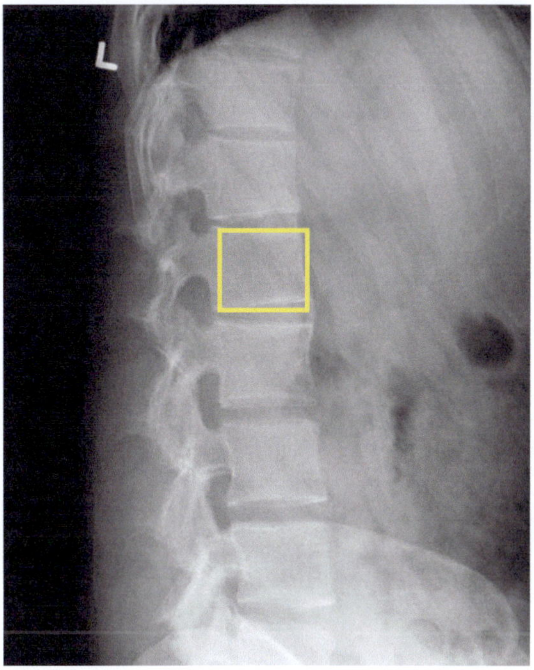

Fig. 67.6 Squaring of the vertebrae and loss of lumbar lordosis

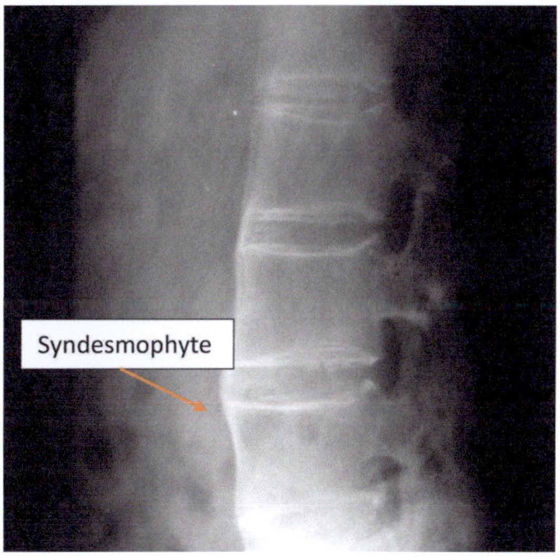

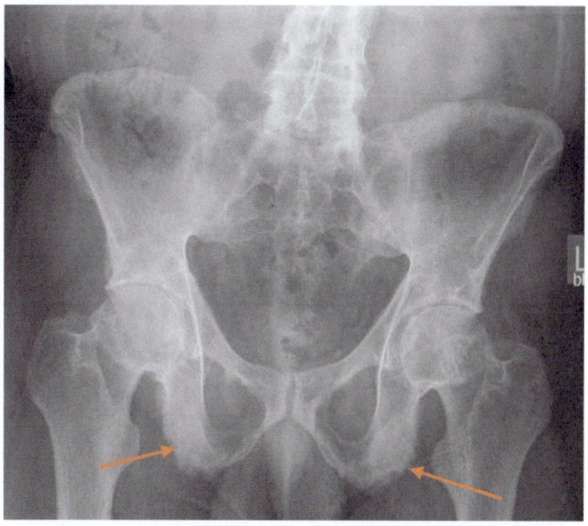

Ischial whiskering with bilateral hip joint arthritis

Fig. 67.7 Plain radiographs showing syndesmophytes formation, bamboo spine/dagger sign, and ischial whiskering

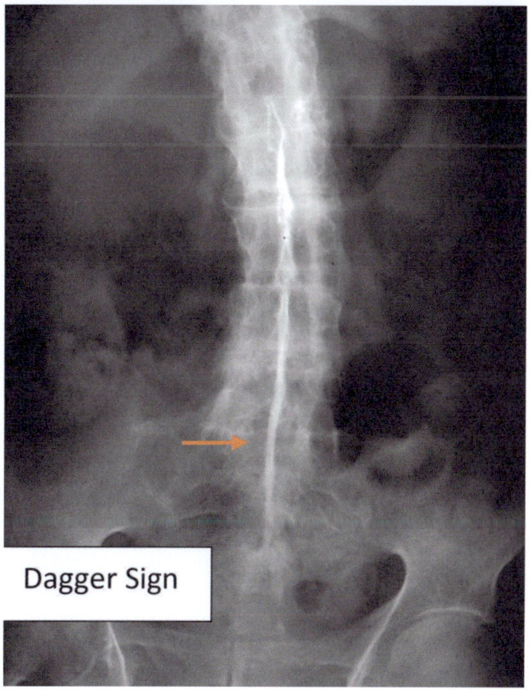

Fig. 67.8 X-ray lumbar spine AP view suggesting Dagger sign

- *Bamboo spine, dagger sign, trolley track* appearance (Fig. 67.8).
- *Romanus sign/shiny corner sign:* sclerosis of margins of vertebral body (Fig. 67.9).

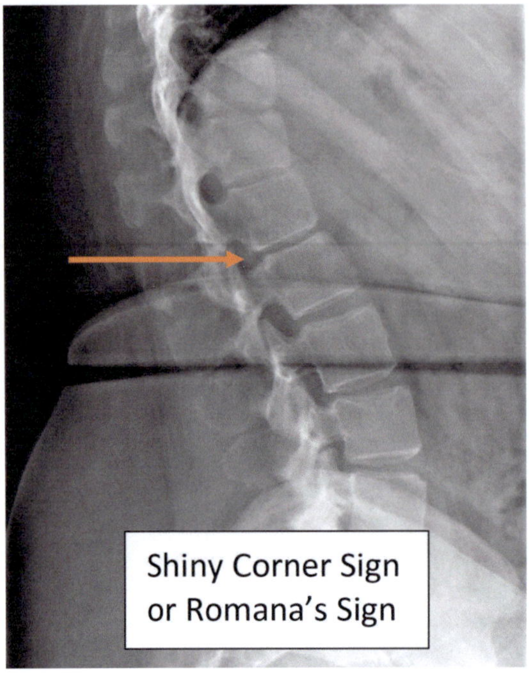

Fig. 67.9 X-ray lumbar spine lateral view showing irregularity and erosion involving the anterior and posterior edges of the vertebral endplates of L1–L2 vertebrae

67.9 Treatment

No cure for AS, although treatments and medications can reduce symptoms and pain.

67.9.1 Lifestyle Modifications

Lifestyle modifications such as quitting smoking, maintaining a healthy weight, and avoiding positions that strain the back can help reduce pain and improve mobility.

67.9.2 Physical Therapy

- Low intensity aerobic exercise
- Transcutaneous electrical nerve stimulation (TENS)
- Thermotherapy
- Proprioceptive neuromuscular facilitation (PNF)
- Hydrotherapy
- Physical therapy can help improve joint mobility and muscle strength
- Exercises that focus on stretching and strengthening the back and abdominal muscles can help improve posture and reduce pain

67.9.3 Medical Management

The medical management of ankylosing spondylitis (AS) typically involves the use of nonsteroidal anti-inflammatory drugs (NSAIDs), disease-modifying antirheumatic drugs (DMARDs), and biologic agents.

Here are some of the common drugs and doses used in AS:

1. Nonsteroidal anti-inflammatory drugs (NSAIDs):
   Ibuprofen: 1200–2400 mg/day in divided doses
   Naproxen: 1000–1500 mg/day in divided doses
   Celecoxib: 200 mg twice daily
2. Disease-modifying antirheumatic drugs (DMARDs):
   Sulfasalazine: starting dose of 500 mg twice daily, increased by 500 mg/week up to a maximum of 2 g twice daily
   Methotrexate: starting dose of 7.5–15 mg once weekly, increased by 2.5–5 mg/week up to a maximum of 25 mg/week
3. Biologic agents:
   Adalimumab: It is a monoclonal antibody that specifically targets tumor necrosis factor alpha (TNF-alpha)

Dose: 40 mg subcutaneously every other week or 80 mg every other week for the first dose

Etanercept: It is a fusion protein that acts as a tumor necrosis factor (TNF) inhibitor by binding to and inhibiting TNF-alpha

Dose: 50 mg subcutaneously once weekly or 25 mg subcutaneously twice weekly

Infliximab: It is a monoclonal antibody that specifically targets tumor necrosis factor alpha (TNF-alpha)

Dose: 5 mg/kg intravenously at weeks 0, 2, and 6, then every 6–8 weeks thereafter

It is important to note that the dosages and frequencies of these medications depending on the patient's condition, medical history, and response to treatment may vary.

#Extra-Edge

The Bath Ankylosing Spondylitis Disease Activity Index (BASDAI) is used to assesses the need for additional therapy.

BASDAI is a self-reported questionnaire that consists of six questions related to the patient's pain, stiffness, and other symptoms over the past week. The questions are scored on a 0–10 scale, with 0 indicating no disease activity and 10 indicating the highest level of disease activity.

The six questions in BASDAI are as follows:

1. How severe is your fatigue/tiredness?
2. How severe is your spinal pain or neck pain?
3. How severe is your peripheral joint pain/swelling?
4. How severe is your enthesitis (inflammation of tendons and ligaments)?
5. How severe is your morning stiffness?
6. How severe is your ability to perform daily activities?

The total BASDAI score ranges from 0 to 50, with higher scores indicating more severe disease activity. A score of 4 or higher indicates active disease, and a reduction in BASDAI score by 2 or more points is considered clinically meaningful.

The Bath Ankylosing Spondylitis Functional Index (BASFI) is used to establish a current baseline and subsequent response to therapy.

BASFI is a self-reported questionnaire that consists of ten questions related to the patient's ability to perform daily activities. The questions are scored on a 0–10 scale, with 0 indicating no difficulty in performing the activity and 10 indicating the highest level of difficulty.

The ten questions in BASFI are as follows:

1. Getting up from bed
2. Getting up from a chair
3. Putting on socks or stockings
4. Bending forward to pick up small objects
5. Reaching up to a high shelf
6. Sitting for long periods
7. Standing still for long periods
8. Walking on flat ground
9. Climbing stairs
10. Looking over either shoulder

The total BASFI score ranges from 0 to 100, with higher scores indicating more severe functional impairment. A reduction in BASFI score by 2 or more points is considered clinically meaningful.

Bottom of form

67.9.4 Surgery

In severe cases of AS, arthroplasty or joint replacement surgery of the knees and hip joint remains the only options. Surgical interventions are challenging as giving anesthesia in these cases are difficult. This is due to changes in the upper airway which can lead to difficulties in intubating the airway, and calcification of ligaments makes administering spinal and epidural anesthesia equally challenging in these cases (Table 67.3).

#Extra-Edge

Flexible fiber-optic method of intubation is often used during induction by general anesthesia.

#Extra-Edge

Multiple Choice Questions

1. All are true for ankylosing spondylitis except,
   (a) Starts with sacroiliac joint involvement
   (b) Enthesitis is common
   (c) Common in males
   (d) Plain radiograph is most sensitive
2. Which of the following is not extra-articular manifestation of ankylosing spondylitis?
   (a) Anterior uveitis
   (b) Aortic valvular diseases
   (c) Pulmonary fibrosis
   (d) Dilated cardiomyopathy
3. An young male with low back pain, morning stiffness, and reduced chest expansion is likely to be diagnosed with?
   (a) Rheumatoid arthritis
   (b) Gout

Table 67.3 Differences between ankylosing spondylitis and ankylosing hyperostosis/diffuse idiopathic skeletal hyperostosis (DISH)

	Ankylosing spondylitis	Ankylosing hyperostosis/diffuse idiopathic skeletal hyperostosis (DISH)
Age	Young	Elderly
Sacroiliitis	Always present	Absent
Chest expansion	Marked but not reliable	Mild restriction
Tenderness	Sacroiliac	Dorsolumbar
Syndesmophytes	Present (marginal)	Present (extra-marginal)
ESR	High	Normal to mild rise

   (c) Pseudogout
   (d) Ankylosing spondylitis
4. Which joint is rarely involved in ankylosing spondylitis?
   (a) Hip
   (b) Knee
   (c) Shoulders
   (d) Ankle
5. Scleritis with autoimmune joint disorders are seen with?
   (a) Ankylosing spondylitis
   (b) Gout
   (c) Reactive arthritis
   (d) Rheumatoid arthritis

Answers: 1. (d), 2. (d), 3. (d), 4. (d), 5. (d)

References for Further Reading

1. https://www.statpearls.com/ArticleLibrary/viewarticle/17609#:~:text=Ankylosing%20spondylitis%20(AS)%20is%20a,digits%2C%20and%20entheses%20are%20characteristic.
2. https://www.webmd.com/ankylosing-spondylitis/what-is-ankylosing-spondylitis
3. https://pubmed.ncbi.nlm.nih.gov/33754220/
4. https://www.ncbi.nlm.nih.gov/pmc/articles/PMC6804882/
5. https://pubmed.ncbi.nlm.nih.gov/35928330/

Soft Tissue Affections of Upper Limb and Lower Limb

68

Sanny Kumar Singh and Ranjit Kumar Singh

68.1 Subacromial Bursitis

Subacromial bursitis is a common cause of shoulder pain, resulting from inflammation of the subacromial bursa—a fluid-filled sac located between the supraspinatus tendon and the acromion, which helps reduce friction during shoulder movement. The condition often develops due to repetitive overhead activity, trauma, or associated rotator cuff tendinopathy. Patients typically present with dull, aching pain over the lateral or anterolateral aspect of the shoulder, which may radiate to the deltoid region. The pain is often aggravated by overhead movements, reaching across the body, or activities like combing hair, lifting objects, or dressing. Night pain is common, especially when lying on the affected side. A characteristic finding is a painful arc of movement, particularly during abduction between 60 and 120 degrees.

On examination, there may be localized tenderness below the acromion, and special tests such as Neer's and Hawkins–Kennedy tests are often positive, reproducing the symptoms. Passive range of motion is usually preserved, distinguishing it from adhesive capsulitis, while strength may be slightly reduced due to pain but typically without true muscle weakness unless there is a coexisting rotator cuff tear. Diagnosis is mainly clinical, but imaging such as ultrasound or MRI can confirm bursal inflammation or rule out other pathologies in persistent or unclear cases.

Treatment is primarily conservative and includes rest from aggravating activities, ice application, and nonsteroidal anti-inflammatory drugs (NSAIDs) to reduce pain and inflammation. Physiotherapy is crucial and focuses on stretching tight shoulder structures, improving posture, and strengthening the rotator cuff and scapular stabilizers to restore normal biomechanics and prevent recurrence. If symptoms are severe or unresponsive to initial treatment, a corticosteroid injection into the subacromial space may provide significant short-term relief, though repeated injections are discouraged due to risks such as tendon weakening and skin atrophy. Surgical intervention, such as arthroscopic bursectomy or subacromial decompression, is considered only in chronic cases that fail to improve after at least 3 to 6 months of conservative management. Prognosis is generally excellent with timely diagnosis and appropriate rehabilitation, with most patients achieving full recovery and return to normal activities within a few weeks to a few months.

S. K. Singh (✉)
Department of Orthopaedics, Postgraduate Institute of Medical Education & Research, Chandigarh, India

R. K. Singh
Department of Orthopaedics, Nalanda Medical College & Hospital, Patna, Bihar, India

V. Kumar et al. (eds.), *A Quick Guide to Essential Orthopedics*,
https://doi.org/10.1007/978-981-95-2676-5_68

68.2 Bicipital Tendonitis

Bicipital tendonitis, also referred to as biceps tendinopathy, describes inflammation or degeneration of the long head of the biceps tendon as it passes through the bicipital groove of the humerus. This condition is frequently observed in individuals involved in repetitive overhead activities, such as swimming, tennis, or weight lifting, and may also develop secondary to rotator cuff dysfunction or shoulder instability. Patients often report aching anterior shoulder pain that intensifies with overhead movements or lifting and may extend down the anterior arm. Pain can be triggered by actions like throwing, pushing, or carrying heavy objects. Clinical examination typically reveals tenderness over the bicipital groove, particularly when the arm is externally rotated and slightly abducted. Provocative tests such as Speed's test (resisted forward flexion with forearm supinated) and Yergason's test (resisted supination with elbow flexed) commonly reproduce the reported pain. Passive range of motion generally remains intact, and strength tends to be normal unless there is significant pain or a partial tear. Diagnosis is mainly clinical but can be supported by musculoskeletal ultrasound or MRI if uncertainty exists or if associated pathology, such as rotator cuff tears, is suspected. Management is usually conservative and includes rest from aggravating activities, application of ice, and use of NSAIDs to control symptoms. A structured physiotherapy program focusing on stretching the shoulder capsule and strengthening the rotator cuff and scapular stabilizers may help address muscle imbalances and decrease stress on the biceps tendon. Ultrasound-guided corticosteroid injections into the bicipital groove can be considered for short-term symptom relief in persistent cases, though their use should be limited due to potential risk of tendon weakening. In chronic or unresponsive cases, particularly those involving structural damage such as tendon subluxation, partial tear, or rupture, surgical interventions like biceps tenodesis or tenotomy may be indicated. With suitable management, most patients demonstrate improvement and resume activity within several weeks to months.

68.3 Olecranon Bursitis

Olecranon bursitis is the inflammation of the bursa located over the posterior aspect of the elbow, between the olecranon process and the overlying skin. It can be caused by repeated minor trauma (as seen in occupations or activities involving prolonged leaning on the elbows), acute injury, infection, inflammatory arthropathies like gout or rheumatoid arthritis, or may be idiopathic. Clinically, patients typically present with swelling over the tip of the elbow, which may be painless or associated with mild to moderate discomfort, especially during elbow flexion. The swelling is soft, fluctuant, and mobile, and in noninfectious cases, the overlying skin is usually normal in color and temperature. In septic bursitis, signs such as erythema, warmth, tenderness, and systemic symptoms like fever may be present. Active and passive range of motion of the elbow remains largely unaffected, which helps distinguish it from intra-articular pathology.

Diagnosis is primarily clinical, though aspiration of the bursal fluid is indicated when infection or crystal arthropathy is suspected. Analysis includes cell count, Gram stain, culture, and crystal examination. Imaging is rarely needed unless underlying bone involvement is suspected. Treatment depends on the underlying cause. For noninfectious bursitis, conservative management includes activity modification, compression, ice application, and NSAIDs. Aspiration may relieve discomfort, but recurrence is common. If symptoms persist or cause functional limitation, corticosteroid injection may be considered, although repeated injections are discouraged. Septic bursitis requires prompt aspiration and appropriate antibiotic therapy, and in some cases, repeated drainage or surgical bursectomy may be necessary. Surgical intervention may also be considered in chronic, recurrent, or refractory noninfectious cases.

68.4 Tenosynovitis of Flexor Tendons

Tenosynovitis of the flexor tendons refers to inflammation of the synovial sheath that surrounds the flexor tendons of the hand, most commonly affecting the fingers and thumb. It can result from repetitive strain, overuse, trauma, infection, or inflammatory conditions such as rheumatoid arthritis. A common form is stenosing tenosynovitis, also known as "trigger finger," in which thickening of the tendon or its sheath causes difficulty in tendon gliding through the A1 pulley, leading to painful catching or locking of the digit in flexion. Infectious flexor tenosynovitis is a surgical emergency, often caused by penetrating injuries introducing bacteria (commonly *Staphylococcus aureus*), and is characterized by Kanavel's four cardinal signs: fusiform swelling of the digit, finger held in flexion, tenderness along the flexor tendon sheath, and pain on passive extension. In noninfectious cases, patients typically report localized pain, swelling, and stiffness over the affected tendon, often worsened with movement or gripping. Diagnosis is mainly clinical, though ultrasound may assist in detecting fluid in the sheath or guiding injections.

Treatment of noninfectious tenosynovitis includes rest, splinting, activity modification, NSAIDs, and physiotherapy. In cases of trigger finger, corticosteroid injections into the tendon sheath are commonly effective, especially in early stages. Surgical release of the A1 pulley may be considered in recurrent or persistent cases. In infectious tenosynovitis, urgent surgical drainage and debridement, along with intravenous antibiotics, are required to prevent tendon necrosis and preserve hand function. Early recognition and appropriate treatment are critical, as delayed management can lead to tendon rupture, adhesions, or permanent loss of motion. With timely and appropriate therapy, the prognosis is generally good.

68.5 De Quervain's Tenosynovitis

De Quervain's tenosynovitis is a painful inflammatory condition affecting the tendons of the first dorsal compartment of the wrist—specifically, the abductor pollicis longus (APL) and extensor pollicis brevis (EPB) tendons. It is most commonly seen in individuals who perform repetitive thumb movements or wrist ulnar deviation, such as new mothers, factory workers, or people frequently using smartphones. Patients typically present with pain and swelling over the radial side of the wrist near the base of the thumb, which worsens with gripping, lifting, pinching, or thumb motion. The hallmark clinical sign is a positive Finkelstein's test, in which the patient experiences sharp pain when the thumb is flexed into the palm and the wrist is deviated ulnarly. Tenderness over the radial styloid and sometimes crepitus may be noted on examination. Diagnosis is primarily clinical and imaging is rarely required, although ultrasound may reveal tendon sheath thickening or fluid collection. Treatment is initially conservative and includes activity modification, rest, splinting of the thumb and wrist (thumb spica splint), application of ice, and NSAIDs for pain relief. In cases not responding to initial measures, a corticosteroid injection into the tendon sheath often provides significant symptomatic improvement. If conservative treatment fails after 6–8 weeks or symptoms are recurrent, surgical release of the first dorsal compartment may be considered to relieve tendon entrapment. Prognosis is excellent with early diagnosis and appropriate therapy, and most patients return to normal activities with complete resolution of symptoms.

68.6 Carpal Tunnel Syndrome Secondary to Synovitis

Carpal tunnel syndrome (CTS) secondary to synovitis refers to median nerve compression at the wrist caused by inflammation and thickening of the synovial tissue surrounding the flexor tendons within the carpal tunnel. This is commonly associated with inflammatory arthropathies such as rheumatoid arthritis, lupus, or gout. Synovial proliferation reduces the space within the tunnel and increases pressure on the median nerve, leading to sensory and motor symptoms. Patients typically present with numbness, tingling, or burning pain in the thumb, index, middle, and radial half of the ring finger, often worse at night or with repetitive hand use. They may also report hand weakness, clumsiness, or dropping objects.

On examination, positive Tinel's sign (tingling on percussion over the carpal tunnel), Phalen's test (wrist flexion reproducing symptoms), and thenar muscle atrophy in advanced cases may be noted. In inflammatory CTS, joint swelling, warmth, and morning stiffness may also be present. Diagnosis is clinical but can be supported by nerve conduction studies and ultrasound or MRI, which may show thickened synovium and median nerve compression. Management focuses on controlling the underlying synovitis with disease-modifying antirheumatic drugs (DMARDs) or corticosteroids, along with wrist splinting, activity modification, and NSAIDs for symptom relief. Local corticosteroid injection into the carpal tunnel may reduce synovial inflammation and relieve nerve compression. In severe or refractory cases, surgical decompression through carpal tunnel release may be required, often combined with synovectomy to remove inflamed synovial tissue. Early treatment is crucial to prevent permanent nerve damage and preserve hand function.

68.7 Trigger Finger

Trigger finger, also known as stenosing tenosynovitis, is a condition in which the flexor tendon of a finger or thumb becomes irritated and thickened, leading to difficulty in smooth gliding through the A1 pulley at the base of the digit. This results in painful catching, locking, or clicking during finger movement. The condition commonly affects the ring finger and thumb and is more frequent in middle-aged adults, females, and individuals with systemic conditions such as diabetes mellitus or rheumatoid arthritis. Patients typically report discomfort or stiffness in the affected finger, particularly in the morning, and may notice a palpable nodule or tenderness at the base of the finger. In more advanced cases, the digit may lock in flexion and require passive manipulation to extend. On examination, triggering is observed during active finger motion, and localized tenderness over the A1 pulley is present. Diagnosis is clinical and does not usually require imaging.

Initial treatment is conservative and includes activity modification, NSAIDs, splinting of the affected finger (especially at night), and stretching exercises. In cases not responding to conservative therapy, a corticosteroid injection into the flexor tendon sheath near the A1 pulley is often effective, particularly in early stages. If symptoms persist despite one or two injections, or if the finger is persistently locked, surgical release of the A1 pulley is considered. This is typically a minor procedure with a high success rate. The prognosis is excellent in most cases, especially with early recognition and appropriate treatment.

68.8 Trochanteric Bursitis

Trochanteric bursitis, also termed greater trochanteric pain syndrome (GTPS), refers to inflammation of the bursa overlying the greater trochanter of the femur. It often occurs due to repetitive microtrauma, direct injury, biomechanical stress (e.g., from leg-length discrepancy or altered gait), or as part of underlying conditions such as osteoarthritis, lumbar spine disorders, or iliotibial (IT) band syndrome. It is more prevalent in middle-aged women and runners. Patients typically present with lateral hip pain, localized over the greater trochanter, which may radiate to the lateral thigh but does not extend below the knee. Pain is aggravated by prolonged standing, lying on the affected side, climbing stairs, or crossing the legs. On examination, there is tenderness on palpation over the greater trochanter, and pain may be reproduced with resisted abduction, hip rotation, or active stretching of the hip abductors. Unlike intra-articular hip pathology, trochanteric bursitis does not significantly affect passive range of motion.

Diagnosis is primarily clinical, but imaging such as ultrasound or MRI may help confirm bursitis or rule out gluteal tendinopathy or partial tears. X-rays are usually normal but may be used to exclude bony abnormalities. Treatment is initially conservative, including activity modification, weight loss, NSAIDs, and physiotherapy focusing on stretching of the iliotibial band and strengthening of gluteal muscles. Local corticosteroid injection into the trochanteric bursa is effective for persistent cases and offers substantial pain relief, though repeated injections are discouraged due to potential soft tissue atrophy. Shock wave therapy and platelet-rich plasma (PRP) injections are emerging options with some evidence for benefit in chronic cases. Surgical intervention, such as bursectomy or IT band release, is rarely required and reserved for recalcitrant symptoms despite prolonged conservative care. The prognosis is generally excellent with appropriate nonoperative management, though recurrence can occur if biomechanical contributors are not addressed.

68.9 Prepatellar Bursitis

Prepatellar bursitis is the inflammation of the bursa located between the skin and the patella, commonly referred to as "housemaid's knee" due to its association with prolonged kneeling. It may result from acute trauma (e.g., a direct blow), chronic repetitive microtrauma, infection, or inflammatory conditions such as gout or rheumatoid arthritis. It is more frequently observed in individuals whose occupations involve frequent kneeling, such as plumbers, carpenters, and wrestlers. Patients typically present with anterior knee swelling that is soft, fluctuant, and localized over the patella. Pain may range from mild discomfort to significant tenderness, particularly with pressure on the knee or full flexion. The overlying skin may appear normal in noninfectious cases, while erythema, warmth, and systemic symptoms (fever, chills) suggest septic bursitis, which occurs in a notable proportion of cases, especially if there is skin breakdown. Knee joint movement is usually preserved, and the absence of deep joint pain helps distinguish it from intra-articular pathology. Diagnosis is mainly clinical, but aspiration of the bursal fluid is recommended when infection or crystal arthropathy is suspected. Fluid analysis should include Gram stain, culture, cell count, and crystal examination. Imaging (ultrasound or MRI) is rarely needed unless complications are suspected.

Treatment of noninfectious bursitis includes activity modification, avoiding kneeling, compression, NSAIDs, and ice application. Aspiration can relieve pressure and discomfort, and corticosteroid injections may be considered for persistent symptoms, though repeated use is discouraged. Septic bursitis requires immediate aspiration, appropriate antibiotic therapy based on culture sensitivity, and occasionally surgical drainage if the infection does not respond to conservative treatment. Surgical bursectomy is rarely needed but may be indicated in chronic, recurrent, or nonresolving cases. With appropriate care, the majority of patients recover fully, and preventive strategies such as using knee pads or avoiding prolonged kneeling can help reduce recurrence.

68.10 Pes Anserine Bursitis

Pes anserine bursitis is an inflammatory condition of the bursa located between the pes anserinus tendon insertion (formed by the sartorius, gracilis, and semitendinosus muscles) and the medial aspect of the proximal tibia, just below the knee joint. It is commonly seen in middle-aged women, overweight individuals, and athletes involved in running or activities requiring repetitive knee flexion. Contributing factors include obesity, knee osteoarthritis, malalignment (genu valgum), tight hamstrings, and improper training techniques. Clinically, patients complain of medial knee pain that is aggravated by climbing stairs, rising from a seated position, or during prolonged walking. The pain is typically localized about 4–5 cm below the medial joint line and may be accompanied by tenderness and mild swelling over the insertion of the pes anserine tendons. Unlike intra-articular pathology, joint range of motion is typically preserved, and there is no joint effusion.

Diagnosis is largely clinical, although ultrasound may reveal bursal fluid or inflammation, and MRI can help exclude other conditions such as medial meniscus injury in cases of diagnostic uncertainty. Management is primarily conservative and involves activity modification, NSAIDs, ice application, and stretching and strengthening of the hamstrings and quadriceps. Addressing biomechanical issues—such as improper footwear, valgus deformity, or tight musculature—is essential to prevent recurrence. Physical therapy focusing on correcting gait abnormalities, posture, and flexibility is key to long-term relief. Corticosteroid injections into the bursa may be used in persistent cases to reduce inflammation and pain. Surgical intervention is rarely required and is reserved for chronic, refractory cases that do not respond to extensive conservative measures. Prognosis is excellent, with most patients achieving symptom resolution through nonoperative treatment and lifestyle modifications.

68.11 Baker's Cyst

Baker's cyst, or popliteal cyst, is a fluid-filled swelling that forms in the popliteal fossa, usually as a result of distension of the gastrocnemio-semimembranosus bursa. It is not a true cyst but rather a communication between the knee joint and the bursa, often associated with underlying intra-articular knee pathology. Common causes include osteoarthritis, rheumatoid arthritis, meniscal tears, and other joint effusions that increase intra-articular pressure, forcing synovial fluid into the bursa. Baker's cysts are more common in adults over 40 and may also occur in children, although usually without joint pathology in the pediatric population.

Clinically, patients may present with a posterior knee swelling that is soft, fluctuant, and located between the medial head of the gastrocnemius and the semimembranosus tendon. The swelling may vary in size and is often more prominent when standing and reduced when the knee is flexed. Associated symptoms include tightness, discomfort, or aching pain behind the knee, particularly with full flexion or extension. In some cases, the cyst can rupture, leading to leakage of fluid into the calf, causing sudden pain, swelling, and redness—a presentation that can mimic deep vein thrombosis (DVT), and is often referred to as a "pseudothrombophlebitis syndrome." On examination, a Baker's cyst may be palpable as a smooth, soft mass in the posteromedial knee, and transillumination may be positive if the cyst is superficial. Ultrasound is the first-line imaging modality used to confirm the presence of the cyst, distinguish it from DVT, and detect associated joint effusion or meniscal pathology. MRI is more sensitive and can help identify underlying intra-articular lesions.

Management depends on the severity of symptoms and the presence of underlying joint disease. Asymptomatic cysts often require no treatment and may resolve spontaneously. Symptomatic cysts are initially managed conservatively with NSAIDs, ice application, compression, physiotherapy, and treatment of the primary joint disorder. Aspiration of the cyst under ultrasound guidance may provide temporary relief, and corticosteroid injection into the joint or cyst may reduce inflammation and recurrence. However, recurrence is common if the underlying pathology is not addressed. Surgical excision of the cyst is rarely indicated but may be considered for persistent, painful, or recurrent cysts, particularly when mechanical symptoms are present or when associated intra-articular conditions require arthroscopy. With appropriate management, the prognosis is generally good, although recurrence is possible, especially in patients with chronic inflammatory or degenerative joint disease.

68.12 Posterior Tibial Tendinitis

Posterior tibial tendinitis is an overuse inflammatory condition affecting the posterior tibial tendon, which plays a crucial role in supporting the medial longitudinal arch and inverting the foot. This tendon runs behind the medial malleolus and inserts into the navicular and midfoot bones. Tendinitis occurs due to repetitive stress, commonly in runners, athletes, dancers, and individuals with flatfeet or improper footwear. It is also associated with obesity, hypertension, diabetes, and inflammatory arthropathies. Patients typically present with medial ankle and foot pain, which may radiate along the arch and worsen with weight-bearing or activity, especially walking or running. In early stages, the tendon is inflamed but intact, while chronic or untreated cases can lead to posterior tibial tendon dysfunction (PTTD) and progressive adult-acquired flatfoot deformity.

On examination, there may be swelling and tenderness posterior to the medial malleolus, pain with resisted foot inversion, and difficulty performing a single-leg heel raise. In more advanced stages, collapse of the arch, hindfoot valgus, and forefoot abduction may be observed. Diagnosis is primarily clinical, supported by ultrasound or MRI to assess tendon integrity and rule out partial or full-thickness tears. X-rays may be useful in later stages to evaluate structural deformity. Management depends on the severity and stage of the condition. Early-stage tendinitis is treated conservatively with rest, ice application, NSAIDs, activity modification, and immobilization using a walking boot or brace. Once pain subsides, a structured rehabilitation program including stretching, strengthening of the tibialis posterior and intrinsic foot muscles, and use of custom orthotics to support the arch is crucial. Corticosteroid injections are generally avoided near the posterior tibial tendon due to the risk of tendon rupture. In refractory cases or when significant tendon degeneration or rupture occurs, surgical intervention may be needed, ranging from tendon debridement and repair to osteotomies or tendon transfer procedures. With timely diagnosis and appropriate management, early-stage posterior tibial tendinitis usually resolves well, but delayed treatment can lead to permanent deformity and functional impairment.

68.13 Achilles Tendinitis

Achilles tendinitis is an overuse injury characterized by inflammation or degeneration of the Achilles tendon, which connects the gastrocnemius and soleus muscles to the calcaneus. It commonly affects runners, athletes, and individuals engaged in repetitive jumping or high-impact sports, but may also result from sudden increases in activity, improper footwear, or poor training techniques. There are two main types: insertional tendinitis, which occurs at the tendon's attachment to the calcaneus, and noninsertional tendinitis, affecting the midportion of the tendon. Patients typically present with posterior heel or lower calf pain, which develops gradually and worsens with activity, particularly running or climbing stairs. Stiffness is often prominent in the morning or after prolonged rest.

On examination, there is tenderness along the tendon, often with swelling or nodularity, and pain is exacerbated by resisted plantar flexion or passive dorsiflexion. In noninsertional tendinitis, a palpable thickening or nodular swelling may be felt 2–6 cm above the calcaneal insertion. Thompson's test is used to assess for complete rupture, which presents as a sudden "pop" during activity and inability to plantar flex. Diagnosis is largely clinical, but ultrasound or MRI may be used to assess tendon structure and confirm tendinosis or partial tearing. X-rays can show calcifications in insertional tendinitis or a Haglund's deformity.

Initial management is conservative and includes rest, ice application, NSAIDs, and activity modification, such as reducing running intensity and avoiding uphill climbs. Heel lifts and eccentric calf-strengthening exercises are central to rehabilitation. A walking boot or orthosis may be used for severe cases. Corticosteroid injections are generally avoided due to the risk of tendon rupture. If symptoms persist beyond 6 months despite conservative care, surgical intervention may be considered, including debridement of degenerated tissue or tendon repair. With early recognition and proper management, most cases of Achilles tendinitis resolve within weeks to months, but chronic cases may lead to tendinosis and increased risk of rupture if neglected.

68.14 Plantar Fasciitis

Plantar fasciitis is the most common cause of inferior heel pain, accounting for approximately 10% of running-related injuries and a significant number of visits to orthopedic and primary care clinics. The condition results from repetitive microtrauma and degeneration of the plantar fascia, a thick band of connective tissue that runs from the medial calcaneal tuberosity to the metatarsal heads, supporting the medial longitudinal arch of the foot. Despite the "-itis" suffix, chronic plantar fasciitis is better characterized as a fasciosis, involving collagen degeneration, fibroblast proliferation, and neovascularization rather than acute inflammation. It is most prevalent in middle-aged adults, though it can affect younger individuals, particularly runners, military recruits, and occupational workers who spend long hours standing or walking. Risk factors include obesity, tight Achilles tendons, limited ankle dorsiflexion, pes planus (flatfeet), pes cavus (high arches), prolonged standing, and inappropriate footwear with poor arch support.

Clinically, patients report sharp, stabbing pain in the medial aspect of the heel, especially during the first steps in the morning or after periods of prolonged sitting. This "start-up pain" typically decreases with ambulation but may return or worsen after extended activity. On physical examination, there is localized tenderness over the medial calcaneal tuberosity and along the proximal plantar fascia. The windlass test, which passively dorsiflexes the toes while the patient stands on tiptoes or the examiner extends the great toe, can reproduce the pain. Passive ankle dorsiflexion may also elicit discomfort due to tension on a tight Achilles tendon.

Diagnosis is primarily clinical. Plain radiographs are not routinely required but may be used to rule out alternative diagnoses such as calcaneal stress fractures or to identify calcaneal spurs, which may coexist but are not causative. Ultrasound can show thickening (>4 mm), hypoechogenicity, and increased vascularity of the fascia. MRI may be reserved for refractory or atypical cases.

Initial management is nonoperative and includes rest, ice application, NSAIDs, and activity modification to reduce repetitive strain. A structured physical therapy program emphasizing plantar fascia and gastrocnemius–soleus stretching, eccentric strengthening, and soft tissue massage is highly effective. Use of arch supports, heel cups, night splints, and supportive footwear is essential in off-loading the fascia and promoting healing. Weight loss should be encouraged when appropriate. For patients with persistent symptoms beyond 6–8 weeks, corticosteroid injections may provide short-term relief but carry risks such as plantar fascia rupture or fat pad atrophy. Other modalities include shock wave therapy, platelet-rich plasma (PRP) injections, and custom orthotics. Surgical release of the plantar fascia is rarely necessary and reserved for severe, recalcitrant cases. With timely and appropriate conservative management, more than 90% of patients achieve significant symptom improvement within 6–12 months.

68.15 Retrocalcaneal Bursitis

Retrocalcaneal bursitis is an inflammatory condition of the bursa located between the posterior aspect of the calcaneus and the anterior surface of the Achilles tendon, just superior to its insertion. This bursa serves as a cushion to reduce friction between the tendon and the bone. Inflammation of the retrocalcaneal bursa is often caused by repetitive stress, overuse, or mechanical irritation and is commonly seen in runners, athletes, and individuals who wear poorly fitting or rigid footwear. It may also occur secondary to underlying conditions such as Haglund's deformity, rheumatoid arthritis, spondyloarthropathies, or insertional Achilles tendinopathy. Patients typically present with posterior heel pain and swelling that is worsened by walking, running, or wearing tight shoes. The pain is localized just anterior to the Achilles tendon insertion and can be distinguished from Achilles tendinitis, which causes pain more proximally. On physical examination, there is tenderness on palpation of the soft area between the Achilles tendon and the calcaneus, often with visible swelling or erythema. The "two-finger squeeze test"—squeezing the bursa between the thumb and index finger on either side of the Achilles tendon—may reproduce pain. Passive dorsiflexion of the ankle or resisted plantar flexion may also exacerbate symptoms.

Diagnosis is primarily clinical, but lateral ankle X-rays may be done to identify bony abnormalities such as Haglund's deformity. Ultrasound or MRI can confirm the diagnosis by visualizing fluid accumulation and bursal inflammation and can help rule out Achilles tendon pathology. Initial treatment is conservative and includes rest, ice application, NSAIDs, heel lifts or cushioned footwear, and activity modification to reduce pressure on the bursa. A short course of immobilization with a walking boot may be necessary in severe cases. Physical therapy focusing on Achilles stretching, eccentric strengthening, and correction of biomechanical contributors is important for long-term recovery. Corticosteroid injections into the bursa are used cautiously due to the risk of Achilles tendon rupture. In chronic or refractory cases, especially with structural deformity, surgical bursectomy or resection of Haglund's deformity may be considered. With appropriate management, prognosis is generally excellent.

Part IX

Degenerative Disorders

Osteoarthritis

69

Arghya Kundu Choudhury and Mazhar Ali

69.1 Introduction

Osteoarthritis (OA) is recognized as the most prevalent joint disorder encountered in clinical settings and stands among the foremost causes of disability on a global scale. Radiological manifestations of OA become apparent in the majority of individuals by the age of 65, with approximately 80% of people over 75 exhibiting radiographic changes. The disease spectrum ranges from being entirely asymptomatic to presenting as disabling monoarthritis or polyarthritis. The hallmark symptom is mechanical pain. Although OA can affect any synovial joint, the hands, knees, and hips are most frequently involved.

69.2 Etiology

The precise cause of primary OA remains incompletely elucidated, with evidence pointing to a multifactorial origin involving both genetic predisposition and environmental influences. Epigenetic mechanisms are estimated to contribute between 30% and 65% to OA susceptibility. Advancing age represents the most significant risk factor, associated with diminished joint resilience against mechanical stress, sarcopenia, and enhanced bone turnover.

The female sex demonstrates a higher prevalence, potentially due to anatomical variations in joint alignment, ligament laxity, impact of pregnancy, and differences in bone mineral density. Notably, the postmenopausal period correlates with an increased risk, suggesting estrogen's involvement in joint health and pain sensitivity modulation. Anatomical abnormalities, including congenital deformities or joint malalignment, predispose to abnormal biomechanics and subsequent OA development. Modifiable risk elements comprise occupational hazards involving repetitive joint use, obesity, metabolic syndrome, smoking, vitamin D insufficiency, muscle weakness, and reduced bone density.

69.3 Pathogenesis

OA is a degenerative condition of synovial joints marked by progressive cartilage deterioration, culminating in pain, stiffness, and impaired mobility. Its pathogenesis involves a dynamic interplay of mechanical forces, inflammatory mediators, and oxidative stress.

At the microscopic level, OA is characterized by alterations in cartilage composition, notably

A. Kundu Choudhury (✉)
Department of Hip, Knee and Robotic Joint Replacement, Sarvodaya Hospital and Research Centre, Faridabad, Haryana, India

M. Ali
Department of Orthopaedics & Spine Surgery, Nishtar Medical University, Multan, Punjab, Pakistan

V. Kumar et al. (eds.), *A Quick Guide to Essential Orthopedics*,
https://doi.org/10.1007/978-981-95-2676-5_69

the depletion of proteoglycans and collagen fibers, leading to reduced cartilage strength and elasticity. Beyond cartilage degradation, OA also involves the synovial membrane, subchondral bone, and periarticular ligaments. Synovial inflammation promotes the release of catabolic enzymes, further accelerating cartilage loss.

Subchondral bone undergoes changes, resulting in sclerosis and the development of osteophytes —osseous projections around joint margins—which exacerbate mechanical dysfunction and discomfort. Additionally, ligamentous structures and periarticular tendons may suffer involvement, contributing to joint instability and mechanical derangement.

69.4 Classification

69.4.1 Idiopathic (Primary) OA

69.4.1.1 Localized (Monoarticular/ Pauciarticular)

- Hand: distal interphalangeal (DIP; Heberden's nodes), proximal interphalangeal (PIP; Bouchard's nodes), first carpometacarpal (CMC) joint.
- Hip: less common in the Indian population.
- Knee: predominant.
- Spine: involving apophyseal or intervertebral joints.

69.4.1.2 Generalized (Polyarticular)

Generalized (polyarticular) OA involves three or more of the aforementioned joint sites.

69.4.2 Secondary OA

- Traumatic.
- Congenital/developmental: dysplasia, varus/ valgus deformities, Perthes disease.
- Infectious: tubercular arthritis (notably the knee and hip), often presenting with a triad of flexion, valgus deformity, external rotation, and posterior tibial subluxation.
- Inflammatory: rheumatoid arthritis, seronegative spondyloarthropathies.
- Metabolic: hemochromatosis, ochronosis (alkaptonuria), Gaucher disease.

69.5 Clinical Features

The classical symptomatology of OA includes joint pain exacerbated by activity and relieved with rest. Pain typically intensifies by late afternoon or evening and may also manifest upon awakening. Two principal pain patterns are identified:

A dull, throbbing ache that progressively becomes more persistent and predictable, frequently accompanied by stiffness after periods of immobility—termed the "gelling phenomenon."

Brief, intense, and unpredictable pain episodes that can be distressing and disrupt daily routines.

Based on clinical progression, OA is categorized into:

- Early OA: intermittent sharp, mechanical pain restricting strenuous activities.
- Moderate OA: increasingly constant pain, occasional joint locking (especially knees), and impaired function.
- Advanced OA: persistent dull pain interspersed with sudden, severe exacerbations, leading to social and recreational withdrawal.

Additional signs include joint tenderness, stiffness, audible crepitus, restricted range of motion, effusion, deformity, and instability.

69.5.1 Common Joint Involvement

- Monoarticular: knee most commonly, followed by the hip.
- Polyarticular: DIP involvement predominates.
- Overall most frequent: DIP joints.

Special Note Quadriceps muscle weakness, particularly affecting the vastus medialis, is a prevalent finding in knee OA.

Primary OA Knee The medial compartment typically bears excess load due to an altered mechanical axis, accelerating degeneration and resulting in bilateral varus deformities.

69.6 Diagnostic Evaluation

69.6.1 Preferred Investigation

Plain radiographs (anteroposterior [AP] and lateral views) of the affected joints remain the cornerstone.

69.6.2 Kellgren–Lawrence Grading System

Grade	Radiographic findings
0	No detectable radiographic changes
1	Doubtful joint space narrowing, possible osteophyte formation
2	Definite osteophytes, possible joint space narrowing
3	Multiple moderate osteophytes, definite joint space narrowing, subchondral sclerosis, and possible bony end deformity
4	Extensive osteophytes, severe joint space loss, pronounced sclerosis, and marked deformity (Fig. 69.1)

69.6.3 Key Radiological Features

Asymmetric joint space narrowing
Subchondral sclerosis
Subchondral cysts
Osteophyte formation and joint deformity

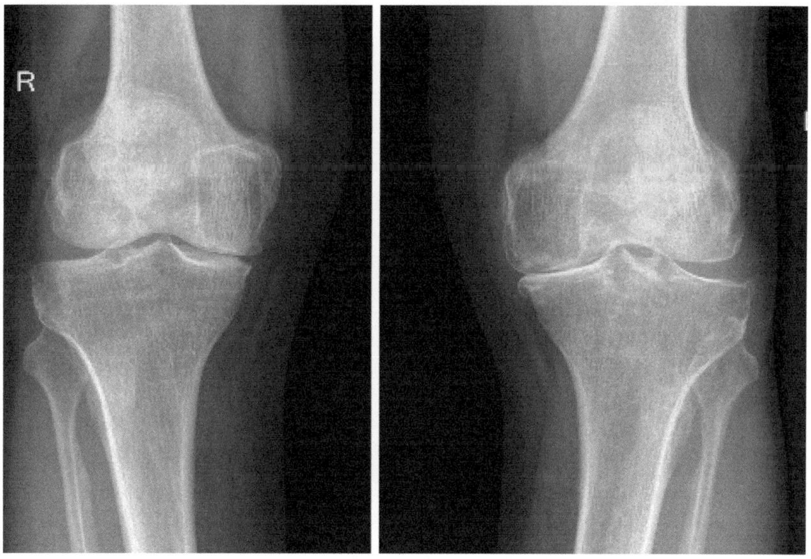

Fig. 69.1 Plain radiograph depicting AP view of bilateral OA knees (Kellgren–Lawrence grade 4, with bilateral varus deformity)

69.7 Differential Diagnosis

- Rheumatoid arthritis
- Gout
- Pseudogout
- Septic arthritis
- Hemochromatosis
- Fibromyalgia
- Lyme disease
- Ankylosing spondylitis
- Psoriatic arthritis
- Parvovirus-associated arthritis
- Neuropathic arthropathy

69.8 Treatment

69.8.1 Management Principles

Treatment strategies are individualized based on disease severity and joint involvement. Nonpharmacological measures, such as weight reduction and physiotherapy, are foundational. Use of braces, splints, walking aids, and lifestyle modifications should be prioritized.

69.8.2 Pharmacological Interventions

First-line: topical or oral nonsteroidal anti-inflammatory drugs (NSAIDs) (aceclofenac preferred currently). Oral NSAIDs should be used cautiously in patients with cardiovascular disease or those predisposed to gastrointestinal complications.

Adjuncts: intra-articular corticosteroid injections for moderate to severe pain unresponsive to oral agents. These provide transient relief but should be used judiciously due to the risk of cartilage damage.

Other agents: duloxetine, muscle relaxants, glucosamine, chondroitin sulfate, intra-articular hyaluronic acid, platelet-rich plasma (PRP) injections, and opioids. Certain therapies like acetaminophen and topical capsaicin have limited efficacy. Novel therapies under investigation include biologics, stem cell therapies, and cannabinoids.

69.8.3 Rehabilitation

Muscle strengthening, range-of-motion exercises, and low-impact aerobic training are effective. Complementary modalities include cryotherapy, heat application, therapeutic ultrasound, transcutaneous electrical nerve stimulation (TENS), and neuromuscular electrical stimulation (NMES).

69.8.4 Surgical Options

High tibial osteotomy (HTO): medial opening wedge osteotomy in younger patients to realign weight-bearing axis (Fig. 69.2).

Unicondylar knee arthroplasty: indicated for isolated medial compartment OA with an intact anterior cruciate ligament (Fig. 69.3).

Total joint arthroplasty: total knee or total hip replacement in elderly individuals for restoring pain-free joint mobility (Fig. 69.4).

Fig. 69.2 Postoperative AP (**a**) and lateral (**b**) radiographs depicting high tibial osteotomy

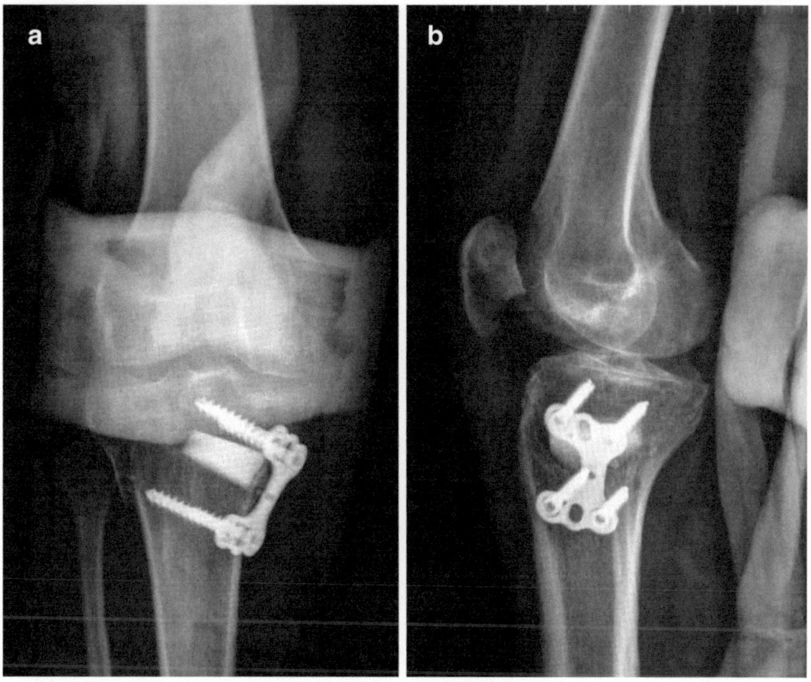

Fig. 69.3 (**a**) AP view and (**b**) lateral view radiographs showing postoperative medial unicondylar knee arthroplasty in a patient

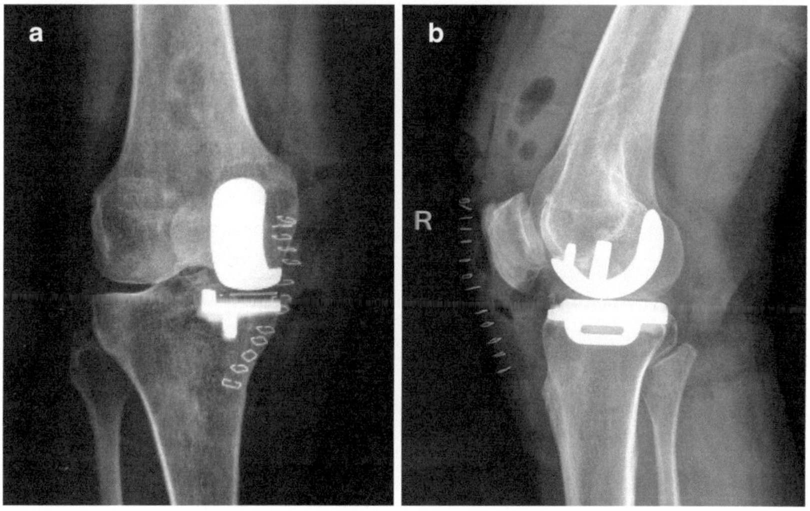

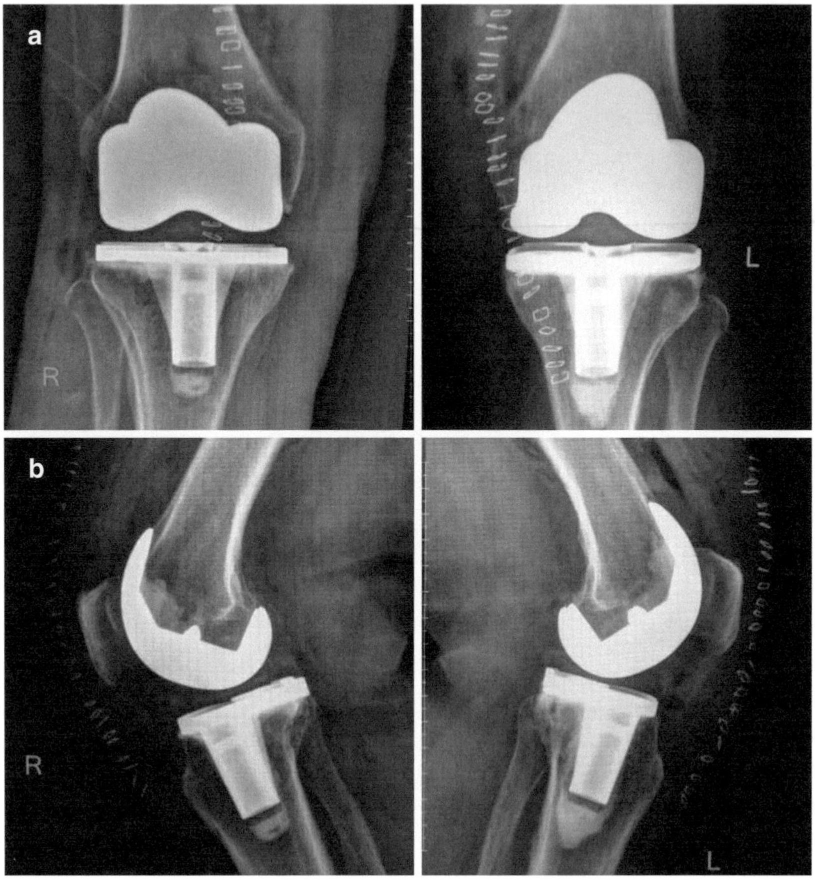

Fig. 69.4 Postoperative AP (**a**) and lateral (**b**) radiographs depicting bilateral total knee replacement

Multiple Choice Questions

1. Which of the following statements is incorrect?
   (a) Thickening of the synovial membrane is one of the earliest features of knee osteoarthritis
   (b) Knee osteoarthritis is more common than hip osteoarthritis in India
   (c) Metacarpophalangeal (MCP) joint is usually spared in osteoarthritis
   (d) Hip arthrodesis if done for osteoarthritis leads to pain-free condition but with reduced range of motion
2. Pain and arthritis of the distal interphalangeal joint is seen in
   (a) Osteoarthritis
   (b) Rheumatoid arthritis
   (c) Seronegative spondyloarthropathy
   (d) Psoriatic arthropathy
3. Arthritis involving the DIP, PIP, and first carpometacarpal joints with sparing of MCP joints and wrists is seen with
   (a) Rheumatoid arthritis
   (b) Seronegative spondyloarthropathy
   (c) Osteoarthritis
   (d) Psoriatic arthropathy
4. Which of the following bursae always communicates with the knee joint cavity?
   (a) Prepatellar
   (b) Deep infrapatellar
   (c) Superficial infrapatellar
   (d) Suprapatellar
5. Which of the following arthritic conditions can lead to loose body formation?
   (a) Rheumatoid arthritis

(b) Osteoarthritis
(c) Systemic lupus erythematosus (SLE) arthropathy
(d) Reactive arthritis

Answers: 1. (a), 2. (a), 3. (c), 4. (d), 5. (b)

References for Further Reading

1. https://www.ncbi.nlm.nih.gov/books/NBK482326/#:~:text=It%20can%20be%20classified%20into,devastating%20and%20permanently%20disabling%20disorder.
2. https://www.ncbi.nlm.nih.gov/books/NBK507884/
3. https://my.clevelandclinic.org/health/diseases/5599-osteoarthritis
4. https://pubmed.ncbi.nlm.nih.gov/36150676/
5. https://pubmed.ncbi.nlm.nih.gov/32722615/

Spondylosis and Lumbar Canal Stenosis

70

Aaditya Keerti Mongia and Ruchit Khera

Canal stenosis or spinal stenosis is a term used to describe various disease conditions that result in narrowing of the central spinal canal, or intervertebral foramina, leading to compression of nerve roots.

70.1 Aetiology

Spinal canal stenosis is most commonly seen secondary to degenerative spinal diseases. Any pathology leading to narrowing of the spinal canal leads to reduction in space available for thecal sac, thereby resulting in compression of nerve roots producing symptoms which are commonly related to activity.

Various causes of spinal canal stenosis are listed in Table:

Acquired	Congenital
Chronic prolapsed intervertebral disc	Skeletal dysplasia
Hypertrophic ligamentum flavum	Achondroplasia
Facet arthropathy—hypertrophy	Spinal deformities
Degenerative disease	Trefoil-shaped canal [1]
Post-traumatic	

A. K. Mongia (✉)
Assistant Professor Gautam Buddha Chikitsa Mahavidyalaya & Associate Director Shiv Chikitsalay, Dehradun, India

R. Khera
Associate Professor, Gautam Buddha Chikitsa Mahavidyalaya, Dehradun, India

70.2 Clinical Features

The incidence of spinal canal stenosis increases with age. Patients are usually elderly males, commonly seen after 50 years of age.

In patients with lumbar canal stenosis (LCS), pain is the most common symptom for which patients seek medical attention. Pain is usually gradual in onset and can be localized to the lower back or radiate to the buttocks, thighs and legs. The pattern of pain may vary from dull aching type to sharp shooting, and at times may be associated with cramping or burning sensations.

Cardinal manifestation of lumbar canal stenosis is neurological claudication. The usual presenting complaint is transient numbness and paraesthesia or aching or heaviness in lower limbs that usually starts after standing upright or walking for a few minutes. Patients get symptomatic relief by squatting or sitting or leaning forwards, i.e. by flexing the spine and this is referred to as 'spinal claudication. Symptoms get aggravated while walking downhill (as the spine goes into extension).

Patients prefer to cycle or walk uphill rather than downhill, as while walking uphill the spine gets flexed, which maximizes the spinal canal capacity and alleviates symptoms.

The distance at which pain starts after beginning to walk is referred to as the 'walking distance', described in number of steps or in terms

V. Kumar et al. (eds.), *A Quick Guide to Essential Orthopedics*,
https://doi.org/10.1007/978-981-95-2676-5_70

of minutes from the start of walking to the onset of pain.

Physical examination commonly reveals mild tenderness in lumbar spine; however, patients usually do not have any neurological deficit. Symptom for the same can be reciprocated by asking the patient to walk.

Distal pulses (dorsalis pedis and posterior tibial and anterior tibial arteries) are palpable, which also differentiate lumbar canal stenosis from vascular claudication.

70.3 Investigations

Plain radiograph of lumbar spine in anteroposterior and lateral views are usually suggestive of features of degenerative disc or spondylolisthesis.

Spinal canal diameter can be measured on plain X-ray; however, it can be more accurately measured using computed tomography (CT) Scan. Gold standard for lumbar canal stenosis is magnetic resonance imaging (MRI), which helps to measure spinal canal diameter, assess associated disc degeneration and also detect impingement on nerve roots.

Canal diameter in about 20% of the normal population is found to be consistent with findings of lumbar canal stenosis, so it is always wise to correlate clinical findings and imaging findings before final diagnosis [2]. Most studies are based on criteria by Verbiest et al., wherein he defined relative spinal stenosis as a diameter between 10 and 12 mm, whereas absolute stenosis was a diameter less than 10 mm [3], but this criteria do not apply to trefoil-shaped LCS [1].

70.4 Treatment

Lumbar canal stenosis can be managed conservatively or surgically. Conservative treatment includes postural correction, bracing and avoiding exacerbating factors.

Medications in the form of analgesics, nonsteroidal anti-inflammatory drugs (NSAIDs) and muscle relaxants have been widely used for conservative management. Epidural injections of local anaesthetic and steroid are also used along with conservative management and physiotherapy. However, there is very little evidence in the literature to support these [4].

70.4.1 Surgical Management

Surgical Management is indicated in patients who fail conservative treatment or in those with severe restriction of activity or neurological deficit. Surgical management mainly includes decompression surgery with or without fusion. Decompression surgery may include one or any among laminotomy, flavectomy, facetectomy or discectomy at one or more relevant levels.

Back pain symptoms are more commonly found in patients with spondylolisthesis or spondylo-degenerative disease, which may also warrant the need for fusion in such patients (Fig. 70.1).

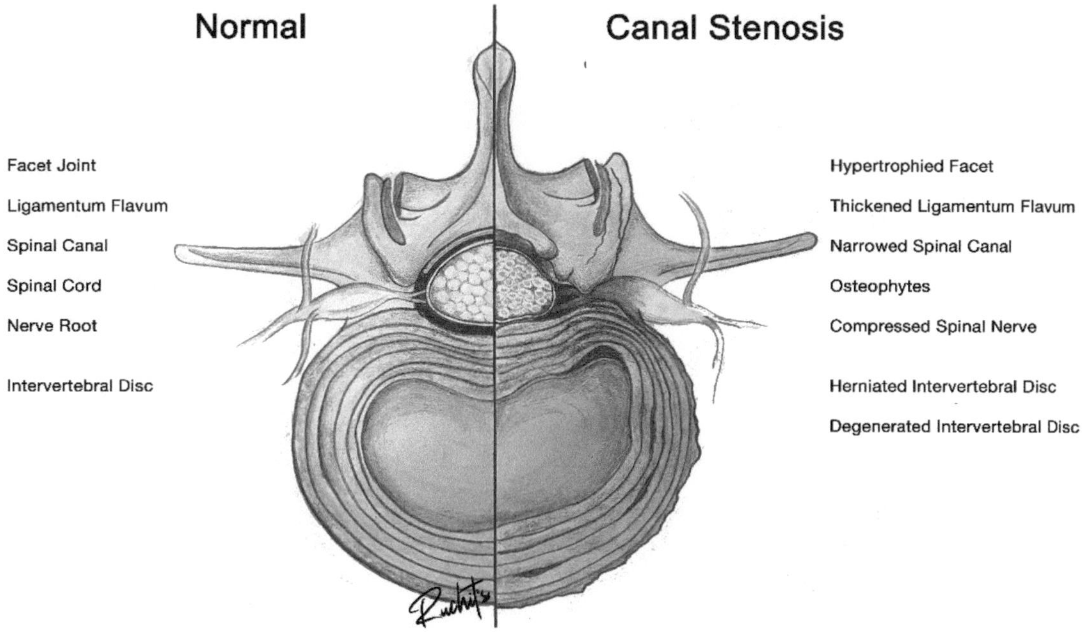

Fig. 70.1 Cross section of normal vs diseased vertebrae and intervertebral disc

Recommended Reading

1. Genevay S. Steven J Atlas, Lumbar Spinal Stenosis. Best Pract Res Clin Rheumatol. 2010;24(2):253–65.
2. Conway J, Tomkins CC, Haig AJ. Walking assessment in people with lumbar spinal stenosis: capacity, performance, and self-report measures. Spine J. 2011 Sep;11(9):816–23.

References

3. Eisenstein S. The trefoil configuration of the lumbar vertebral canal. A study of South African skeletal material. J Bone Joint Surg Br. 1980;62-B(1):73–7.
4. Jarvik JG, Deyo RA. Diagnostic evaluation of low back pain with emphasis on imaging. Ann Intern Med. 2002;137(7):586–97.
5. Verbiest H. Pathomorphologic aspects of developmental lumbar stenosis. Orthop Clin North Am. 1975;6(1):177–96
6. Genevay S, Atlas SJ. Lumbar spinal stenosis. Best Pract Res Clin Rheumatol. 2010;24(2):253–65.

Part X

Metabolic Bone Diseases

71 Rickets and Osteomalacia

Anand Bhushan and Mahesh Prasad

71.1 Introduction

Rickets is a metabolic bone disease of children (before fusion of epiphysis) with clinical features of softening of the bones and deformities. It is caused by deficient or delayed mineralization of osteoid matrix at the growth plate due to inadequate calcium and phosphate deposition occurring prior to physeal closure. The growth plate fails to mineralize while cartilage and osteoid continue to expand. Patients present with characteristic features such as bowing of long bones, ligamentous laxity, brittle bones, and enlargement of costal cartilage.

71.2 Pathophysiology

Three hormones (vitamin D3, parathormone (PTH), and calcitonin) operate collectively to regulate the calcium levels in body fluids, most important being vitamin D, which is responsible for homeostatic maintenance of serum calcium and phosphorus levels and the mineralization of bone. The physiologic form of the vitamin, 1,25(OH)2D3, acts on two main target organs—the intestine and bone. The kidney and the parathyroid glands have also been identified as sites of action. Parathyroid glands secrete PTH which mobilizes calcium from bone and increases urinary excretion of phosphate. Parafollicular cells (C cells) secrete a third hormone, calcitonin, which plays a relatively minor role in impeding bone resorption. A fourth local hormone, parathyroid hormone-related protein (PTHrP), acts on one of the PTH receptors and is vital in skeletal development in utero.

Vitamin D3 is the natural, endogenously produced compound resulting from interaction of ultraviolet light with a cholesterol derivative, 7-dehydrocholesterol,in the deeper layers of the skin. To attain its active form, vitamin D undergoes two successive hydroxylations—first in the liver and second in the kidneys.

Vitamin D3 and its hydroxylated derivatives are transported in the plasma bound to a globulin vitamin D binding proteinor globulin (DBP), which is also known as Gc protein andbinds G-actin. The affinity of DBP for previtamin D3 is low, but for vitamin D3 is high. In the liver, 25-hydroxylase converts vitamin D (cholecalciferol) to 25-hydroxycholecalciferol. The final step occurs in the kidney, where *1α-hydroxylase* adds the second hydroxyl group, and 25-hydroxycholecalciferol is converted to 1,25-dihydroxyvitamin D (calcitriol). PTH and hypophosphatemia cause upregulation of

A. Bhushan (✉)
Big Apollo Spectra Hospital, Patna, India

M. Prasad
Department of Orthopaedics, Patna Medical College & Hospital, Patna, India

V. Kumar et al. (eds.), *A Quick Guide to Essential Orthopedics*,
https://doi.org/10.1007/978-981-95-2676-5_71

1α-hydroxylase, while hyperphosphatemia and calcitriol inhibit this enzyme.

Most calcitriol circulates bound to DBP. Calcitriol (1,25-dihydroxycholecalciferol) is also synthesized in placenta, keratinocytes in the skin, and macrophages. Persons with sarcoidosis and pulmonary alveolar macrophages also produce 1,25-dihydroxycholecalciferol, due to stimulation by interferon γ. Also synthesized in the kidneys is the less active metabolite 24,25-dihydroxycholecalciferol.

The primary function of vitamin D is to maintain calcium and phosphate homeostasis, thereby ensuring normal mineralization of the skeleton. The target areas for vitamin D action include bone, gastrointestinal tract, kidneys, and parathyroid gland (Table 71.1 and 71.2).

71.2.1 Vitamin D–Dependent Type 1 Rickets

Occurring generally during the first year of life, vitamin D–dependent type 1 rickets (VDDR I) is a rare autosomal recessive disease of vitamin D metabolism that occurs due to homozygous inactivating mutations in the CYP27B1 gene, leading to impaired production of the enzyme 1 alpha-

Table 71.1 Metabolism of vitamin D

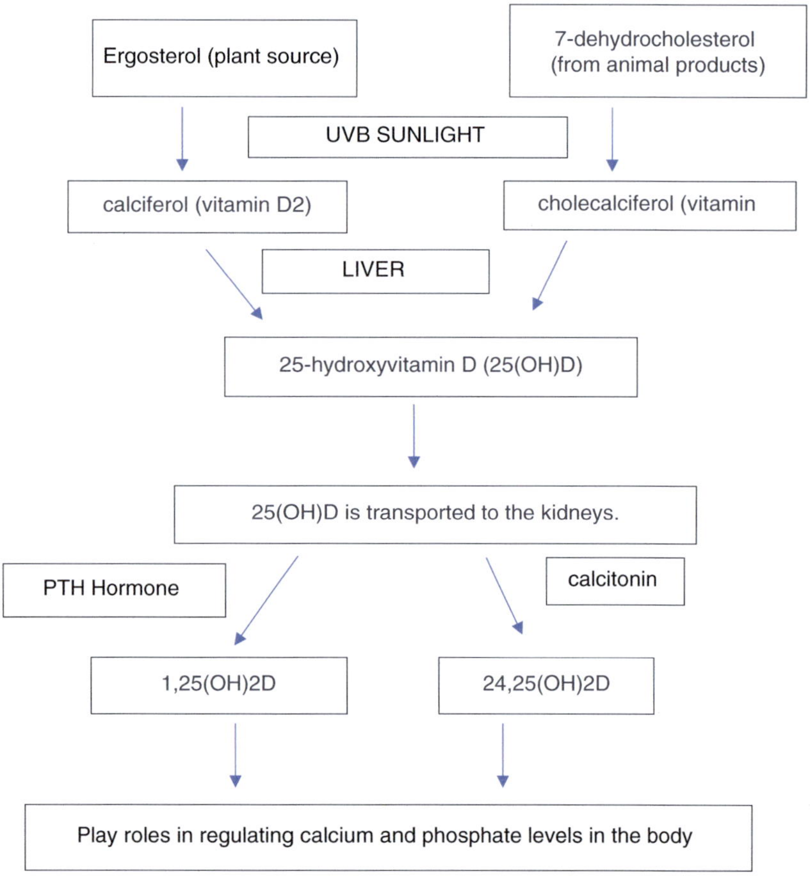

Table 71.2 Etiological classification of rickets

Vitamin D disorders	Nutritional deficiency of vitamin D	
	Vitamin D–dependent rickets type 1	
	Vitamin D–dependent rickets type 2	
	Congenital vitamin D deficiency	
	Secondary vitamin D deficiency	Malabsorption
		Decrease liver 25-hydroxylase
		Increase degradation
		Chronic kidney disease
Renal losses	Autosomal dominant hypophosphatemic rickets	
	Autosomal recessive hypophosphatemic rickets	
	X-linked hypophosphatemic rickets	
	Hereditary hypophosphatemic rickets with hypercalciuria	
	Excess production of phosphatonin	Neurofibromatosis
		Tumor-induced rickets
		McCune-Albright syndrome
		Epidermal nevus
	Dent disease	
	Fanconi syndrome	
	Distal renal tubular acidosis	
Calcium deficiency	Decrease intake	
	Malabsorption	
Phosphorus deficiency	Premature infants (rickets of prematurity)	

hydroxylase, which in turn leads to low serum levels of the active metabolite calcitriol.

71.2.2 Vitamin D–Dependent Type 2 Rickets

Also occurring during infancy, VDDR type 2 (VDDR II), or hereditary vitamin D–resistant rickets, is a rare autosomal recessive disease caused by a defect in the calcitriol vitamin D receptor. The defect causes the body to be irresponsive to calcitriol, resistant to 1,25-dihydroxyvitamin D.

71.2.3 Renal Rickets

The term renal rickets is usually restricted to those with chronic kidney disease. Chronic kidney disease results in the deficiency of the enzyme 1 alpha-hydroxylase, which decreases the production of 1,25 hydroxyvitamin D (calcitriol).

71.2.4 Hypophosphatemic Rickets

The main defect in these forms of rickets is the increased loss of phosphate through the urine due to various genetic mutations, mostly X-linked dominant.

71.3 Clinical Features

Clinical findings of rickets are highly variable and depend on the etiology and severity of the disorder, as well as the age at the time of presentation. Most children will have stunted skeletal growth, and they present with swollen and tender joints. In advanced cases, they may present with irritability, weakness, and bony deformities. During the first 6 months of life, rickets can present with tetany or convulsions.

71.3.1 Head

- Craniotabes—softening of cranial bones, a sensation similar to pressing a ping pong ball on applying pressure on the occiput or the parietal bones
- Frontal bossing
- Delayed dentition and tooth caries
- Delayed closure of fontanel
- Craniosynostosis

71.3.2 Chest

- Rachitic rosary—widening of osteochondral junction, feels like beads of a rosary
- Harrison's groove—occurs due to pulling of softened ribs during inspiration by the diaphragm. Softened ribs also predispose to atelectasis and pneumonia because of decreased air entry
- Pectus carinatum (pigeon breast)—sternum projects forward

71.3.3 Spine

- Scoliosis (uncommon)
- Kyphosis (rachitic cat back)
- Accentuation of lumbar lordosis

71.3.4 Limbs and Joints

- Bone pain and tenderness
- Coxa vara
- Genu valgum or varum
- Windswept deformity
- Bowing of tibia, femur, radius, and ulna
- Widening of wrist, elbow, knee, and ankle because of enlargement of ends of long bones
- Rachitic saber shins
- Sausage-like enlargement of ends of phalanges and metacarpals, with regular constrictions corresponding to the joints string of pearls deformity
- Double malleoli sign

71.3.5 General

- Failure to thrive
- Protuberant abdomen
- Apathy, listlessness, and irritability
- Proximal muscle weakness
- Ligament laxity
- Symptoms of hypocalcemia—tetany, seizures, and stridor due to laryngeal spasm
- Bilateral lamellar cataract (vitamin D deficiency in early infancy)

The clinical features also vary depending on the type of deficiency:

- X-linked hypophosphatemic rickets predominantly have lower extremity changes.
- Rickets associated with decreased serum calcium has symptoms of hypocalcemia, e.g., dietary vitamin D deficiency, vitamin D–dependent rickets (VDDR) type I and II, chronic kidney disease, and dietary calcium deficiency.

71.4 Radiological Signs

- Radiographs
  - Common findings on xrays

71.4.1 Findings

On anteroposterior (AP) and lateral radiographic views of the affected bone, rickets is characterized by:

Generally, all bones appear more radiolucent, with coarsened trabecular patterns. The most conspicuous abnormalities are found at the growth plate regions of long bones. These consist of a widened growth plate with irregular, frayed, and cupped metaphyseal margins (*paintbrush metaphyses*), particularly in long bones with fastest-growing growth plates, like proximal humerus, distal radius and ulna, and distal femur.

Widened growth plate is due to continued hypertrophy of cartilage cells.

Due to absent mineralization the metaphysis is soft; hence, with axial pressure, the epiphysis is pushed into metaphysis causing cupping.

Irregular calcification leads to fraying of the metaphysis, giving "trees on plateau top" appearance.

- Bowing deformities of the long bones, especially the femur and tibia.
- Epiphyses also appear frayed at the borders.
- Bowing deformities and shortening of the long bones are, however, more pronounced in early rickets. Changes in the shaft appear a few weeks later than metaphysis. Best seen in the rapidly growing distal ends of the radius and ulna (more so in the ulna).

Sometimes sharply defined radiolucent transverse zones are seen, known as *Umbau zones* (*Looser's zones*). The circumflex artery pulsating against soft bone may produce Looser's zone in proximal humerus.

The radiographic findings in vitamin D–resistant rickets are similar to those in infantile rickets.

As the effects of weight bearing become more important, scoliosis and vertebral end plate deformities may develop in older children. This contributes to an overall decrease in height of the child.

Triradiate-shaped pelvis due to protrusion of the hip and spine into the soft pelvis.

Fractures: Trivial trauma may result in fracture of the weakened, undermineralized bone in long-standing cases of rickets.

71.4.2 Findings of Healing Rickets

Evidence of healing is seen within 2–3 weeks of adequate therapy and total recalcification is usually complete in 2 months.

- Reappearance of the dense zone of provisional calcification and is seen as a transverse line of increased density.
- Increase in cupping of the healing metaphysis is seen compared to the active stage of rickets.
- Recalcification of the subperiosteal osteoid produces a thick envelope of cortex that surrounds the shaft.
- The epiphyseal ossification center becomes sharply defined in the healing stage.

When the patient is on intermittent or inadequate treatment, the process of calcification and repair is irregular. Patchy sclerosis of the metaphysis is seen, sometimes with alternating sclerotic and lucent bands (Table 71.3).

Table 71.3 Characteristics of different types of rickets

	Family history	Myopathy	Growth defect	Serum Ca	Serum P	Alkaline phosphatase	Urine Ca	Urine P	Osteitis fibrosa	Others
Vitamin D deficiency	–	+	+/–	Low	Low	High	Low	Low	+/–	Dietary deficiency or malabsorption
Renal tubular	+	–	++	N	Low	High	Low	High	+	Amino aciduria
Renal glomerular	–	+	++	Low	High	High	Low	Low	++	Renal failure anemia

N Normal, *Ca* Calcium, *P* Phosphorus

71.5 Treatment

Vitamin D deficiency remains the most common cause of rickets globally. The core treatment of nutritional vitamin D deficiency rickets is adequate intake of vitamin D, calcium, and phosphorus.

Vitamin D can be administered by the following methods:

- *Stoss therapy*: 300,000–600,000 IU of vitamin D is administered orally or intramuscularly as 2–4 doses over 1 day.
- *Alternate therapy*: high-dose vitamin D, with doses ranging from 2000–5000 IU/day over 4–6 weeks.

After completion of therapy, daily vitamin D intake of 400 IU/day is to be maintained, typically given as a supplement. Also, of paramount importance is adequate dietary calcium and phosphorus intake, common sources for which are milk, formula diets, and other dairy products.

With early diagnosis and high compliance of treatment, the prognosis of nutritional rickets is excellent. The radiological signs of improvement start appearing within a few months, and the laboratory parameters also normalize within a few weeks. If the improvement is not seen, same dose may be repeated once, before diagnosing the patient with refractory rickets.

When diagnosed late or neglected, children present with severe deformities and may sustain permanent deformities. An orthopedic intervention may only be required to correct these residual deformities but is undertaken only after the bone disease is healed.

As a prevention method to nutritional rickets, a dose of multivitamin containing 200–400 IU of vitamin D should be administered daily to breastfed children, and for others, the diet should ensure adequate vitamin D intake.

71.5.1 Vitamin D-Dependent Type 1 Rickets

As expected, these children will not respond to high doses of cholecalciferol but respond to physiologic doses of calcitriol or 1α-hydroxyvitamin D (1–2 μg daily). Adequate intake of dietary calcium (30–75 mg/kg per day of elemental calcium) should be maintained.

71.5.2 Vitamin D-Dependent Type 2 Rickets

Because VDDR II is a hereditary disease resistant to 1,25-dihydroxyvitamin D, no completely proven treatment is available. Despite its difficulty, the most plausible way is to saturate the normal receptors through megadoses of calcitriol and calcium.

71.5.3 Renal Rickets

Because patients with chronic kidney disease cannot convert the calcidiol into the active form calcitriol, vitamin D supplementation alone is therefore ineffective for renal rickets. Instead, a low-phosphate diet, dietary phosphate binders, and oral administration of 1-alfacalcidol or calcitriol is advised, along with maintaining normal 25 hydroxyvitamin D level. Bicarbonate supplements (*Shohl's solution*—citric acid, sodium citrate) is given in renal tubular acidosis.

71.5.4 Hypophosphatemic Rickets

Phosphate supplementation (elemental phosphorus in 3–5 doses of 20–60 mg/kg per day) remains the cornerstone of management. *Joule's solution*—Dibasic sodium phosphate, phosphoric acid—is commonly given.

Orthopedic Treatment Orthopedic treatment is required for the correction of deformities and can be either conservative or operative.

(a) *Conservative methods:* Mild deformities usually correct spontaneously as rickets heals. Specially designed splints can be used for the correction of deformities, e.g., mermaid splints for correction of knee deformities.
(b) *Operative methods:* After 6 months of starting medical treatment, if moderate or severe deformities persists, surgery may be required. Corrective osteotomies (*multilevel osteotomy*) using a variety of fixation devices including K-wires, plates, intramedullary nails, and/or external fixation are performed.

71.6 Osteomalacia

71.6.1 Introduction

The term osteomalacia per se literally means "soft bones." It is principally a metabolic bone disease with defective mineralization of bone (osteoid) and results in a large amount of unmineralized osteoid. It is a qualitative defect as opposed to a quantitative defect like osteoporosis. Unlike rickets which is found in children (open physis) and occurs due to deficient mineralization at the cartilage of growth plates, osteomalacia is found in adults (closed physis). It is usually due to prolonged deficiency of vitamin D.

Diagnosis is made on the basis of serum labs, clinical features, and radiographic findings. The mainstay of treatment is vitamin D supplementation and resolution of the underlying etiology.

71.6.2 Pathophysiology

Osteoclasts (bone-resorbing cells) and osteoblasts (bone-forming cells responsible for formation of osteoid matrix in which inorganic salts are deposited to form mineralized bone) function in coordination for bone remodeling. This process is influenced directly or indirectly by hormones, i.e., parathyroid hormone (PTH) and calcitonin, which act in response to serum calcium levels. Hypocalcemia caused by vitamin D deficiency stimulates the secretion of PTH by the parathyroid glands which in turn mobilizes calcium from the bones to maintain normal serum calcium levels and thus leading to osteomalacia (Table 71.4).

71.6.3 Symptoms

Patients suffer from nonspecific symptoms such as:

Generalized bone pain, usually in lower spine, pelvis, or lower extremities
Muscle pain
Proximal muscle weakness, wasting and fatigue
Muscle spasms
Arthralgias and myalgias
Deformities, commonly at the spine, limbs, and pelvis in long-term osteomalacia
Sometimes, fractures of long bones, ribs, and vertebrae and hypocalcemic seizures or tetany may also be seen

71.6.4 Physical Examination

On inspection: Patient walks with a waddling gait due to hip pain and thigh weakness. There is also difficulty in rising from a chair and climbing stairs.

71.6.5 Investigations

Findings in cases of osteomalacia include:

Hypophosphatemia or hypocalcemia
High bone alkaline phosphatase and low bone mineral density (BMD) less than 80% of the young adult mean
The serum vitamin D level is severely low in patients with nutritional osteomalacia, increased serum PTH and decreased urinary calcium are other sensitive markers.

Table 71.4 Risk factors—the conditions predisposing a patient to osteomalacia

Vitamin D–deficient diets	
Decreased vitamin D production	Cold weather climates reduce sunlight exposure High amount of melanin in dark skin competes with 7-dehydrocholesterol for ultraviolet-B (UVB) light absorption Obesity leads to adipose sequestration, resulting in less calcidiol substrate available for activation Production and storage decrease with age
malabsorption	Crohn disease Cystic fibrosis Celiac disease Cholestasis Surgical alteration (gastric bypass)
Altered metabolism of vitamin D	Chronic kidney disease/renal osteodystrophy (decreased 1 alpha-hydroxylase activity) Nephrotic syndrome (excretion of vitamin D binding–protein [DBP]) Pregnancy (decreased calcidiol)
Hypophosphatemia or hypocalcemia	Renal tubular acidosis/Fanconi syndrome Tumor-induced osteomalacia (commonly due to benign tumors of skin, muscles, paranasal sinuses, and bones of extremities)
Chronic alcoholism	
Tumors (tumor-induced osteomalacia)	
Drugs	Drugs associated with vitamin D deficiency Phenytoin Phenobarbital Rifampin Cholestyramine Cadmium Glucocorticoids Drugs affecting phosphate homeostasis Aluminum-containing phosphate-binding antacids Ifosfamide Drugs affecting bone mineralization Aluminum Etidronate Fluoride

71.6.6 Radiographs

- Osteopenia is the most common sign due to decreased bone mineral content involving all bones
- Coarse, indistinct trabecular pattern: overall decrease in number of bony trabeculae, giving a coarse, mottled appearance
- The cortices of long bones become thin
- Pseudofractures or Looser's zones: Looser's zones are linear radiolucent bands of under-mineralized osteoid that occur in a bilateral and symmetric distribution. They are oriented perpendicular to the long axis of the bone. The characteristic sites include:
  - Axillary margins of scapula
  - Superior and inferior pubic rami
  - Medial femoral necks
  - Posterior margins of the proximal ulna
  - Ribs
- Fractures (especially in the proximal femur/femoral neck)
- Biconcave vertebral bodies
- Trefoil pelvis
- Protrusio acetabuli

71.6.7 Treatment

Primarily, the treatment is nonoperative, with a focus on treating the underlying pathology and replenishing vitamin D and other electrolyte deficiencies. Large doses of oral vitamin D (1000 IU/day) are usually recommended. Supplementation of calcium with a dose of at least 1000 mg must also be given to the patient, as inadequate calcium intake may have contributed to the etiology. Dosage of supplement is 400–800 IU/day of vitamin D for patients on long-term anticonvulsant therapy. Patients with hepatobiliary disease are given supplements of 25(OH) vitamin D, and patients with renal disease are treated with supplements of 1,25(OH)2 vitamin D. Healing of osteomalacia is achieved when there are increases in urinary calcium excretion and bone mineral density.

Multiple Choice Questions

1. All are seen in rickets except
   (a) Craniotabes
   (b) Rachitic rosary
   (c) Bleeding
   (d) Bone deformity
2. Enzyme 1 alpha-hydroxylase is found in which organ?
   (a) Skin
   (b) Liver
   (c) Brain
   (d) Kidney
3. In which of the following conditions in a child is there decreased mineralization of epiphyseal plate?
   (a) Rickets
   (b) Osteoporosis
   (c) Osteomalacia
   (d) Scurvy
4. Mode of inheritance in hypophosphatemic rickets is
   (a) Autosomal dominant
   (b) Autosomal resistant
   (c) X-linked dominant
   (d) X-linked recessive
5. X-ray changes seen in rickets are
   (a) Metaphyseal cupping and fraying
   (b) Calcification of epiphysis
   (c) Metaphyseal widening
   (d) White sclerotic ring around epiphysis
   (e) Osteopenia
6. Osteomalacia is caused due to
   (a) Vitamin C deficiency
   (b) Vitamin D deficiency
   (c) Vitamin E deficiency
   (d) None
7. Osteomalacia is caused by which of the following drugs?
   (a) Valproate
   (b) Carbamazepine
   (c) Aspirin
   (d) Phenytoin
8. Looser's zone is a feature of
   (a) Osteoporosis
   (b) Osteomalacia
   (c) Metastasis
   (d) Scurvy
9. Test for vitamin D deficiency is
   (a) ALP level
   (b) Vitamin D level
   (c) Calcium level
   (d) Phosphate level
10. Osteomalacia is associated with
   (a) Decrease in osteoid volume
   (b) Decrease in osteoid surface
   (c) Increase in osteoid maturation time
   (d) Increase in mineral apposition rate

Answers: 1. (c), 2. (d), 3. (a), 4. (c), 5. (a, c, e), 6. (b), 7. (d), 8. (b), 9. (b), 10. (c)

References

1. Holick MF. Vitamin D deficiency. N Engl J Med. 2007;357(3):266.
2. Takeda E, Yamamoto H, Taketani Y. Vitamin D-dependent rickets type I and type II. Acta PaediatrJpn. 1997;39:508–13.
3. Sahay M, Sahay R. Renal rickets-practical approach. Indian J Endocrinol Metab. 2013;17:S35–44.
4. Imel EA, Econs MJ. Approach to the hypophosphatemic patient. J Clin Endocrinol Metab. 2012;97:696–706.

5. Chanchlani R, Nemer P, Sinha R, Nemer L, Krishnappa V, Sochett E, Safadi F, Raina R. An overview of rickets in children. Kidney Int Rep. 2020;5(7):980–90.
6. Rokan Z, Kealey WD. Osteomalacia: a forgotten cause of fractures in the elderly. BMJ Case Rep. 2015 Feb;09:2015.
7. Rosen CJ. Clinical practice. Vitamin D insufficiency. N Engl J Med. 2011;364(3):248–54.
8. Fukumoto S, Ozono K, Michigami T, Minagawa M, Okazaki R, Sugimoto T, Takeuchi Y, Matsumoto T. Pathogenesis and diagnostic criteria for rickets and osteomalacia—proposal by an expert panel supported by the Ministry of Health, Labour and Welfare, Japan, the Japanese Society for Bone and Mineral Research, and the Japan Endocrine Society. J Bone Miner Metab. 2015 Sep;33(5):467–73.
9. Zimmerman L, McKeon B. Osteomalacia. [Updated 2022 Apr 28]. In: StatPearls [Internet]. Treasure Island: StatPearls Publishing; 2023.
10. Minisola S, Colangelo L, Pepe J, Diacinti D, Cipriani C, Rao SD. Osteomalacia and vitamin D status: a clinical update 2020. JBMR Plus. 2020;5(1):e10447. https://doi.org/10.1002/jbm4.10447. PMID: 33553992; PMCID: PMC7839817

Osteoporosis

72

Anand Bhushan and Ranjit Kumar Singh

72.1 Introduction

Osteoporosis is both a qualitative and quantitative defect of bone, i.e., an equivalent loss of matrix and minerals, that usually affects all the bones of the body. It results in increased bone fragility, and hence susceptibility to fracture. Osteoporosis is by far the commonest metabolic bone disease. It is a silent disease and usually presents only after a fracture, which causes important secondary health problems and sometimes even death.

72.2 Etiopathogenesis

There is a balance between bone tissue loss by resorption and rebuilding by formation to maintain a normal amount of bone tissue in the body. If the resorption rate is more than formation rate, there will be a net bone loss. Menopause and advancing age commonly cause an imbalance that leads to net bone loss. Also, the peak bone mass (PBM) majorly depends on genetic factors, health during growth, nutrition, endocrine status, gender, and physical activity. The resultant bone is an architecturally weakened structure with reduced mass, which further increases the risk of fracture.

72.2.1 Risk Factors

- Advancing age
- Female gender
- Estrogen insufficiency, sex steroid deficiency
- Alcoholism and smoking
- Sedentary lifestyle
- Low dietary calcium
- Use of glucocorticoids

A. Bhushan (✉)
Big Apollo Spectra Hospital, Patna, India

R. K. Singh
Nalanda Medical College & Hospital,
Patna, Bihar, India

V. Kumar et al. (eds.), *A Quick Guide to Essential Orthopedics*,
https://doi.org/10.1007/978-981-95-2676-5_72

72.2.2 Classification of Osteoporosis (Tables 72.1 and 72.2)

Table 72.1 Classification of osteoporosis

Primary	Type 1	Postmenopausal
	Type 2	Senile or involutional
	Type 3	"Postclimacteric," it is not a part of the original classification, but is similar to type 1 osteoporosis but occurring in males
Secondary	Hormonal	Hypogonadism, thyrotoxicosis, Cushing's syndrome, hyperprolactinemia, and diabetes mellitus
	Drugs	Steroids, phenobarbital, anticonvulsants, anticoagulants, cytotoxic agents, etc.
	Nutritional	Calcium deficiency, vitamin C and vitamin D deficiency, malabsorption, alcohol intake, and malnutrition
	Metabolic diseases	Osteogenesis imperfecta, homocystinuria, Marfan syndrome, etc.
	Chronic liver and renal disease	
	Miscellaneous	Multiple myeloma, rheumatoid arthritis, mastocytosis, thalassemia, Wilson's disease, hemochromatosis, etc.

Table 72.2 Classification of primary osteoporosis

	Type 1	Type 2
	Postmenopausal	Senile
Etiology	Estrogen withdrawal	Age-related reduced bone turnover
Age	Above 50	Above 75
Female-to-male ratio	5:2	2:1
Bone involvement	Mainly trabecular bone	Proportionately involves both trabecular and cortical bone
Turnover	Usually high-turnover osteoporosis	Usually low-turnover osteoporosis
Fracture site	Predominantly vertebral	Predominantly proximal femur fracture
PTH level	Normal to low	Increased

72.3 Clinical Features and Diagnosis

Between fractures, most patients are free of symptoms. Pain usually results from collapse of vertebra, especially in the dorsal and lumbar regions, typically acute in nature, and may radiate along the distribution of the respective intercostal nerve and into the abdomen. These may occur even with trivial trauma. The collapse fractures usually cause anterior wedging of the vertebrae and result in loss of height with kyphosis (*dowager's or widow's hump*). Scoliosis is also common. Recurrent episodes of vertebral collapse at different levels result in increasing spine deformity with loss of height.

Sometimes, the first clinical event is a low-energy fracture of the distal radius (Colles' fracture), the hip, or the ankle.

Once the clinical diagnosis has been established, before initiating treatment, the patient should be tested to rule out underlying secondary causes of osteoporosis (e.g., hyperparathyroidism, malignant disease, or hypercortisolism).

72.4 Various Modalities for the Detection of Osteoporosis

- Standard radiography
- Radiogrammetry
- Photodensitometry
- Compton scattering
- Neutron activation analysis
- Single- and dual-photon absorptiometry
- Dual-energy X-ray absorptiometry
- Quantitative computed tomography
- Quantitative ultrasound
- Magnetic resonance imaging
- Multidetector computed tomography

72.5 Radiographs

Key signs include increased bony radiolucency, cortical thinning, insufficiency fractures, and altered trabecular patterns. Compression fractures of the vertebral bodies, wedging at multiple levels, or biconcave distortion of the vertebral end plates (codfish vertebra) are typical of severe osteoporosis. Singh's index is used for osteoporosis grading.

72.6 DEXA Scan

The diagnosis should be followed by assessment of bone mineral density (BMD), commonly measured by dual-energy X-ray absorptiometry (DEXA) scan of the spine and hips, using the lower value of the two. It measures BMD from L2 to L4 and compiles scores. In the hip, it measures BMD from femoral neck, trochanter, and intertrochanteric region and compiles scores. In otherwise healthy women above the age of 50 years, anything more than 2 SD below the average for the relevant population group may be taken as indicative of osteoporosis.

It is then matched to the DEXA scan of a 30-year-old individual, and the T-score is calculated. According to WHO, T-scores of 0 to −1 are normal, −1 to −2.5 indicate osteopenia, and less than −2.5 is categorized as osteoporosis.

The z-score is a comparison between age-, race-, and sex-matched populations, wherein z-score of −1 = T-score of −2.5.

72.7 Investigations to Rule Out Secondary Osteoporosis

- Complete blood count (CBC)
- Serum creatinine, calcium, phosphorus, and magnesium
- Alanine aminotransferase (ALT), aspartate aminotransferase (AST), and alkaline phosphatase (AP)
- Thyroid-stimulating hormone (TSH) and free T4
- Vitamin D (V-D) (25(OH)D)
- Parathyroid hormone (PTH)
- Total testosterone and gonadotropins in younger men
- Biochemical bone turnover markers (BTMs)

72.8 Prevention and Treatment

The principal goal of treatment is prevention. Bone densitometry is used to identify women who can be at more than usual risk of suffering a fracture at menopause, and prophylactic treatment of this group can be initiated.

Women approaching menopause are advised to take adequate levels of dietary calcium and vitamin D, to maintain a high level of physical activity and avoid smoking and alcohol.

72.9 Drugs Used in Osteoporosis

1. *Inhibit resorption*: bisphosphonates, denosumab, calcitonin, estrogen, selective estrogen receptor modulators (SERMs), gallium nitrate
2. *Stimulate formation*: teriparatide (PTH analog), calcium, calcitriol, fluorides
3. *Both actions*: strontium ranelate

Drugs that decrease bone resorption reach a plateau in 2–3 years since bone formation also decreases. However, drugs promoting bone formation can increase BMD throughout the duration of treatment.

Calcium should be given at 1500 mg/day dosage and vitamin D 400–800 IU/day. In patients with vitamin D deficiency, initial treatment with the active metabolite 1,25-dihydroxyvitamin D3 (short half-life: 4 hours; expensive) followed by long-lasting, less expensive vitamin D2 or D3 is done.

Hormone replacement therapy (HRT) with estrogen (or a combination of estrogen and progesterone) is the mainstay of bone loss prevention in osteoporotic postmenopausal women.

SERMs—raloxifene selectively stimulates estrogen receptor in bone, thus used in treatment.

Bisphosphonates are regarded as the preferred medication for postmenopausal osteoporosis. They act by binding to the surface of hydroxyapatite crystals, thereby reducing osteoclastic bone resorption and the general rate of bone turnover. It is not metabolized and excreted intact in urine. Its half-life is ~10 years, and cessation of treatment does not lead to rapid bone loss unlike HRT.

First-generation drug, etidronate, inhibits both bone resorption and formation, hence approved for treating Paget's disease and hypercalcemia but not osteoporosis. Second- and third-generation drugs like alendronate and risedronate inhibit resorption 1000 times more than bone formation, hence used in treating postmenopausal and steroid-induced osteoporosis. They can be administered orally in once-weekly doses for both prevention and treatment of osteoporosis. Gastrointestinal side effects are a bother and suitable precautions should be taken.

For patients who cannot tolerate the drug, pamidronate has been given intravenously at 3-month intervals.

Recent advances in drug treatment for reducing osteoclastic activity and bone resorption, interrupting the RANKL–RANK interaction, which is essential for prompting osteoclastogenesis, are the novel treatment recently developed. *Denosumab*, an antibody to RANKL, an effective new line of treatment for postmenopausal osteoporosis.

72.10 Management of Fractures

Femoral neck and other long-bone fractures may need operative treatment.

Analgesic treatment for painful vertebral fractures with partial rest and assistance with personal care for about 6 weeks.

For support and pain relief, spinal orthoses are provided, but they cannot correct any structural deformity. Occasionally, operative measures are called for to treat severe compression fractures.

Multiple Choice Questions

1. True about osteoporosis is
   (a) Hereditary has no role
   (b) Alcohol abuse is not a risk factor
   (c) Normally, bone loss slows down after menopause
   (d) Inactivity increases the risk
2. Most common site of osteoporosis is
   (a) Humerus
   (b) Scapula
   (c) Vertebra
   (d) Flat bone
3. Osteoporotic vertebral fracture most commonly occurs at which level
   (a) Cervical

(b) Dorsolumbar
(c) Dorsal
(d) Lumbosacral

4. Gold standard investigation for diagnosis of osteoporosis
(a) Single bone densitometry
(b) DEXA
(c) Quantitative CT
(d) Histomorphometry of bone

5. Kyphotic deformity is most commonly associated with
(a) Osteoporosis
(b) Trauma
(c) Ankylosing spondylitis
(d) Rickets

6. As per WHO criteria, osteoporosis is defined as T-score
(a) Equal to or below −1.0
(b) Equal to or below −1.5
(c) Equal to or below −2.0
(d) Equal to or below −2.5

Answers: 1. (d), 2. (c), 3. (b), 4. (b), 5. (a), 6. (d)

References

1. Sözen T, Özışık L, Başaran NÇ. An overview and management of osteoporosis. Eur J Rheumatol. 2017;4(1):46–56. https://doi.org/10.5152/eurjrheum.2016.048. Epub 2016 Dec 30. PMID: 28293453; PMCID: PMC5335887.
2. NIH Consensus Development Panel on Osteoporosis Prevention, Diagnosis, and Therapy. Osteoporosis prevention, diagnosis, and therapy. JAMA. 2001;285:785–95. [PubMed] [Google Scholar].
3. Cosman F, de Beur SJ, LeBoff MS, Lewiecki EM, Tanner B, Randall S, et al. Clinician's guide to prevention and treatment of osteoporosis. Osteoporos Int. 2014;25:2359–81. https://doi.org/10.1007/s00198-014-2794-2. [PMC free article] [PubMed] [Google Scholar].
4. Tannenbaum C, Clark J, Schwartzman K, Wallenstein S, Lapinski R, Meier D, et al. Yield of laboratory testing to identify secondary contributors to osteoporosis in otherwise healthy women. J Clin Endocrinol Metab. 2002;87:4431–7. https://doi.org/10.1210/jc.2002-020275. [PubMed] [Google Scholar].
5. Watts NB, Bilezikian JP, Camacho PM, Greenspan SL, Harris ST, Hodgson SF, et al. American Association of Clinical Endocrinologists Medical Guidelines for clinical practice for the diagnosis and treatment of postmenopausal osteoporosis. Endocr Pract. 2010;16(Suppl 3):1–37. https://doi.org/10.4158/10024.GL. [PMC free article] [PubMed] [Google Scholar].
6. LeBoff M, Greenspan S, Insogna K, et al. The clinician's guide to prevention and treatment of osteoporosis. Osteoporos Int. 2022;33:2049–102. https://doi.org/10.1007/s00198-021-05900-y.

73 Hyperparathyroidism

Anand Bhushan and Rajeev Anand

Hyperparathyroidism (HPT) is a medical condition defined by excessive secretion of parathyroid hormone (PTH), which disrupts calcium balance in the body. PTH naturally facilitates calcium release from bones into the bloodstream and drives significant bone remodeling. Dysregulation of parathyroid function leads to altered calcium homeostasis, resulting in increased renal calcium reabsorption, phosphaturia, enhanced production of 1,25-dihydroxyvitamin D3 (promoting intestinal calcium absorption), and elevated bone turnover, all of which contribute to characteristic physiological abnormalities.

HPT is categorized into three types: *Primary, Secondary, and Tertiary.*

73.1 Primary Hyperparathyroidism

Primary HPT arises from excessive, unregulated PTH production due to abnormalities in one or more parathyroid glands.

Causes include:

1. *Parathyroid adenoma*: the most common cause, accounting for approximately 85% of cases
2. *Parathyroid hyperplasia*: may occur independently or as part of multiple endocrine neoplasia (MEN) syndromes
3. *Parathyroid adenocarcinoma*: rare

73.2 Secondary Hyperparathyroidism

Secondary HPT, more prevalent than primary HPT, develops as a compensatory response to chronic hypocalcemia.

Causes include:

1. *Chronic renal failure*: The leading cause where reduced renal function leads to elevated serum phosphate levels, which suppress serum calcium, prompting hypertrophy of parathyroid chief cells. Additionally, impaired renal production of active 1,25-dihydroxyvitamin D further lowers serum calcium.
2. *Malabsorption disorders or dietary deficiencies* causing hypocalcemia may contribute to secondary HPT.

A. Bhushan (✉)
Big Apollo Spectra Hospital, Patna, India

R. Anand
Patna Medical College & Hospital, Patna, Bihar, India

V. Kumar et al. (eds.), *A Quick Guide to Essential Orthopedics*,
https://doi.org/10.1007/978-981-95-2676-5_73

73.3 Tertiary Hyperparathyroidism

Tertiary HPT emerges in patients with prolonged secondary HPT, where the parathyroid glands develop autonomous function, leading to severe hypercalcemia, hyperphosphatemia, and elevated PTH levels. Unlike secondary HPT, which is characterized by hypocalcemia, tertiary HPT is distinguished by *hypercalcemia.*

73.4 Pathophysiology

PTH plays a critical role in regulating calcium and phosphate transport in bones, kidneys, and intestines. Serum ionized calcium levels tightly control PTH synthesis and release. Approximately 99% of the body's calcium is stored in the skeleton.

- PTH mobilizes body's calcium store to maintain serum levels.
- PTH also reduces phosphate reabsorption in the kidneys' proximal and distal tubules, lowering plasma phosphate concentrations, which helps stabilize serum calcium.
- Additionally, PTH enhances renal calcium reabsorption and, in conjunction with low serum calcium and phosphate, stimulates 1,25-dihydroxyvitamin D production to boost intestinal calcium and phosphorus absorption (Fig. 73.1).

Cortical bone experiences heightened turnover, leading to increased resorption, greater cortical porosity, and cortical thinning. In cancellous bone, reduced osteoclastic resorption and osteoblastic activity result in diminished bone formation and thinner structural units.

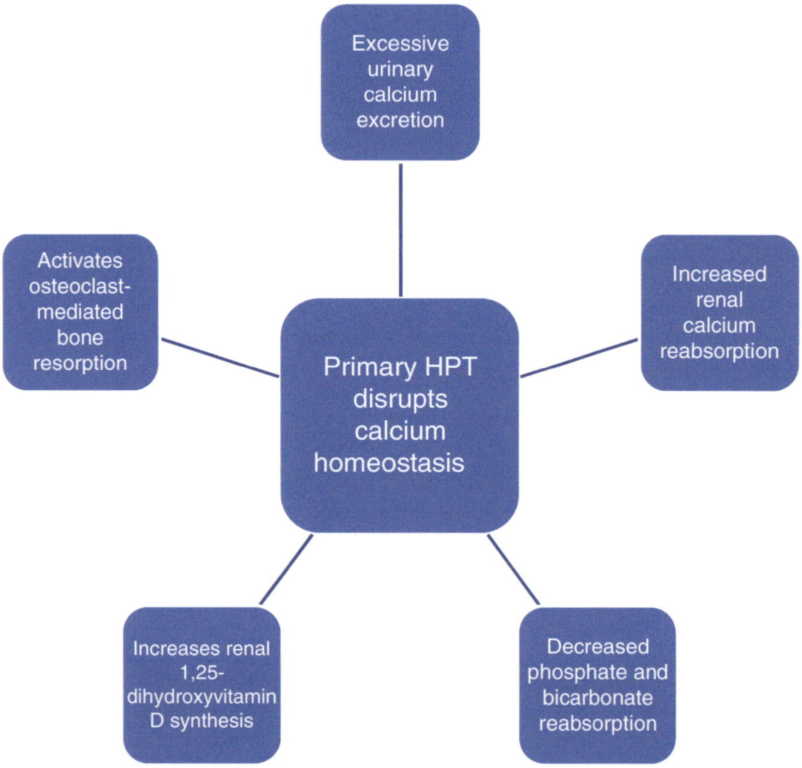

Fig. 73.1 Primary HPT pathophysiology: excessive PTH disrupts calcium homeostasis, prompting increased renal calcium reabsorption, decreased phosphate and bicarbonate reabsorption, and excessive urinary calcium excretion. It also activates osteoclast-mediated bone resorption and increases renal 1,25-dihydroxyvitamin D synthesis, enhancing intestinal calcium and phosphate uptake

In *secondary HPT*, bone loss occurs from a progressively reduced bone mass, though periosteal bone formation during aging may increase the bone's cross-sectional area.

73.5 Clinical Manifestations

Primary HPT symptoms stem from hypercalcemia, driven by increased intestinal calcium absorption, elevated bone turnover, and enhanced renal tubular calcium reabsorption. Historically, patients presented with *reduced bone mineral density (BMD) or fragility fractures.* However, in recent years, routine screening has led to more asymptomatic cases. Women are more commonly affected than men, with peak incidence between ages 20 and 60.

Symptoms, when present, may include fatigue, muscle weakness, polyuria, nausea, constipation, heartburn, anorexia, or vague complaints such as memory impairment, difficulty concentrating, or low mood.

73.5.1 Complications

1. *Nephrolithiasis* is the most common complication.
2. *Hypertension:* second most common.
3. *Peptic ulcers.*
4. *Pancreatitis.*
5. *Psychiatric issues.*
6. *Cardiovascular complications.*

73.6 Biochemical Findings

- In *primary HPT,* serum calcium levels are elevated, while phosphate levels are reduced, and PTH levels are either high or inappropriately normal. To ensure accuracy, serum calcium should be corrected for albumin levels or measured as ionized calcium, as certain medications (e.g., hydrochlorothiazide or lithium) can falsely elevate calcium levels. These drugs should be discontinued for 3 months before retesting.
- In *secondary HPT*, plasma calcium is normal or low, with serum phosphate levels elevated in chronic renal failure or reduced in malabsorption states.
- *Pseudohyperparathyroidism* refers to hypercalcemia caused by malignancy without skeletal metastases or primary HPT (Table 73.1).

Table 73.1 Summary of HPT biochemical findings

	Primary	Secondary	Tertiary
S. Ca^{2+}	Increased	Normal/decreased	Increased
PO_4	Decreased	Increased/decreased	Increased/decreased
ALP	Normal/increased	Increased	Increased
PTH	Normal/increased	Increased	Increased+

73.7 Diagnostic Imaging

1. *Technetium-99 m (Tc99m) sestamibi scintigraphy and ultrasonography* are used for localization of parathyroid adenomas and to help identify nodular goiter.
2. *A 24-hour urinary calcium excretion test* is essential to rule out familial hypocalciuric hypercalcemia (Fig. 73.2).

Radiographic findings in HPT include bone resorption with reduced density, prominent trabecular patterns, loss of cortical definition, subperiosteal resorption, a "*salt-and-pepper*" skull appearance, distal clavicle tapering, and brown tumors.

Subperiosteal resorption, a hallmark of HPT, is commonly observed at the *radial margins* of the middle and proximal phalanges of the second and third fingers, the medial metaphysis of the humerus and tibia, the undersurface of the distal clavicle, and the trochanters.

Subligamentous resorption may occur at ligament and tendon attachment sites, such as the trochanters, humeral and ischial tuberosities, and calcaneus.

Other findings include a granular skull appearance, *rugger jersey spine* (ill-defined bands of increased bone density near vertebral endplates), and destructive arthropathy in long-term dialysis patients.

Brown tumors, resulting from hemorrhagic giant cell proliferations, commonly affect the mandible, pelvis, ribs, and femora.

Soft tissue changes may include nephrocalcinosis, renal calculi, chondrocalcinosis, and calcification in periarticular tissues or visceral organs.

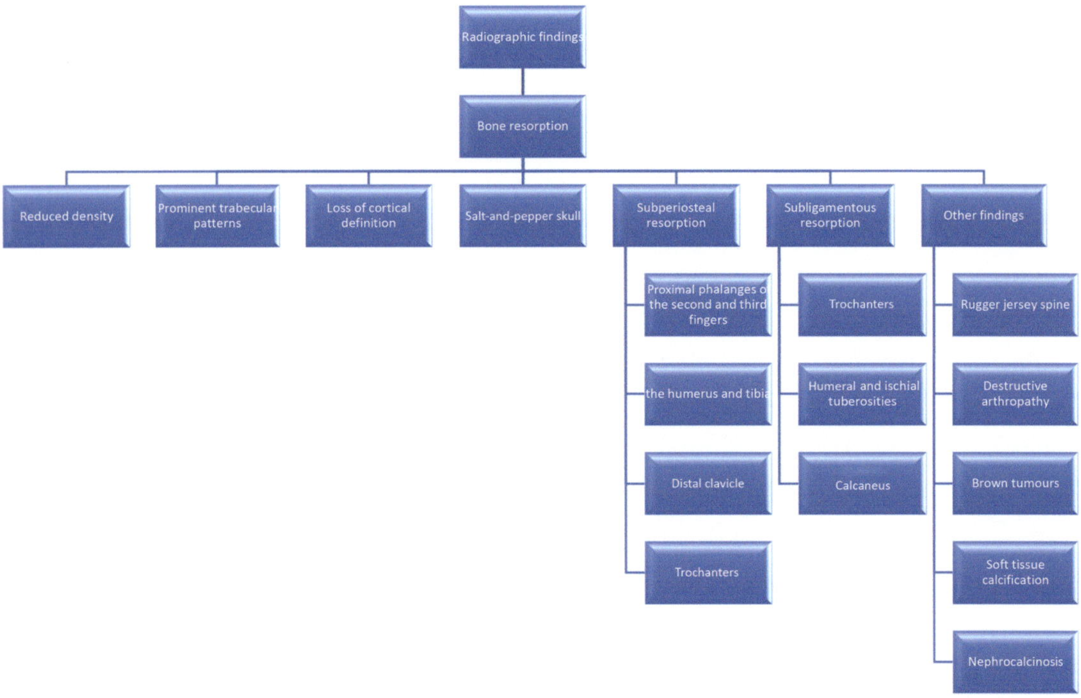

Fig. 73.2 Radiographic findings in HPT

73.8 Treatment Approaches (Fig. 73.3)

Parathyroidectomy remains the definitive treatment for *primary HPT*:

- Normalizes parathyroid function
- Improves BMD
- Reduces fracture risk
- Lowers renal stone formation
- Enhances renal function

Medical management indications include:

- Patients unsuitable for surgery
- Those with mild asymptomatic disease
- Those with osteoporosis or progressive BMD loss who do not meet surgical criteria

Medical management includes:

1. *Adequate hydration*—critical to prevent acute hypercalcemia and hypercalcemic crises. Thiazide diuretics should be avoided due to their effect on urinary calcium reabsorption, and chronic lithium therapy should be discontinued, as it elevates PTH levels.
2. *Calcium* intake in primary HPT should align with general population guidelines and not be restricted.
3. *Vitamin D* levels should be maintained between 50 and 75 nmol/L using daily cholecalciferol doses of 600–1000 IU, with careful monitoring of serum and urinary calcium.
4. In postmenopausal women with mild asymptomatic HPT, *hormone replacement therapy (estrogen) or selective estrogen receptor modulators* (e.g., *raloxifene*) may improve BMD and provide skeletal protection.
5. *Bisphosphonates*, used at doses similar to those for osteoporosis, offer skeletal protection in mild primary HPT without lowering serum calcium. *Denosumab* also supports skeletal health at the spine and hip but does not reduce serum calcium.
6. *Cinacalcet*, a calcimimetic agent, is approved for primary HPT with hypercalcemia when surgery is not feasible, *as well as for secondary HPT in dialysis patients and parathyroid cancer.* It effectively lowers PTH and serum calcium but does not protect bone health. Combining cinacalcet with bisphosphonates provides both skeletal protection and calcium reduction.

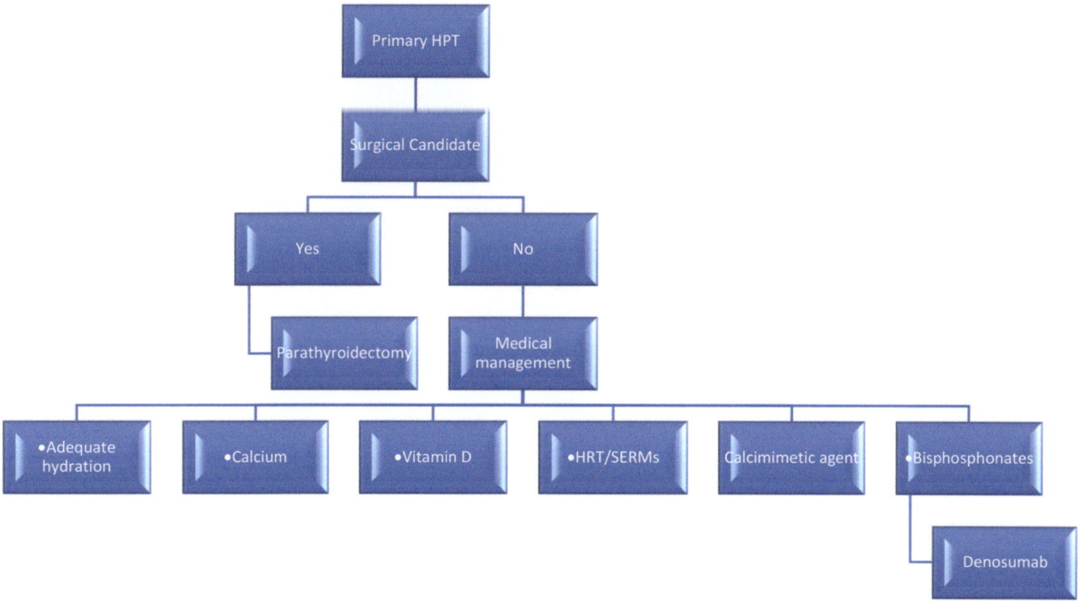

Fig. 73.3 Treatment flowchart for primary HPT

Table 73.2 Summary of treatment options for HPT

	Primary HPT	Secondary HPT	Tertiary HPT
Parathyroidectomy[a]	+++	+	+
Adequate hydration	++	++	++
Calcium/vitamin D	++	++	++
HRT (estrogen)/SERMs[b]	+	+/−	+/−
Bisphosphonates	+	−	−
Calcimimetic agent	+	+	−
Noncalcemic vitamin D analogs	−	++	−

[a]Parathyroidectomy is indicated for tertiary HPT or severe HPT in end-stage renal disease unresponsive to medical therapy
[b]In postmenopausal women

In *secondary HPT* associated with end-stage renal disease, key treatments include *noncalcemic vitamin D analogs* (e.g., *22-oxacalcitriol, paricalcitol, doxercalciferol*) and calcimimetic agents that reduce PTH secretion by binding to parathyroid calcium-sensing receptors.

Hyperphosphatemia management involves dietary phosphate restriction (800–1000 mg/day, though compliance is challenging) and phosphate binders, which are initiated when phosphate levels rise (Table 73.2).

References

1. Dandurand K, Ali DS, Khan AA. Primary hyperparathyroidism: a narrative review of diagnosis and medical management. J Clin Med. 2021;10(8):1604. https://doi.org/10.3390/jcm10081604. PMID: 33918966; PMCID: PMC8068862.
2. van der Plas WY, Noltes ME, van Ginhoven TM, Kruijff S. Secondary and tertiary hyperparathyroidism: a narrative review. Scand J Surg. 2020;109(4):271–8. https://doi.org/10.1177/1457496919866015. Epub 2019 Jul 31. PMID: 31364494.
3. Institute of Medicine; Committee to Review Dietary Reference Intakes for Calcium and Vitamin. In: Ross AC, Yaktine AL, Del Valle HB, editors. Reference Intakes for Calcium and Vitamin D. Washington, DC: The National Academic Press; 2011.
4. Keutgen XM, Buitrago D, Filicori F, Kundel A, Elemento O, Fahey TJ 3rd, Zarnegar R. Calcimimetics versus parathyroidectomy for treatment of primary hyperparathyroidism: retrospective chart analysis of a prospective database. Ann Surg. 2012;255:981–5.
5. Kidney Disease: Improving Global Outcomes (KDIGO) CKDMBD Update Work Group. KDIGO clinical practice guideline for the diagnosis, evaluation, prevention and treatment of chronic kidney disease mineral and bone disorder (CKD-MBD). Kidney Int Suppl. 2017;7:1–59.

Fluorosis

74

Anand Bhushan and Mahesh Prasad

Fluorine is essential for the mineralization of human bones and formation of dental enamel. Around 96% of the fluorine in the body is present in the bones and teeth. Drinking water and foods such as cheese, tea, and sea fishes are the main sources. The recommended level of fluoride in drinking water in India is 0.5 to 0.8 mg/l. As per World Health Organization (WHO), the upper concentration in drinking water at 1.5 mg/l.

Fluorine is often called a double-edged sword. At very low concentration, ~1 ppm or less, it reduces the incidence of dental caries. However, slightly higher levels, ~2–4 ppm or more, can precipitate mottled tooth enamel; 8 ppm results in skeletal anomalies in 10% of individuals, and >100 ppm causes growth disturbances, kidney damage, or death. Fluorosis is most commonly the result of drinking contaminated water (mostly underground water) in certain geographic areas, especially India and China (endemic fluorosis).

74.1 Pathology

Fluorine is absorbed through the gastrointestinal tract and is deposited as fluorapatite crystals in bone lattice, which are resistant to osteoclastic resorption. It stimulates osteoblastic activity, leading to calcium retention and secondary hyperparathyroidism.

Subperiosteal new bone accretion and osteosclerosis are characteristic pathological features, seen most markedly in the vertebrae, ribs, pelvis, forearm, and leg bones. Hyperostosis at the bony attachments of ligaments, tendons, and fascia also occurs. Tensile strength of skeleton is reduced, and bones fracture more easily. In advanced stages, the spinal vertebrae get fused and presents with associated neurological symptoms.

Skeletal fluorosis is usually not recognized until the disease reaches an advanced stage.

Tooth enamel is principally made up of hydroxyapatite (87%) which is crystalline calcium phosphate. Fluorosis of dental enamel occurs when excess fluoride is ingested during the first 7 years of life (years of tooth calcification).

A. Bhushan (✉)
Big Apollo Spectra Hospital, Patna, India

M. Prasad
Department of Orthopaedics, Patna Medical College & Hospital, Patna, India

V. Kumar et al. (eds.), *A Quick Guide to Essential Orthopedics*,
https://doi.org/10.1007/978-981-95-2676-5_74

74.2 Clinical Features

Manifestations can be stress fractures, back pain, bone pain, joint stiffness, flexion contractures, deformities, and cervical myeloradiculopathy. Spastic paraparesis and quadriparesis may develop in advanced cases with grossly reduced anteroposterior diameter of the spinal canal, narrowing of the intervertebral foramina, sclerosis of the vertebral column, and ossification of the spinal ligaments.

Other manifestations are:

- Hypothyroidism
- Anemia
- Secondary hyperparathyroidism
- Bone loss
- Obesity
- Diabetes
- Insulin resistance
- Hypertension
- Atherosclerosis
- Cardiovascular disease

Neonatal skeletal fluorosis occurs in babies born to mothers with high intake of fluoride during pregnancy.

74.3 Phases of Skeletal Fluorosis

- Preclinical phase—asymptomatic—slight increase in bone mass on X-ray
- Phase I—musculoskeletal sporadic pain, joint stiffness, osteosclerosis of pelvis and spine
- Phase II—degenerative and destructive—chronic arthritic symptoms, calcification of ligaments/interosseous membranes, increased osteosclerosis of cancellous bone with or without long bone osteoporosis
- Phase III—crippling fluorosis—limitation of joint movement, calcification of ligaments, muscle wasting, neurological defects, metabolic bone disease (rickets, osteomalacia, osteoporosis, and secondary HPT), pseudofractures

74.4 Diagnosis

The diagnosis is usually made based on the characteristic imaging features.

74.5 Imaging Features

Earliest radiological changes appear within 6 months of continuous exposure to >2.5 mg/day. Involvement of the axial skeleton is characteristic. Osteosclerosis, osteophytosis, and ossification of ligamentous (most evident on the pelvis and spine) and fascial attachments are characteristic X-ray features. Interosseous membrane calcification is the most characteristic radiographic finding of fluorosis. Sparing of the skull distinguishes fluorosis from Paget's disease.

Urinary fluoride (normal 0.2 mg/L to 1.0 mg/L) is the most accurate screening test. Definitive diagnosis is made through quantitative measurement of dry-ashed bone fluoride (normal 0 μg/g to 140 μg/g).

74.6 Treatment

Prevention appears to be the only solution as there is no definitive medical treatment for skeletal fluorosis other than removing the source and managing the symptoms. This is achieved by the provision of safe drinking water having fluoride content <0.5 ppm. The defluoridation techniques like "Nalgonda" technique (most popular; consists of flocculation, sedimentation, and filtration of by the addition of aluminum sulfate/chloride combined with lime), adsorption on activated alumina, electrocoagulation, and reverse osmosis can be adopted to make the water drinkable.

Although there is no cure, there are many components of the disease that are treatable.

About 1–2 gm of elemental calcium should be given per day with vitamin supplements. Juvenile skeletal fluorosis is seen more commonly in children with inadequate calcium in the diet. It is imperative to ensure adequate calcium and vitamin D intake in all individuals, especially growing children, as they decrease fluoride toxicity. Osteomalacia with insufficiency fractures may need vitamin D supplementation.

Nonsteroidal anti-inflammatory drugs (NSAIDs) and physiotherapy can be used for symptomatic relief.

Neurological manifestations in severe skeletal fluorosis are due to compression of the spinal cord and nerve roots by the osteophytosis.

Decompression laminectomy may be needed in advanced stages for compression myelopathy.

Multiple Choice Questions

1. Most of the systemic fluoride is retained in which of the following?
   (a) Kidneys
   (b) Mineralized tissues
   (c) Blood plasma
   (d) Oral mucosa
2. Dental Fluorosis can begin at levels over _____ ppm.
   (a) 2 ppm
   (b) 8 ppm
   (c) 4 ppm
   (d) 1.7 ppm
3. Skeletal fluorosis is seen in drinking water fluoride levels over
   (a) 2 ppm
   (b) 8 ppm
   (c) 20 ppm
   (d) 40 ppm
4. Increased bone density occurs in
   (a) Cushing's syndrome
   (b) Hypoparathyroidism
   (c) Fluorosis
   (d) Hyperthyroidism
5. Which is the diagnostic radiological finding of fluorosis?
   (a) Sclerosis of sacroiliac joint
   (b) Interosseous membrane ossification
   (c) Osteosclerosis of vertebral body
   (d) Ossification of ligament of knee joints

Answers: 1. (b), 2. (a), 3. (c), 4. (c), 5. (b)

References

1. Joseph AJ, Rajan R, Paul JS, Cherian KE, Kapoor N, Jebasingh F, Asha HS, Nicolaï T, Thomas P. The continuing crippling challenge of skeletal fluorosis – case series and review of literature. J Clin Transl Endocrinol Case Rep. 2022;24:100114. https://doi.org/10.1016/j.jecr.2022.100114.
2. Everett ET. Fluoride's effects on the formation of teeth and bones, and the influence of genetics. J Dent Res. 2011;90(5):552–60.
3. Kurdi MS. Chronic fluorosis: the disease and its anaesthetic implications. Indian J Anaesth. 2016;60(3):157–62.
4. Dubey S, Agarwal M, Gupta AB. Recent developments in defluoridation of drinking water in India. In: Singh VP, Yadav S, Yadava RN, editors. Environmental pollution [Internet]. Singapore: Springer Singapore; 2018. [cited 2021 Dec 10]. pp. 345–56.
5. Patel PP, Patel PA, Zulf MM, Yagnik B, Kajale N, Mandlik R, et al. Association of dental and skeletal fluorosis with calcium intake and serum vitamin D concentration in adolescents from a region endemic for fluorosis. Indian J Endocrinol Metab. 2017;21(1):190–5.
6. Wang Y, Yin Y, Gilula LA, Wilson AJ. Endemic fluorosis of the skeleton: radiographic features in 127 patients. AJR Am J Roentgenol. 1994;162(1):93–8.
7. Krishnamachari KA. Skeletal fluorosis in humans: a review of recent progress in the understanding of the disease. Prog Food Nutr Sci. 1986;10(3–4):279–314.

Gout

75

Anand Bhushan and Rajeev Anand

75.1 Introduction

Gout is a metabolic disorder, which typically presents with recurring attacks of a red, painful, hot, and swollen joint. Gout is often known as "*the disease of kings*" or "*rich man's disease*." There is a disturbance in the metabolism of urates, resulting in the deposition of monosodium urate (MSU) crystals within the joints along with soft tissues. Although hyperuricemia is the main pathology, gout does not occur in all hyperuricemic patients, and there are other factors like genetic predisposition which has a role to play in the incidence. Only 5% of people with uric acid level more than 9 mg/dL develop gout.

Men in the age group of 40–50 years are most commonly affected.

75.2 Etiopathogenesis

Serum uric acid level is maintained by the balance between its production, either from purine intake in the diet or endogenous production by cellular turnover, and its excretion by the kidneys and gastrointestinal tract (GIT). The cause of gout is chronically high blood levels of uric acid (urate), i.e., hyperuricemia which leads to deposition of the urate crystals. A gout attack is caused when uric acid crystallizes at excessive concentrations and deposits in the tendons, joints, and surrounding tissues. The pathological threshold is considered to be 6.8 mg/dL. Increased production is responsible for only 10% of cases of gout, while the remaining 90% are caused by its renal underexcretion.

Other factors like synovial fluid pH, water concentration, electrolyte levels, and synovial components such as proteoglycans and collagen may affect the solubility of uric acid in the joint. Deposition of urate crystals in the joint initiates the inflammatory process cascade by being engulfed by the synovial phagocytic cells.

Gout can be of two types:

(a) Primary—occurs due to inborn defects, either in the metabolism of purine or in the secretion of urates by the renal tubules
(b) Secondary—caused by any acquired disorders that result in the increased turnover of nucleic acids, e.g., myeloproliferative disorders

Regular consumers of beer or sugar-sweetened beverages, people who consume purine-rich foods like liver, shrimp, or anchovies, or people who are overweight are more likely to develop gout. Male gender and age are the other risk factors (Table 75.1).

A. Bhushan (✉)
Big Apollo Spectra Hospital, Patna, India

R. Anand
Patna Medical College & Hospital, Patna, Bihar, India

V. Kumar et al. (eds.), *A Quick Guide to Essential Orthopedics*,
https://doi.org/10.1007/978-981-95-2676-5_75

Table 75.1 Pathogenesis of hyperuricemia

Overproduction 10%	Dietary purine	Meat (beef, pork, lamb)
		Seafood (shrimps, tuna)
		Beer
	Endogenous purine synthesis	Malignancy
		Tumor lysis syndrome
	Purine salvage	HGPRT deficiency
		PRPS deficiency
	Purine breakdown	Glycogen storage disease
Underexcretion 90%	Urinary excretion	Diuretics
		Renal failure
	Urinary reabsorption	Alcohol
		Genetic defects
Risk factors	Male	
	Age	
	Obesity	
	Hypertension	
	Diabetes mellitus	

75.3 Diagnosis

Most widely all over the world, gout is diagnosed clinically. Definitive diagnosis involves the demonstration of the pathognomonic MSU crystals in synovial fluid by joint fluid aspirate or tophus aspirate. These are needle-shaped and show strong negative birefringence under polarized light microscopy and are considered as the gold standard of diagnosis. The European Alliance of Associations for Rheumatology (EULAR) recommendations advise synovial fluid analysis to exclude other causes, mainly septic arthritis.

75.4 Clinical Presentations

Clinically, four stages are seen:

1. Asymptomatic gout—presence of hyperuricemia, discovered accidently.
2. Acute gouty arthritis (within hours)—usually monoarticular peripheral acute arthritis, most commonly involving the first metatarsophalangeal (MTP) joint, known as *podagra*. Gout has a predilection for the lower limb, e.g., tarsal and metatarsal joints, ankles, knees, wrists, metacarpophalangeal (MCP) joints, as well as interphalangeal joints of the hands.
3. Intercritical gout (hours to days)—symptom-free period between acute attacks. However, without proper treatment newer attacks can be more frequent and more severe.
4. Chronic tophaceous gout—deposition of MSU crystals (tophi) in tendons, ligaments, cartilage, bone, and other soft tissues including synovium or in the subcutaneous tissues or the skin in a para-articular location in cases which are untreated.
   Kidney injury, tophi, and kidney stones are other potential outcomes of hyperuricemia.

Gout attacks generally come on suddenly, frequently at night.

1. Intense joint pain—although it can damage any joint, gout typically impacts the big toe. The elbows, wrists, fingers, ankles, and knees are other joints that are frequently involved.
2. Residual discomfort—some joint discomfort may remain from a few days to a few weeks. Ensuing episodes are often more prolonged and more likely to involve more joints.
3. Inflammatory redness—affected joints develop swelling, tenderness, warmth, and redness.
4. Limited mobility—unable to move the joints normally, as gout worsens.

75.4.1 Complications

Recurrent gout—some individuals might get gout frequently each year. Medications may help prevent gout attacks in those with recurrence.

Advanced gout—if left untreated, it can erode a joint and eventually destroy it. Deposits of urate crystals develop under the skin as tophus nodules. Tophi can appear at various sites including the elbows, feet, fingers, hands, and Achilles tendons. Tophi are often asymptomatic, but during gout bouts, they can swell and become tender.

Renal stones—there might be deposition of uric acid crystals in the urinary tract, leading to kidney stones. These are generally managed medically. In advanced cases, surgical intervention might be required.

Laboratory studies show elevated erythrocyte sedimentation rate (ESR), leukocytosis, and hyperuricemia. However, during an acute attack, blood uric acid levels could be surprisingly normal. Also, hyperuricemia is mostly asymptomatic and does not necessitate the diagnosis of gout. The analysis of synovial fluid should include assessing leukocyte count, chemistry, culture, and sensitivity. In acute gout, synovial fluid leukocytic count may exceed 50.000 cells/μL in some cases, mostly polymorphs. In gout, glucose level is normal in contrast to septic arthritis, in which bacteria consume glucose, leading to low levels. Septic arthritis should be ruled out in gouty cases, as both may be present in the same joint. So, culture and sensitivity along with Gram stain are crucial to confirm the diagnosis.

Urinary uric acid of more than 800 mg/24 h indicates increased production of uric acid and requires a drug that prevents uric acid production such as xanthine oxidase inhibitors rather than a uricosuric agent.

75.5 Imaging Features

Radiography is of high significance and is the most widely used imaging method in gout. General features include dense soft tissue tophi, preservation of joint space, bone erosions (marginal, periarticular overhanging margin sign, intraosseous), normal bone density, periosteal new bone formation, secondary degenerative joint changes, chondrocalcinosis, and avascular necrosis.

Ultrasonography has an increased role for the diagnosis and management of gout in recent times. It can detect joint effusion, changes in synovitis, synovial proliferation, hypervascularization, and bone erosions. Articular cartilage *double contour sign,* occurring due to crystal deposition on the surface of the cartilage, is a very specific ultrasonographic feature of gout.

Computed tomography (CT) is the best technique for the assessment and characterization of crystal arthropathies. Also, it is helpful in assessing erosions in chronic gout; however, it is not helpful in the diagnosis of acute gout.

Dual-energy CT (DECT) is a quick, highly accurate, noninvasive method to visualize urate crystals and early erosions, even before the radiographs. It is superior to all other modalities in detecting urate deposition anywhere in the area imaged. It, however, cannot detect the crystal deposition on the surface of the cartilage, which is detected by ultrasonography.

The role of magnetic resonance imaging (MRI) is limited; however, it is useful for evaluation of gout at unusual sites.

75.6 Treatment

The treatment of gout mainly depends on urate-lowering therapy, aimed at correcting hyperuricemia. The focus should also be on the prevention of acute flares, patient education, diet, and lifestyle changes.

75.7 Treatment of Acute Flares

Colchicine, glucocorticoids, and nonsteroidal anti-inflammatory medications (NSAIDs) are effective in acute flares. Evidence does not support the use of one NSAIDs (indomethacin, celecoxib, naproxen, etc.) over others, and the selection should be based on the patient's prior response and concerns over specific side effects. They are usually used in high doses for the shortest possible interval until the acute attack is controlled.

The anti-inflammatory potential of glucocorticoids is well established, and they should be continued until the acute attack has fully resolved and should be gradually tapered down to stop.

The recommended dose of colchicine for an acute flare is 1.2 mg, followed by 0.6 mg one hour later. It should be used with caution in patients with chronic kidney disease.

Intra-articular steroid injections are very efficient and are recommended in the management of mono- or pauciarticular flares.

75.8 Treatment of Chronic Gout and Prevention of Flares

The principle of treatment of gout includes target to lower the urate levels. It can be reduced after the acute attack subsides, by changing one's lifestyle. The serum uric acid target should be below 6 mg/dL in all gouty patients and below 5 mg/dL in severe gout patients, to allow more rapid dissolution of the crystal load.

Patient education regarding the disease, its curable nature, and the importance and methods of urate-lowering targets is an important aspect of the treatment. Recommended diet and lifestyle changes include weight loss in obese patients, avoidance of beer, sugar sodas, restriction of meat and seafood intake, and increased intake of skimmed milk, along with increased physical activity.

Uric acid inhibitors (e.g., allopurinol) or uricosuric agents (helps to remove uric acid through urine) (e.g., Probenecid) offer long-term protection in people who experience recurrent attacks. It may be preventive to take vitamin C and consume low-fat dairy products in the diet (Fig. 75.1).

Xanthine oxidase inhibitors, either allopurinol or febuxostat, are commonly recommended as the initial agents. They inhibit the production of urate and reduce hyperuricemia caused by both overproduction or underexcretion. Treatment should be started with allopurinol first, and only if it is not tolerated or ineffective, febuxostat is recommended as there are concerns of cardiac risks associated with febuxostat.

Allopurinol is a purine analog and competitively inhibits xanthine oxidase and other enzymes as well in the pathway. The recommended dose is 300–400 mg. The major side effects are allopurinol hypersensitivity syndrome with drug rash with eosinophilia and systemic symptoms (DRESS).

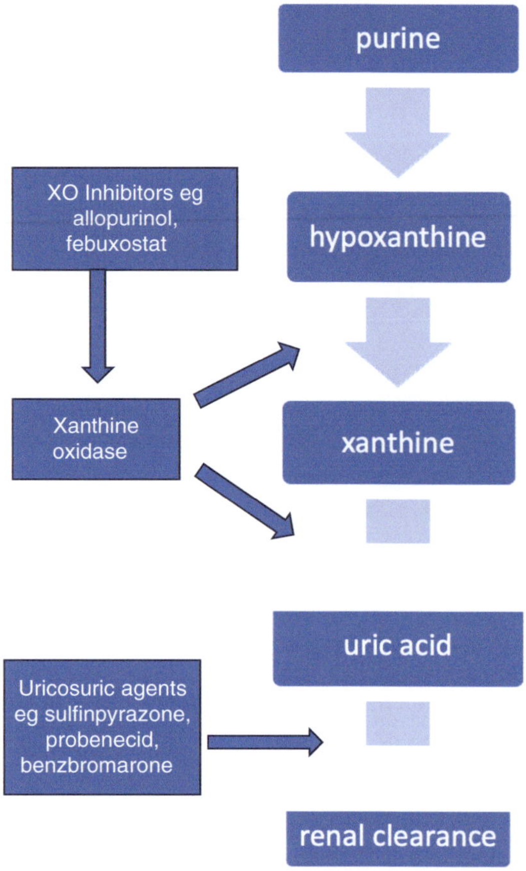

Fig. 75.1 Mechanism of action of urate-lowering agents

Febuxostat is a nonpurine, noncompetitive inhibitor of both the oxidized and reduced forms of xanthine oxidase but does not inhibit other enzymes. It is approved in gout patients with normal renal function or mild to moderate chronic kidney disease and is recommended in doses of 40, 80, and 120 mg.

Uricosuric agents (probenecid and lesinurad) reduce the reabsorption of uric acid from the proximal tubule by inhibiting renal transporters. Probenecid is used as an add-on to xanthine oxidase therapy or when xanthine oxidase inhibitors are contraindicated. It has an increased risk of renal stone formation and should not be used in patients with a history of renal stones.

Multiple Choice Questions

1. Accumulation of which of the following causes gout?
   (a) Cholesterol
   (b) Blood urea
   (c) Synovial fluid
   (d) Uric acid
2. Most common site of a gout attack is
   (a) Knee
   (b) Foot
   (c) Ankle
   (d) Big toe
3. Which of the following is not the first-line treatment of gout?
   (a) NSAID
   (b) Corticosteroid
   (c) Aspirin
   (d) Colchicine
4. Most commonly, uric acid is eliminated through
   (a) Sweat
   (b) Urine
   (c) Breathing
   (d) Liver metabolism
5. In patients with gout, which of the following should be avoided in food?
   (a) Alcohol
   (b) Dairy products
   (c) Both
   (d) None

Answers: 1. (d), 2. (d), 3. (c), 4. (b), 5. (a)

References

1. Ragab G, Elshahaly M, Bardin T. Gout: an old disease in new perspective – A review. J Adv Res. 2017;8(5):495–511. https://doi.org/10.1016/j.jare.2017.04.008. Epub 2017 May 10. PMID: 28748116; PMCID: PMC5512152.
2. Dalbeth N, Merriman TR, Stamp LK. Gout Lancet. 2016;388(10055):2039–52. [PubMed] [Google Scholar].
3. Emmerson BT. The management of gout. New Engl J Med. 1996;334(7):445–51. [PubMed] [Google Scholar].
4. McQueen FM, Doyle A, Dalbeth N. Imaging in gout–what can we learn from MRI, CT, DECT and US? Arthritis Res Ther. 2011;13(6):246.
5. Pillinger MH, Mandell BF. Therapeutic approaches in the treatment of gout. Semin Arthritis Rheum. 2020;50(3S):S24–30. https://doi.org/10.1016/j.semarthrit.2020.04.010. PMID: 32620199.

Part XI

Newer Techniques

Total Joint Replacement—Hip and Knee

76

Arghya Kundu Choudhury and Manuj Jain

76.1 Introduction

The surgical procedure in which the diseased joint is replaced and reconstructed with an artificial metallic prosthesis is known as joint replacement.

Total hip replacement (THR)—both the acetabular part is replaced and the femoral component is inserted within the femoral canal or the proximal femur, with a large sized femoral head component [2].

Total knee replacement (TKR)—it is actually a resurfacing procedure in which the diseased bony surfaces are placed with metallic prosthesis [1].

76.1.1 Indications of Total Joint Replacement

1. Relieves pain
2. Provides mobility without compromising joint stability
3. Corrects the deformity in the joint

A. Kundu Choudhury (✉)
Department of Hip, Knee and Robotic Joint Replacement, Sarvodaya Hospital and Research Centre, Faridabad, Haryana, India

M. Jain
Department of Orthopaedics, 166 Military Hospital, Jammu, Jammu and Kashmir, India

76.1.2 Absolute Contraindications of Total Joint Replacement

1. Presence of active joint infection or sepsis
2. Any infective foci in the body

76.2 Total Hip Replacement

76.2.1 Biomechanics

The normal hip joint is best understood, and the forces acting at the hip are classically described by a lever diagram (Fig. 76.1).

The hip centre is the fulcrum that acts between two opposing forces.

Lever arm 1 is the distance from the hip centre to the centre of body weight.

Lever arm 2 is the abductor mechanism, which is the distance from the hip centre to the greater trochanter (the insertion point of the hip abductors).

These two lever arms oppose each other. The body weight lever arm is 2.5 times longer than the abductor muscle lever arm, and so the counteracting forces at the hip by abductors should be 2.5 times greater and stronger than body weight. The greater the body weight, the more force across the hip joint by multiple factors. This is

V. Kumar et al. (eds.), *A Quick Guide to Essential Orthopedics*,
https://doi.org/10.1007/978-981-95-2676-5_76

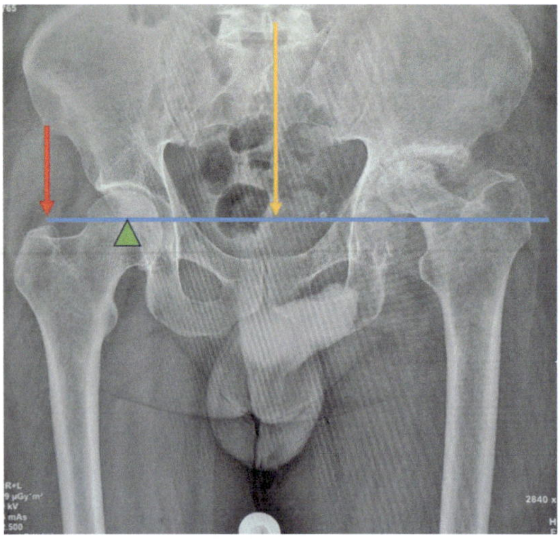

Fig. 76.1 Normal hip joint and the lever arm concept

one theoretical correlation between obesity and hip arthritis.

- Joint reactive forces depend on the activity. The force of walking is 2.5× body weight, the force of jogging is 6× body weight, and the force of running is 8× body weight.

76.2.1.1 So How Does a THR Work?

In progressive hip degeneration, the head begins to collapse, the neck shortens, and the abductor mechanism loses tension causing weakness and pain due to increased joint reactive forces.

These lead to

- Pain
- Lurch during walking because of abductor lever arm shortening and weakness
- Limb length discrepancies (LLD)—head collapse and neck shortening
- Deformities (sagittal—flexion, Coronal—abduction/adduction, Rotational—external/internal)—spasm and shortening of muscle due to pain

Current techniques for hip reconstruction focus on restoring the native anatomy of the hip – placing the acetabular component in a low and medial position to restore the centre of rotation of the hip and selecting a femoral stem with adequate head/neck sizes that will restore vertical and horizontal offset (maximizing tension of the abductors) and normalize the leg lengths.

76.2.1.2 Types of Hip Replacement

1. *Total hip replacement*—both parts of the hip joint, the acetabulum and the femoral head, are replaced by prosthesis components.
2. *Hemiarthroplasty*—only one part of the hip joint, the femoral head, is replaced by a prosthesis. It can be of two types:
   - Bipolar—where the modularity is more, allowing increased stability and movement
   - Unipolar—one single composite prosthesis—Austin Moore prosthesis
3. *Hip resurfacing*—only the diseased femoral head part and the acetabular surface are replaced with a metallic prosthesis.

76.2.1.3 Types of Prosthesis [3]

1. Based on the type of fixation:
   - *Cemented THR/cemented hemiarthroplasty*—bone cement is used for fixation of the prosthesis with the native prepared femoral bone.
   - *Uncemented THR/uncemented hemiarthroplasty*—prosthesis is fixed in the bony surface prepared without any cement, and with time osteointegration occurs between the prosthesis and the patient's native bone.
2. Based on the type of bearing surface:
   - *Hard on Hard Bearing Surface*
     - *Metal on metal*—both articulating surfaces are made of metal; the femoral head and the liners are made of metal. Obsolete nowadays.
     - *Ceramic on ceramic* – Both articulating surfaces, the femoral head and the liners, are made of ceramics (alumina/zirconia ceramic compounds). Least chances of generation of wear particles and aseptic loosening in the long term.
   - *Hard on Soft Bearing Surface*
     - *Metal on poly*—the femoral head is metallic, the acetabular component is also metallic, and the liner in between is

made of highly crosslinked polyethylene.
- *Ceramic on poly*—the acetabular component is metallic, the femoral head is made of ceramics, and the liner in between is made of highly crosslinked polyethylene (Fig. 76.2).

76.2.2 Parts of the Prosthesis

1. *Acetabular component or acetabular shell*—the part of the shell which fits over the acetabular surface.
2. *Liner*—the articulating surface which fits over the acetabular shell and articulates with the femoral head.
3. *Femoral head*—the head fits over the adequately selected femoral neck, which connects the femoral stem and articulates with the liner.
4. *Articulating femoral stem*—the femoral canal is prepared, and a stem is broached in the femoral canal, which forms the femoral component in a THR prosthesis.

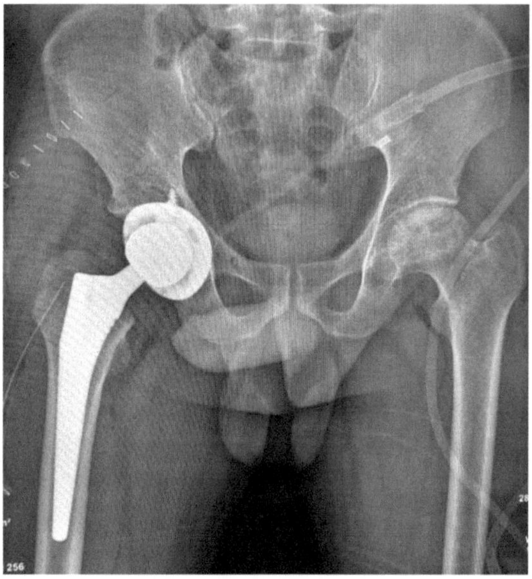

Fig. 76.2 Post-operative radiograph showing uncemented right THR

76.2.3 Indications

- Primary osteoarthritis (OA)—rare in India
- Secondary osteoarthritis—majority of cases:
  (a) Inflammatory arthritis—rheumatoid arthritis, ankylosing spondylitis, psoriatic arthropathy
  (b) Osteonecrosis of the femoral head/avascular necrosis of the femoral head
  (c) Post-traumatic arthritis
  (d) Post-tubercular or tubercular arthritis
  (e) Post-septic sequelae
  (f) Developmental—neglected dysplastic hip

76.2.4 Contraindications

- Active infection in the joint
- Any septic foci in the body or the skin overlying the surgical site
- Particular metallic hypersensitivity
- Renal insufficiency in patients receiving a metal-on-metal prosthesis

76.2.5 Complications

- *Periprosthetic joint infections (PJI)*—septic or infectious occurrence after THR, with biofilm formation over the prosthesis. Biofilm is a microcolony of infective pathogens which rests over the prosthesis surface surrounded by a protective coating formed mostly by the polysaccharide matrix (85%) and the organism or cells (15%).
- *Dislocation of the components*—usually because of malpositioning of the components.
- *Aseptic loosening*—due to wear particles formed by motion in the joints; these are engulfed by macrophages which activates an inflammatory cascade and osteoclastic overactivity.
- *Thromboembolism-related complications*—deep venous thrombosis and pulmonary embolism.

- *Cemented THR—cement-related complications*—due to bone cement particles released into the bloodstream, which can lead to pulmonary embolism.
- *Aseptic lymphocyte-dominant vasculitis-associated lesion (ALVAL)* is a histological entity denoting a chronic inflammatory response to metal particles (cobalt and chromium ions) from a metal-on-metal prosthesis, resulting in swelling around the hip prosthesis. Usually, it is associated with aseptic loosening of the prosthesis.
  - *Stiffness of the joint.*
  - *Mortality.*
  - *Limb length discrepancies.*
  - *Periprosthetic fractures.*

76.2.5.1 Revision Hip Arthroplasty

With more and more primary arthroplasties in India, incidence of revision surgeries is also increasing. All arthroplasties fail eventually after a lifespan, even with the best available implants.

- *Septic Revision Hip Arthroplasty Secondary to PJI*

Usually a two-stage procedure is selected. First stage—component removal and implantation of an antibiotic-loaded cement spacer in the joint. Followed by adequate debridement and collection of specific local tissues for pathogenic organism culture. This is followed by a course of culture-specific antibiotics and monitoring of blood parameters—erythrocyte sedimentation rate (ESR)/C-reactive protein (CRP). Once the parameters normalize to baseline values, second-stage reimplantation of THR components is done. Revision scenarios are often challenging, with a wide variety of metallic prostheses required for adequate reconstruction.

- *Aseptic Loosening*

Usually a single-stage procedure is selected after adequate work up to rule out any causes of infectious pathology.

76.3 Total Knee Replacement

Usually, the diseased surface of the knee joints is replaced when the joint articular cartilages are completely denuded, causing the subchondral bone to be exposed and constantly rubbed against each other, generating severe pain.

76.3.1 Knee Replacement Components

1. *Femoral component*—fixes over the resected distal femur, including both condyles. Usually, it comprises of cobalt-chromium metallic alloys.
2. *Tibial component*—the base plate which fixes over the resected surface of the proximal tibia. It is usually made of titanium alloys.
3. *Insert*—has a central post and it fixes with the tibial base plate and articulates with the femoral components, allowing flexion and extension. It is usually made of highly crosslinked polyethylene.

76.3.2 Types of Knee Replacements

1. *Total Knee Replacement and Unicondylar or Partial Knee Replacement*
   - *Total Knee Replacement*
     Both condyles of the femur and the proximal tibia are resurfaced by a metal-backed prosthesis with or without patellar resurfacing (Fig. 76.3).
   - *Partial Knee Replacement*
     Only the diseased or degenerative condyle of the femur and the tibia is replaced with a metal surface.

     In case of varus knee with only *anteromedial compartment OA* with *sufficient anterior cruciate ligament (ACL)* integrity, a medial unicondylar replacement or partial medial knee replacement is preferred (Fig. 76.4).
2. *Based on the Types of Prosthesis Selection*

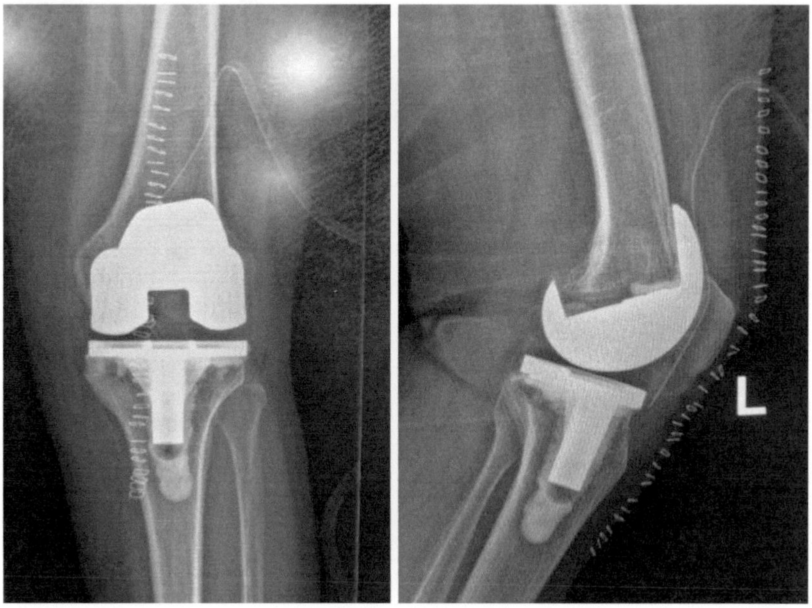

Fig. 76.3 Post-operative X-ray showing cemented left knee TKR—AP view and lateral view

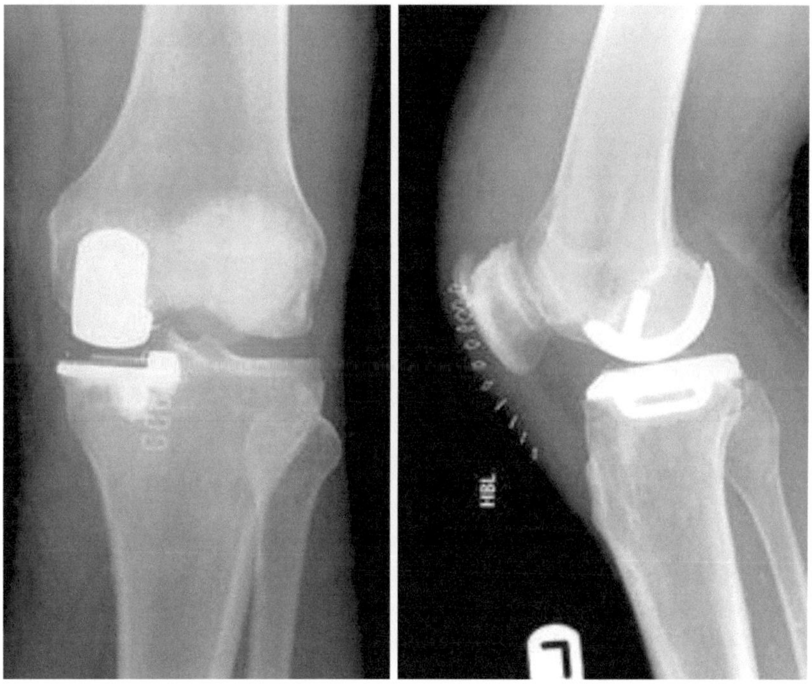

Fig. 76.4 Post-operative X-ray showing partial knee replacement or medial unicondylar knee replacement—AP view and lateral view

- *Posterior-Stabilized Total Knee Replacement (PS-TKR)*
  The posterior-stabilized total knee arthroplasty (PS-TKA) is designed with the goal of mechanical alignment. It relies on tibial and femoral cuts that are perpendicular to the mechanical axis.
  It sacrifices the posterior cruciate ligament (PCL) in order to get the cam-post to function properly.
  The PS-TKA uses a cam on the femur to engage the back of the tibial post (at 40–90° flexion) to push the femur over the tibial contact point posteriorly during knee flexion. This is 'posterior rollback' and it is essential for the knee to achieve deep flexion because terminal flexion occurs when the posterior femoral cortex impinges on the posterior tibial plateau. By allowing the femur to rollback, it creates more offset before impingement occurs, enabling a deeper flexion.
- *Cruciate-Retaining TKR*
  The PCL ligament is retained and carefully balanced.
  The cruciate-retaining total knee arthroplasty (CR-TKA) design utilizes the native PCL to prevent anterior translation of the femur during knee flexion, and therefore does not have the cam-post mechanism. The PCL is a knee stabilizer in flexion and it helps in balancing the knee during flexion and retains more or less native knee kinematics.

3. *Based on the Fixation Types*
   - *Cemented TKR*—Bone cement is used for fixation of the prosthesis with the native prepared femoral and tibial bone surfaces.
   - *Uncemented TKR*—prosthesis is fixed in the bony surface prepared without any cement, and with time osteointegration occurs between the prosthesis and the patient's native bone.

76.3.3 Indications

- Primary osteoarthritis (majority of cases in India) with degenerative changes and varus or valgus knee deformities
- Secondary osteoarthritis:
  1. Inflammatory arthritis—rheumatoid arthritis, ankylosing spondylitis, psoriatic arthropathy
  2. Osteonecrosis of the distal femoral condyles
  3. Post-traumatic arthritis
  4. Post-tubercular or tubercular arthritis
  5. Haemophilic arthritis of the knee

76.3.4 Contraindications

- Active infection in the joint
- Any septic foci in the body or the skin overlying the surgical site
- Particular metallic hypersensitivity

76.3.5 Complications

- *Femoral Cam Jump*

The PS-TKA can dislocate, the cam jumps the post, if the flexion gap is too loose and the knee is placed under varus stress. Poly wear at the cam-post interface is a concern based on implant retrieval analysis. It appears that wear severity is highly dependent on ligament balancing.

This can lead to more and more anterior post wear and in long term can lead to aseptic loosening.

- *Patellar Clunk Syndrome*

Patellar clunk syndrome is usually seen with the PS-TKA because suprapatellar scar tissue can get caught within the cam or the box as the knee goes into extension, around 30–45° (the patella starts travelling proximally and the prominent scar tissue catches the lip). Treatment requires arthroscopic tissue removal.

- *Instability*

In a PS-TKA design, more of the distal femur bone cut is required for adequate balancing when the PCL is sacrificed, and this can lead to flexion gap looseness and, in turn, can affect the stability.

- *Patella Baja*

More bony resection from the distal femur can lead to joint line elevation. Up to 8-mm joint line elevation is acceptable; after this, it can affect the patellofemoral joint tracking and stability and lead to patella baja (low-lying or low-riding patella).

- *Patellofemoral Joint Overloading*

Patellar osteophytes are resected and peripatellar denervation is usually with an electrocautery coagulation and this is known as patelloplasty. If this is not adequately performed, it can lead to patellofemoral crepitus and overloading of the joint.

- *Anterior Knee Pain*
  - *Stiffness of the Joint*—limited range of motion in the post-operative period, often requiring manipulation under anaesthesia or arthroscopic scar tissue removal.
  - *Aseptic Loosening*—macrophage–osteoclast activity leads to aseptic prosthesis loosening.

    Management needs revision TKR—same principle like revision THR, in a single sitting or two-stage surgery.
  - *Periprosthetic Joint Infection and Implant Loosening*—acute or peri-operative PJI (<2 weeks) and chronic PJI (>2 weeks) can occur due to bloodstream-related microorganism forming matured biofilm over the prosthesis.

    Revision TKR is performed in such settings—same principle like THR, *a two-stage revision is preferably performed.*
  - *Periprosthetic Fractures*

Multiple Choice Questions

1. A 49-year-old lady with proven anteromedial compartment primary knee osteoarthritis with intact ACL integrity and correctable varus deformity. Management of choice will be
   (a) Unicompartmental knee replacement
   (b) High tibial osteotomy
   (c) Total knee replacement
   (d) Patellofemoral joint replacement
2. A post-TKR patient is developing fever after 48 h of surgery with excessive discharge from her knee wounds. Which one of the following is not an ideal next step in management?
   (a) Send swab from discharge for culture
   (b) IV antibiotics escalation
   (c) Irrigation and debridement
   (d) Revision knee replacement
3. Metal-on-metal bearings for total hip arthroplasty (THA) or resurfacing should be avoided in which of the following clinical situations?
   (a) A history of significant alcohol use
   (b) A history of renal insufficiency
   (c) A history of hepatitis
   (d) Thalassemia
4. Use of a metal-on-metal bearing compared with the use of a metal-on-crosslinked polyethylene (PE) bearing of the same diameter will result in which of the following?
   Smaller wear particles
   (a) Smaller wear particles
   (b) Increased volumetric wear
   (c) Increased linear wear
   (d) Decreased incidence of dislocation
5. Rakesh, a 25-year-old male underwent ceramic-on-ceramic left total hip replacement

for avascular necrosis of femoral head in case of sickle cell anaemia. Enthusiasm for ceramic-on-ceramic implants has recently been somewhat tempered by reports of reproducible noise, particularly squeaking. It has been a source of dissatisfaction requiring revision. The onset of squeaking usually occurs more than

(a) 1 year after implantation
(b) 5 years after implantation
(c) 10 years after implantation
(d) 15 years after implantation

Answers: 1. (a), 2. (d), 3. (b), 4. (a), 5. (a)

References

1. https://www.ncbi.nlm.nih.gov/books/NBK507914/.
2. https://www.ncbi.nlm.nih.gov/books/NBK507864/.
3. https://pubmed.ncbi.nlm.nih.gov/29097396/.

77 Partial Knee Replacement

Bismaya Sahoo and Mazhar Ali

77.1 Introduction

Partial knee replacement (PKR) is a surgical procedure in which a part of the arthritic knee is replaced. It can be unicondylar knee arthroplasty (UKA) or a patellofemoral arthroplasty (PFA).

77.2 UKA [1]

It may be medial or lateral condylar arthroplasty. Medial condyle arthroplasty is most commonly done.

77.3 Indications

- Elderly, thin individuals with unicompartmental disease
- Younger individuals with isolated medial compartment arthritis
- Younger individuals with higher body mass index (BMI)

77.4 Indications for PFA

- Age less than 65 years
- Isolated patellofemoral arthritis with no malalignment of the patellar mechanism
- Pain during daily activities localized to the patellofemoral joint and not responded to non-steroidal anti-inflammatory medications or injections
- Post-traumatic arthritis, primary patellofemoral osteoarthritis, and patellofemoral dysplasia without malalignment
- Alternative to patellectomy

77.5 Contraindications

- Inflammatory arthritis
- Flexion contracture of 15 degrees or more
- Preoperative arc of motion of less than 90 degrees
- Angular deformity of more than 10 degrees from the mechanical axis for varus knees or 5 degrees for valgus knees
- Significant cartilaginous erosion in the weight-bearing areas of the opposite compartment
- Anterior cruciate ligament deficiency
- Collateral ligament insufficiency
- Obesity (a relative contraindication to UKA)

B. Sahoo (✉)
Department of Orthopedics, All India Institute of Medical Sciences, Kalyani,
Kalyani, West Bengal, India

M. Ali
Department of Orthopaedics & Spine Surgery,
Nishtar Medical University, Multan, Punjab, Pakistan

V. Kumar et al. (eds.), *A Quick Guide to Essential Orthopedics*,
https://doi.org/10.1007/978-981-95-2676-5_77

77.6 Types of Implants

- Fixed bearing—a type in which round femoral component articulates with a relatively flat tibial articular surface (Fig. 77.1)
- Mobile bearing—a type in which polyethylene insert can rotate short distances within the metal tibial component (Fig. 77.2)

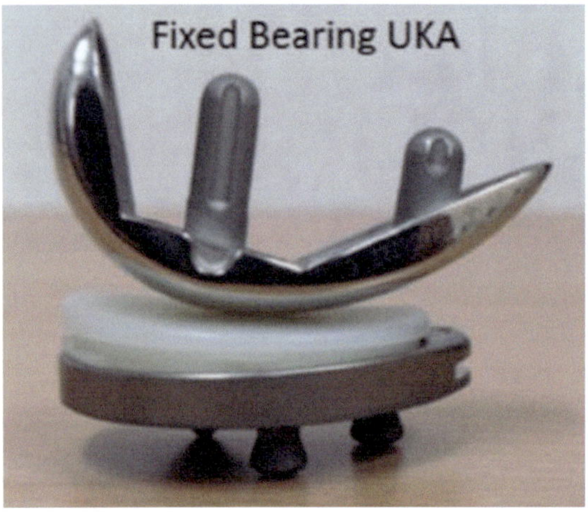

Fig. 77.1 Fixed bearing UKA

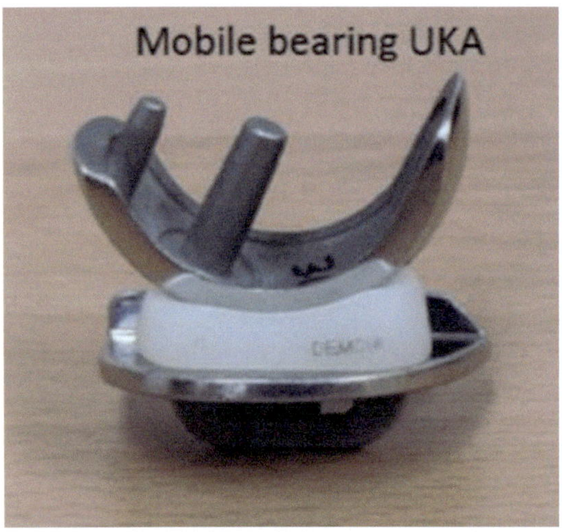

Fig. 77.2 Mobile bearing UKA

77.7 Advantages

- Shorter rehabilitation time
- Greater average postoperative range of motion
- Preservation of the proprioceptive function of the cruciate ligaments, which give a more natural-feeling knee
- Shorter hospital stay
- Less blood loss
- Less invasive procedure that has a good likelihood of lasting the patient's lifetime

77.8 Complications

- *Thromboembolism*: Deep vein thrombosis (DVT) is the most significant complication post-arthroplasty. Age >40 years, diabetes, hypertension, obesity, myocardial infarction, and estrogen use are some of the risk factors associated with it.
- Infection: It is the most dreaded complication of knee replacement, accounting for 2–3%. Risk factors include skin ulceration, previous knee surgery, use of a hinged-knee prosthesis, obesity, concomitant urinary tract infection, steroid use, renal failure, diabetes mellitus, poor nutrition, malignancy, and psoriasis.
- Neurovascular complications: It is a rare but severe complication accounting for 0.03–0.2% cases. Peroneal nerve palsy is seen in about 1–2% cases.
- Other complications that can occur following UKA include bearing dislocation, aseptic loosening, polyethylene wear, periprosthetic fracture, progression of arthritis to the contralateral compartment, infection, bone-implant impingement, retention of cement debris in the joint, ankylosis of the knee, recurrent hematoma in the knee, and persistent pain.

77.9 Future Prospects

UKA has the potential to become the preferred operation for the treatment of limited degenerative knee disease. More recently, the development and use of robot-assisted technology has made performing UKA technically less demanding. With robotic assistance, UKA component placement may become more accurate and precise [2, 3].

Multiple Choice Questions

1. Partial knee replacement is contraindicated in all of the following except:
   (a) Flexion contracture >15 degrees
   (b) Cruciate ligament deficiency
   (c) Obesity
   (d) Collateral ligament deficiency
2. Partial knee replacement includes all of the following except:
   (a) Medial compartment arthroplasty
   (b) Lateral compartment arthroplasty
   (c) Patellofemoral arthroplasty
   (d) Bicondylar arthroplasty
3. Patellofemoral arthritis is indicated in:
   (a) Age <65 years
   (b) Malaligned patella
   (c) Patellar dysplasia
   (d) Unicondylar osteoarthritis
4. Advantages of partial knee replacement are all except:
   (a) Less blood loss
   (b) Less invasive
   (c) Less postop range of motion
   (d) Less rehabilitation time
5. Most dreaded complication of partial knee replacement is:
   (a) Deep vein thrombosis
   (b) Infection
   (c) Foot drop
   (d) Periprosthetic fracture

Answers: 1. (c), 2. (d), 3. (a), 4. (c), 5. (b)

References

1. Frederick M. Azar, James H. Beaty, S. T. Canale, Willis C. Campbell Campbell's operative orthopaedics, 14, 3, Ch.7, Arthroplasty of the knee, Elsevier, Philadelphia
2. Plate J, Mofidi A, Mannava S, Lorentzen C, Smith B, Seyler T, McTighe T, Jinnah R. Unicompartmental knee arthroplasty: past, present, future. Reconstr Rev. 2012;2(1) https://doi.org/10.15438/rr.v2i2.15.
3. Lang JE, Mannava S, Floyd AJ, Goddard MS, Smith BP, Mofi di A, Seyler TM, Jinnah RH. Robotic systems in orthopaedic surgery. J Bone Joint Surg Br. 2011;93(10):1296–9.

78 Shoulder, Elbow and Ankle Replacement

Tushar Gupta and Roop Bhushan Kalia

78.1 Shoulder Arthroplasty

Various pathologies of the shoulder joint may warrant the replacement of a part or all components of the shoulder joint. The various types, indications, contraindications and complications are discussed as follows:

78.2 Shoulder Hemiarthroplasty

The humeral articular surface is replaced with a stemmed humeral component.

78.2.1 Indications

1. Glenohumeral arthritis if:
   - Rotator cuff is deficient
   - Glenoid bone stock is inadequate
2. Rotator cuff arthropathy
3. Osteonecrosis without glenoid involvement
4. Proximal humerus fractures with significant destruction (Fig. 78.1)

78.2.2 Contraindications

1. Infection
2. Neuropathic joint
3. Unmotivated patient
4. Coracoacromial ligament deficiency

78.2.3 Radiographs

1. True (Grashey) anteroposterior (AP) of shoulder
2. Axillary view
3. CT scan—glenoid version and glenoid bone stock
4. MRI—evaluation of rotator cuff

78.2.4 Complications

1. Progressive glenoid arthrosis
2. Tuberosity displacement/malunion
3. Joint overstuffing
4. Subcutaneous (anterosuperior) escape

T. Gupta (✉) · R. B. Kalia
Department of Orthopedics, All India Institute of Medical Sciences, Rishikesh, Uttarakhand, India

V. Kumar et al. (eds.), *A Quick Guide to Essential Orthopedics*,
https://doi.org/10.1007/978-981-95-2676-5_78

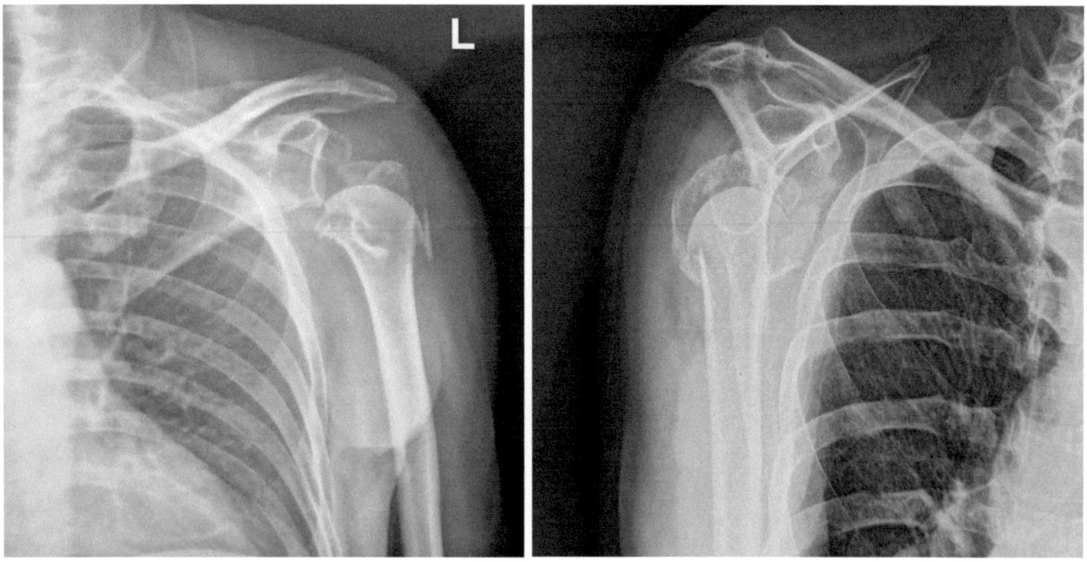

Fig. 78.1 Old proximal humerus fracture with significant destruction

78.3 Total Shoulder Arthroplasty (TSA)

Replacement of the humeral head and glenoid resurfacing. An intact and functional rotator cuff with adequate glenoid stock is essential for performing a successful TSA.

78.3.1 Indications

1. Pain (anterior to posterior), especially at night, affecting the activities of daily living
2. Glenoid chondral wear to bone
3. Posterior humeral head subluxation

78.3.2 Contraindications

1. Insufficient glenoid bone stock
2. Rotator cuff arthropathy
3. Deltoid dysfunction
4. Irreparable rotator cuff (hemiarthroplasty or reverse total shoulder arthropathy is preferable)
5. Brachial plexus palsy

78.3.3 Preoperative Radiology

1. Radiographs
   - True AP: extent of arthritis and presence of superior migration of humerus
   - Axillary view: presence of posterior wear of glenoid
2. CT scan—to determine glenoid version and glenoid bone stock
3. MRI—to evaluate rotator cuff condition

78.3.4 Instrumentation

1. Glenoid component
2. Humerus component with stem

78.3.5 Complications

1. Glenoid loosening—most common (MC) cause of TSA failure
2. Vascular injury—MC arcuate artery (branch of the anterior humeral circumflex artery)
3. Humeral stem loosening
4. Malposition of components

5. Improper soft tissue balancing
6. Iatrogenic rotator cuff injury
7. Stiffness
8. Infection
9. Neurologic injury—MC axillary nerve
10. Periprosthetic fracture

78.4 Reverse Shoulder Arthroplasty (RSA)

This uses a convex glenoid hemispheric ball and a concave humerus articulating cup to reconstruct the glenohumeral joint (Fig. 78.2). Shifting the centre of rotation inferiorly and medially gives the deltoid a mechanical advantage and hence used in the following conditions:

78.4.1 Indications

1. Rotator cuff tear arthropathy
2. Comminuted four-part proximal humerus fractures
3. Prior failed shoulder arthroplasty

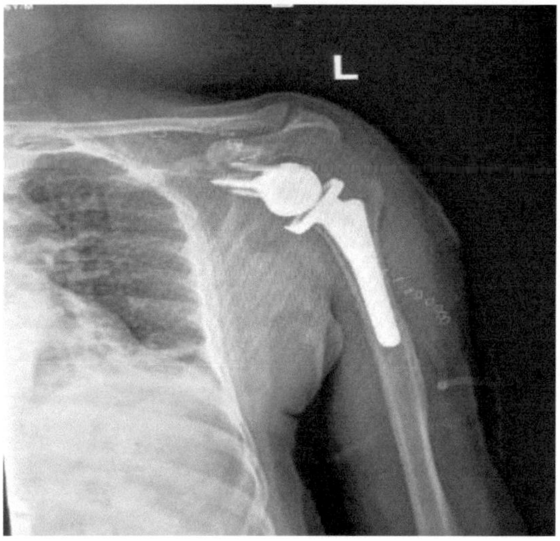

Fig. 78.2 Post-operative X-ray of RSA

78.4.2 Favourable Candidates

1. Low functional demand patients
2. Physiological age >70 years
3. Sufficient glenoid bone stock
4. Working deltoid muscle
5. Intact axillary nerve

78.4.3 Contraindications

1. Axillary nerve dysfunction
2. Deltoid deficiency
3. Acromion deficiency
4. Glenoid osteoporosis
5. Active infection

78.4.4 Complications

1. Scapular notching
2. Dislocation
3. Glenoid loosening
4. Deep infection
5. Acromial or scapular spine fractures
6. Neurapraxia of axillary nerve

78.5 Elbow Arthroplasty

Elbow arthroplasty is a one-stop solution to preserve motion and render patients with debilitating elbow pathologies, inflammatory and post-traumatic arthritis, pain-free. Although with modern times, several types of elbow arthroplasties have been described; however, the following types are of common relevance:

Type of elbow arthroplasty	Radial head excision	Radial head arthroplasty	Total elbow arthroplasty
Indications	• Rheumatoid arthritis isolated to the radiocapitellar joint • Unreconstructable radial head fracture in a ligamentously stable elbow	• Unreconstructable radial head fracture (Fig. 78.3) • Radial head malunion or nonunion • Radiocapitellar arthritis	• Rheumatoid arthritis • Post-traumatic arthritis • Intra-articular distal humeral fractures in the elderly with poor bony quality
Instrumentation	None	Radial head prosthesis (Fig. 78.4)	Ulnar and humeral components with stems
Complications	• Progressive degenerative changes in ulnohumeral joint • Radial shortening • Wrist pain	• Capitellar degeneration	• Aseptic loosening • Infection • Instability • Wound healing • Ulnar neuropathy • Triceps insufficiency • Bone loss • Periprosthetic fracture

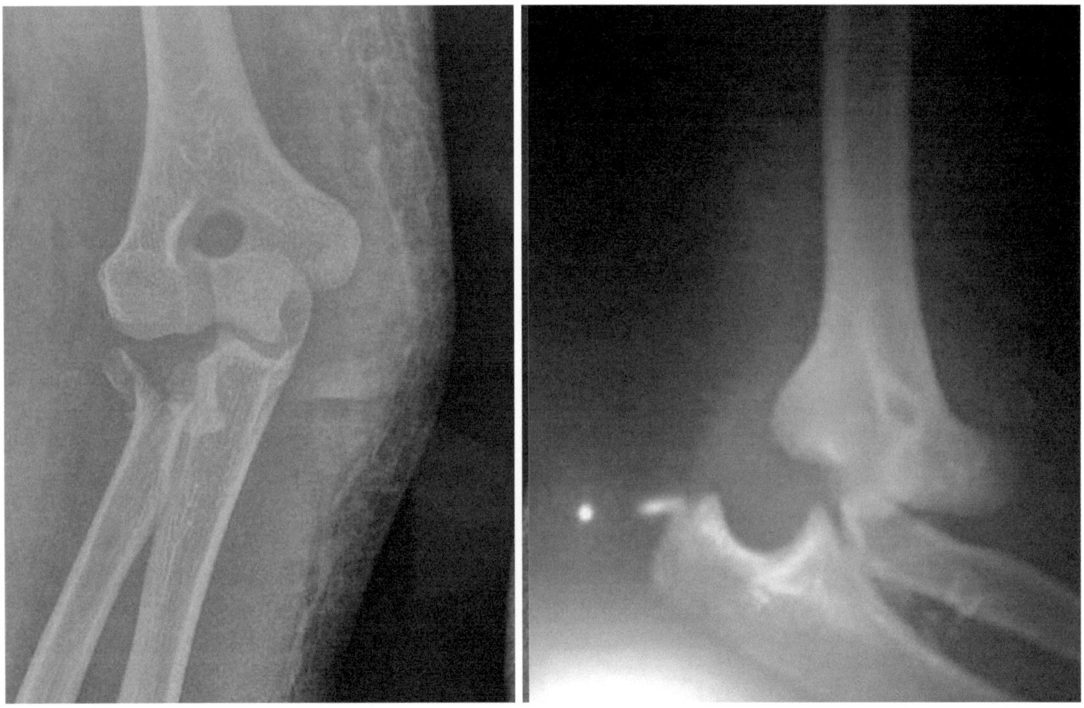

Fig. 78.3 Chronic elbow dislocation with complex radial head fracture

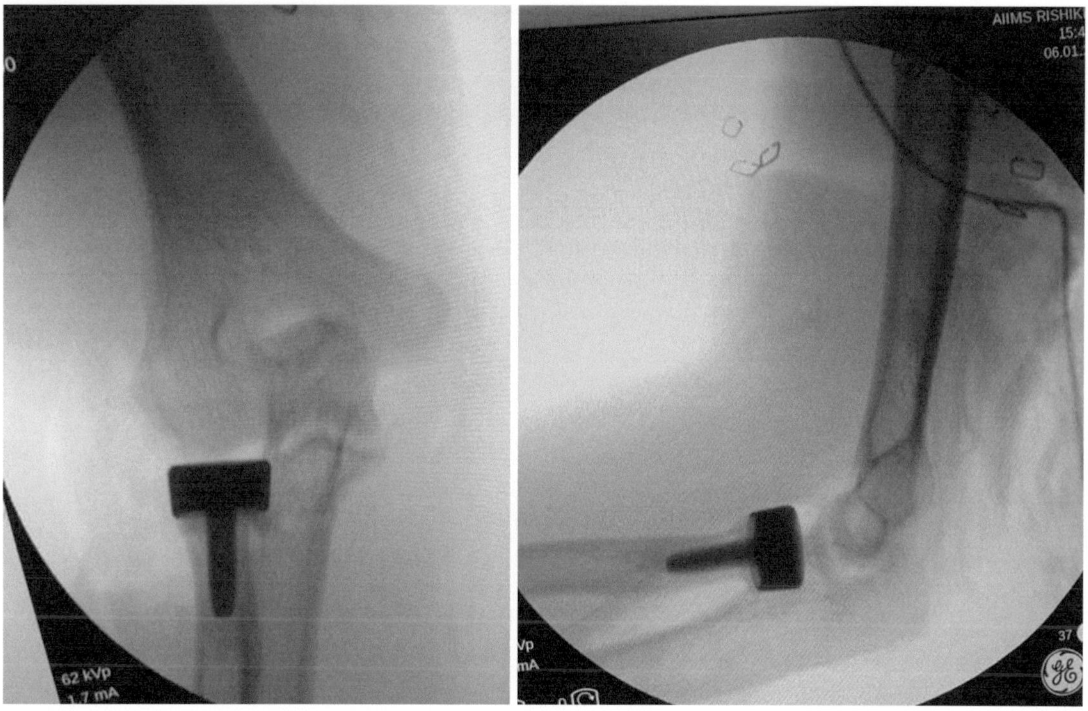

Fig. 78.4 Radial head arthroplasty performed for the case

78.6 Ankle Arthroplasty

78.6.1 Aim

1. Resolution of pain
2. Gain of functional range of motion
3. To restore mechanical alignment to the ankle

78.6.2 Indications

1. End-stage ankle arthritis—unilateral or bilateral

78.6.3 Contraindications

1. Active infection
2. Peripheral vascular disease
3. Charcot arthropathy
4. Severe osteoporosis/insufficient bone stock
5. Inadequate soft tissue envelope
6. Osteonecrosis of the talus
7. Peripheral neuropathy

78.6.4 Components Used

1. Tibial component
2. Talar component
3. Intervening polyethylene mobile-bearing meniscus

78.6.5 Favourable Candidates

1. Older (middle- to old-aged), low demand, reasonably mobile patient with no significant comorbidities
2. Normal or low body mass index
3. Well-aligned and stable hindfoot
4. Good soft tissue condition

78.6.6 Radiographs Required

1. Weight-bearing AP and lateral views of the ankle—extent of arthritis
2. MRI of the ankle—presence of osteonecrosis, amount of involvement, bone loss and size of subchondral cysts

78.6.7 Complications

1. Delayed wound healing
2. Superficial wound infection
3. Deep wound infection
4. Sensory deficits
5. Intraoperative fracture
6. Component loosening
7. Subsidence
8. Osteolysis

Multiple Choice Questions

1. All of the following are contraindications of ankle arthroplasty except:
   (a) Charcot arthropathy
   (b) Infection
   (c) Arthritis
   (d) Osteonecrosis of the talus
2. All of the following are contraindications of reverse shoulder arthroplasty except:
   (a) Axillary nerve dysfunction
   (b) Deltoid deficiency
   (c) Acromion deficiency
   (d) Rotator cuff arthropathy
3. Which is the most common cause of total shoulder arthroplasty failure?
   (a) Glenoid loosening
   (b) Humeral stem loosening
   (c) Malposition of components
   (d) Improper soft tissue balancing
4. Which of the following preoperative factors is a contraindication to total shoulder arthroplasty?
   (a) Eccentric posterior glenoid erosion
   (b) Full thickness supraspinatus tear
   (c) Inflammatory arthritis
   (d) Preganglionic brachial plexus injury
5. Most common complication of total ankle arthroplasty is:
   (a) Delayed wound healing
   (b) Superficial wound infection
   (c) Deep wound infection
   (d) Component loosening

Answers: 1. (c), 2. (d), 3. (a), 4. (d), 5. (a)

Further Reading

Sanchez-Sotelo J. Total shoulder arthroplasty. Open Orthop J. 2011;5:106–14. https://doi.org/10.2174/1874325001105010106. PMID: 21584206; PMCID: PMC3093753.

Hermena S, Rednam M. Reverse shoulder arthroplasty. [Updated 2022 Oct 1]. In: StatPearls [Internet]. Treasure Island (FL): StatPearls Publishing; 2023. Available from: https://www.ncbi.nlm.nih.gov/books/NBK574545/.

Misra A, Kapur R, Maffulli N. Complex proximal humeral fractures in adults–a systematic review of management. Injury. 2001;32(5):363–72. https://doi.org/10.1016/s0020-1383(00)00242-4.

Little CP, Graham AJ, Carr AJ. Total elbow arthroplasty: a systematic review of the literature in the English language until the end of 2003. J Bone Joint Surg Br. 2005;87(4):437–44. https://doi.org/10.1302/0301-620X.87B4.15692.

Haddad SL, Coetzee JC, Estok R, Fahrbach K, Banel D, Nalysnyk L. Intermediate and long-term outcomes of total ankle arthroplasty and ankle arthrodesis. A systematic review of the literature. J Bone Joint Surg Am. 2007;89(9):1899–905. https://doi.org/10.2106/JBJS.F.01149.

Introduction to Arthroscopy

79

Kshitij Gupta and Manuj Jain

79.1 What Is Arthroscopy?

Arthroscopy is the culmination of the Greek words "*arthro*" (joint) and "*skopein*" (to look). It is a minimally invasive approach to the joint for diagnosis as well as therapeutics, which has revolutionized orthopedic surgeries decreasing patient morbidities while expanding our horizons. During the past decades, improvements in lens systems and fiber optics have enabled us to make miniaturized scopes and instruments, making arthroscopy possible for virtually all joints including endoscopy in spine surgeries. The aim of this chapter is to provide students with an insight into the ever-expanding world residing inside the small confines of our joints.

79.2 Arthroscopy vs. Conventional Arthrotomy

Arthroscopic techniques have kept orthopedic surgeries at the cutting edge of medicine. With the help of newer instruments and latest technologies, these minimally invasive surgeries have replaced the conventional open surgeries for the management of intra-articular problems. Arthroscopy has several advantages over its conventional counterparts, justifying its popularity in recent times. Some of them are:

- Lesser postoperative morbidity
- Earlier return to work
- Reduced hospital stay
- Smaller incisions
- Reduced operative time
- Less intense inflammatory reaction
- Absence of secondary effects like neuroma formation, scars, functional imbalances
- Reduced complication rates
- Improved follow-up evaluations with relook/second-look surgeries in case of persistent symptoms
- Ability to perform surgeries not possible through open arthrotomies, e.g., certain meniscal tears are not accessible through open procedures and require arthroscopic repair.

Every technique has got its own pros and cons. Similarly, arthroscopic procedures have got certain disadvantages which include:

K. Gupta (✉)
Department of Orthopedics, All India Institute of Medical Sciences, Rishikesh, Uttarakhand, India

M. Jain
Department of Orthopaedics, 166 Military Hospital, Jammu, Jammu and Kashmir, India

V. Kumar et al. (eds.), *A Quick Guide to Essential Orthopedics*,
https://doi.org/10.1007/978-981-95-2676-5_79

- A steep learning curve
- Difficulty operating through small holes within the limited confines of the joint
- Possible damage to articular cartilage
- Specialized setup required for these surgeries can be quite expensive

79.2.1 Indications and Contraindications of Arthroscopic Surgery

Many intra-articular and periarticular conditions can be managed with arthroscopy. Although knee and shoulder are the most commonly scoped joints, arthroscopy can be performed on almost any joint including the hip, ankle, elbow, and wrist. Some of the indications of arthroscopy are:

General Indications
- Diagnostic scopy
- Joint debridement and lavage
- Removal of loose bodies
- Synovial biopsy or synovectomy

Knee Joint
- Meniscal repair or resection
- Anterior cruciate ligament (ACL) and posterior cruciate ligament (PCL) reconstruction
- Chondral defect repair, including microfracture

Shoulder Joint
- Rotator cuff repair or debridement
- Labral/superior labrum anterior and posterior (SLAP) and instability repair
- Subacromial decompression
- Acromioclavicular (AC) joint pathology
- Biceps tenotomy/tenodesis

Hip Joint
- Management of femoroacetabular impingement (FAI) lesions
- Labral tears
- Iliopsoas tendon pathology

Ankle Joint
- Osteochondral defect of the talus
- Microfracture of osteochondral defect
- Anterior talofibular ligament (ATFL)/anterior inferior tibiofibular ligament (AITFL) impingement

Wrist Joint
- Triangular fibrocartilage complex (TFCC) injuries
- Interosseous ligament injuries
- Assistance for anatomic reduction of fractures

There are very few contraindications of arthroscopic surgeries, which include:

- Risk of joint sepsis through skin infection or remote infection seeding.
- Partial or complete ankylosis of the joint is a relative contraindication.
- Major collateral ligamentous or capsular disruption can lead to fluid extravasation into the soft tissues and is a relative contraindication.

79.3 Instruments Used in Arthroscopy

The basic instrument kit consists of the following: arthroscopes (30° and 70°); probe; scissors; basket forceps; grasping forceps; arthroscopic knives; motorized meniscus cutter and shaver; electrosurgical, laser, and radiofrequency (RF) instruments; and miscellaneous equipment.

79.3.1 Arthroscope

An arthroscope is an optical instrument connected with cameras and a fiber-optic cable to the screen. The 30° and 70° scopes are the most common ones used in the arthroscopic surgeries. The 70° scopes are used to view around the corners of the joint. The scope's field of view changes based on the size of the scope. The 1.9-mm scope has a 65° field of view, the 2.7-mm scope a 90° field of view, and the 4.0-mm scope, a 115° field of view. Wider viewing angles make orientation by the observer much easier. Rotation of angled scopes allows much larger area to be viewed (Fig. 79.1).

79.3.2 Probe

The probe is the most common and important instrument used in diagnostic as well as operative arthroscopy. It is a blunt-tipped instrument angled at 90° at the end. It is used to probe and palpate the intra-articular structures and gives the surgeon a feel of what he is seeing (Fig. 79.2).

79.3.3 Scissors

Arthroscopic scissors are 3–4 mm in diameter with straight or hooked jaw design. Hooked scissors are preferred as they tend to hook the tissues and pull the tissue between the cutting edges rather than pushing the material away, which happens with straight scissors. It is used to cut structures like meniscus/labrum (Fig. 79.3).

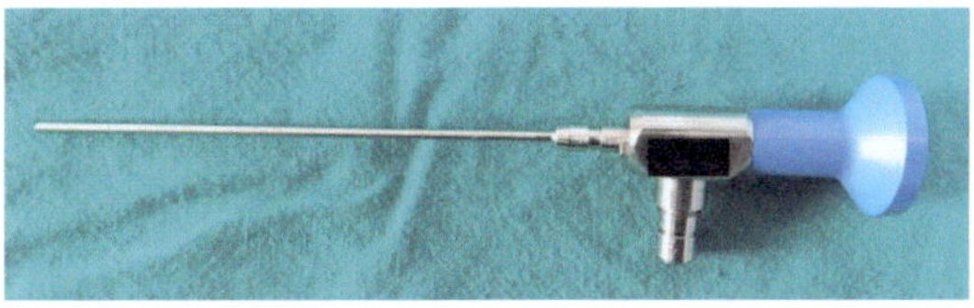

Fig. 79.1 Arthroscope

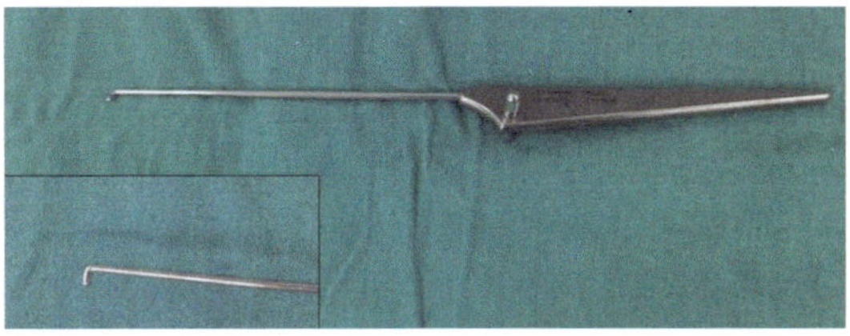

Fig. 79.2 Probe

79.3.4 Basket Forceps

Basket or punch biopsy forceps are used for biting tissues into very small pieces. It has an open base that allows the tissue to drop freely within the joint, which can then be easily removed by the suction irrigation system (Fig. 79.4).

79.3.5 Grasping Forceps

Grasping forceps as the name suggests, are used for holding and retrieving intra-articular structures, or holding tissues in tension for cutting. They have serrated or sharp teeth to hold the structures between them with a ratchet lock to secure the held tissue (Fig. 79.5).

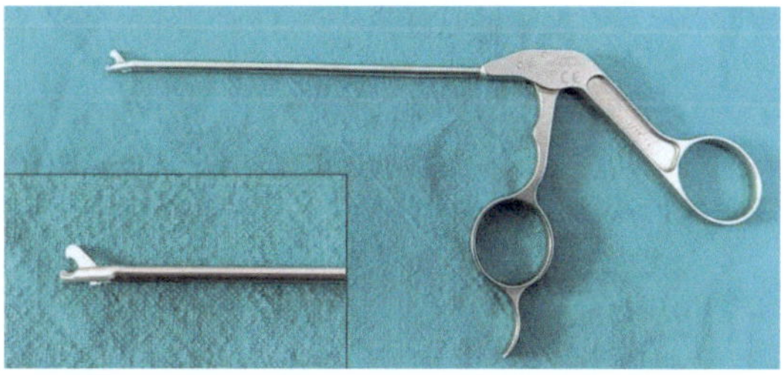

Fig. 79.3 Arthroscopic scissors

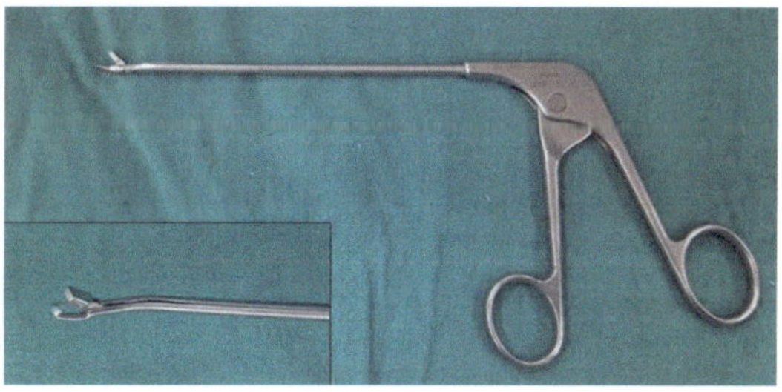

Fig. 79.4 Basket forceps

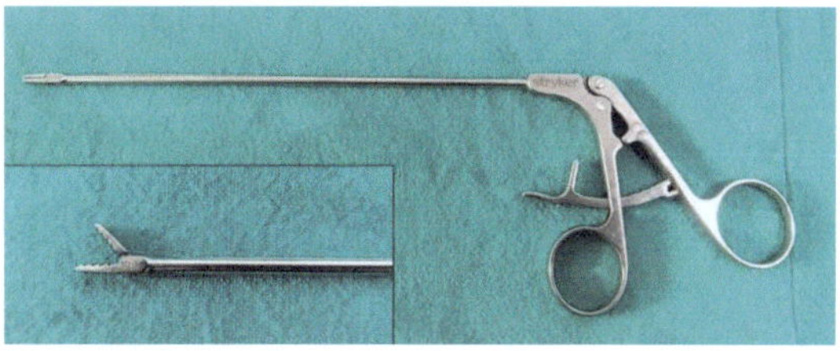

Fig. 79.5 Grasping forceps

79.3.6 Knife Blades

Arthroscopic knives are used for cutting things. There are a variety of designs available. Blades are usually encased in a retractable sheath, so that the blade is exposed only when needed, reducing the risk of damage to other structures.

79.3.7 Motorized Shavers

Motorized shavers consist of an outer hollow sheath and a rotating inner cannula with corresponding windows. The inner cannula window has sharp edges functioning as cutters with the tissue being drawn into the window using the suction system attached to the shaver (Fig. 79.6).

79.3.8 Electrocautery and Radiofrequency Instruments

Electrocautery and radiofrequency instruments have been used as tools for cutting and achieving hemostasis inside the joint. Although they are very useful, a few reported complications include articular damage, osteonecrosis, and tissue damage caused by the irrigant (Fig. 79.7).

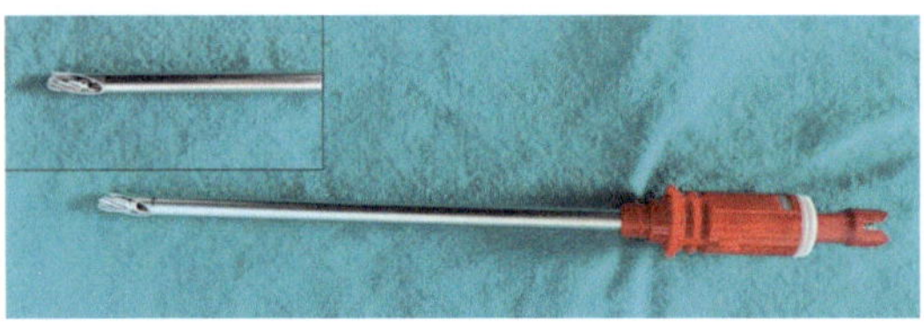

Fig. 79.6 Motorized shaver

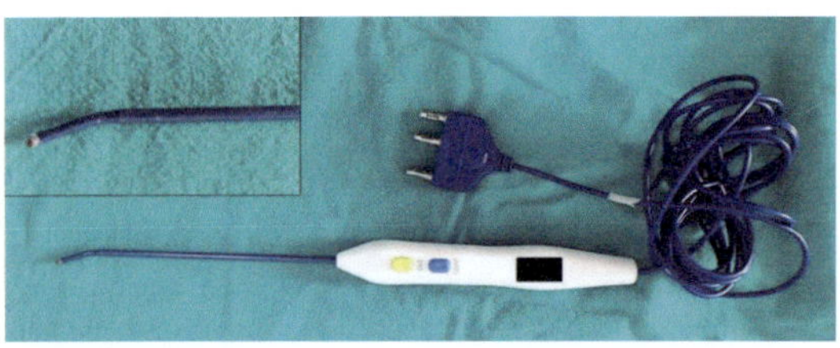

Fig. 79.7 Arthroscopic radiofrequency (RF)

Note: Triangulation Technique Triangulation is a basic technique for operative arthroscopy. It involves using instruments through a portal other than the viewing portal and bringing the instrument into the field of view so that the instrument tip and the arthroscope form the apex of a triangle. It is advisable to start with the arthroscope away from the intended structure, placing the instrument into the field of view and advancing the scope as well as the instrument toward the intended structure. This simultaneously zooms in on the structure as the instrument is advanced forward keeping everything within the field of view.

79.4 Irrigation System

Irrigation and distension of the joint are necessary for arthroscopic procedures. They created space within the joint and keep the field of view clear. Inflow is maintained either through the arthroscopic sheath or a separate portal. Ringer's lactate is the preferred solution instead of isotonic saline. Inflow and pressure can be changed by using pumps or by changing the elevation of the solution. For the knee, a pressure of around 45–60 mm Hg is needed, created by elevating the solution 3 feet above the joint level. Addition of epinephrine (1 mg/L of saline) can help reduce bleeding, keeping the field of view clear.

79.5 Tourniquet

For arthroscopy of distal joints, tourniquet is almost always applied and inflated as needed. Its main function is to reduce the flow of blood to the limb, providing a clear field of view. Contraindications to the use of a tourniquet include a history of thrombophlebitis and significant peripheral vascular disease. There are no major disadvantages of using a tourniquet under specified duration of 90–120 min. Other than providing a clear field of view to the operating surgeon, studies have failed to conclusively prove any improvement in functional outcome for the patient.

Table 79.1 Standard arthroscopic portals for different joints

Portal	Function	Location and technique	Complication
Portals of knee			
Anterolateral	Primary viewing portal	Lateral to patellar tendon over soft spot on joint line Made in flexion	
Anteromedial	Primary instrumentation portal	Medial to patellar tendon over soft spot on joint line Made in flexion	
Posteromedial	Visualize posterior horn and PCL	1 cm above joint line, behind medial collateral ligament (MCL)	Risk of injury to saphenous nerve
Posterolateral	Visualize posterior horn and PCL	1 cm above joint line, between lateral collateral ligament (LCL) and biceps tendon	Risk of injury to common peroneal nerve
Portals of shoulder			
Posterior	Primary viewing portal	2 cm inferior and 1 cm medial to posterolateral corner of acromion, directed toward coracoid tip	Risk of injury to axillary nerve and suprascapular nerve
Anterior	Viewing and subacromial decompression	Lateral to coracoid process, anterior to AC joint	Risk of injury to cephalic vein and musculocutaneous nerve
Lateral	Subacromial decompression	1–2 cm distal to lateral edge of acromion	
Anteroinferior	Anterior labral repair	Slightly inferior to coracoid	

79.6 Arthroscopic Portals

The most common portals used in knee and shoulder arthroscopy, along with their function and location, are presented in Table 79.1. In the knee, anterolateral portal is the first one to be made as the primary viewing portal and Anteromedial portal is the primary instrumentation portal. While in shoulder, posterior portal is the first portal to be made, and all other portals are made under visualization from the posterior portal with the help of a spinal needle.

Multiple Choice Questions

1. Which one is the standard viewing portal used for knee arthroscopy?
   (a) Anteromedial
   (b) Anterolateral
   (c) Posteromedial
   (d) Posterolateral
2. Which of the following is NOT an advantage of arthroscopy over conventional arthrotomy?
   (a) Lesser blood loss
   (b) Early return to work
   (c) Lesser hospital stay
   (d) Easy to learn
3. Arthroscopy cannot be used for which of the following knee procedures?
   (a) Anterior cruciate ligament reconstruction
   (b) Meniscal repair
   (c) Lateral collateral ligament repair
   (d) Microfracture for cartilage defect
4. Which is the primary viewing portal for shoulder arthroscopy?
   (a) Posterior
   (b) Anterior
   (c) Lateral
   (d) Anteroinferior

5. Which arthroscopic instrument allows the surgeon to palpate intra-articular structures with minimal risk of damage?
   (a) Arthroscopic knife
   (b) Arthroscope
   (c) Probe
   (d) Basket forceps

Answers: 1. (b), 2. (d), 3. (c), 4. (a), 5. (c)

80 Introduction to Endoscopy in Spine

Nikhil Goyal

80.1 Introduction

Minimally invasive spinal surgery (MISS) has gained significant interest in recent years, driven by surgeons, patients, healthcare economics, and industry. One particular technique, spinal endoscopy, has emerged as a promising option for the management of various spinal pathologies. While initial technological limitations hindered its widespread use previously, better knowledge of minimally invasive surgical corridors and better instrumentation have led to the expansion of spinal endoscopic techniques in current times [1].

80.2 Uses

Spinal endoscopy can be used for degenerative diseases, traumatic fractures, tumors, and infections in the cervical, thoracic, and lumbar spine. The most robust clinical data supports the efficacy of endoscopic spinal decompressions, but spinal instrumentation and fusion can also be performed using endoscopic techniques [2].

80.3 Techniques

In endoscopic lumbar spine surgery, two approaches are used: transforaminal and interlaminar.

In transforaminal approach, discectomy and decompression are done through the intervertebral foramen between the exiting and traversing roots.

In interlaminar approach, discectomy is done in between the two laminae of the superior and inferior vertebrae. In cases of anatomical constraints for the transforaminal approach like L5-S1 disc and cases with upward migration of disc into the canal, interlaminar approach is used [3].

80.4 Advantages

- Minimal bony and soft tissue dissection
- Preserved anatomy, hence lower risk of segmental instability
- Better visualization of anatomical structures can help minimize iatrogenic damage
- Decreased blood loss
- Reduced postoperative pain, earlier mobilization, and return to work
- Improved cosmesis

N. Goyal (✉)
Department of Orthopedics, All India Institute of Medical Sciences, Rishikesh, India

V. Kumar et al. (eds.), *A Quick Guide to Essential Orthopedics*,
https://doi.org/10.1007/978-981-95-2676-5_80

80.5 Disadvantages

- Steep learning curve:
  During the initial learning curve, higher rates of recurrence and treatment failure may be observed compared to conventional techniques. The variability in complication rates is primarily related to the acquisition of the specific skills required for endoscopic procedures. Therefore, surgeon experience plays a pivotal role in minimizing complications and achieving outcomes comparable to other minimally invasive spine surgery (MISS) techniques.

  Complications can include:

- Dural tears
- Nerve root injury
- Injury to vascular structures
- Perforation of peritoneal sac and abdominal structures
- Iatrogenic facet damage causing instability
- Wrong side or level surgery
- Postoperative discitis
- Postoperative hematoma formation
- Cerebrospinal cyst formation

Multiple Choice Questions

1. Which approach can be used during spine endoscopy for lumbar disc herniation?
   (a) Transforaminal approach
   (b) Translaminar approach
   (c) Interforaminal approach
   (d) Intralaminar approach
2. Spinal endoscopy can be used in which of the following conditions?
   (a) Traumatic pathology
   (b) Tumors
   (c) Degenerative conditions
   (d) All of the above
3. Which of the following is a disadvantage of spinal endoscopy?
   (a) Long operative time
   (b) High blood loss
   (c) Steep learning curve
   (d) Slow rehabilitation
4. A national-level football player has come to you with L4-L5 prolapsed intervertebral disc (PIVD) requiring operative intervention. You have planned an endoscopic discectomy. Which of the following complications you will not take consent for?
   (a) Nerve root injury
   (b) Wrong-level surgery
   (c) Spinal instability
   (d) Need for blood transfusion
5. Interlaminar approach for spine endoscopy is best suited for:
   (a) L4-L5 discectomy
   (b) L5-S1 discectomy
   (c) L3-L4 discectomy
   (d) L1-L2 discectomy

Answers: 1. (a), 2. (d), 3. (c), 4. (d), 5. (b)

References

1. Lee CH, Choi M, Ryu DS, Choi I, Kim CH, Kim HS, Sohn MJ. Efficacy and safety of full-endoscopic decompression via interlaminar approach for central or lateral recess spinal stenosis of the lumbar spine: a meta-analysis. Spine (Phila Pa 1976). 2018;43(24):1756–64.
2. Ahn Y. Endoscopic spine discectomy: indications and outcomes. Int Orthop. 2019;43(4):909–16.
3. Choi G, Pophale CS, Patel B, Uniyal P. Endoscopic spine surgery. J Korean Neurosurg Soc. 2017;60(5):485–97.

MIX
Papier aus verantwortungsvollen Quellen
Paper from responsible sources
FSC® C105338

If you have any concerns about our products,
you can contact us on
ProductSafety@springernature.com

In case Publisher is established outside the EU,
the EU authorized representative is:
Springer Nature Customer Service Center GmbH
Europaplatz 3, 69115 Heidelberg, Germany

Printed by Libri Plureos GmbH
in Hamburg, Germany